Atlas of Cytopathology
A Pattern Based Approach

CHRISTOPHER J. VANDENBUSSCHE

ERIKA F. RODRIGUEZ

DEREK B. ALLISON

M. LISA ZHANG

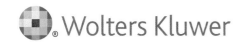
. Wolters Kluwer

Philadelphia • Baltimore • New York • London
Buenos Aires • Hong Kong • Sydney • Tokyo

Acquisitions Editor: Keith Donnellan
Development Editor: Ariel S. Winter
Editorial Coordinator: Tim Rinehart
Marketing Manager: Julie Sikora
Production Project Manager: Kim Cox
Design Coordinator: Holly McLaughlin
Manufacturing Coordinator: Beth Welsh
Prepress Vendor: TNQ Technologies

9 8 7 6 5 4 3 2 1

Printed in China

Library of Congress Cataloging-in-Publication Data

ISBN-13: 978-1-4963-9704-1

Cataloging-in-Publication data available on request from the Publisher.

---

shop.lww.com

To Cherry and Josephine.
Christopher J. VandenBussche, MD, PhD

To Fausto, Olivia, and Melissa.
Erika F. Rodriguez, MD, PhD

To Catherine, my wife, hero, and best friend.
To Wesley and Avery, the world is yours for the taking!
Derek B. Allison, MD

To Alan, my forever best friend and biggest supporter.
M. Lisa Zhang, MD

The challenges of cytopathology are difficult to capture in a textbook; in reality, most melanoma cells do not contain pigment, air-drying artifacts alter cytomorphology, and benign respiratory cells may obscure lung carcinoma cells. Specimens of borderline adequacy leave one to question whether a definitive diagnosis can be made. Most cytopathology textbooks present us with ideal cells—the best cells photographed from the best specimens. In reality, these ideal cells may not be seen, nor are they required for a proper diagnosis. In many instances, ideal cells may even be insufficient for a diagnosis if not seen in a particular pattern or context.

This atlas presents more than 1500 representative high-quality images. Rather than focus on obscure diagnoses, numerous images from frequently seen diagnoses are included to cover the different preparations, artifacts, and limitations seen during a cytopathology sign out. The most commonly encountered pitfalls are also provided, as well as advice on when and how to hedge.

Rather than focus strictly on single cells, this atlas acknowledges the importance of pattern recognition in cytopathology. The different cell populations and background material seen in a specimen may form a pattern that leads to a specific diagnosis. An experienced cytopathologist must learn to absorb microscopic fields full of cells, as examining each individual cell in a specimen is not possible.

The text is high yield and focused on checklists, key features, diagnostic pearls and pitfalls, frequently asked questions, and sample notes, all further described below.

- Each chapter opens with a "Chapter Checklist" that outlines the enclosed structure and allows the reader to quickly hone in on select patterns and pertinent differential considerations. Similar "Checklists" are found throughout the chapter to neatly organize complicated topics.
- "The Unremarkable X": Depending on the type of specimen, normal background cells may or may not be commonly seen. In instances where background cells are present, they may contain changes that can confound a diagnosis. In instances where background cells are unexpected, they may be mistaken as lesional cells. This section provides a description of the normal background cells that may be seen in each specimen type.
- The "Pearls & Pitfalls" sections include lessons from real life sign out experience with an emphasis on important diagnostic clues, mimics, and hazards.
- The "Frequently Asked Questions" sections stem from our busy consult service and teaching sessions. In this section, we discuss real-life diagnostic dilemmas and offer diagnostic tips and tools to sort through commonly encountered sign-out challenges.
- All major topics close with a "Key Features" section that summarizes the essential elements of the subtopic for handy reference.
- A "Sample Note" section accompanies the more challenging topics. In these sections, an example cytopathology report is included with the top-line diagnoses, including pertinent discussion and salient references. These "Notes" offer a template of how to synthesize complicated topics and are based on real-life cases and interactions with clinicians. The select references are included for those interested in further reading but can also be included in pathology reports to help guide clinical management.
- "Self-Assessment Questions" appear as an appendix at the end of the book and as an interactive "Quiz" online to emphasize important teaching points. These sections offer the reader experience and confidence with high-yield teaching topics. Questions are in the format of the board-type examinations and can also serve as useful board preparatory materials.

ACKNOWLEDGMENTS

The authors thank Dr. Morgan Cowan for reviewing select chapters and Dr. Austin McCuiston for test-driving the chapter questions.

CONTENTS

FINE-NEEDLE ASPIRATION OF THE THYROID

1

CHAPTER OUTLINE

PAUCICELLULAR PATTERN

CHECKLIST: Etiologic Considerations for the Paucicellular Pattern

☐ Benign Follicular Nodule/Colloid Nodule
☐ Nondiagnostic (Insufficient Cellularity)
☐ Nondiagnostic (Cyst Fluid Only)
☐ Cystic Follicular Nodule
☐ Cystic Papillary Thyroid Carcinoma

The paucicellular pattern is defined by a lack of adequate follicular cells obtained during fine-needle aspiration (FNA) of a thyroid nodule. More specifically, according to The Bethesda System for Reporting Thyroid Cytopathology (TBSRTC), there must be at least six groups present, with each group containing at least 10 follicular cells across an entire specimen for the material to be considered adequate for classification into a diagnostic category.[1] If, however, the specimen contains abundant colloid, numerous lymphocytes, or any atypical cells, the follicular cell adequacy criteria does not have to be met. Paucicellular specimens may be comprised of predominantly blood, colloid, cyst contents, or ultrasound gel. Nondiagnostic specimens are associated with a significantly increased risk of malignancy on follow-up than benign specimens (Table 1.1).

BENIGN FOLLICULAR NODULE/COLLOID NODULE

A colloid nodule is essentially a benign follicular nodule containing abundant colloid and rare to absent follicular cells. Owing to the extremely low risk of malignancy associated with this finding, a colloid nodule is considered to be benign and adequate for evaluation, despite the lack of at least six groups each containing at least 10 follicular epithelial cells. Colloid is often blue/violet in color on Diff-Quik stained preparations and orange/pink or green/blue in color on Pap stained preparations (Figures 1.1-1.7). The texture of the colloid

TABLE 1.1: The Bethesda System for Reporting Thyroid Cytopathology

Diagnostic Category	ROM	Predicted ROM Due to NIFTP Reclassification	Common Clinical Management
Nondiagnostic or Unsatisfactory	5-10%	5-10%	Repeat FNA with ultrasound guidance
Benign	0-3%	0-3%	Clinical and ultrasound follow-up
Atypia of Undetermined Significance (Aus) or Follicular Lesion of Undetermined Significance (FLUS)	10-30%	6-18%	Repeat FNA, molecular testing, or lobectomy based on ultrasound characteristics
Follicular Neoplasm (FN) or Suspicious for a Follicular Neoplasm (SFN)	25-40%	10-40%	Molecular testing or lobectomy based on ultrasound characteristics
Suspicious for Malignancy	50-75%	45-60%	Near-total thyroidectomy or lobectomy
Malignant	97-99	94-96%	Near-total thyroidectomy or lobectomy

FNA, fine-needle aspiration; NIFTP, noninvasive follicular thyroid neoplasm with papillary-like nuclear features; ROM, Rate of malignancy.
Adapted and modified from Tables 1.2 and 1.3 in *The 2017 Bethesda System for Reporting Thyroid Cytopathology. 2nd ed.: Springer International Publishing*; 2017.

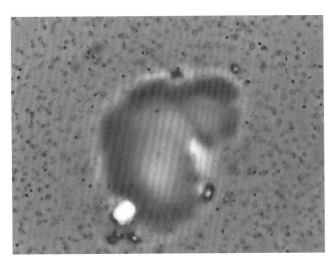

Figure 1.1. Benign colloid. Blue, watery colloid is present in the background of this smear while a denser, darker blue blob of colloid is present in the center of the field (Diff-Quik stain).

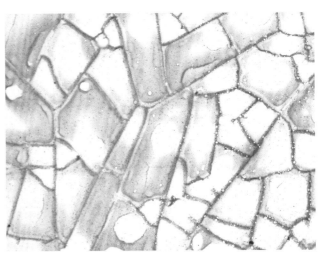

Figure 1.2. Benign colloid. Benign colloid. Thin, watery watery, blue colloid that has cracked to create a mosaic pattern (Diff-Quik stain).

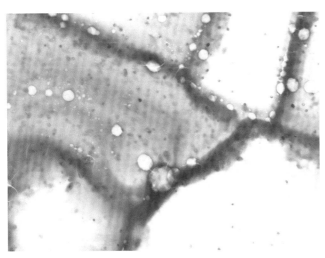

Figure 1.3. Benign colloid. High-power view of the previous case (Figure 1.2) showing a mosaic pattern of colloid with cracks and bubbles (Diff-Quik stain).

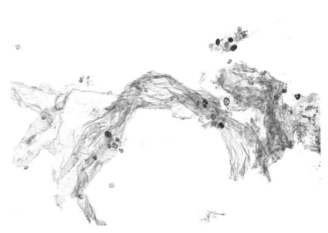

Figure 1.4. Benign colloid. On ThinPrep preparations, watery colloid can fold in on itself and crinkle in a way reminiscent of tissue paper (Pap stain).

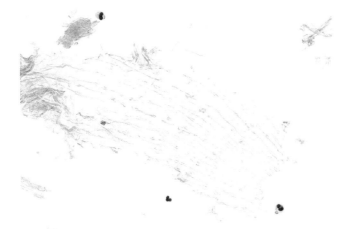

Figure 1.5. Benign colloid. On ThinPrep preparations, thin colloid can fold in on itself to result in a tissue paper–like appearance (Pap stain).

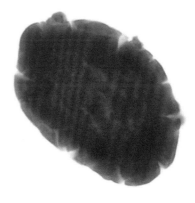

Figure 1.6. Benign colloid. Colloid can be dense and take on a hyaline appearance. When dense, it can crack on liquid-based preparations and form hard edges at the periphery to create a "flower-like arrangement" (Pap stain).

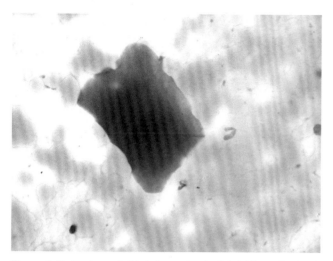

Figure 1.7. Benign colloid. A dense chunk of dark blue colloid with rough edges (Diff-Quik stain).

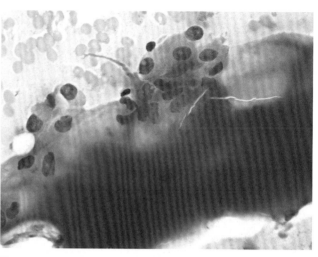

Figure 1.8. Malignant colloid. Classic "bubblegum" colloid is thick, sticky, and ropey. In this case, note the adjacent malignant cells with papillary thyroid carcinoma nuclear features, including nuclear elongation, enlargement, and irregular nuclear borders (Diff-Quik stain).

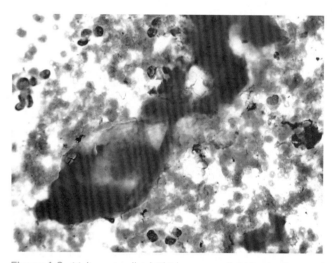

Figure 1.9. Malignant colloid. Thick, ropey colloid in a background of malignant cells with papillary thyroid carcinoma nuclear features: enlargement and irregular nuclear borders (Diff-Quik stain).

can provide a clue to the nature of the lesion. Watery colloid may be difficult to distinguish from thickened serum but may crack, creating a mosaic pattern, or form large bubbles. In contrast, benign thick colloid has a dense appearance and often appears as amorphous "specks" aligned in the direction of smearing in conventional smears. In liquid-based preparations, colloid can have a delicate "tissue paper" appearance or form globules containing perpendicular cracks (sometimes mistaken for psammoma bodies). These features contrast to those of colloid typically seen in papillary thyroid carcinoma (PTC), which forms dense "bubblegum" globules (Figures 1.8 and 1.9).

SAMPLE NOTE: COLLOID NODULE

Benign colloid nodule. See note.

Note: The specimen consists of abundant watery colloid only. If the lesion is well-sampled, even in the absence of at least six groups of at least 10 follicular cells per group, samples like this one are adequate for evaluation and best considered benign.

KEY FEATURES of "Benign Colloid"

* Colloid stains blue/violet in color on Diff-Quik.

* Colloid appears orange/pink or green/blue on the Pap stain.

* Watery colloid may form cracks or bubbles.

* Dense colloid forms amorphous globules or specks aligned in the direction of slide smearing.

* Colloid on liquid-based preparations has a delicate "tissue paper" appearance or forms round globules with perpendicular cracks.

NONDIAGNOSTIC (INSUFFICIENT CELLULARITY)

FNAs of thyroid nodules that lack abundant colloid, atypical follicular cells, numerous lymphocytes, and at least six groups of at least 10 benign follicular cells are considered to be nondiagnostic. These criteria are designed to avoid false-positive diagnoses by ensuring that a sufficient number of follicular cells are present and evaluable to render an accurate diagnosis. For FNAs that are considered nondiagnostic, the recommendation is to repeat the FNA because 10% of these nodules are actually malignant on follow-up.[2-4] It is important to note, however, that the rate of malignancy (ROM) in nondiagnostic FNAs also depends on the characteristics of the nodule. For example, solid nodules have a higher ROM than nodules that are >50% cystic.

> **FAQ:** How is a nodule managed if both the initial and repeat FNAs are nondiagnostic?
>
> ---
>
> **Answer:** Although repeating an FNA after an initial nondiagnostic diagnosis results in a diagnostic category 60-80% of the time, the remainder will again be nondiagnostic.[5-8] Because most of these nondiagnostic nodules are benign on follow-up, two successive nondiagnostic interpretations may be considered benign, as long as there are no worrisome features on the clinical examination or ultrasound. If worrisome features are present, close follow-up, repeat FNA, or even surgery may be warranted.

NONDIAGNOSTIC (CYST FLUID ONLY)

Aspirates that are comprised of cystic contents are considered to be inadequate if the number of follicular epithelial cells does not meet the criteria of TBSRTC.[1] Cystic degeneration is fairly common in benign follicular nodules and, when aspirated, yields predominantly watery fluid and vacuolated macrophages, which are often stippled with hemosiderin that can be identified due to its characteristic green cytoplasmic appearance on the Pap stain and small, blue to purple appearance on the Diff-Quik stain (Figures 1.10-1.14). Owing to the fact that PTCs can be cystic, this diagnosis cannot be excluded without adequate cytologic evaluation of the follicular cell component. Therefore, TBSRTC recommends that these aspirates be classified as nondiagnostic with a note that informs the clinician that only cyst fluid was present.[1] This recommendation comes from the fact that nodules that are nondiagnostic due to the presence of only cyst fluid have a much lower ROM than cases that are nondiagnostic due to simply insufficient cellularity.[9] If no worrisome features are identified on ultrasound of a cystic lesion with cyst fluid only, a repeat FNA may not be necessary.

SAMPLE NOTE: CYST FLUID ONLY

Nondiagnostic. Cyst fluid only. See note.

Note: The specimen consists of cyst fluid and vacuolated macrophages only. The specimen is considered inadequate for evaluation owing to a lack of at least six groups of 10 follicular cells per group. Because of the low risk of malignancy in cystic nodules with this FNA appearance, however, correlation with the ultrasound findings is recommended to determine whether or not the size and complexity of this cystic nodule requires a repeat FNA.

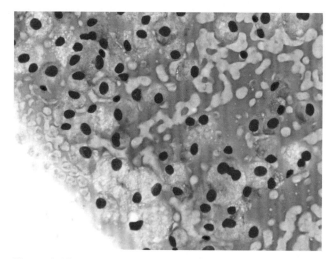

Figure 1.10. Cyst fluid. In the thyroid, the presence of vacuolated macrophages is associated with cystic degeneration. Note the numerous vacuolated macrophages in this image, an indicator that cyst contents were aspirated (Diff-Quik stain).

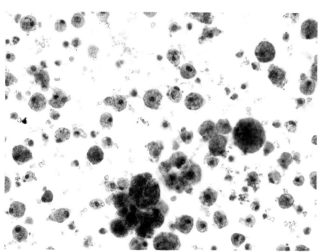

Figure 1.11. Cyst fluid. Hemorrhage is common during cystic degeneration. As a result, hemosiderin-laden macrophages are commonly seen on fine-needle aspiration (FNA) of cystic thyroid nodules, which have an abundance of green cytoplasmic material on the Pap stain (Pap stain).

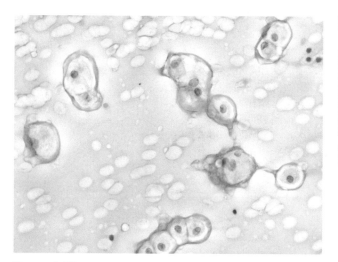

Figure 1.12. Cyst fluid. Note the numerous vacuolated macrophages in this field in a background of watery colloid, indicative of secondary cystic degeneration (Pap stain).

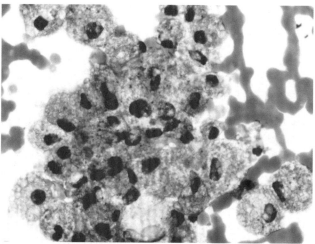

Figure 1.13. Cyst fluid. These vacuolated macrophages contain blue cytoplasmic granules, which represent an accumulation of hemosiderin (Diff-Quik stain).

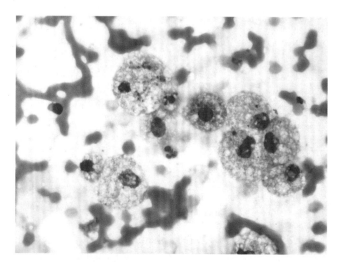

Figure 1.14. Cyst fluid. This high magnification view shows vacuolated macrophages with a minimal amount of hemosiderin accumulation in their cytoplasm (Diff-Quik stain).

CYSTIC FOLLICULAR NODULE

Cystic degeneration is a common feature in follicular nodules, especially those present in patients with multinodular goiter. In addition to cyst fluid containing macrophages with or without hemosiderin, these aspirates show scattered benign follicular cells and cyst-lining cells. Cyst-lining cells may appear as streaming cells with "stretched" cytoplasm containing bipolar processes and have enlarged and elongated nuclei, occasional nuclear grooves, pale chromatin, rare intranuclear cytoplasmic inclusions, and prominent nucleoli (Figures 1.15-1.19). Owing to overlap with atypical features seen in PTC, rare cases may result in an indeterminate diagnosis, such as AUS or even SPTC.[10]

CYSTIC PAPILLARY THYROID CARCINOMA

A major potential pitfall in a paucicellular specimen is to miss a small number of atypical follicular epithelial cells that will trigger a partial or complete thyroidectomy. The main purpose of the cellularity criteria is to ensure that enough cells are sampled to detect atypia. Therefore, if atypia is present, the minimum cellularity requirement for adequacy

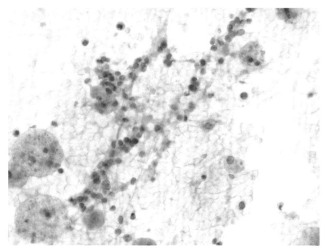

Figure 1.15. Cystic follicular nodule. Scattered, small follicular epithelial cells are seen together with vacuolated macrophages containing pigment, indicating secondary cystic degeneration of a follicular thyroid nodule (Pap stain).

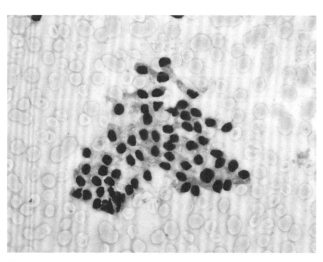

Figure 1.16. Cystic follicular nodule. Cyst-lining follicular epithelial cells are present with abundant, elongated cytoplasm with small vacuoles and mildly atypical nuclei (Diff-Quik stain).

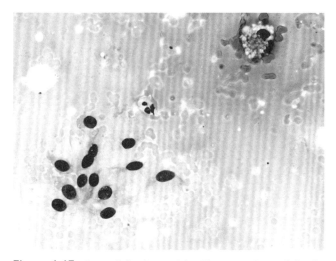

Figure 1.17. Cystic follicular nodule. These cyst-lining follicular epithelial cells have elongated bipolar cytoplasmic processes and oval nuclei. Note the vacuolated macrophage which further supports that these changes are most likely reparative secondary to cyst formation (Diff-Quik stain).

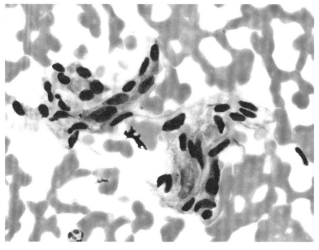

Figure 1.18. Cystic follicular nodule. These cyst-lining cells demonstrate reparative changes, including enlarged and elongated nuclei, subtle nuclear grooves, and elongated cytoplasmic processes (Diff-Quik stain).

is not necessary.[11] PTC can undergo cystic change; however, the amount of cystic change, and resultant cellularity, varies from case to case. To this point, as many as 10% of PTCs are nearly completely cystic.[10,12] For a case to be considered adequate in this scenario, the atypia must be consistent with conventional PTC nuclear changes; however, these cases also display several features consistent with the cystic nature of the lesion. Cystic PTCs are predominantly composed of thin, watery cyst fluid with scattered hemosiderin-laden macrophages and neoplastic cells with atypical nuclear features and abundant, hypervacuolated cytoplasm reminiscent of macrophages (Figures 1.20-1.25). Owing to

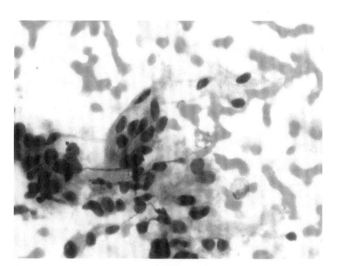

Figure 1.19. Cystic follicular nodule. Separate field (Diff-Quik stain).

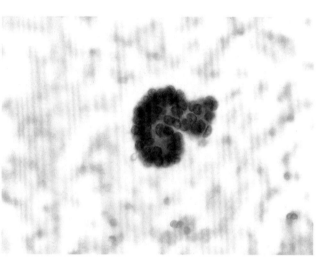

Figure 1.20. Cystic papillary thyroid carcinoma (PTC). Owing to the abundance of cystic fluid in these nodules, cellularity is often scant in comparison to conventional PTC. Note the rare, single aggregate of malignant follicular epithelial cells showing nuclear enlargement, overlap, irregular nuclear membranes, and pale chromatin (Pap stain).

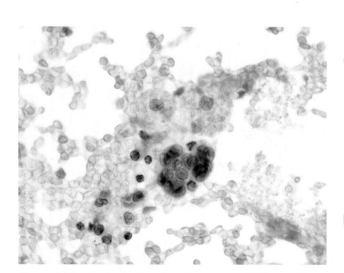

Figure 1.21. Cystic papillary thyroid carcinoma (PTC). In addition to the malignant cells showing nuclear enlargement, overlap, irregular nuclear membranes, and nuclear clearing, hemosiderin-laden macrophages can be seen, indicating the cystic nature of this lesion (Pap stain).

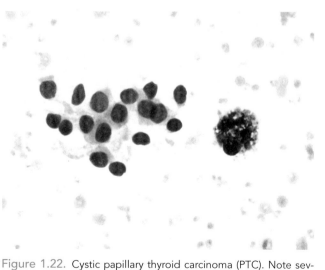

Figure 1.22. Cystic papillary thyroid carcinoma (PTC). Note several follicular epithelial cells with nuclear enlargement, elongation, and slightly irregular nuclear contours with abundant elongated cytoplasm and a background hemosiderin-laden macrophage. This level of atypia is indeterminate for PTC due to the overlap of these features with reparative changes seen in cyst-lining cells. In other fields, however, clearly malignant cells were identified, suggesting that these cells are most likely also malignant (Diff-Quik stain).

the enlarged, hypervacuolated cytoplasm, cystic PTC cells often have decreased N/C ratios compared to those seen in conventional PTC. The main entity in the differential diagnosis is a cystic follicular nodule with cyst-lining cells, which typically lack nuclear membrane irregularities and intranuclear pseudoinclusions (though rarely intranuclear pseudoinclusions may be seen).

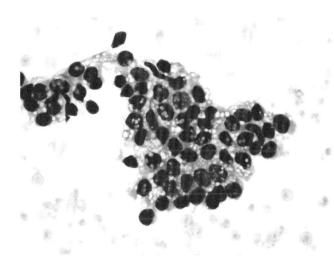

Figure 1.23. Cystic papillary thyroid carcinoma (PTC). This small sheet contains follicular epithelial cells with abundant cytoplasmic vacuoles and enlarged nuclei containing irregular nuclear membranes and nuclear overlap (Diff-Quik stain).

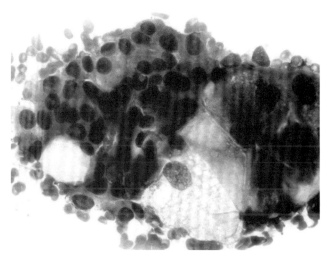

Figure 1.24. Cystic papillary thyroid carcinoma (PTC). The field contains a group of malignant follicular epithelial cells displaying nuclear enlargement, nuclear overlap, nuclear folding, and intranuclear pseudoinclusions. Even though the cytoplasm is more abundant and variably vacuolated, resulting in a decreased N/C ratio, the remaining nuclear features are consistent with a PTC (Diff-Quik stain).

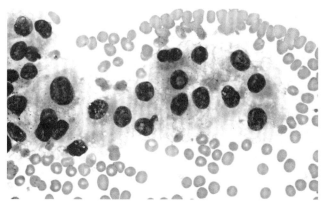

Figure 1.25. Cystic papillary thyroid carcinoma (PTC). Note the intranuclear pseudoinclusion, which is considered to be one of the most specific features of malignancy (Diff-Quik stain).

MACROFOLLICULAR PATTERN

CHECKLIST: Etiologic Considerations for the Macrofollicular Pattern

☐ Normal Thyroid/Benign Follicular Nodule

The macrofollicular pattern consists of variably sized, nonoverlapping follicles and fragmented sheets of follicular epithelial cells. The terminology "macro" may at first seem confusing because it is not a statement about the overall size of the sheet of cells, which becomes fragmented upon aspiration. Macrofollicular, more accurately, is the pattern of normal, unremarkable follicular epithelium as it appears secondary to FNA sampling. The shape of the follicles is largely a product of the amount of colloid that has distended the follicle and can vary considerably. The macrofollicular pattern is the most commonly encountered pattern in thyroid FNA.[13] It is important to interpret the findings in this pattern in the context of the clinical scenario and ultrasound findings to ensure that adequate sampling of the targeted lesion was obtained. As a result, some basic familiarity with the recent guidelines from the American College of Radiology Thyroid Imaging, Reporting and Data System (TI-RADS),[14] as shown in Tables 1.2 and 1.3, can be helpful to synthesize all the information.

NORMAL THYROID/BENIGN FOLLICULAR NODULE

Normal thyroid is most often inadvertently aspirated when a nodule is difficult to sample, either due to the size or location of the nodule. Normal thyroid is usually less cellular than the benign, hyperplastic counterpart—a benign follicular nodule—but is otherwise indistinguishable on the cytomorphologic appearance alone. In most cases, the macrofollicular pattern is indicative of a benign follicular nodule, which is essentially an adenomatoid nodule seen in patients with multinodular goiter or, less commonly, lymphocytic thyroiditis or a follicular adenoma. This pattern is frequently representative of a benign follicular nodule because FNA represents targeted sampling of a nodule and not unremarkable thyroid. In both normal thyroid and a benign follicular nodule, the follicular epithelial cells should be evenly spaced and well-organized within a tissue fragment, and possess scant to moderate amounts of cytoplasm, round nuclei with coarse chromatin, and inconspicuous nucleoli (Figures 1.26-1.35). The macrofollicular pattern is most notably distinguished from the microfollicular pattern—which reveals predominantly small follicles (<15 cells) that are uniform and crowded instead of forming sheets—and the papillary pattern, which contains papillary-shaped monolayer sheets of follicular cells. Even if a few microfollicles are present, a benign diagnosis should be rendered if the majority of the lesion shows bland nuclear features and is predominately macrofollicular.

FAQ: How is a nodule diagnosed as benign on FNA managed clinically?

Answer: The management of a benign diagnosis on thyroid FNA is largely dependent on the ultrasound characteristics of the nodule. According to the 2015 American Thyroid Association Guidelines,[5] nodules that have a very low suspicion should be considered benign owing to the fact that radiographic surveillance has little utility. If desired, FNA can be repeated greater than 2 years after the initial benign diagnosis, and if a second benign diagnosis is rendered, ultrasound surveillance is no longer indicated. For nodules that are of low to intermediate suspicion, a repeat FNA should be done 1-2 years after the initial diagnosis; however, if there is evidence of increased growth or other changes in the radiographic characteristics, a repeat sample may be obtained sooner. Finally, for nodules with a benign diagnosis but high suspicion based on the ultrasound findings, a repeat ultrasound and FNA should be done within 1 year.

TABLE 1.2: Radiographic Ultrasound Characteristics Used to Compile the ACR TI-RADS Score

Composition (Choose 1)	Points	Echogenicity (Choose 1)	Points	Shape (Choose 1)	Points	Margin (Choose 1)	Points	Echogenic Foci (Choose All Apply)	Points
Cystic or almost completely cystic	0	Anechoic	0	Wider than tall	0	Smooth	0	None or large comet-tail artifact	0
Spongiform	0	Hyperechoic or isoechoic	1	Taller than wide	3	Ill-defined	0	Macro-calcifications	1
Mixed cystic and solid	1	Hypoechoic	2			Lobulated or irregular	2	Peripheral (rim) calcifications	2
Solid or almost completely solid	2	Very hypoechoic	3			Extra-thyroidal extension	3	Punctate echogenic foci	3

ACR TI-RADS, American College of Radiology Thyroid Imaging, Reporting and Data System.
Adapted from Figure 1 of the recent guidelines from the Tessler FN, Middleton WD, Grant EG, et al. ACR thyroid imaging, reporting and data system (TI-RADS): white paper of the ACR TI-RADS committee. *J Am Coll Radiol.* 2017;14(5):587-595.

TABLE 1.3: Utilizing the TI-RADS Score

Category	ACR TI-RADS Score[a]	Interpretation	Recommendation	Rate of Malignancy
TR1	0	Benign	No FNA	0.3%
TR2	2	Not suspicious	No FNA	1.5%
TR3	3	Mildly suspicious	FNA if ≥2.5 cm Follow if ≥1.5 cm	1.7-4.8%
TR4	4-6	Moderately suspicious	FNA if ≥1.5 cm Follow if ≥1.0 cm	5.9-12.8%
TR5	7 or more	Highly suspicious	FNA if ≥1.0 cm Follow if ≥0.5 cm	20.7-68.4%

[a]The ACR TI-RADS (TR) score is compiled by adding the points assigned in each of five ultrasound characteristic categories, including composition, echogenicity, shape, margin, and echogenic focus as outlined in Table 1.2.
ACR TI-RADS, American College of Radiology Thyroid Imaging, Reporting and Data System; FNA, fine-needle aspiration.
Table compiled from data retrieved from Middleton WD, Teefey SA, Reading CC, et al. Multiinstitutional analysis of thyroid nodule risk stratification using the American College of Radiology thyroid imaging reporting and data system. *AJR Am J Roentgenol.* 2017;208(6):1331-1341; Rosario PW, da Silva AL, Nunes MB, Borges MAR. Risk of malignancy in thyroid nodules using the American College of Radiology thyroid imaging reporting and data system in the NIFTP era. *Horm Metab Res.* 2018;50(10):735-737.

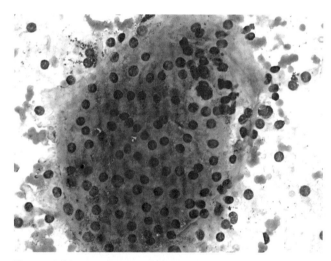

Figure 1.26. Benign macrofollicle. Follicular cells can be seen at evenly spaced intervals with round, bland nuclei and abundant blue cytoplasmic granules (Diff-Quik stain).

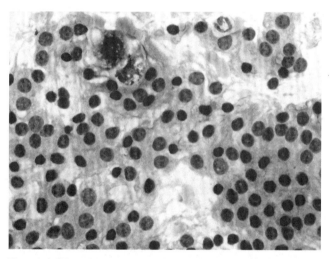

Figure 1.27. Benign macrofollicle. This flat sheet contains evenly spaced follicular cells with round, uniform nuclei (Diff-Quik stain).

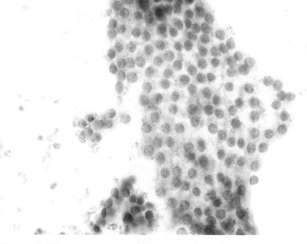

Figure 1.28. Benign macrofollicle. The follicular cells in this fragment are evenly spaced and have round, uniform nuclei (Pap stain).

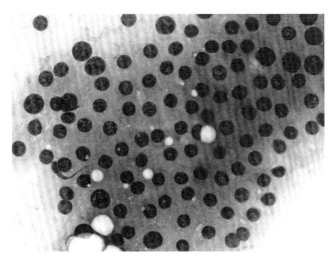

Figure 1.29. Benign macrofollicle. The presence of air bubbles may cause "pseudo" intranuclear pseudoinclusions when they occur over the nucleus. Remember that true intranuclear pseudoinclusions must have the same color and characteristic as the cytoplasm (Diff-Quik stain).

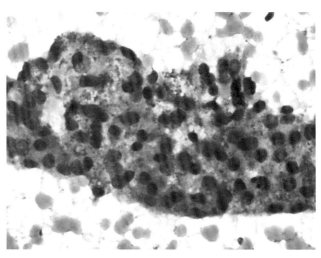

Figure 1.30. Benign macrofollicle. In some cases, macrofollicles can appear slightly irregular due to the smearing process and result in what may appear as disorganized with nuclear overlap (Diff-Quik stain).

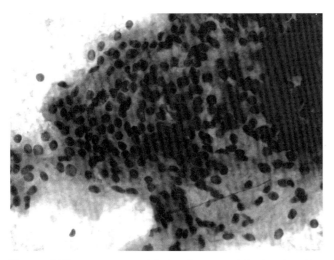

Figure 1.31. Benign macrofollicle. This macrofollicular sheet has a syncytial appearance and the nuclei appear slightly disorganized and enlarged. Mild nuclear contour irregularities can be seen. The remainder of the specimen contained colloid and bland-appearing follicular cells (Diff-Quik stain).

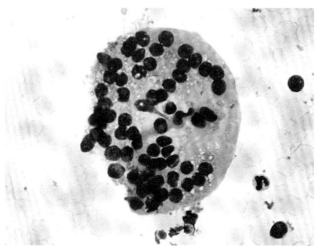

Figure 1.32. Benign macrofollicle. This fragment of follicular cells has a syncytial appearance and may be mistaken for a multinucleated giant cell (Diff-Quik stain).

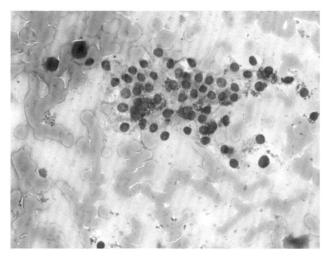

Figure 1.33. Benign macrofollicle. In some cases, macrofollicles may get slightly disrupted during aspiration or smearing, resulting in slight fragmentation. Still, these cells are relatively evenly spaced and contain bland nuclei. Note the presence of colloid globules and blue cytoplasmic granules in this case which help support a benign diagnosis (Diff-Quik stain).

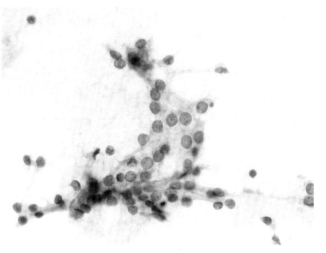

Figure 1.34. Benign macrofollicle. This disrupted macrofollicle consists of bland follicular cells that are small, uniform, and non-overlapping (Pap stain).

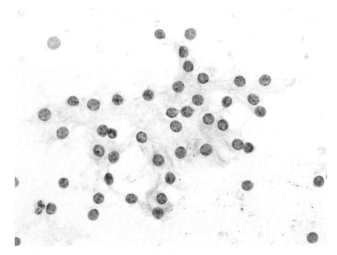

Figure 1.35. Benign macrofollicle. This disrupted fragment is most likely benign due to the presence of small and uniform follicular cells that lack crowding and nuclear atypia (Pap stain).

MICROFOLLICULAR PATTERN

CHECKLIST: Etiologic Considerations for the Microfollicular Pattern

☐ Atypia of Undetermined Significance (AUS) with Architectural Atypia

☐ Suspicious for a Follicular Neoplasm/Follicular Neoplasm

☐ Suspicious for Papillary Thyroid Carcinoma, Papillary Thyroid Carcinoma, and Noninvasive Follicular Thyroid Neoplasm with Papillary-like Nuclear Features (NIFTP)

☐ Parathyroid Tissue

The microfollicular pattern is the hallmark architectural pattern of follicular neoplasms and most commonly correlates with a follicular adenoma or a follicular carcinoma upon surgical resection. Although no well-established, specific criteria exist to define a microfollicle, most experts would agree that microfollicles are composed of relatively uniform, round groups of less than 15 follicular epithelial cells that are crowded and show overlap with little to no colloid present. According to The Bethesda System, the follicular cells should be arranged in a circle that is at least two-thirds complete. The differential diagnosis for the microfollicular pattern includes both follicular and papillary neoplasms, as well as benign and neoplastic parathyroid lesions.

ATYPIA OF UNDETERMINED SIGNIFICANCE (AUS) WITH ARCHITECTURAL ATYPIA

For lesions containing scant follicular cells with predominantly microfollicular architecture, a diagnosis of Atypia of Undetermined Significance (AUS) should be made (Figures 1.36-1.42). In rare instances, one pass may contain only microfollicular architecture while other passes lack microfollicular architecture, suggesting that the lesion may have only been sampled on one pass. The presence of colloid and/or additional follicular cells without microfollicular architecture is reassuring and strongly suggests the nodule in question is benign. The differential diagnosis includes an adenomatoid nodule, follicular adenoma, follicular variant of PTC, NIFTP, and follicular carcinoma. As a result, the American Thyroid Association recommends that a diagnosis of AUS should be managed by repeating an FNA or by performing molecular testing.[5] In most circumstances, the diagnostic dilemma for this categorical diagnosis is whether there is sufficient cellularity to justify a diagnosis of suspicious for a follicular neoplasm/follicular neoplasm (SFN/FN), which may trigger a thyroid lobectomy.

FAQ: What does "architectural atypia" actually mean?

Answer: Architectural atypia, in contrast to cytologic atypia, refers to a scant specimen that is comprised of predominantly microfollicles. Microfollicles are small follicular structures containing 15 or less follicular cells. They are often scattered in the field parallel to the direction a slide was smeared in conventional smear preparations. Microfollicles usually form ring-like structures and several microfollicles may be attached together to form larger fragments. When a pronounced microfollicular architecture is seen, it raises concern for a follicular adenoma, follicular carcinoma, or other lesions with a microfollicular architecture mentioned above.

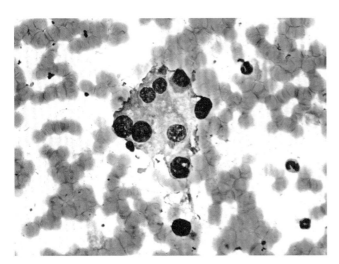

Figure 1.36. Atypia of Undetermined Significance (AUS) with architectural atypia. Relatively uniform round group of follicular cells that lack significant cytologic atypia. Overall, this specimen was scant and contained a few of these similarly appearing groups (Diff-Quik stain).

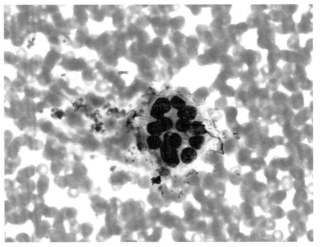

Figure 1.37. Atypia of Undetermined Significance (AUS) with architectural atypia. This small group of follicular cells possess small and round nuclei in a fairly scant specimen lacking macrofollicles and colloid (Diff-Quik stain).

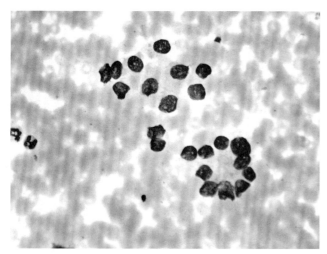

Figure 1.38. Atypia of Undetermined Significance (AUS) with architectural atypia. Two microfollicles can be seen: one with slightly overlapping nuclei, and another that is slightly disrupted. The cells contain a minimal degree of atypia, including some slight elongation and nuclear membrane irregularities. The notable microfollicles in an otherwise fairly scant specimen was most in keeping with categorization as AUS secondary to architectural atypia (Diff-Quik stain).

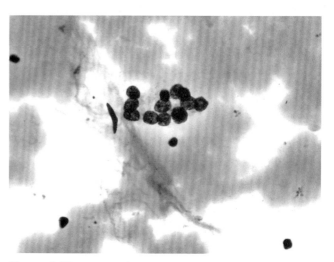

Figure 1.39. Atypia of Undetermined Significance (AUS) with architectural atypia. It is the microfollicular pattern, rather than the cytologic features that are atypical in this case (Diff-Quik stain).

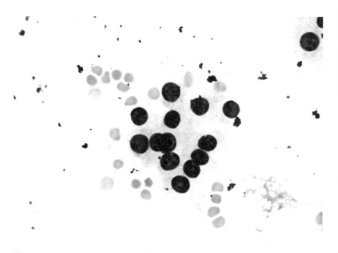

Figure 1.40. Atypia of Undetermined Significance (AUS) with architectural atypia. Bland, monotonous follicular cells with round nuclei and small chromocenters are present, consistent with a microfollicle (Diff-Quik stain).

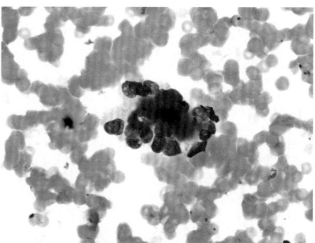

Figure 1.41. Atypia of Undetermined Significance (AUS) with architectural atypia. A microfollicle is present with follicular cells arranged around central, dense colloid (Diff-Quik stain).

SUSPICIOUS FOR A FOLLICULAR NEOPLASM/FOLLICULAR NEOPLASM (SFN/FN)

The microfollicular pattern is the hallmark architectural change present in follicular neoplasms on FNA. Even though follicular adenomas are more likely to have a macrofollicular pattern, it is well-established that many of them show a predominant microfollicular architecture and cannot be separated from a follicular carcinoma on cytomorphology alone. Samples are typically cellular with only scant colloid and consist of relatively monomorphic follicular epithelial cells arranged in crowded, round groups of less than 15 cells. The follicular cells often overlap and usually contain round nuclei and with slight hyperchromasia (Figures 1.43-1.47). In some settings, some nuclear variability and nucleoli are present;

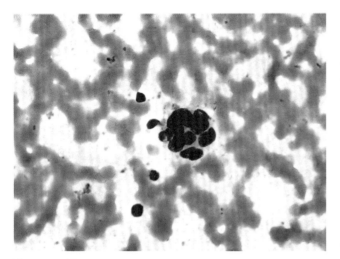

Figure 1.42. Atypia of Undetermined Significance (AUS) with architectural atypia. Small three-dimensional group of bland, round follicular cells forming a microfollicle (Diff-Quik stain).

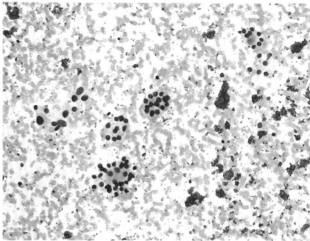

Figure 1.43. Suspicious for a Follicular Neoplasm (SFN). The smear is cellular and comprised predominantly of microfollicles with bland cytologic features. Note the presence of a microfollicle with scant colloid in the center and at the top right portion of the image. Furthermore, note the presence of ultrasound gel at the top left and to the right of this field. This material is purple and coarsely granular and should not be misinterpreted as colloid (Diff-Quik stain).

however, most features of PTC should be absent. Distinguishing follicular carcinoma from follicular adenoma requires evaluation for capsular and lymphovascular invasion on surgical specimen.

FAQ: What is the role of molecular testing in thyroid FNA?

Answer: Molecular testing is primarily used to inform clinical management in the context of indeterminate FNA diagnoses: AUS and SFN/FN. Several commercially available tests are commonly used that analyze a variety of genes and genomic alterations: Afirma Gene Sequence Classifier, ThyGenX, and ThyroSeq. The relative strengths of these panels has historically been in the negative predictive value (positive predictive values vary among the different panels); however, as our understanding of the molecular alterations in thyroid neoplasms grows, these panels may play an increasingly important role in informing management, as long as cost can be contained moving forward. See Table 1.4 for a list of some of the more common molecular alterations in thyroid neoplasms and the associated clinical significance.

SUSPICIOUS FOR PAPILLARY THYROID CARCINOMA, PAPILLARY THYROID CARCINOMA, AND NONINVASIVE FOLLICULAR THYROID NEOPLASM WITH PAPILLARY-LIKE NUCLEAR FEATURES (NIFTP)

PTC variants can display a wide range of architectural and cytomorphological patterns; however, regardless of the variant, the diagnosis is made based on well-defined, "classic" nuclear features and not based on the presence of papillae or the presence of a macro- or microfollicular pattern. In fact, papillae are entirely absent in NIFTP and the follicular variant of PTC, and these lesions are composed of small- to medium-sized, uniform, round follicles containing cells with the nuclear features (Figures 1.48-1.53). As a result, it is important to always identify atypical nuclear features, even when a microfollicular pattern is present. Thankfully, the management for the lesions in this differential diagnosis—SFN/FN, NIFTP, follicular variant of PTC, and PTC—is surgical and requires at least a thyroid lobectomy. The Suspicious for Malignancy category is used when diffuse atypia is seen,

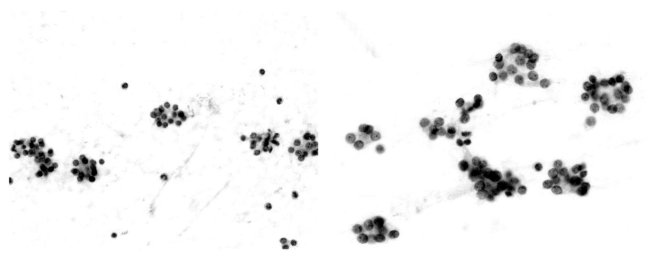

Figure 1.44. Suspicious for a Follicular Neoplasm (SFN). Microfollicles often form a linear arrangement in the direction upon which the slide was smeared. The major difference between this diagnosis and Atypia of Undetermined Significance (AUS) with architectural atypia is the increased cellularity of the specimen in SFN (Pap stain).

Figure 1.45. Suspicious for a Follicular Neoplasm (SFN). Another view from the same case highlights the predominant microfollicular architecture in the specimen (Pap stain).

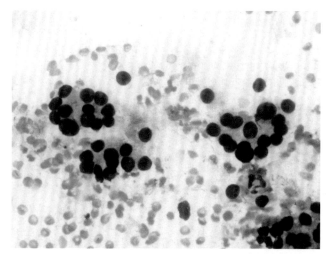

Figure 1.46. Suspicious for a Follicular Neoplasm (SFN). This specimen was highly cellular and comprised of many small, crowded groups and microfollicles, as seen above (Diff-Quik stain).

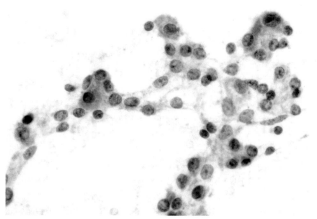

Figure 1.47. Suspicious for a follicular neoplasm. The smear was cellular and comprised of loosely cohesive microfollicles. Upon aspiration, these groups may become slightly disrupted (Pap stain).

but is insufficient for a definitive diagnosis of malignancy. The category is most often used when there is concern for papillary thyroid carcinoma, in which case the term Suspicious for Papillary Thyroid Carcinoma is used.[1] See the "Papillary Thyroid Carcinoma" and the "Noninvasive Follicular Thyroid Neoplasm with Papillary-like Nuclear Features" sections under the "Papillary Pattern" for more information.

PARATHYROID TISSUE

Parathyroid gland can be mistakenly sampled if located directly on the surface or within the thyroid gland (intrathyroidal). It is not uncommon for normal or enlarged parathyroid gland tissue to be mistaken for a thyroid nodule on the physical examination or ultrasound. As a result, inadvertent sampling of parathyroid tissue during FNA may lead to a misdiagnosis. FNA of parathyroid tissue often reveals round to oval single and overlapping cells that can resemble thyroid follicular cells. In addition, parathyroid cells can cluster and form crowded groups that resemble the microfollicles seen in follicular neoplasms, making the distinction between the two on cytomorphology alone nearly impossible (Figures 1.54-1.57). The presence of colloid would favor sampling of the thyroid; however, parathyroid adenomas may contain a colloid-like material.[40]

TABLE 1.4: Common Molecular Alterations Thyroid Neoplasms of Follicular Cell Origin

Diagnosis	Commonly Affected Genes	Common Molecular Alterations	Significance
Follicular neoplasms (FTA, FTC, and PTC-EFV/NIFTP)	NRAS, HRAS, KRAS	NRAS p.Q61R most common in FTA, FTC, and PTC-EFV, followed by HRAS mutations	RAS mutations are markers of thyroid neoplasms with a follicular architecture[17]; higher prevalence in iodine deficiency[18]; believed to promote tumor progression in carcinomas[19]
	PAX8/PPARG rearrangements	Most frequent rearrangement is PAX8-PPARG (20-50% FTCs and much lower in FTAs)[20]	Posited to be an initiating event in thyroid neoplasms with a follicular architecture[20]; more likely in young female patients with local invasion and lower rates of distant metastases[21,22]
Papillary thyroid carcinoma (PTC)	BRAF	p.V600E (most frequent alteration found in approximately 45% of PTCs)[23,24]	Diagnostic for malignancy; predictive of a clinical response to kinase inhibitors[25,26]
	RET–PTC	Rearrangements with a variety of partners (detected in 5-25% of PTCs)[27]	Strong association with radiation exposure[28,29] and found in younger patients with aggressive clinical behavior[30]
	NTRK1/3	Rearrangements with several partners[30]	ETV6-NTRK3 fusion has been seen in 15% of radiation-induced PTC[31] and found in younger patients with aggressive clinical behavior[30]
Hurthle cell neoplasms	Mitochondrial DNA	Mutations in the MT-ND genes encoding complex I (>70% of cases)[32]	Mutations linked to accumulation of defective mitochondria and the resultant sensitivity to hypoxia and oncocytic morphology[33]
Poorly differentiated thyroid carcinoma (PDTC)/anaplastic thyroid carcinoma (ATC)	TP53	Mutations in 10-35% of PDTCs and 40-80% of ATCs[34]	Inactivation is a final step in tumor progression and indicates a poor prognosis[34]
	TERT	Promoter mutations (C288T is the most common)[35]	Often coexists with BRAF p.V600E[35] and is a powerful negative prognostic marker, promoting progression from PTC to a PDTC or ATC[36]
	PI3K–PTEN–AKT pathway	Any pathway dysregulation is seen in 11% of PDTCs and 39% of ATCs[34]	Associated with tumor progression but may respond to treatment with AKT or mTOR inhibitors[38,39]

FTA, follicular thyroid adenoma; FTC, follicular thyroid carcinoma; PTC-EFV, papillary thyroid carcinoma-encapsulated follicular variant; NIFTP, noninvasive follicular thyroid neoplasm with papillary-like nuclear features.
Adapted and modified from Tables 2, 3, and 4 from Acquaviva G, Visani M, Repaci A, et al. Molecular pathology of thyroid tumours of follicular cells: a review of genetic alterations and their clinicopathological relevance. Histopathology. 2018;72(1):6-31.

PAPILLARY PATTERN

CHECKLIST: Etiologic Considerations for the Papillary Pattern

☐ Papillary Thyroid Carcinoma (PTC)

☐ Multinodular Goiter (Papillary Hyperplasia)

☐ Chronic Lymphocytic Thyroiditis (CLT)

☐ Hyalinizing Trabecular Tumor

☐ Noninvasive Follicular Thyroid Neoplasm with Papillary-like Nuclear Features (NIFTP) and Follicular Variant of Papillary Thyroid Carcinoma

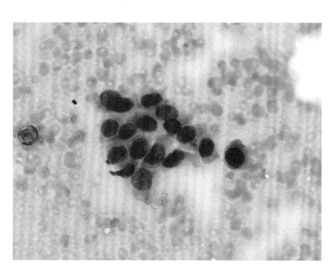

Figure 1.48. Atypia of Undetermined Significance (AUS) with nuclear atypia. These follicular cells are enlarged and oval to elongated in shape and demonstrate some irregularity in their nuclei. These cells, however, do not contain well-pronounced nuclear atypia to warrant a more serious diagnosis, nor are they arranged in a microfollicular pattern (Diff-Quik stain).

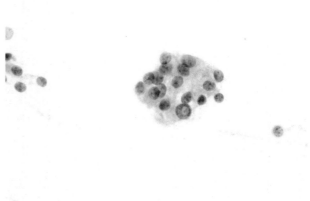

Figure 1.49. Suspicious for Papillary Thyroid Carcinoma (SPTC). This specimen was comprised of predominantly microfollicles, although certain atypical nuclear features are present, including nuclear enlargement, nuclear overlap, fine chromatin, and an intranuclear pseudo-inclusion. On follow-up, this nodule contained vascular and capsular invasion and was diagnosed as a minimally invasive, follicular variant of PTC (Pap stain).

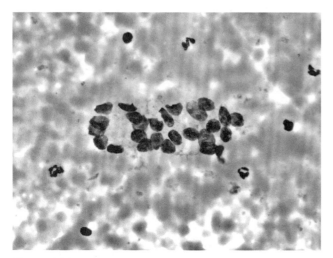

Figure 1.50. Suspicious for Papillary Thyroid Carcinoma (SPTC). A separate smear from the same case of minimally invasive follicular variant of PTC (Figure 1.49) showing follicular cells with nuclear overlap, nuclear membrane irregularities, and nuclear grooves (Diff-Quik stain).

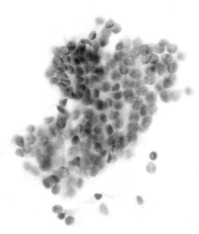

Figure 1.51. Suspicious for Papillary Thyroid Carcinoma (SPTC). This crowded group of cells is comprised of five to six cohesive microfollicles with cells displaying nuclear overlap, nuclear grooves, and chromatin clearing. On follow-up, this case met the criteria for a noninvasive follicular thyroid neoplasm with papillary-like nuclear features (Pap stain).

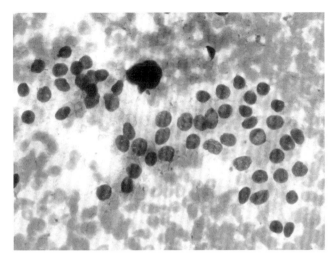

Figure 1.52. Suspicious for Papillary Thyroid Carcinoma (SPTC). Disrupted and disorganized microfollicles can be seen comprised of enlarged follicular cells with oval nuclei, irregular nuclear membranes, and nuclear grooves. Note the dark and dense colloid in the middle of the field. On follow-up, this case was consistent with a noninvasive follicular thyroid neoplasm with papillary-like nuclear features (NIFTP). These cases typically have less pronounced nuclear atypia and lack intranuclear pseudoinclusions (Diff-Quik stain).

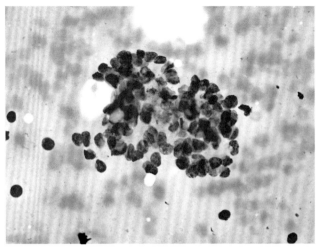

Figure 1.53. Suspicious for Papillary Thyroid Carcinoma (SPTC). Separate field, showing slightly more pronounced nuclear atypia (Diff-Quik stain).

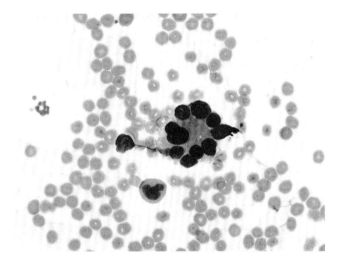

Figure 1.54. Parathyroid tissue with a microfollicular architecture (Diff-Quik stain).

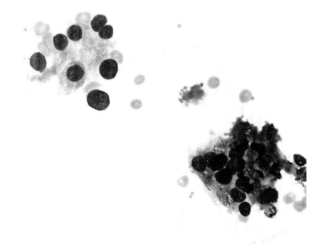

Figure 1.55. Parathyroid tissue with a microfollicular architecture (Diff-Quik stain).

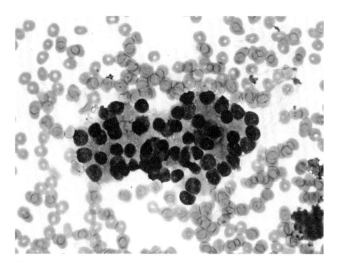

Figure 1.56. Parathyroid tissue with a microfollicular architecture. Several cohesive microfollicles are present and comprised of bland, overlapping cells with slightly bubbly and granular cytoplasm (Diff-Quik stain).

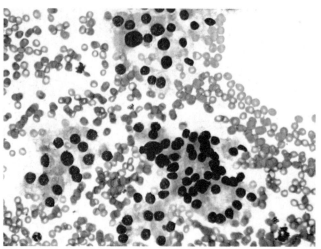

Figure 1.57. Parathyroid tissue with a microfollicular architecture. Several loosely cohesive groups forming microfollicles are present and show some nuclear size variation. The cells have fine, granular cytoplasm, which are common findings in parathyroid adenomas. These lesions, however, are virtually indistinguishable from a thyroid follicular nodule (Diff-Quik stain).

The papillary pattern can apply to specimens containing a papillary architecture as well as specimens containing cells with atypical nuclear features found in papillary thyroid carcinoma. Specimens containing papillary architecture contain monolayer fragments with papillary shapes and/or true papillae with central fibrovascular cores lined by follicular cells. When this architecutre is seen, the differential diagnosis includes papillary hyperplasia—as seen in multinodular goiter—and PTC. The nuclear atypia seen in PTC consists of the following: large, oval nuclei with irregular nuclear membranes, nuclear overlap and crowding, longitudinal nuclear grooves, intranuclear pseudoinclusions, and fine, pale chromatin. A number of diagnostic entities may contain several of these features resulting in diagnostic dilemmas.

KEY FEATURES of "Papillary Thyroid Carcinoma Nuclear Changes"
- The neoplastic cells have nuclei that are enlarged (2-3× normal follicular cells), oval to elongated, and crowded.
- The nuclear membranes are thickened and irregular.
- The nuclei are folded, forming longitudinal grooves (coffee bean nuclei).
- The chromatin is pale and powdery.
- Intranuclear pseudoinclusions may be identified, and are the most specific single feature for PTC.
- When identified, nucleoli are small and peripherally placed.

FAQ: What if I identify a few atypical nuclear features in follicular cells, but the atypical cells are only present in a fibrin clot?

Answer: Benign follicular cells can become entrapped in a fibrin clot and become artificially crowded, irregularly shaped, enlarged, and elongated.[41] Such atypia is commonly seen when cells are found within a clot and should not be overinterpreted. If possible, a diagnosis should rely more heavily on the appearance of cells seen outside of clot material. Blue cytoplasmic granules on the Diff-Quik stain, if present, are more common in benign follicular cells, which may be a helpful clue.[42]

PAPILLARY THYROID CARCINOMA

Papillary thyroid carcinoma (PTC) is the most common malignant thyroid neoplasm, accounting for roughly 80% of cases in the United States.[43] Fortunately, PTC generally carries an excellent prognosis with a 10-year survival rate >90%.[43] The classic type of PTC—the most common form—usually demonstrates both a papillary architecture (Figures 1.58-1.68) and nuclear atypia (Figures 1.69-1.80). When both nuclear atypia and papillary architecture are present, a malignant diagnosis can be rendered with confidence. In many instances, however, not all features are present—either due to sampling limitations or the fact that the PTC may show variant features. For example, there are multiple PTC variants that may have strikingly different cytologic and architectural features; however, variant classification is often neither possible nor necessary on FNA.[44] Fortunately, patient triage is the same regardless of the variant.

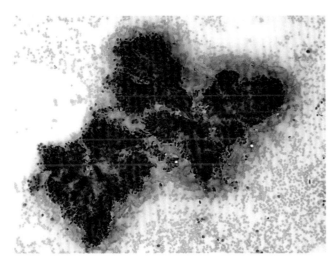

Figure 1.58. Papillary thyroid carcinoma (PTC). A low magnification view displaying branching papillary structures with inner stalks containing magenta fibrovascular cores and papillary tufts comprised of overlapping follicular cells. These complex papillary structures are diagnostic for PTC (Diff-Quik stain).

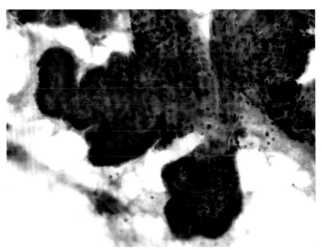

Figure 1.59. Papillary thyroid carcinoma (PTC). These papillary structures contain fibrovascular cores and cellular tufts. Although these features are diagnostic for PTC, they are rarely identified in fine-needle aspiration (FNA) samples (Pap stain).

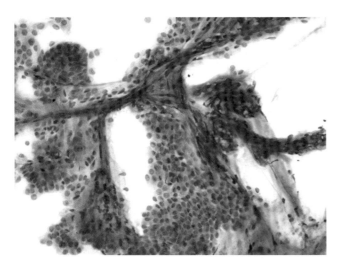

Figure 1.60. Papillary thyroid carcinoma (PTC). True papillae contain fibrovascular cores, such as those seen here. Note the complex nature of these fragments, indicative of a complex papillary process that is diagnostic for PTC (Diff-Quik stain).

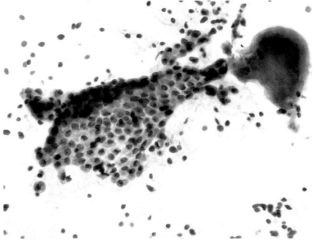

Figure 1.61. Papillary thyroid carcinoma (PTC). The malignant cells form a monolayer sheet that has a papillary architecture (Pap stain).

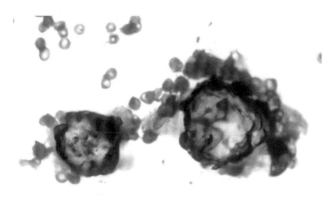

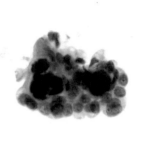

Figure 1.62. Papillary thyroid carcinoma (PTC). Two psammoma bodies with layered lamellations can be seen in this field. Although generally regarded as specific findings for PTC, they are only 50% specific for PTC (see text for further discussion) (Diff-Quik stain).

Figure 1.63. Papillary thyroid carcinoma (PTC). The follicular cells seen here have atypical nuclear features and are arranged in a somewhat microfollicular pattern around dark concretions. These may represent psammoma bodies, although definitive classification is precluded by the inability to appreciate lamellations (Pap stain).

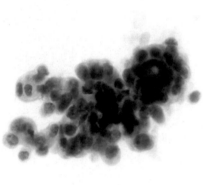

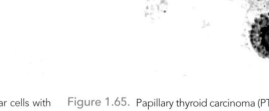

Figure 1.64. Papillary thyroid carcinoma (PTC). Follicular cells with atypical nuclear features surround a psammoma body (Pap stain).

Figure 1.65. Papillary thyroid carcinoma (PTC). This cell block preparation shows several psammoma bodies with surrounding malignant PTC cells, likely forming at the tips of papillae that are undergoing ischemia (H&E stain).

In general, FNA of a PTC will yield a cellular specimen comprised of follicular cells present singly and/or in fragments of various sizes. Large, flat "monolayer" fragments are two-dimensional sheets of follicular cells that may fold and overlap in some areas; a monolayer architecture is especially concerning for PTC. On occasion, papillary fragments with fibrovascular cores may be seen. Colloid, if present, is typically scant and forms dense globules known as "bubblegum" colloid. PTC nuclei often overlap and are typically at least twice the size of those seen in normal follicular cells, resulting in an increased nuclear to cytoplasmic (N/C) ratio. The nuclei and can be round, oval, or elongated. The nuclear membranes are thick and may have irregular contours and/or longitudinal nuclear grooves, which results in a "coffee bean" appearance. The chromatin is often pale, and small nucleoli may be present at the periphery of the nucleus. The most specific feature is the presence of round intranuclear pseudoinclusions, which should have the same color and appearance as the cytoplasm. Psammoma bodies that are typically indicative of ischemic necrosis that occurs

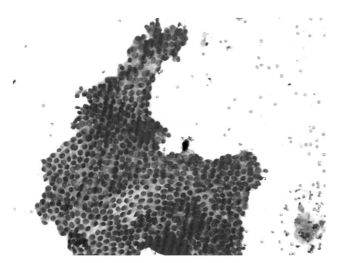

Figure 1.66. Papillary thyroid carcinoma (PTC). This monolayer sheet is comprised of many enlarged follicular cells (compare to red blood cells in the background) with round to oval nuclei. The cellularity in this monolayer sheet and its overall appearance is highly suggestive of PTC (Diff-Quik stain).

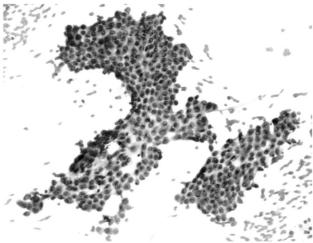

Figure 1.67. Papillary thyroid carcinoma (PTC). This cellular smear is comprised of large, monolayer sheets containing many large, overlapping, follicular cells with nuclear atypia (Pap stain).

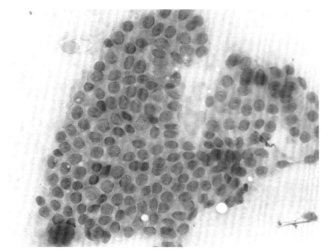

Figure 1.68. Papillary thyroid carcinoma (PTC). The monolayer sheet is comprised of enlarged follicular cells with elongated nuclei, nuclear grooves, and several intranuclear pseudoinclusions. Also, note the chunky, thick "bubblegum" colloid at the lower left corner. (Diff-Quik stain).

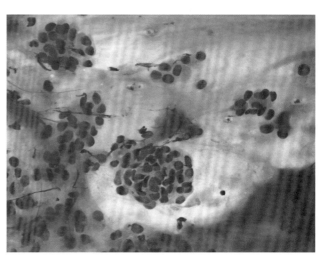

Figure 1.69. Papillary thyroid carcinoma (PTC). The smear is cellular and comprised of small groups of atypical cells caught in dark blue, sticky "bubblegum" colloid (Diff-Quik stain).

at the tips of rapidly growing papillae. Psammoma bodies may indicate that neoplastic, as opposed to hyperplastic, papillae are present in the nodule. However, psammoma bodies may be difficult to aspirate owing to the fact that psammoma bodies are hard concretions of calcium that may not easily pass through the needle. Even in the most obvious cases, each individual malignant cell may only possess a few of the characteristic cytomorphologic nuclear features of PTC. In the context of the entire case, however, most features will, to some degree, be present, and an accurate diagnosis of PTC can be made. Multinucleated giant cells may be more common in cases of PTC but are also commonly seen in benign nodules with a background of lymphocytic thyroiditis.[45] Because many of these features in isolation are nonspecific, most cytopathologists will reserve a definitive malignant diagnosis for cases with overt papillary architecture or readily identifiable intranuclear pseudoinclusions. The remainder of cases will either be classified as Suspicious for Papillary Thyroid Carcinoma or Atypia of Uncertain Significance (AUS) according to the TBSRTC.[1]

PEARLS & PITFALLS

The presence of one or even a few atypical nuclear features must be interpreted with caution, including intranuclear pseudoinclusions. For example, intranuclear pseudoinclusions can also be found in Hurthle cells, medullary thyroid carcinoma (MTC), and hyalinizing trabecular tumor (HTT).[46-48] Therefore, a diagnosis should be made based on a constellation of features. Furthermore, a number of changes may mimic intranuclear pseudoinclusions ("pseudo" intranuclear pseudoinclusions), such as the presence of degenerative nuclear vacuoles, fixation artifacts, and red blood cells overlying the nucleus, resulting in a round, seemingly unstained portion of a nucleus.[1] A true intranuclear pseudoinclusion, however, should have the same texture and staining characteristics as the cytoplasm of the malignant cell because it is the result of invagination of the cytoplasm into the nucleus.

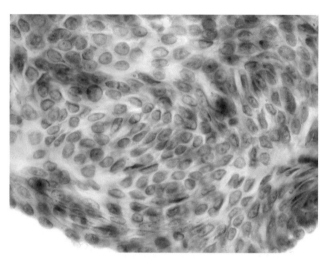

Figure 1.70. Papillary thyroid carcinoma (PTC). Crowded, elongated follicular cells with nuclear grooves, moderate nuclear membrane irregularities, small peripheral nucleoli, and chromatin clearing form a swirling pattern sometimes seen in PTC (Pap stain).

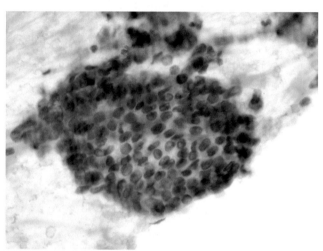

Figure 1.71. Papillary thyroid carcinoma (PTC). Overlapping and elongated follicular cells with nuclear membrane irregularities, nuclear grooves, and pale chromatin are present in a monolayer sheet. Furthermore, several suspected intranuclear pseudoinclusions are present in the center of this sheet. The lack of evenly spaced follicular cells with round, bland nuclei are not consistent with a benign process (Pap stain).

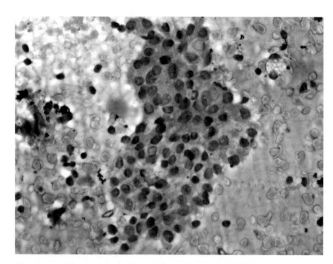

Figure 1.72. Papillary thyroid carcinoma (PTC). This fragment is disorganized and contains large cells with nuclear grooves, irregular nuclear membranes, and an intranuclear pseudoinclusion. Note the vacuolated macrophage at the upper right (Diff-Quik stain).

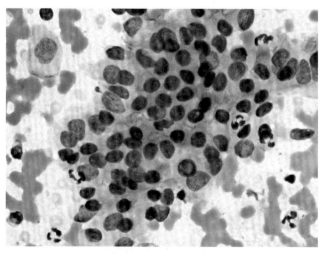

Figure 1.73. Papillary thyroid carcinoma (PTC). This field contains many of the atypical nuclear features seen in PTC, including a prominent intranuclear pseudoinclusion (Diff-Quik stain).

FAQ: How do I handle a specimen that contains psammoma bodies but is otherwise lacking features diagnostic of PTC?

Answer: One should be careful and not immediately diagnose a PTC based on the presence of psammoma bodies alone. Multinodular goiter and Hurthle cell neoplasms can show dystrophic, nonlamellated calcifications that mimic psammoma bodies. In fact, if taken in isolation, the presence of psammoma bodies on FNA is associated with a positive predictive value of 50%.[49] As a result, one must rely on the constellation of features of PTC to render an accurate diagnosis.

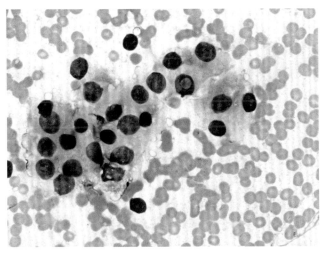

Figure 1.74. Papillary thyroid carcinoma (PTC). Although these cells contain abundant cytoplasm, note the enlarged nuclei and the well-formed intranuclear pseudoinclusion characteristic of PTC (Diff-Quik stain).

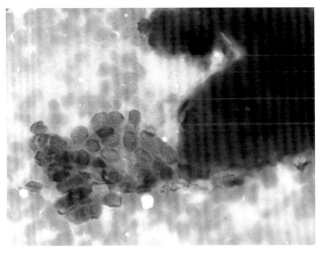

Figure 1.75. Papillary thyroid carcinoma (PTC). While the presence of colloid might suggest a benign process, the cells in this small fragment have elongated nuclei, irregular nuclear contours, and nuclear enlargement (Diff-Quik stain).

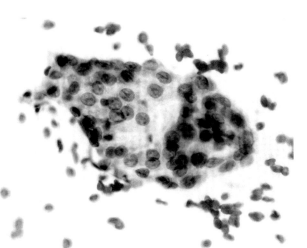

Figure 1.76. Papillary thyroid carcinoma (PTC). Note the pale, powdery chromatin, nuclear grooves, and small, punctate nucleoli that are classic of PTC (Pap stain).

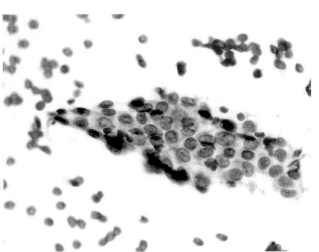

Figure 1.77. Papillary thyroid carcinoma (PTC). Separate field from the prior case (Figure 1.76). These cells are enlarged and elongated and contain nuclear grooves, pale and powdery chromatin, and small, mostly peripheral, punctate nucleoli (Pap stain).

SAMPLE NOTE: ATYPIA OF UNDETERMINED SIGNIFICANCE (AUS)

Atypical of Undetermined Significance (AUS). See note.

Note: The specimen consists of bland follicular cells and colloid; however, there are several calcifications present in the sample that may represent psammoma bodies. Although this finding is nonspecific and can be seen in conditions other than PTC, the positive predictive value for PTC based on this finding alone has been reported to be 50%. Therefore, this sample is best classified as atypical and indeterminate.

Reference:
Ellison E, Lapuerta P, Martin SE. Psammoma bodies in fine needle aspirates. *Cancer.* 1998;84(3):169-175.

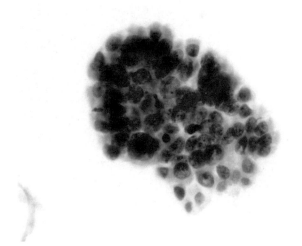

Figure 1.78. Papillary thyroid carcinoma (PTC). This fragment likely represents the tip of a papillary fragment and is composed of enlarged (compared with the lymphocyte in the center of the field) follicular cells showing significant overlap, irregular nuclear membranes, and powdery chromatin (Pap stain).

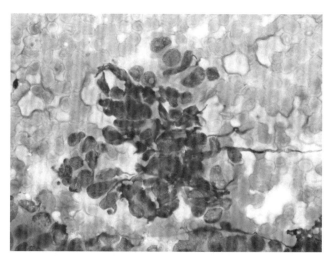

Figure 1.79. Papillary thyroid carcinoma (PTC). A crushed and crowded group of atypical follicular cells contain prominent intranuclear pseudoinclusions. The crushed cells demonstrate chromatin smearing, which might be mistaken for lymphoid tangles (Pap stain).

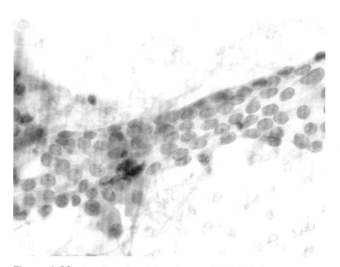

Figure 1.80. Papillary thyroid carcinoma (PTC). This fragment contains streaming malignant PTC cells with the pale, powdery chromatin and small, peripheral, punctate nucleoli. Note the presence of several intranuclear pseudoinclusions (Pap stain).

MULTINODULAR GOITER (PAPILLARY HYPERPLASIA)

Multinodular goiter represents an increase in the size of the thyroid secondary to stimulation by excess thyroid-stimulating hormone (TSH). As these follicular cells become stimulated, hyperplasia develops and results in a nodular pattern of growth with occasional hyperplastic papillae and cells with reactive atypia (Figures 1.81-1.83). Most often, however, these papillae are simple and nonbranching in nature, as opposed to the complex, atypical branching papillae that are characteristic of PTC. Furthermore, the cells lining the hyperplastic papillae in multinodular goiter lack atypical nuclear features and can show Hurthle cell metaplasia, characterized by an abundance of fine, granular cytoplasm (pale purple on the Diff-Quik stain and orange or green on the Pap stain) and large, round nuclei. Owing to the stimulation by TSH, the follicular cells make abundant colloid which should be present in the FNA material. Furthermore, the cellularity in most of these cases is usually low secondary to the abundant colloid, and most cases will have a predominantly macrofollicular pattern (see the "Normal Thyroid/Benign Follicular Nodule" section in the "Macrofollicular Pattern").

PEARLS & PITFALLS

Degenerative features secondary to cyst formation or hemorrhage are not uncommon in multinodular goiter and may result in some degree of atypia. This atypia, however, is usually focal and subtle in comparison to the well-developed nuclear atypia seen in malignant cases of PTC. Flame cells, characterized by magenta/pink, marginal cytoplasmic vacuoles, may also help indicate a reactive, hyperplastic lesion versus a malignant lesion consistent with PTC. It is always important to remember, however, that a patient with multinodular goiter can still have PTC.

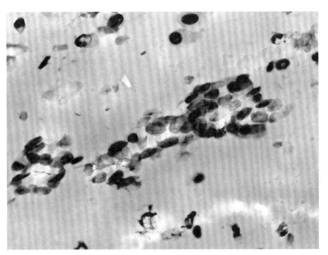

Figure 1.81. Atypia of Undetermined Significance (AUS) with cytologic atypia. Cells caught in a clot may be artificially elongated, crowded, and folded, as seen in this patient who had a multinodular goiter on follow-up (Diff-Quik stain).

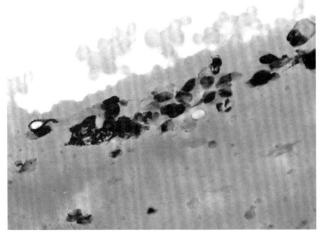

Figure 1.82. Atypia of Undetermined Significance (AUS) with cytologic atypia. Same case from prior Figure 1.81 showing artificial nuclear atypia in follicular cells trapped in a clot (Diff-Quik stain).

CHRONIC LYMPHOCYTIC THYROIDITIS

Chronic lymphocytic thyroiditis (CLT) is an autoimmune disease that leads to destruction of the follicular cells and the formation of germinal centers within the thyroid parenchyma. In CLT, these disrupted follicular cells immediately adjacent to germinal centers can show several features that mimic PTC: focal nuclear enlargement, longitudinal nuclear grooves, prominent nucleoli, and fine, pale chromatin.[50] However, these nuclei are typically round and uniform and lack intranuclear pseudoinclusions (Figures 1.84-1.91). In addition, CLT is classically associated with Hurthle cell metaplasia which is characterized by large, polygonal cells with abundant granular cytoplasm and large nuclei. In some instances, multinucleated giant cells may be seen. A mix of benign follicular cells and Hurthle cells in the

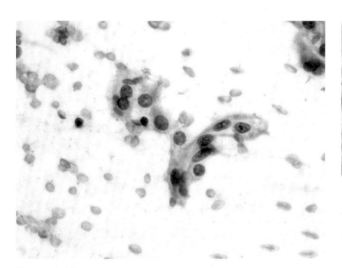

Figure 1.83. Reactive atypia. A benign follicular nodule, such as that seen in a nodular goiter, can undergo cystic change and result in reactive atypia, including nuclear enlargement (compared with the lymphocytes in this field), nuclear elongation, and abundant cytoplasm that may contain elongated projections. In some cases, these features may be difficult to definitively classify as benign (Pap stain).

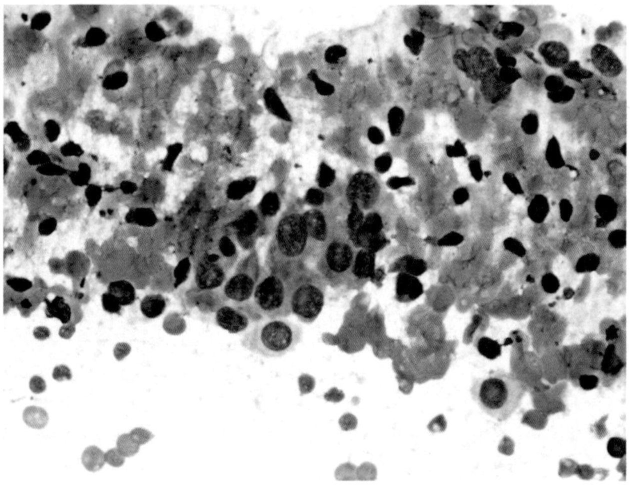

Figure 1.84. Benign adenomatoid nodule in a background of chronic lymphocytic thyroiditis (CLT). Note the abundant lymphocytes admixed with follicular epithelial cells that appear slightly disrupted with minimal cytologic atypia (Diff-Quik stain).

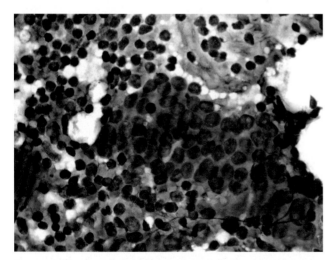

Figure 1.85. Atypia of Undetermined Significance (AUS) with cytologic atypia in a background of chronic lymphocytic thyroiditis (CLT). Note the scattered lymphocytes and lymphoid tangles admixed with crowded, enlarged follicular cells with irregular nuclear membranes. This level of atypia is not uncommon in cases of CLT and may warrant an atypical diagnosis (Diff-Quik stain).

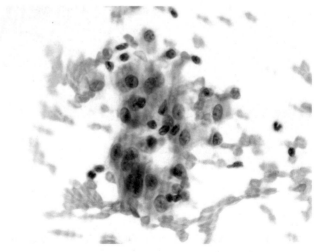

Figure 1.86. Atypia of Undetermined Significance (AUS) with cytologic atypia in a background of chronic lymphocytic thyroiditis (CLT). Scattered lymphocytes surround this irregular group of follicular cells with nuclear enlargement, overlap, irregular borders, pale chromatin, and small, punctate nucleoli. These features may be reactive secondary to CLT; however, patients with CLT may also develop papillary thyroid carcinoma (Pap stain).

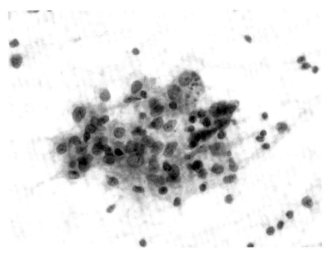

Figure 1.87. Atypia of Undetermined Significance (AUS) with cytologic atypia in a background of chronic lymphocytic thyroiditis (CLT). A separate field from the prior case showing the degree of atypia in a background of lymphocytes (Pap stain).

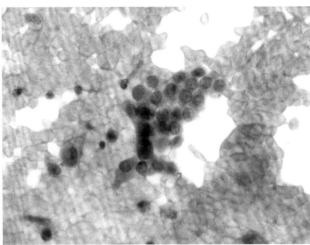

Figure 1.88. Atypia of Undetermined Significance (AUS) with cytologic atypia in a background of chronic lymphocytic thyroiditis (CLT). Scattered lymphocytes are present adjacent to these enlarged follicular cells with atypical nuclei (Pap stain).

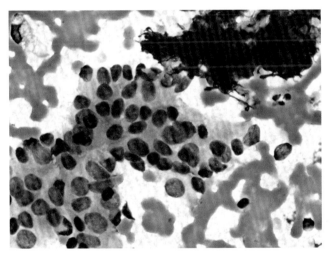

Figure 1.89. Atypia of Undetermined Significance (AUS) with cytologic atypia in a background of chronic lymphocytic thyroiditis (CLT). Note the enlarged, elongated, and overlapping follicular cells adjacent to the crushed lymphocytic aggregate, hinting that these findings might be simply reactive in nature (Diff-Quik stain).

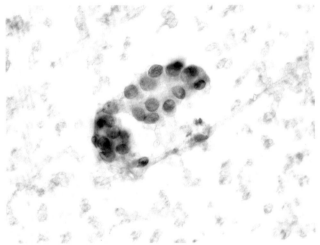

Figure 1.90. Atypia of Undetermined Significance (AUS) with cytologic atypia and microfollicular atypia. The cells are slightly irregular with pale chromatin and small, punctate, peripherally located nucleoli. On follow-up, this nodule was found to be a noninvasive follicular thyroid neoplasm with papillary-like nuclear feature (NIFTP) (Pap stain).

presence of germinal centers is virtually diagnostic of CLT. Because patients with CLT do have an increased risk for both PTC and lymphoma, it is prudent to closely scrutinize all aspirated material. In some cases, a definitive diagnosis is not possible.

HYALINIZING TRABECULAR TUMOR

Hyalinizing trabecular tumor (HTT), formerly referred to as hyalinizing trabecular adenoma, is a rare, benign neoplasm characterized by prominent hyalinization within trabeculae formed by follicular cells. HTT is often associated with bloody but cellular aspirates comprised of cohesive clusters of cells with wispy cytoplasm, as well as single cells with naked nuclei. In HTT, nuclei are elongated with irregular contours, nuclear grooves, and intranuclear pseudoinclusions. The hallmark feature of HTT, however, is the presence of dense hyaline material in the center of follicular cells aggregates.[51] This hyaline material appears magenta on the Diff-Quik stain and pale pink to red on the Pap stain. On FNA, most cases of HTT are diagnosed as either PTC or medullary thyroid carcinoma (MTC).[52] HTT is a known mimic of PTC owing to the presence of several well-developed atypical

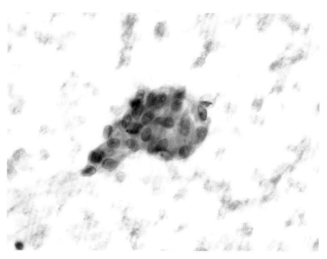

Figure 1.91. Atypia of Undetermined Significance (AUS) with cytologic atypia and microfollicular atypia. This image is a separate field from the prior case that was diagnosed as noninvasive follicular thyroid neoplasm with papillary-like nuclear features (NIFTP) on follow-up. Note the nuclear elongation, nuclear grooves, pale chromatin, and punctate, peripheral nucleoli (Pap stain).

nuclear features, including nuclei with irregular nuclear membranes, longitudinal nuclear grooves, and prominent intranuclear pseudoinclusions—often with more pseudoinclusions than a typical case of PTC. Furthermore, dystrophic calcifications may be present, which may be psammomatous or nonpsammomatous. These features make it extremely difficult to distinguish HTT from PTC on FNA. Both HTT and MTC can have cells with similar cytology and both lack colloid. Furthermore, the hyaline material characteristic of HTT may mimic the amyloid characteristic of MTC. Immunostains for calcitonin (positive in MTC and negative in HTT) and thyroglobulin (negative in MTC and positive in HTT) can distinguish between these tumors if cell block material is available.[51]

NONINVASIVE FOLLICULAR THYROID NEOPLASM WITH PAPILLARY-LIKE NUCLEAR FEATURES (NIFTP) AND FOLLICULAR VARIANT OF PAPILLARY THYROID CARCINOMA

Noninvasive follicular thyroid neoplasm with papillary-like nuclear features (NIFTP) is the updated nomenclature for the entity previously referred to as "noninvasive follicular variant of PTC". Owing to its indolent behavior after lobectomy, the entity now classified as NIFTP no longer represents a thyroid malignancy, which does have an impact on the rate of malignancy of TBSRTC categories.[53] On surgical resection, NIFTP is mainly distinguished from an invasive follicular variant of PTC by the lack of capsular or vascular invasion. This fact means that definitively diagnosing NIFTP by FNA is not possible. About half of the cases of NIFTP are diagnosed as follicular neoplasms by FNA, about a quarter are diagnosed as AUS, and less than 5% are categorized as a malignant lesion.[53-55] On FNA, NIFTP contains a predominantly microfollicular pattern that usually does not contain monolayer sheets and lacks true papillae and psammoma bodies. The nuclear features of NIFTP resemble that of PTC; however, they are usually more subtle and often lack intranuclear pseudoinclusions.[56] As a result, very few of these cases are diagnosed as PTC on FNA.

KEY FEATURES of Noninvasive Follicular Thyroid Neoplasm With Papillary-like Nuclear Features (NIFTP) as Seen on FNA

- The smears are cellular and composed of follicular cells in a microfollicular architecture.
- Nuclear features are similar to that of PTC but are often more subtle with a lack of intranuclear pseudoinclusions.
- The specimen must lack true papillae, psammoma bodies, tumor necrosis, elevated mitotic rate, and cytomorphologic characteristics of a variant of PTC.

SAMPLE NOTE: SUSPICIOUS FOR PAPILLARY THYROID CARCINOMA

Suspicious for Papillary Thyroid Carcinoma. See note.

Note: The specimen consists of numerous microfollicles with papillary-type nuclear features scattered throughout the specimen, including nuclear enlargement, nuclear overlap, irregular nuclear membranes, nuclear grooves, and pale chromatin. The absence of intranuclear pseudoinclusions, overt papillary configurations, and psammoma bodies, as well as the patchy nuclear atypia in this case, does not justify a definitive malignant diagnosis. The differential diagnosis includes PTC (such as classic variant), follicular variant of PTC, and NIFTP, as well as benign entities which can show focal nuclear atypia.

HURTHLE CELL PATTERN

CHECKLIST: Etiologic Considerations for the Hurthle Cell Pattern

☐ Chronic Lymphocytic Thyroiditis (CLT)

☐ Multinodular Goiter

☐ Hurthle Cell Neoplasms

☐ Papillary Thyroid Carcinoma (PTC), Oncocytic and Warthin-like Variants

The Hurthle cell pattern is characterized by the presence of enlarged, polygonal follicular cells with abundant, fine, granular cytoplasm, indicative of an abundance of mitochondria. On a Diff-Quik stain, the granular cytoplasm may appear blue or gray while on a Pap stain, the cytoplasm is green or orange; on an H&E stain, the cytoplasm is pink. Typically, these cells have enlarged, round or oval, central or eccentric nuclei with or without prominent nucleoli. Occasionally, Hurthle cells may be confused with macrophages on liquid-based preparations secondary to the formation of pseudovacuoles that look similar to the vacuoles of macrophages.[37] The Hurthle cell pattern may be present in a variety of thyroid processes. Hurthle cell change may be metaplastic, as seen in CLT and multinodular goiter, or neoplastic, as seen in a Hurthle cell adenoma (HCA), Hurthle cell carcinoma (HCC), or Warthin-like PTC.

CHRONIC LYMPHOCYTIC THYROIDITIS

Chronic lymphocytic thyroiditis (CLT), as previously described (see the "Papillary Pattern"), is an autoimmune disease that leads to damage of the thyroid follicular cells. As a result, lymphohistiocytic aggregates are present and the follicular cells can undergo a metaplastic change and accumulate abundant mitochondria in the cytoplasm, giving the cells a Hurthle cell appearance (Figures 1.92-1.104).[58] As is also seen with Hurthle cell neoplasms, CLT is usually associated with scant or absent colloid. It is important to analyze all available material and look for other diagnostic clues for CLT, such as benign-appearing follicular cells and interspersed polymorphous lymphocytes and lymphohistiocytic aggregates (germinal centers), which would be highly unusual in a Hurthle cell neoplasm. Follicular cells in CLT may also have some degree of reactive atypia, including the presence of nuclear grooves and pale chromatin. As a result, some cases may be difficult to distinguish between a Warthin-like variant of PTC, which is characterized by Hurthle cells with sometimes subtle nuclear atypia and large papillary fragments filled with a lymphoplasmacytoid infiltrate. The presence of these papillae, however, would strongly favor PTC. Finally, the clinical history can be extremely helpful. A patient with a history of lymphocytic thyroiditis is much more likely to have a nodule composed of hyperplastic Hurthle cells as opposed to a Hurthle cell neoplasm or a rare oncocytic or Warthin-like variant of PTC; however, patients with CLT can certainly develop PTC.

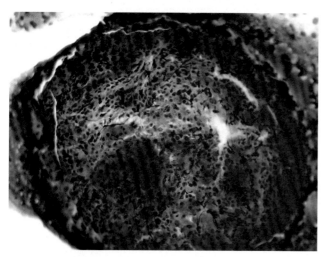

Figure 1.92. Benign, consistent with chronic lymphocytic thyroiditis (CLT). Colloid surrounds a cellular aggregate of abundant crushed and intact lymphocytes admixed with Hurthle cells (Diff-Quik stain).

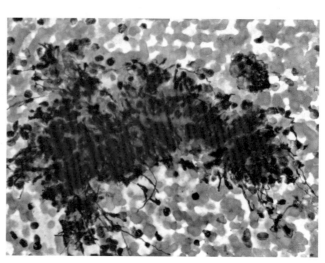

Figure 1.93. Benign, consistent with chronic lymphocytic thyroiditis (CLT). A large cluster of crushed lymphocytes, as seen in this view, is highly indicative of CLT (Diff-Quik stain).

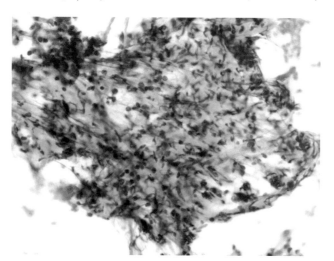

Figure 1.94. Benign, consistent with chronic lymphocytic thyroiditis (CLT). The field contains a large lymphohistiocytic aggregate, highly suggestive of CLT (Pap stain).

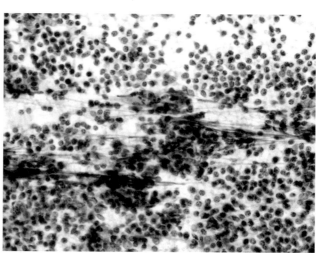

Figure 1.95. Benign, consistent with chronic lymphocytic thyroiditis (CLT). The smear is comprised of numerous dispersed, polymorphous lymphocytes and lymphoid tangles in this patient with CLT (Pap stain).

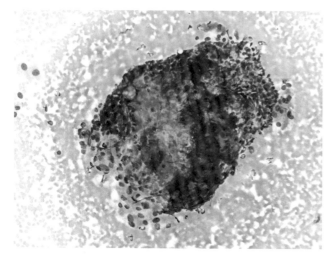

Figure 1.96. Benign, consistent with chronic lymphocytic thyroiditis (CLT). This view shows an aggregate comprised of numerous crushed lymphocytes and follicular cells with abundant, granular cytoplasm and large nuclei, consistent with Hurthle cell metaplasia (Diff-Quik stain).

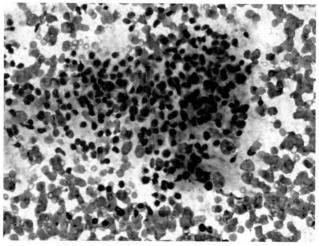

Figure 1.97. Benign, consistent with chronic lymphocytic thyroiditis (CLT). Note the numerous polymorphous lymphocytes and rare, larger cells most likely representing Hurthle cells (Diff-Quik stain).

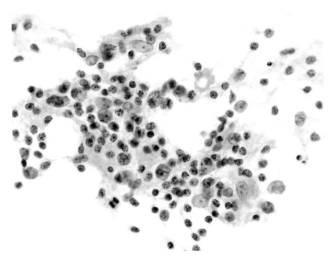

Figure 1.98. Benign, consistent with chronic lymphocytic thyroiditis (CLT). Separate smear from the prior case diagnosed as consistent with CLT. Note the polymorphous lymphocytes and admixed larger cells, most likely representing Hurthle cells (Pap stain).

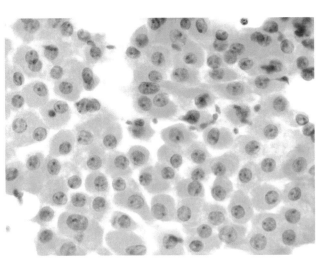

Figure 1.99. Benign, consistent with chronic lymphocytic thyroiditis (CLT). A third smear from this case of CLT shows sheets of Hurthle cells with the characteristic finely granular abundant cytoplasm and large, round nuclei (Pap stain).

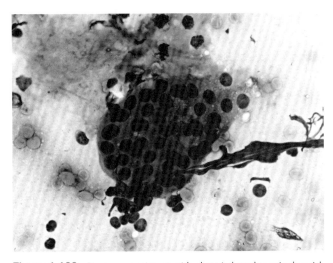

Figure 1.100. Benign, consistent with chronic lymphocytic thyroiditis (CLT). A cluster of follicular cells with Hurthle cell features is seen in a background of lymphocytes and lymphoid tangles (Diff-Quik stain).

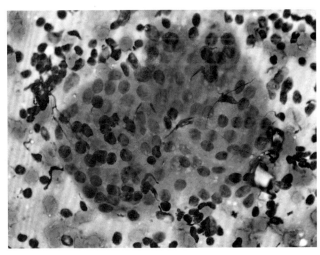

Figure 1.101. Benign, consistent with chronic lymphocytic thyroiditis (CLT). Polymorphous lymphocytes are seen within and also in the background of this sheet of Hurthle cells (Diff-Quik stain).

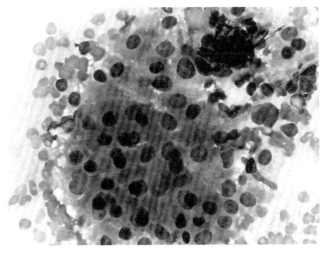

Figure 1.102. Benign, consistent with chronic lymphocytic thyroiditis (CLT). Alternate field (Diff-Quik stain).

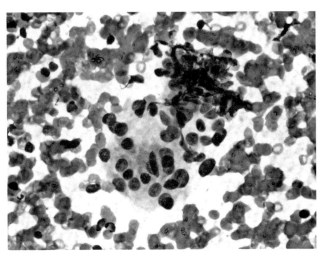

Figure 1.103. Benign, consistent with chronic lymphocytic thyroiditis (CLT). A small group of follicular epithelial cells with Hurthle cell features is adjacent to lymphoid tangles and background lymphocytes (Diff-Quik stain).

KEY FEATURES of Chronic Lymphocytic Thyroiditis

- The background consists predominantly of polymorphous lymphocytes.
- Lymphohistiocytic aggregates may be seen.
- When present, thyroid follicular cells demonstrate diffuse Hurthle cell metaplasia.
- Colloid is typically absent or scant.
- Multinucleated giant cells may be seen.

MULTINODULAR GOITER

Multinodular goiter, as previously described (see the "Papillary Pattern"), occurs secondary to follicular cell hyperplasia, leading to an enlarged thyroid gland. Multiple etiologies and multiple features can be seen on FNA cytology, including Hurthle cell metaplasia, resulting in large, polygonal cells with abundant, finely granular oncocytic cytoplasm and large, round nuclei (Figures 1.105-1.109). In fact, Hurthle cells have been reported to be present

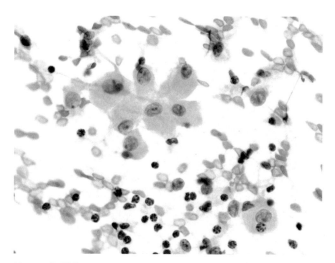

Figure 1.104. Benign, consistent with chronic lymphocytic thyroiditis (CLT). Hurthle cells loosely cluster together in a background of polymorphous lymphocytes (Pap stain).

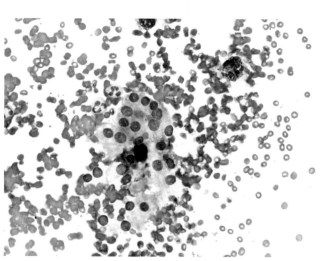

Figure 1.105. Benign, consistent with an adenomatoid nodule. In this patient with a multinodular goiter, several fields contained small groups of follicular epithelium showing Hurthle cell metaplasia. Note the globule of blue colloid in the center of the field and the pigmented, vacuolated macrophages in the background, suggesting cystic degeneration (Diff-Quik stain).

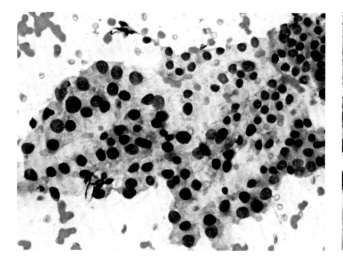

Figure 1.106. Benign, consistent with an adenomatoid nodule. Separate field from the same patient as the prior Figure 1.105 showing sheets of follicular epithelial cells with abundant cytoplasm that may appear "Hurthleoid" (Diff-Quik stain).

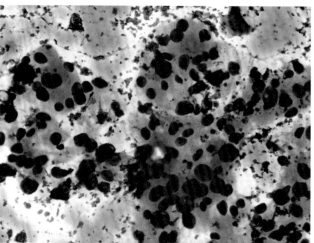

Figure 1.107. Benign, consistent with an adenomatoid nodule. In this field, numerous follicular cells with finely granular cytoplasm and variably sized nuclei are present. In other fields, however, abundant colloid and macrofollicles were present. The overall best explanation for this finding is focal Hurthle cell metaplasia in a benign adenomatoid nodule. Also, note the abundant magenta ultrasound gel in the background (Diff-Quik stain).

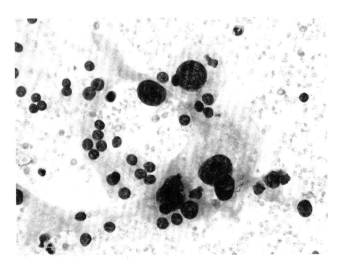

Figure 1.108. Atypia of Undetermined Significance (AUS) with Hurthle cell features. Note the enlarged cells with abundant cytoplasm, resulting in a relatively normal N/C ratio. The presence of prominent nucleoli caused this case to be flagged as atypical. On follow-up, however, this patient was found to have a benign nodular goiter (Diff-Quik stain).

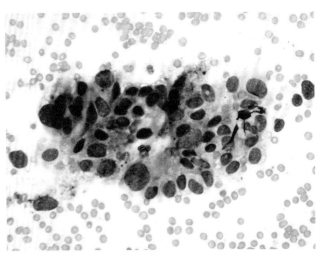

Figure 1.109. Atypia of Undetermined Significance (AUS) with Hurthle cell features. This additional field from the prior patient (Figure 1.108) shows Hurthle cells of varying size and shape. Note the "pseudo" intranuclear inclusion, which lacks the characteristics of the cytoplasm. Also, note the blue cytoplasmic granules, which may be a clue that these cells are benign (Diff-Quik stain).

in as many as 50% of cases of multinodular goiter.[59] In an FNA of a multinodular goiter, these cells should comprise only a fraction of the follicular cells present, with the majority of the specimen containing abundant colloid and scattered follicular cells in a macrofollicular pattern. In fact, the presence of colloid strongly favors against a Hurthle cell neoplasm. Finally, multinodular goiter can occasionally show dystrophic, nonlamellated calcifications that mimic psammoma bodies. The key to recognizing that these are pseudopsammoma bodies is to appreciate the lack of concentric circles most easily seen at the edge of the calcified body.

HURTHLE CELL NEOPLASMS

A diagnosis of Follicular Neoplasm/Suspicious for a Follicular Neoplasm (FN/SFN), Hurthle cell type is recommended when nearly all sampled cells show Hurthle cell change, which should eliminate the majority of nonneoplastic cases that have focal Hurthle cell metaplasia. However, 10-26% of these cases will subsequently be found to be hyperplastic nodules or lymphocytic thyroiditis. Anywhere from 15-45% will be malignant.[60-62] These specimens tend to be hypercellular and contain predominantly single, isolated Hurthle cells that are occasionally in three-dimensional, syncytial groups (Figures 1.110-1.118). There should be little to no colloid and rare to absent lymphocytes. Hurthle cell neoplasms are most often comprised of monomorphic Hurthle cells that exhibit less nuclear size and shape variability than metaplastic Hurthle cells. However, less commonly, neoplastic Hurthle cells may show bizarre nuclear atypia and pleomorphism. Additionally, large nucleoli and/or transgressing vessels are more likely to be seen in Hurthle cell neoplasms than metaplastic Hurthle cells.[58] Cases with papillary nuclear features in any part of the specimen should be excluded from this category because they may represent the oncocytic variant of PTC.[1] The distinction between a benign HCA and a malignant HCC is dependent on lymphovascular and capsular invasion identified on surgical specimens, precluding definitive classification on FNA. Interestingly, unlike follicular carcinoma, which is more commonly associated with vascular metastases, nodal metastases occur in 20-30% of patients with the HCC.[63,64]

PEARLS & PITFALLS

It is important to maintain a broad differential diagnosis and consider entities that can occur in or around the thyroid that are not of follicular origin. For the Hurthle cell pattern, several entities that may have a "Hurthleoid" or oncocytoid appearance include medullary carcinoma of the thyroid, parathyroid adenoma, granular cell tumor, and metastatic renal cell carcinoma. For the listed entities, the patient's clinical history is invaluable; however, immunostains can very easily resolve the diagnostic dilemma in most cases. For this reason, using the needle rinse to make a cell block can be very beneficial. Medullary carcinoma of the thyroid should be positive for calcitonin; parathyroid adenoma should be positive for parathyroid hormone; granular cell tumor will be positive for S100; and metastatic renal cell carcinoma will be negative for TTF-1 (and positive for PAX-8).

PAPILLARY THYROID CARCINOMA, ONCOCYTIC AND WARTHIN-LIKE VARIANTS

Despite the many variants of PTC, all forms share the same characteristic nuclear features. Both the oncocytic and the Warthin-like variants are no different.[65] In both entities, the malignant cells have Hurthle cell features and are enlarged and polygonal with abundant, finely granular oncocytic cytoplasm. Although nuclear atypia can be subtle, the nuclei will often have an irregular contour with grooves and rare pseudoinclusions, pale chromatin, and peripheral nucleoli. The oncocytic variant can show papillary or microfollicular patterns (Figures 1.119-1.124) while the Warthin-like variant is characterized by large papillae lined by neoplastic cells and distended by a lymphoplasmacytic infiltrate resembling a Warthin tumor of the parotid gland (Figures 1.125 and 1.126).[66] Interestingly, the majority of both variants arise in patients with a history of lymphocytic thyroiditis.[66-68]

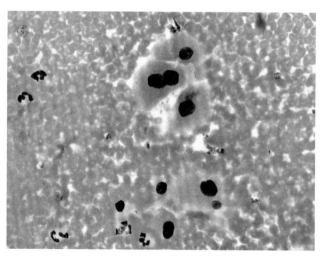

Figure 1.110. Suspicious for a Follicular Neoplasm (SFN), Hurthle cell type. The specimen consisted of a pure population of Hurthle cells with abundant, finely granular cytoplasm and large nuclei with slightly irregular nuclear contours, binucleation, and occasional nucleoli. This latter finding, although very nonspecific, may be more common in Hurthle cell neoplasms versus Hurthle cell metaplasia (Diff-Quik stain).

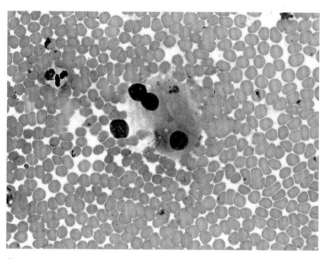

Figure 1.111. Suspicious for a Follicular Neoplasm (SFN), Hurthle cell type. A possible intranuclear pseudoinclusion is seen in one of the cells. Since the color of the inclusion does not match that of the cytoplasm, this may represent a "pseudo" pseudoinclusion (Diff-Quik stain).

DISCOHESIVE PATTERN

CHECKLIST: Etiologic Considerations for the Discohesive Pattern

☐ Poorly Differentiated Thyroid Carcinoma (PDTC)

☐ Anaplastic Thyroid Carcinoma (ATC)

☐ Hurthle Cell Neoplasm

☐ Medullary Thyroid Carcinoma (MTC)

☐ Lymphoma

☐ Parathyroid Tissue

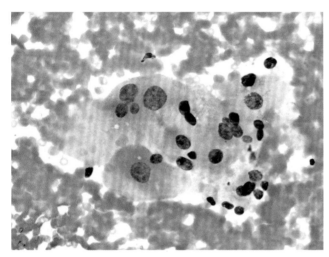

Figure 1.112. Suspicious for a Follicular Neoplasm (SFN), Hurthle cell type. These Hurthle cells are admixed with several admixed lymphocytes, which may bring up chronic lymphocytic thyroiditis in the differential diagnosis. This case, however, was comprised of an abundance of discohesive Hurthle cells, some with prominent nucleoli and multinucleation. On follow-up, this nodule was diagnosed as a Hurthle cell adenoma (Diff-Quik stain).

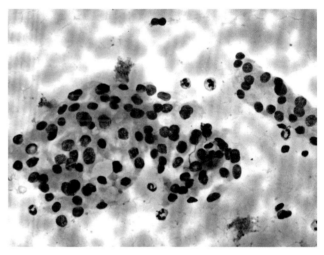

Figure 1.113. Suspicious for a Follicular Neoplasm (SFN), Hurthle cell type. Sheet of Hurthle cells showing some variation in size and shape. On follow-up, this case was diagnosed as a Hurthle cell adenoma (Diff-Quik stain).

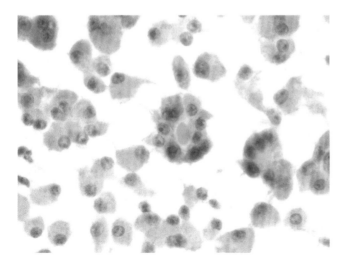

Figure 1.114. Suspicious for a Follicular Neoplasm (SFN), Hurthle cell type. Cellular specimen comprised of small clusters of discohesive Hurthle cells with prominent nucleoli. On follow-up, this specimen was diagnosed as a Hurthle cell carcinoma (Pap stain).

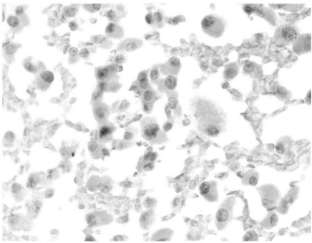

Figure 1.115. Suspicious for a Follicular Neoplasm (SFN), Hurthle cell type. An alternate field from the prior patient with Hurthle cell carcinoma showing multiple, discohesive Hurthle cells (Pap stain).

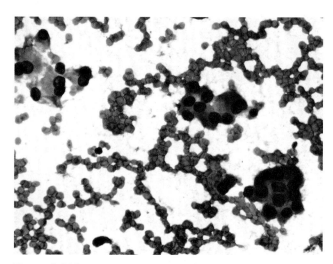

Figure 1.116. Suspicious for a Follicular Neoplasm (SFN), Hurthle cell type. This third field from the prior patient with Hurthle cell carcinoma shows multiple small groups of Hurthle cells with prominent nucleoli (Diff-Quik stain).

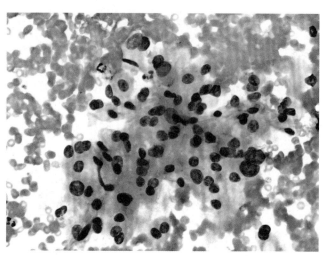

Figure 1.117. Suspicious for a Follicular Neoplasm (SFN), Hurthle cell type. A group of Hurthle cells that demonstrate fairly significant nuclear size and shape variation, as well as prominent nucleoli. Follow-up was consistent with a Hurthle cell carcinoma (Diff-Quik stain).

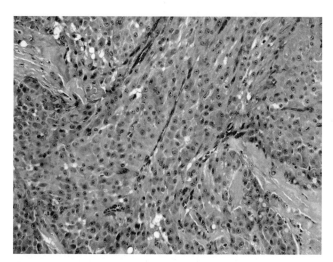

Figure 1.118. Hurthle cell carcinoma. Note the sheets of Hurthle cells that can be seen dissecting the capsule of this nodule on this resection specimen (H&E).

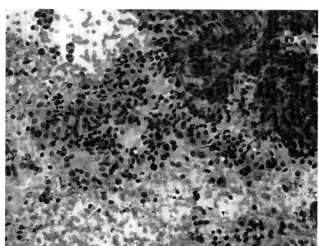

Figure 1.119. Papillary thyroid carcinoma (PTC), oncocytic variant. Multiple scattered single cells and cells arranged in groups are present with abundant, blue cytoplasm. Note the papillary fragment at the top right portion of the field (Diff-Quik stain).

On occasion, thyroid FNAs will reveal highly cellular smears comprised of predominantly discohesive cells in the absence of colloid or cystic features. The differential diagnosis for this pattern ranges from benign parathyroid tissue to a medullary thyroid carcinoma (MTC). Furthermore, lymphomas, most commonly B-cell lymphomas, may occur; patients with a history of CLT are at least 60 times more likely to develop lymphoma of the thyroid than the general population.[69-71] As a result, the presence of a discohesive pattern on FNA should also warrant careful consideration of diagnoses that are not of a follicular epithelial origin.

POORLY DIFFERENTIATED THYROID CARCINOMA

Poorly differentiated thyroid carcinoma (PDTC) is a rare malignancy derived from the follicular cells of the thyroid without obvious papillary, follicular, or anaplastic features (Figures 1.127-1.130). PDTC is frequently associated with regional and distant metastases at the time of presentation and carries a 5-year survival of approximately 60%.[72] According to the histopathologic Turin criteria, (1) the growth pattern should be insular, solid, or trabecular;

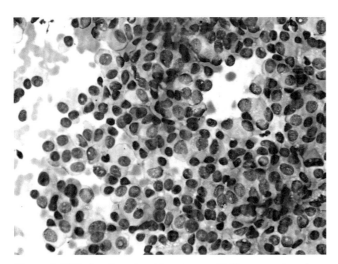

Figure 1.120. Papillary thyroid carcinoma (PTC), oncocytic variant. The field is cellular and comprised of malignant cells with abundant oncocytic cytoplasm, limiting the amount of nuclear overlap that is typically seen in PTC cases; however, note the disorganization and the presence of intranuclear pseudoinclusions (Diff-Quik stain).

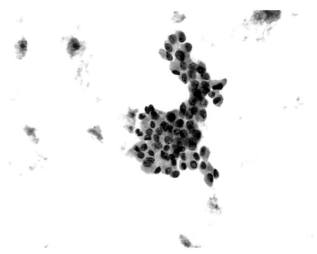

Figure 1.121. Papillary thyroid carcinoma (PTC), oncocytic variant. This ThinPrep specimen shows a cluster of malignant cells with subtle nuclear atypia and abundant oncocytic cytoplasm (Pap stain).

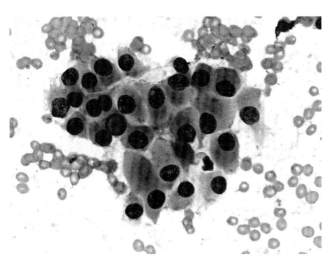

Figure 1.122. Papillary thyroid carcinoma (PTC), oncocytic variant. Note the abundant oncocytic cytoplasm and the intranuclear pseudoinclusions (Diff-Quik stain).

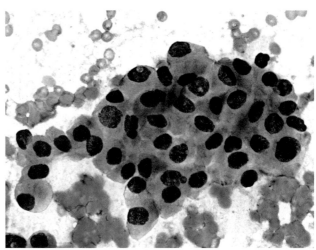

Figure 1.123. Papillary thyroid carcinoma (PTC), oncocytic variant. Separate field from the prior case (Figure 1.122) showing additional atypical nuclear features, such as nuclear elongation and nuclear membrane irregularity (Diff-Quik stain).

(2) the tumor should contain at least increased mitotic activity (≥3 per 10 high-power field), tumor necrosis, or convoluted nuclei; and (3) the tumor should lack features diagnostic of PTC.[73] It is no surprise that these criteria, which are fairly restrictive, cannot be similarly applied on small FNA samples. As a result, a definitive diagnosis of PDTC cannot be made on FNA but may be suggested. These tumors have scant to absent colloid and are highly cellular and composed primarily of discohesive cells in a background of disorganized clusters and microfollicles. The malignant cells are often monotonous and round with scant cytoplasm, increased N/C ratios, and hyperchromatic nuclei with small nucleoli. Some cells may appear plasmacytoid while others may show more nuclear variation and atypia; however, the presence of significant nuclear pleomorphism is more suggestive of an anaplastic carcinoma. In some cases, nuclear overlap, grooves, and intranuclear pseudoinclusions may raise the possibility of a PTC; however, the presence of individual cells, mitotic figures, or necrosis would strongly favor PDTC. In other cases, it may be difficult to distinguish PDTC from MTC. In these cases, the clinical history, such as an elevated calcitonin level, or positive immunostaining for TTF-1 would favor an MTC or PDTC, respectively.

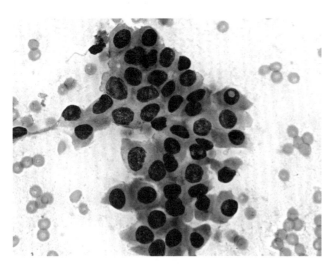

Figure 1.124. Papillary thyroid carcinoma (PTC), oncocytic variant. Third field from the same patient (Figures 1.122 and 1.123) showing intranuclear pseudoinclusions, as well as some nuclear overlap, nuclear membrane irregularity, and nuclear grooves (Diff-Quik stain).

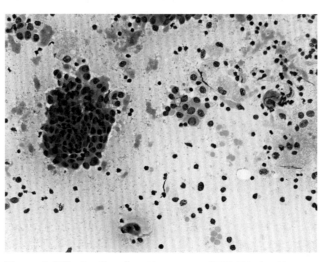

Figure 1.125. Papillary thyroid carcinoma (PTC), Warthin-like variant. A swirling cluster of oncocytic cells with nuclear crowding can be seen adjacent to a separate small group of oncocytic epithelium displaying a prominent intranuclear pseudoinclusion. Note the background lymphocytes that would typically be absent in an oncocytic variant of PTC (Diff-Quik stain).

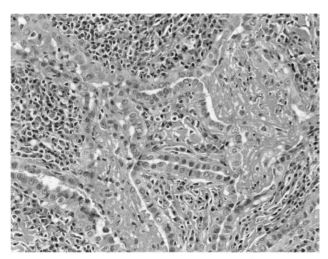

Figure 1.126. Papillary thyroid carcinoma (PTC), Warthin-like variant. This field is from the surgical follow-up from the same case (Figure 1.125) showing oncocytic epithelium lining papillary fragments filled with a lymphoplasmacytic infiltrate, reminiscent of a Warthin tumor of the parotid gland (H&E).

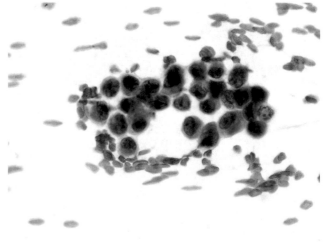

Figure 1.127. Poorly differentiated thyroid carcinoma. A loose aggregate of malignant cells displays irregular nuclei with clefts, prominent nucleoli, clumpy chromatin, and no definitive evidence of papillary differentiation or undifferentiation. This diagnosis is essentially one of exclusion. Follow-up was consistent with a poorly differentiated thyroid carcinoma in this case (Pap stain).

KEY FEATURES of Poorly Differentiated Thyroid Carcinoma

- The smears are cellular and comprised of abundant discohesive cells, disorganized clusters, and microfollicles.

- The carcinoma cells are monotonous, round cells with scant cytoplasm that may appear vacuolated and degenerative (can also appear plasmacytoid).

- The carcinoma cells demonstrate an increased N/C ratio with hyperchromatic nuclei that may be round or convoluted, coarse to finely granular chromatin, and prominent nucleoli.

- Abundant mitotic figures and necrosis are common.

- Features diagnostic of PTC are absent.

- The carcinoma cells lack the significant nuclear pleomorphism seen in ATC.

ANAPLASTIC THYROID CARCINOMA

Anaplastic thyroid carcinoma (ATC) is a devastating carcinoma with one of the worst prognoses of all malignancies. Despite the fact that it represents <5% of thyroid carcinomas, it accounts for approximately half of the mortality in this organ with a 1-year survival of only 28%.[74] Because of the abysmal prognosis, recognizing this entity on FNA is crucial because surgery and radiation are typically reserved for palliative efforts rather than for a surgical cure. On FNA, the samples are typically composed of abundant discohesive, large squamoid (epithelioid form), spindled (sarcomatoid form), or multinucleated (giant cell form) tumor cells with marked nuclear pleomorphism and bizarre atypia (Figures 1.131-1.138). The nuclei have irregular nuclear membranes, coarse chromatin, and prominent nucleoli with or without intranuclear pseudoinclusions. Mitotic figures are abundant, and necrosis is common. Colloid is typically absent in the anaplastic regions; however, many of these tumors appear to arise in the background of

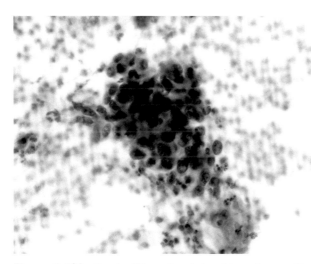

Figure 1.128. Poorly differentiated thyroid carcinoma. Clearly malignant cells are present with abnormal nuclear features that are not concordant with papillary thyroid carcinoma. The background contained abundant necrotic debris and mixed inflammation (Pap stain).

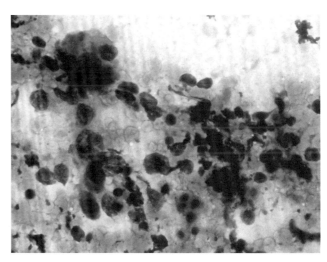

Figure 1.129. Poorly differentiated thyroid carcinoma. This field consists of malignant cells showing variable nuclear shape and size in a background of necrosis. Although there are some features of papillary thyroid carcinoma (PTC), including focal nuclear elongation and nuclear grooves, the level of atypia in this case and the background necrosis favor a poorly differentiated thyroid carcinoma in this sample (Diff-Quik stain).

Figure 1.130. Poorly differentiated thyroid carcinoma. Single, malignant cells are seen with varying amounts of cytoplasm and anisonucleosis, raising the possibility of an anaplastic thyroid carcinoma. On surgical resection, however, the degree of atypia was most in keeping with a poorly differentiated thyroid carcinoma (Diff-Quik stain).

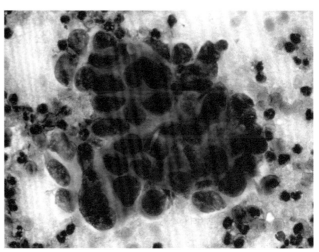

Figure 1.131. Anaplastic thyroid carcinoma. Note the bizarre nuclear atypia and nuclear size and shape variation (Diff-Quik stain).

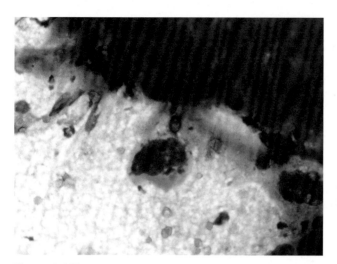

Figure 1.132. Anaplastic thyroid carcinoma. Note the single cell in the center of the frame with an enlarged and bizarre nucleus and dense, squamoid cytoplasm (Diff-Quik stain).

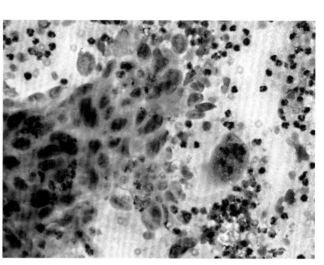

Figure 1.133. Anaplastic thyroid carcinoma. A loose aggregate of malignant cells is adjacent to a single cell with bizarre atypia in an inflammatory and necrotic background (Diff-Quik stain).

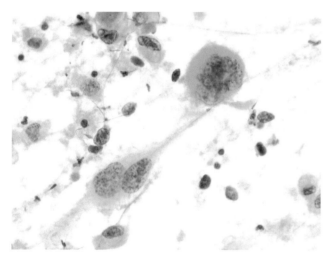

Figure 1.134. Anaplastic thyroid carcinoma. These highly a typical bizarre cells have dense, elongated cytoplasmic processes in a necrotic background (Pap stain).

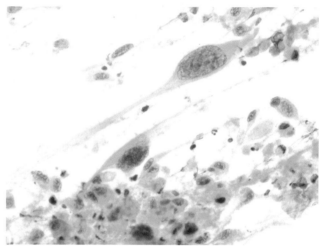

Figure 1.135. Anaplastic thyroid carcinoma. Separate field from the same case as Figure 1.134 displaying enlarged single cells with macronuclei and elongated cytoplasmic processes in a necrotic background (Pap stain).

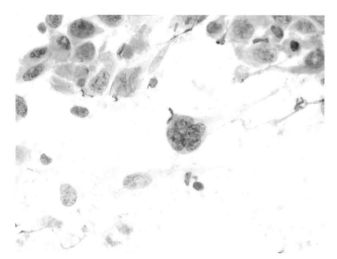

Figure 1.136. Anaplastic thyroid carcinoma. Separate field from the same case as the two prior Figures 1.134 and 1.135 showing multinucleation in a malignant cell (Pap stain).

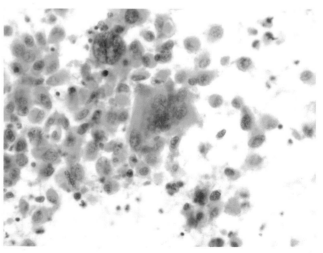

Figure 1.137. Anaplastic thyroid carcinoma. Final field from the same patient (Figures 1.134-1.136) displaying smaller epithelioid malignant cells and tumor giant cells in a necrotic background (Pap stain).

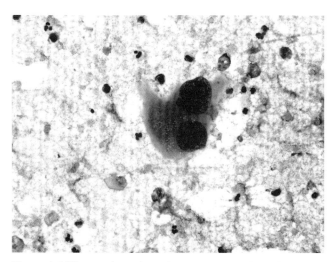

Figure 1.138. Anaplastic thyroid carcinoma. Binucleated cells with macronuclei and granular cytoplasm are present in a necrotic background (Diff-Quik stain).

a differentiated PTC with classic features which may be present in the sample. Multinucleated cells, including osteoclast-like giant cells, which are separate from the tumor giant cells, may be present. The epithelioid form may show squamous differentiation; however, distinguishing between an ATC and a primary squamous cell carcinoma of the thyroid is not incredibly important clinically owing to their similarly devastating clinical outcomes. The main differential diagnosis is to exclude a metastasis with a broad panel of immunostains if cell block material is available. Because of the lack of thyroid differentiation, thyroglobulin and TTF-1 are routinely negative in ATCs; however, PAX-8 will still be positive in approximately 76% of cases.[75]

KEY FEATURES of Anaplastic Thyroid Carcinoma

- The specimen is cellular and is comprised of abundant discohesive cells, dense clusters, and disorganized fragments.
- The carcinoma cells are large and can be squamoid (epithelioid form), spindled (sarcomatoid form), or multinucleated (giant cell form).
- The carcinoma cell nuclei are large and pleomorphic with bizarre atypia, including irregular nuclear membranes, nuclear hyperchromasia, coarse chromatin, and prominent nucleoli.
- Mitotic figures are abundant.
- The background shows necrosis and inflammatory cells.

PEARLS & PITFALLS

It is important to understand that ATC represents an undifferentiated form of thyroid carcinoma that may show no features suggestive of follicular origin. In this case, it may be necessary to exclude a metastasis. Because of the aggressive nature of ATC and the extent of disease on presentation, there will be a high clinical suspicion for a high-grade malignancy during the FNA procedure, and dedicated passes for a cell block preparation or a core biopsy should be obtained. It is important to realize that, unlike well-differentiated thyroid neoplasms, ATC is usually negative for thyroglobulin and TTF-1 by immunochemistry. Fortunately, PAX-8 remains positive in about three-quarters of these cases[75] and, when used in combination with other markers to exclude distant sites of origin, can help make a definitive diagnosis.

HURTHLE CELL NEOPLASMS

Hurthle cell neoplasms, including HCA and HCCs, produce cellular specimens comprised of predominantly discohesive, large, polygonal oncocytic cells with abundant finely granular cytoplasm, large nuclei, and prominent nucleoli (Figures 1.139-1.143). Importantly, rare intranuclear pseudoinclusions, as well as nonconcentric calcified concretions (pseudopsammoma bodies) can be seen and should not be interpreted as features of PTC in this context. PTCs can rarely be of the oncocytic or Warthin-like variants and show abundant malignant Hurthle cells; however, classic PTC nuclear features, despite the PTC subtype, should be present in those cases. Although several entities can show Hurthle cell metaplasia, the discohesive pattern and pure population of Hurthle cells favor a neoplastic process. See the "Hurthle Cell Neoplasms" section under the "Hurthle Cell Pattern" for additional discussion.

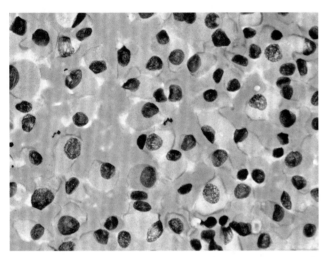

Figure 1.139. Suspicious for a Follicular Neoplasm (SFN), Hurthle cell type. The smear is cellular and shows multiple, dispersed, and monomorphic Hurthle cells. Follow-up revealed a Hurthle cell carcinoma (Diff-Quik stain).

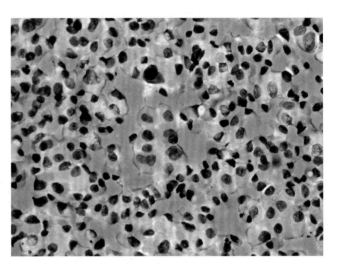

Figure 1.140. Suspicious for a Follicular Neoplasm (SFN), Hurthle cell type. Separate field from the prior specimen (Figure 1.139) containing abundant dispersed Hurthle cells (Diff-Quik stain).

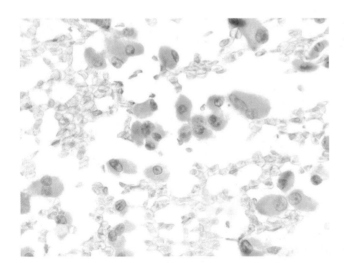

Figure 1.141. Suspicious for a Follicular Neoplasm (SFN), Hurthle cell type. Dispersed Hurthle cells are present with varying amounts of cytoplasm and occasional nucleoli. Follow-up was consistent with a Hurthle cell carcinoma (Pap stain).

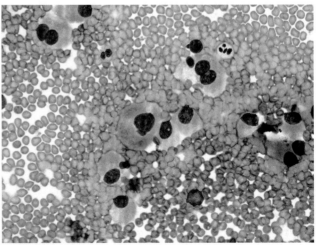

Figure 1.142. Suspicious for a Follicular Neoplasm (SFN), Hurthle cell type. Dispersed Hurthle cells show binucleation and plasmacytoid features. Follow-up revealed a diagnosis of Hurthle cell carcinoma (Diff-Quik stain).

MEDULLARY THYROID CARCINOMA

Medullary thyroid carcinoma (MTC) derives from the parafollicular C cells of the thyroid gland, as opposed to the thyroid follicular cells, and accounts for 5-10% of thyroid cancers with a 5-year survival rate between 60-80%.[76] Activating *RET* mutations are characteristic of this tumor, and although the majority of cases are sporadic, MTC can be associated with multiple endocrine neoplasia (MEN) types 2a and 2b.[77,78] As a result, younger patients may require germline testing for *RET* mutations. If MTC is in the differential diagnosis, an elevated serum calcitonin level can be highly informative. On FNA, MTC will show discohesive, single round, polygonal, spindle, or bipolar cells with eccentric/plasmacytoid nuclei. The cytoplasm may contain red neurosecretory granules on the Diff-Quik stain (Figures 1.144-1.155). The nuclei have a neuroendocrine "salt-and-pepper" chromatin appearance with a moderate degree of pleomorphism. The nuclear atypia seen in PTC will not be present; however, intranuclear pseudoinclusions

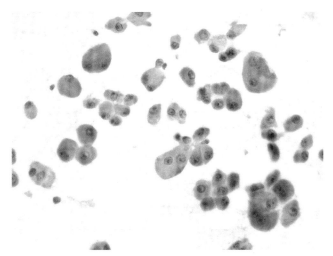

Figure 1.143. Suspicious for a Follicular Neoplasm (SFN), Hurthle cell type. A Pap stain from the same case as Figure 1.142 showing dispersed mononuclear and binucleated Hurthle cells with prominent nucleoli (Pap stain).

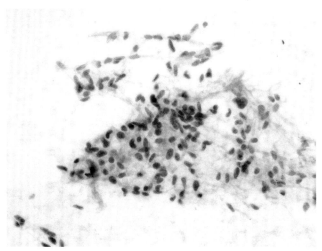

Figure 1.144. Medullary thyroid carcinoma. This field shows a mix of loosely cohesive and single spindled cells with elongated nuclei with smooth contours and speckled chromatin (Pap stain).

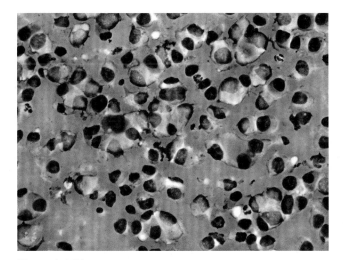

Figure 1.145. Medullary thyroid carcinoma. These dispersed plasmacytoid cells have large nuclei and some cells show multinucleation (Diff-Quik stain).

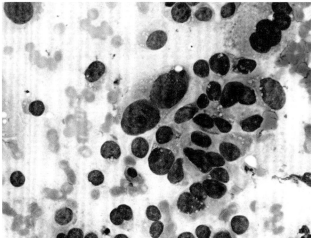

Figure 1.146. Medullary thyroid carcinoma. In this field, the malignant cells are highly variable with some cells being round, elongated, or markedly enlarged. At the top right, there is a "pseudo" pseudoinclusion. This inclusion can be distinguished from the characteristic inclusions seen in papillary thyroid carcinoma (PTC) because it lacks the color and consistency of the cytoplasm (Diff-Quik stain).

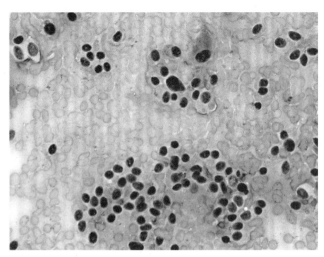

Figure 1.147. Medullary thyroid carcinoma. Malignant cells are dispersed and present in loose clusters with variable amounts of pale cytoplasm with round and oval nuclei. Although most cells are relatively monotonous, a few are markedly enlarged (Diff-Quik stain).

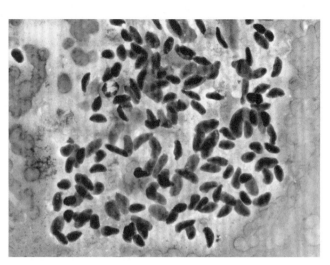

Figure 1.148. Medullary thyroid carcinoma. Dispersed and monotonous spindled cells can be seen with occasional bent nuclei. Note the lack of nuclear atypia seen in cases of papillary thyroid carcinoma (PTC) (Diff-Quik stain).

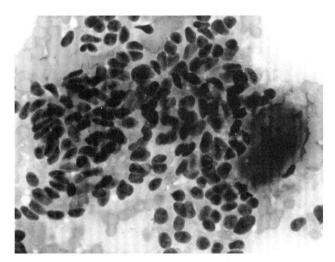

Figure 1.149. Medullary thyroid carcinoma (MTC). A deposit of amorphous amyloid is present next to a loosely cohesive cluster of oval epithelioid cells characteristic of MTC (Diff-Quik stain).

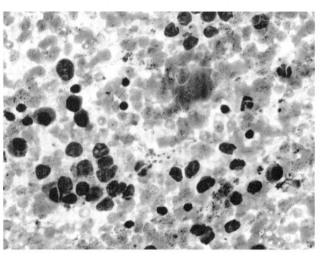

Figure 1.150. Medullary thyroid carcinoma. Compared to the lymphocytes in the background, these dispersed single cells are enlarged and have scant cytoplasm. Note the presence of amorphous magenta amyloid (Diff-Quik stain).

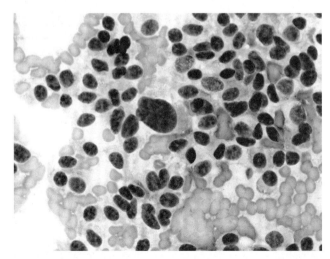

Figure 1.151. Medullary thyroid carcinoma. Predominantly dispersed, monotonous cells with oval and elongated nuclei are adjacent to a markedly enlarged cell with similar chromatin quality, a common finding in this diagnosis (Diff-Quik stain).

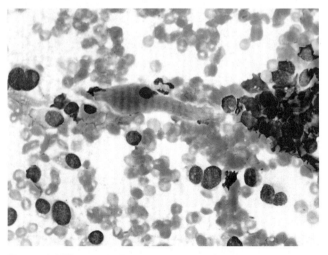

Figure 1.152. Medullary thyroid carcinoma. Malignant epithelioid cells are present as single cells as well as in a small cluster adjacent to amorphous amyloid (Diff-Quik stain).

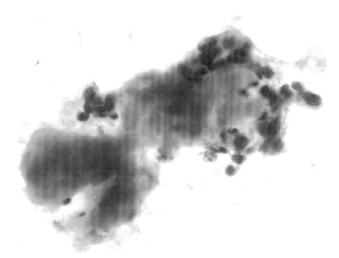

Figure 1.153. Medullary thyroid carcinoma. A large portion of amorphous, chunky amyloid is seen with surrounding malignant cells (Pap stain).

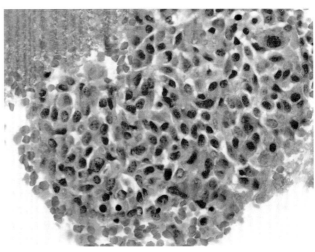

Figure 1.154. Medullary thyroid carcinoma. This cell block preparation shows epithelioid and plasmacytoid malignant cells with pink, finely granular cytoplasm and speckled chromatin (H&E stain).

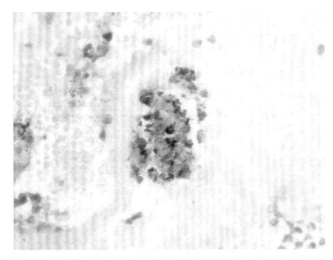

Figure 1.155. Medullary thyroid carcinoma. Cytoplasmic positivity for calcitonin is present in this cell block preparation (calcitonin stain).

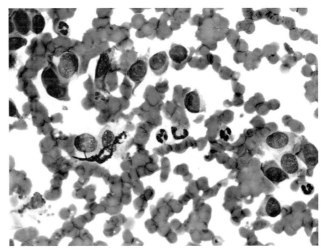

Figure 1.156. Metastatic melanoma. Malignant melanoma cells are often dispersed and can be epithelioid, plasmacytoid, or spindled and mimic medullary thyroid carcinoma (MTC). However, the presence of prominent nucleoli strongly favor a melanoma over MTC (Diff-Quik stain).

are present in many cases and should not be interpreted as a feature diagnostic of PTC.[79] The main entities in the differential diagnosis for MTC include PTC, PDTC, and metastases such as melanoma (Figures 1.156 and 1.157).

KEY FEATURES of Medullary Thyroid Carcinoma

- The smear contains discohesive round, polygonal, spindle, or bipolar cells with ill-defined borders.
- The specimen contains abundant amphophilic and fibrillary cytoplasm which may contain red neurosecretory granules on the Diff-Quik stain.
- Nuclei may be eccentric and result in a plasmacytoid appearance or may be multinucleated.
- Nuclei are round, oval, or elongated in shape and hyperchromatic with "salt-and-pepper" chromatin and inconspicuous nucleoli.
- Intranuclear pseudoinclusions are present in many cases.
- Dense, amorphous amyloid is present in most cases but may be difficult to distinguish from colloid.

PEARLS & PITFALLS

MTC can be a difficult diagnosis to make on FNA. The main entities in the differential diagnosis include PTC, PDTC, and metastatic processes, such as melanoma. For MTC, colloid will be minimal or absent; however, dense, amorphous amyloid is present in the some MTCs and can mimic the appearance of colloid. If a cell block is available, a Congo red stain can be helpful for determining the presence of amyloid while positive staining with calcitonin, chromogranin, and synaptophysin immunostains will confirm the diagnosis and also distinguish it from PDTC. It is important to remember that TTF-1 will also be positive in MTC and is not useful for differentiating between C cell and follicular cell neoplasms.[80] Differentiating between a melanoma and MTC can be extremely difficult on cytomorphology alone because they are both comprised of discohesive cells that can be epithelioid, spindled, plasmacytoid, or bipolar. Furthermore, MTC can undergo melanocytic differentiation and produce melanin pigment. As a result, immunochemistry may be necessary to make the correct diagnosis. Calcitonin is the single most helpful stain because it should be positive in MTC, even if melanocytic differentiation is present and the tumor is staining with one or more "melanoma markers."

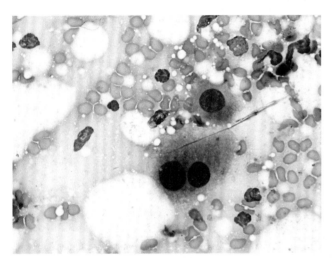

Figure 1.157. Metastatic melanoma. Malignant melanoma cells can also be binucleated and mimic medullary thyroid carcinoma or a Hurthle cell lesion. If nucleoli are not prominent and cytoplasmic pigment is absent, this can be an extremely difficult distinction to make on cytomorphology alone (Diff-Quik stain).

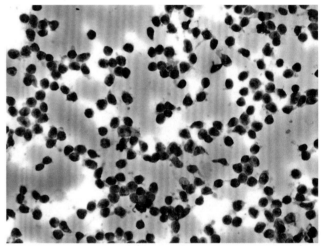

Figure 1.158. Extranodal marginal zone lymphoma. The smears are cellular and comprised of predominantly small, round, monocytoid lymphocytes with pale, light-blue cytoplasm and occasional nucleoli. Although it is extremely difficult to distinguish these cells from a reactive process, the blue cytoplasm is a helpful feature (Diff-Quik stain).

LYMPHOMA

Most primary lymphomas involving the thyroid gland are non-Hodgkin B-cell lymphomas, the majority of which arise in the background of CLT. The two most common lymphoma subtypes are diffuse large B-cell lymphoma (DLBCL) and extranodal marginal zone B-cell lymphomas (EMZL). Furthermore, secondary lymphomatous involvement of the thyroid gland occurs in approximately 20% of patients with disseminated lymphoma. Therefore, it is important to keep lymphoma in the differential diagnosis. Both DLBCL and EMZL reveal highly cellular, discohesive lymphocytes in a background of lymphoglandular bodies. In EMZL, the neoplastic cells are roughly 2× the size of normal lymphocytes and contain a moderate amount of cytoplasm, open chromatin, and small nucleoli (Figures 1.158 and 1.159). In DLBCL, the cells contain a moderate amount of basophilic cytoplasm on Diff-Quik, nuclei at least 3× the size of normal lymphocytes, coarse chromatin, and prominent nucleoli (Figures 1.160 and 1.161). Furthermore, DLBCL is often found in a background of naked nuclei and necrotic debris, which can be a helpful diagnostic clue.

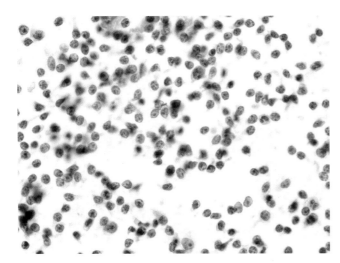

Figure 1.159. Extranodal marginal zone lymphoma. Although this population may appear polymorphous on first glance, the majority of the cells have the same nuclear size, shape, and chromatin characteristics with nucleoli easily identified. Fortunately, flow cytometry was performed and showed a monoclonal B-cell population with lambda restriction (Pap stain).

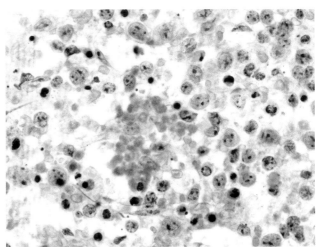

Figure 1.160. Diffuse large B-cell lymphoma. The large cells have scant cytoplasm and multiple small nucleoli, consistent with the centroblastic variant (Pap stain).

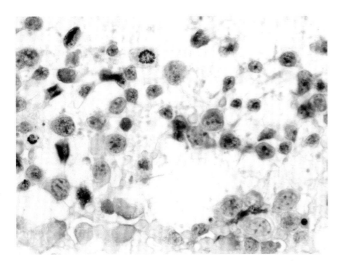

Figure 1.161. Diffuse large B-cell lymphoma. Separate field from the prior case (Figure 1.160) revealing discohesive malignant cells with scant basophilic cytoplasm and small, punctate nucleoli. Note the ring-like mitotic figure at the top center of the field (Pap stain).

PARATHYROID TISSUE

As previously mentioned (see the "Microfollicular Pattern"), parathyroid tissue can be mistakenly sampled if located directly on the surface or within the thyroid gland (intrathyroidal). More commonly, parathyroid tissue mimics thyroid follicular cells with a microfollicular architecture; however, parathyroid tissue smears may show numerous discohesive, naked nuclei (Figures 1.162-1.165). The nuclei are most commonly round to oval and may show mild anisonucleosis. The chromatin typically has a salt-and-pepper appearance, owing to its neuroendocrine-like characteristics.

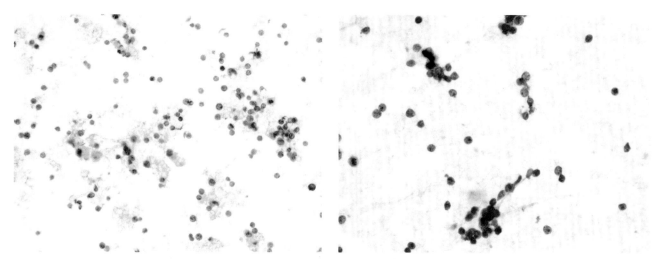

Figure 1.162. Parathyroid tissue. At this low magnification, it can be difficult to distinguish these singly dispersed parathyroid cells from lymphocytes. The key here is to recognize the slightly blue, granular cytoplasm that is present near clustering groups (Pap stain).

Figure 1.163. Parathyroid tissue. This view consists predominantly of cells that have lost the majority of their cytoplasm; however, the more intact cells have more cytoplasm with red granules. The chromatin of these cells is speckled, and nucleoli range from small to prominent in this field (Pap stain).

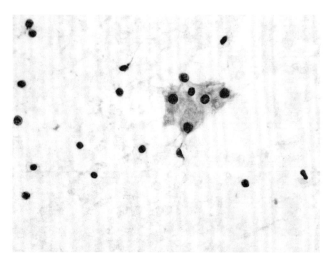

Figure 1.164. Parathyroid tissue. Parathyroid tissue can be present in small sheets, microfollicles, or as discohesive cells. This view shows a microfollicle comprised of cells with abundant granular cytoplasm and nuclei with speckled chromatin. The background also contains nuclei that have been stripped of their cytoplasm (Pap stain).

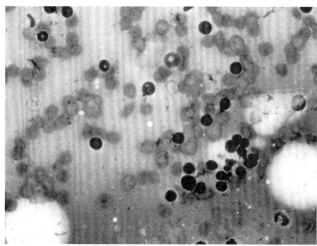

Figure 1.165. Parathyroid tissue. A small microfollicle is present, alongside several scattered naked nuclei with "pseudo" intranuclear pseudoinclusions, which is not uncommonly seen in parathyroid cells. These inclusions can be recognized as artifacts because they are white and of variable size and shape (Diff-Quik stain).

AMORPHOUS PATTERN

CHECKLIST: Etiologic Considerations for the Amorphous Pattern

☐ Amyloid Goiter

☐ Medullary Thyroid Carcinoma (MTC)

☐ Chronic Lymphocytic Thyroiditis (Late Stage)

The amorphous pattern can be seen in a variety of thyroid-based lesions, such as amyloidosis, amyloid-containing MTC, and late-stage CLT. In each of these settings, a careful review of the clinical history and the radiographic findings will significantly help narrow the differential diagnosis.

AMYLOID GOITER

Primary and secondary amyloid deposition in the thyroid gland can lead to diffuse, bilateral goiter. On FNA, amyloid is often seen as glassy, purple to pink or orange amorphous material which can mimic colloid. Fibroblasts, however, are often embedded in amyloid and can be a helpful feature in distinguishing it from colloid. More focal amyloid deposition may be seen in MTC, which may be more difficult to appreciate.

MEDULLARY THYROID CARCINOMA

Medullary thyroid carcinoma (MTC), previously discussed in the "Discohesive Pattern", is a malignant neoplasm arising from the calcitonin-producing parafollicular C cells. On FNA, samples are usually cellular and consist of predominantly single cells and loose clusters that are variably epithelioid, plasmacytoid, or spindled. The nuclei have neuroendocrine-type chromatin, and intranuclear pseudoinclusions are common. Although not a predominant part of the aspirated material, dense, amorphous amyloid is present in the majority of cases (Figures 1.166-1.169). It can often be difficult to distinguish from colloid; however, if a

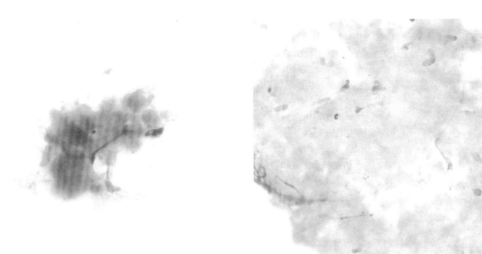

Figure 1.166. Medullary thyroid carcinoma. Amorphous, fluffy amyloid should be distinguished from colloid (Pap stain).

Figure 1.167. Medullary thyroid carcinoma. Amorphous amyloid material is seen with rare admixed crushed cells (Pap stain).

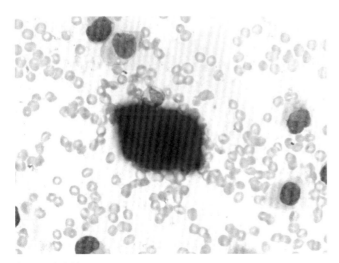

Figure 1.168. Medullary thyroid carcinoma. Discohesive epithelioid to plasmacytoid medullary thyroid carcinoma cells are seen adjacent to a dark blue material which is most likely amyloid; however, colloid can have a similar appearance (Diff-Quik stain).

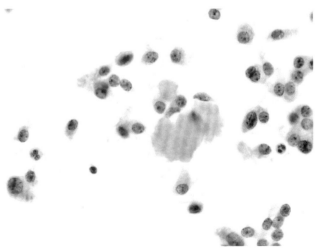

Figure 1.169. Medullary thyroid carcinoma. Small chunks of amorphous amyloid are seen together with malignant cells with speckled chromatin and small nucleoli (Pap stain).

cell block is available, a Congo red stain optimized for formalin-fixed, paraffin-embedded material will produce an apple green appearance with polarized light.

CHRONIC LYMPHOCYTIC THYROIDITIS (LATE STAGE)

Over time, chronic lymphocytic thyroiditis (CLT) can damage the thyroid follicular cells and lead to extensive fibrosis and atrophy, colloquially known as "burnt out" CLT. FNA at this stage is often paucicellular but may also contain abundant, amorphous-appearing collagenous material (Figure 1.170). In the presence of lymphoid follicles, reactive follicular cells, and Hurthle cells, this amorphous material should not confound the diagnosis.

NEAR MISSES

CYST-LINING CELLS INTERPRETED AS PAPILLARY THYROID CARCINOMA

Secondary cystic degeneration and hemorrhage are common findings in patients with multinodular goiter and follicular adenomas. As these secondary cysts form, the follicular epithelium lining the cysts undergoes reparative changes that result in cytologic atypia. On FNA, cyst-lining cells are usually arranged in cohesive sheets that have a streaming appearance. The follicular cells are enlarged and can even appear spindled due to the presence of stretched cytoplasm forming cytoplasmic processes. Like PTC, the cyst-lining cells have enlarged, elongated nuclei that may have nuclear grooves, pale chromatin, and even rare intranuclear cytoplasmic inclusions (Figures 1.171-1.174). These sheets, however, lack nuclear overlap and have more abundant, vacuolated cytoplasm than a typical case of PTC. Owing to some of these overlapping features, however, it may be impossible to distinguish between benign cyst-lining cells and malignant cells from a cystic PTC. As a result, a subset of these cases will be classified as AUS or, if inclusions are present, as Suspicious for PTC.

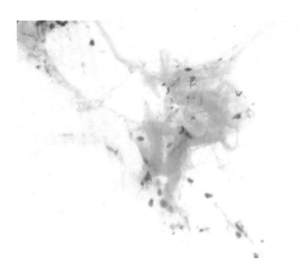

Figure 1.170. Fragments of amorphous collagenous stroma in a patient with long-standing chronic lymphocytic thyroiditis (Pap stain).

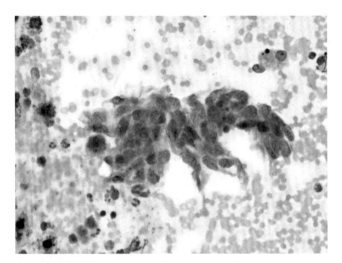

Figure 1.171. Cyst-lining cells versus papillary thyroid carcinoma (PTC). Cyst-lining cells, as shown above, can show reparative changes and appear quite atypical. The above cells are enlarged and appear slightly spindled owing to their elongated nuclei and cytoplasmic processes. Furthermore, the cyst-lining cells above are overlapping and do not have the classic macrofollicular appearance of benign nodules. The presence of vacuolated macrophages at the edges of this field, however, will be a helpful clue that this atypia is reparative in nature (Diff-Quik stain).

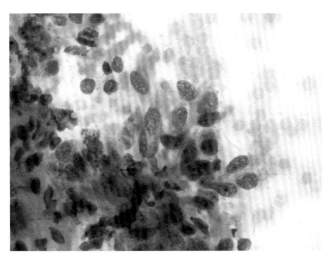

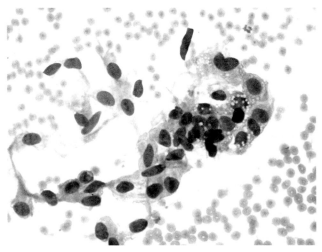

Figure 1.172. Cyst-lining cells versus papillary thyroid carcinoma (PTC). Separate field from the prior case shown in Figure 1.171. These cyst-lining cells appear quite large with oval nuclei, nuclear grooves at the edge, occasional small, punctate nucleoli, and a possible intranuclear pseudoinclusion. Although this degree of atypia can be reparative and seen in cyst-lining cells, a cystic PTC cannot be entirely excluded (Diff-Quik stain).

Figure 1.173. Cyst-lining cells versus papillary thyroid carcinoma (PTC). The above cells show several classic features of cyst-lining cells, including nuclear elongation, bipolar cytoplasmic extensions, and bubbly, vacuolated cytoplasm (Diff-Quik stain).

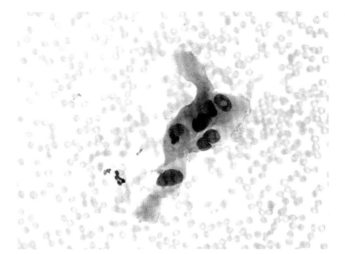

Figure 1.174. Cyst-lining cells versus papillary thyroid carcinoma (PTC). This image is a separate field from the same slide as Figure 1.173. Note the enlarged nuclei and the intranuclear pseudoinclusion. Rarely, cyst-lining cells have been reported to have intranuclear inclusions; however, this finding should at least warrant an atypical diagnosis. On follow-up, this patient was found to have nodular hyperplasia with cystic degeneration, underscoring the fact that cyst-lining atypia can easily be interpreted as cytologic atypia seen in PTC (Diff-Quik stain).

ENLARGED PARATHYROID GLAND INTERPRETED AS SUSPICIOUS FOR A FOLLICULAR NEOPLASM

Enlarged parathyroid glands can easily be mistaken for thyroid nodules on a clinical examination. As a result, it is not uncommon to have an aspiration sample from the parathyroid gland that comes to the cytopathologist as "thyroid." Unfortunately, parathyroid adenomas appear virtually identical to follicular neoplasms by FNA; however, there are a few differences that in some cases may help differentiate these two lesions. For example, definitive colloid material, even if scant in a follicular neoplasm, eliminates parathyroid gland tissue from the differential diagnosis. Second, parathyroid cells are usually smaller than follicular cells, although without doing a side-by-side comparison, recognizing this difference is unrealistic. Finally, parathyroid cells have neuroendocrine-like chromatin, although the chromatin can be variable even within the same case (Figures 1.175-1.177). Fortunately, there are several ancillary tests that can be done to separate these two entities if this differential is entertained. First, parathyroid gland tissue should be positive for antibodies against parathyroid hormone and GATA-3 by immunochemistry while follicular lesions will be negative for both markers.[81] Conversely, follicular neoplasms will be positive for thyroglobulin, TTF-1, and PAX-8 while parathyroid lesions will be negative for all three markers. If material is not available for immunostaining, the cytopathologist can suggest that the clinician order a serum calcium level, which is elevated in the majority of patients with a parathyroid adenoma and is less expensive than repeating an FNA to obtain material for ancillary testing.

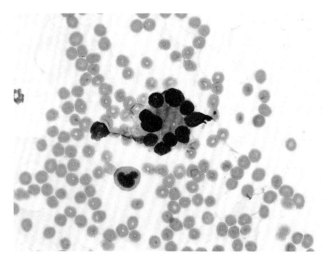

Figure 1.175. Suspicious for a Follicular Neoplasm (SFN) versus parathyroid gland tissue. Cases categorized as Suspicious for a Follicular Neoplasm must be cellular and predominantly comprised of microfollicles, as seen in this case. Parathyroid cells, as shown above, can form microfollicles and appear nearly identical to follicular cells; however, these cells should be smaller. Note how small these cells are when compared to the background red blood cells and the leukocyte (Diff-Quik).

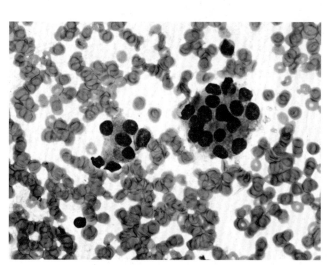

Figure 1.176. Suspicious for a Follicular Neoplasm (SFN) versus parathyroid gland tissue. A separate field from the same patient as in Figure 1.175 showing more parathyroid microfollicles. Note the small cells, as well as the granular cytoplasm that should point you more in the direction of parathyroid cells and away from follicular cells (Diff-Quik stain).

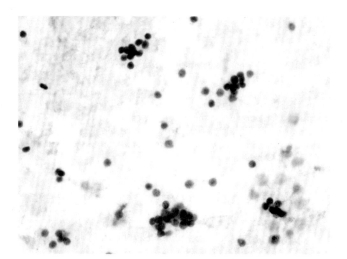

Figure 1.177. Suspicious for a Follicular Neoplasm (SFN) versus parathyroid gland tissue. Cases categorized as Suspicious for a Follicular Neoplasm must be cellular and comprised of predominantly microfollicles. This field shows an alcohol-fixed slide from the same patient as in Figures 1.175 and 1.176. The smear is cellular and comprised of multiple microfollicles. Note the coarse chromatin, small nucleoli, and lack of background colloid (Pap stain).

ONCOCYTIC VARIANT OF PAPILLARY THYROID CARCINOMA

In the oncocytic variant of PTC, the malignant cells contain abundant "Hurthleoid" cytoplasm. As a result, the atypical nuclear features may be difficult to appreciate because the abundant cytoplasm results in a decreased N/C ratio and a decrease in nuclear overlap (Figures 1.178-1.181).[82] Furthermore, Hurthle cells may rarely show intranuclear pseudoinclusions, which decreases the specificity of inclusions in this setting. Therefore, one must rely on a constellation of all of the features of PTC to make

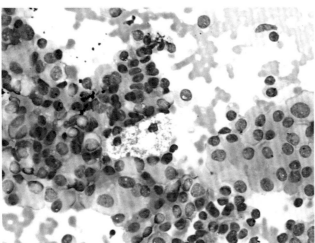

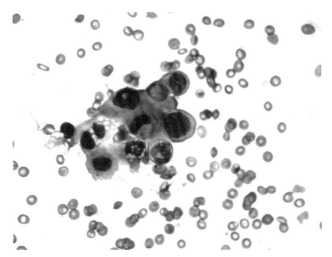

Figure 1.178. Oncocytic variant of papillary thyroid carcinoma (PTC). This field shows a cellular specimen comprised of syncytial groups of cells with abundant granular cytoplasm and absent to focal nuclear atypia. Note the cells on the right which are virtually indistinguishable from the oncocytic cells seen in a Hurthle cell neoplasm. Several cells toward the middle of the field, however, show nuclear elongation, overlapping, and nuclear grooves. It is important to note that the atypical nuclear features may be very subtle in the oncocytic variant of PTC (Diff-Quik stain).

Figure 1.179. Oncocytic variant of papillary thyroid carcinoma (PTC). Small group of large cells with abundant, granular cytoplasm and enlarged nuclei. Contrast the small artifactual vacuoles with the intranuclear pseudoinclusions seen in several of these cells. In contrast to the bubbles, the inclusions have the same color and consistency as the oncocytic cytoplasm. Although inclusions like these may be found in Hurthle cell lesions that are not PTC, their presence is highly concerning (Diff-Quik stain).

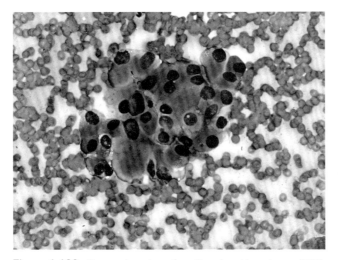

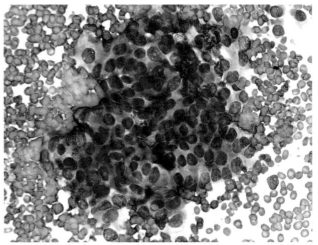

Figure 1.180. Oncocytic variant of papillary thyroid carcinoma (PTC). Cluster of cells with abundant oncocytic cytoplasm and enlarged nuclei with subtle nuclear elongation and nuclear membrane irregularity. Several "pseudo" intranuclear inclusions are present and should not be misinterpreted (Diff-Quik stain).

Figure 1.181. Oncocytic variant of papillary thyroid carcinoma (PTC) mistaken for a Hurthle cell neoplasm. A separate field from the same case as Figure 1.180 showing more diagnostic atypical features for PTC, including nuclear overlap and elongation, nuclear membrane irregularity, nuclear grooves, and an intranuclear pseudoinclusions (bottom center of field) (Diff-Quik stain).

the diagnosis. If the level of atypia is indeterminate for malignancy, many of these lesions will be categorized as SFN with oncocytic features. Unfortunately, this categorization often leads to a thyroid lobectomy instead of the total thyroidectomy a patient with PTC requires. As a result, the patient will need to undergo a second operation for a completion thyroidectomy.

References

1. *The 2017 Bethesda System for Reporting Thyroid Cytopathology.* 2nd ed.: Springer International Publishing; 2017.

2. Haider AS, Rakha EA, Dunkley C, Zaitoun AM. The impact of using defined criteria for adequacy of fine needle aspiration cytology of the thyroid in routine practice. *Diagn Cytopathol.* 2011;39(2):81-86.

3. Gunes P, Canberk S, Onenerk M, et al. A different perspective on evaluating the malignancy rate of the non-diagnostic category of the Bethesda system for reporting thyroid cytopathology: a single institute experience and review of the literature. *PLoS One.* 2016;11(9):e0162745.

4. Chow LS, Gharib H, Goellner JR, Heerden JA. Nondiagnostic thyroid fine-needle aspiration cytology: management dilemmas. *Thyroid.* 2001;11(12):1147-1151.

5. Haugen BR, Alexander EK, Bible KC, et al. 2015 American Thyroid Association Management Guidelines for adult patients with thyroid nodules and differentiated thyroid cancer: the American Thyroid Association guidelines task force on thyroid nodules and differentiated thyroid cancer. *Thyroid.* 2016;26(1):1-133.

6. Orija I, Piñeyro M, Biscotti C, Reddy S, Hamrahian A. Value of repeating a nondiagnostic thyroid fine-needle aspiration biopsy. *Endocr Pract.* 2007;13(7):735-742.

7. Ferreira MA, Gerhard R, Schmitt F. Analysis of nondiagnostic results in a large series of thyroid fine-needle aspiration cytology performed over 9 years in a single center. *Acta Cytol.* 2014;58(3):229-234.

8. Jo VY, Stelow EB, Dustin SM, Hanley KZ. Malignancy risk for fine-needle aspiration of thyroid lesions according to the Bethesda system for reporting thyroid cytopathology. *Am J Clin Pathol.* 2010;134(3):450-456.

9. Takada N, Hirokawa M, Suzuki A, Higuchi M, Kuma S, Miyauchi A. Reappraisal of "cyst fluid only" on thyroid fine-needle aspiration cytology. *Endocr J.* 2017;64(8):759-765.

10. Muller N, Cooperberg PL, Suen KC, Thorson SC. Needle aspiration biopsy in cystic papillary carcinoma of the thyroid. *AJR Am J Roentgenol.* 1985;144(2):251-253.

11. Jaragh M, Carydis VB, MacMillan C, Freeman J, Colgan TJ. Predictors of malignancy in thyroid fine-needle aspirates "cyst fluid only" cases. *Cancer.* 2009;117(5):305-310.

12. Yang GCH, Stern CM, Messina AV. Cystic papillary thyroid carcinoma in fine needle aspiration may represent a subset of the encapsulated variant in WHO classification. *Diagn Cytopathol.* 2010;38(10):721-726.

13. Bommanahalli BP, Bhat RV, Rupanarayan R. A cell pattern approach to interpretation of fine needle aspiration cytology of thyroid lesions: a cyto-histomorphological study. *J Cytol.* 2010;27(4):127-132.

14. Tessler FN, Middleton WD, Grant EG, et al. ACR thyroid imaging, reporting and data system (TI-RADS): white paper of the ACR TI-RADS committee. *J Am Coll Radiol.* 2017;14(5):587-595.

15. Middleton WD, Teefey SA, Reading CC, et al. Multiinstitutional analysis of thyroid nodule risk stratification using the American College of Radiology thyroid imaging reporting and data system. *AJR Am J Roentgenol.* 2017;208(6):1331-1341.

16. Rosario PW, da Silva AL, Nunes MB, Borges MAR. Risk of malignancy in thyroid nodules using the American College of Radiology thyroid imaging reporting and data system in the NIFTP era. *Horm Metab Res.* 2018;50(10):735-737.

17. Nikiforov YE, Nikiforova MN. Molecular genetics and diagnosis of thyroid cancer. *Nat Rev Endocrinol.* 2011;7:569.

18. Shi Y, Zou M, Schmidt H, et al. High rates of RAS codon 61 mutation in thyroid tumors in an iodide-deficient area. *Cancer Res.* 1991;51(10):2690-2693.

19. Garcia-Rostan G, Zhao H, Camp RL, et al. RAS mutations are associated with aggressive tumor phenotypes and poor prognosis in thyroid cancer. *J Clin Oncol.* 2003;21(17):3226-3235.

20. Eberhardt NL, Grebe SKG, McIver B, Reddi HV. The role of the PAX8/PPARgamma fusion oncogene in the pathogenesis of follicular thyroid cancer. *Mol Cell Endocrinol.* 2010;321(1):50-56.

21. Nikiforova MN, Lynch RA, Biddinger PW, et al. RAS point mutations and PAX8-PPARγ rearrangement in thyroid tumors: evidence for distinct molecular pathways in thyroid follicular carcinoma. *J Clin Endocrinol Metab.* 2003;88(5):2318-2326.

22. Sahin M, Allard BL, Yates M, et al. PPARγ staining as a surrogate for PAX8/PPARγ fusion oncogene expression in follicular neoplasms: clinicopathological correlation and histopathological diagnostic value. *J Clin Endocrinol Metab.* 2005;90(1):463-468.

23. Torregrossa L, Viola D, Sensi E, et al. Papillary thyroid carcinoma with rare exon 15 BRAF mutation has indolent behavior: a single-institution experience. *J Clin Endocrinol Metab.* 2016;101(11):4413-4420.

24. Xing M. BRAF mutation in papillary thyroid cancer: pathogenic role, molecular bases, and clinical implications. *Endocr Rev.* 2007;28(7):742-762.

25. Falchook GS, Millward M, Hong D, et al. BRAF inhibitor dabrafenib in patients with metastatic BRAF-mutant thyroid cancer. *Thyroid.* 2015;25(1):71-77.

26. Brose MS, Cabanillas ME, Cohen EEW, et al. Vemurafenib in patients with BRAF(V600E)-positive metastatic or unresectable papillary thyroid cancer refractory to radioactive iodine: a non-randomised, multicentre, open-label, phase 2 trial. *Lancet Oncol.* 2016;17(9):1272-1282.

27. Cancer Genome Atlas Research Network. Integrated genomic characterization of papillary thyroid carcinoma. *Cell.* 2014;159(3):676-690.

28. Prescott JD, Zeiger MA. The RET oncogene in papillary thyroid carcinoma. *Cancer.* 2015;121(13):2137-2146.

29. Nikiforov YE, Rowland JM, Bove KE, Monforte-Munoz H, Fagin JA. Distinct pattern of RET oncogene rearrangements in morphological variants of radiation-induced and sporadic thyroid papillary carcinomas in children. *Cancer Res.* 1997;57(9):1690-1694.

30. Bongarzone I, Vigneri P, Mariani L, Collini P, Pilotti S, Pierotti MA. RET/NTRK1 rearrangements in thyroid gland tumors of the papillary carcinoma family: correlation with clinicopathological features. *Clin Cancer Res.* 1998;4(1):223-228.

31. Leeman-Neill RJ, Kelly LM, Liu P, et al. ETV6-NTRK3 is a common chromosomal rearrangement in radiation-associated thyroid cancer. *Cancer.* 2014;120(6):799-807.

32. Gasparre G, Porcelli AM, Bonora E, et al. Disruptive mitochondrial DNA mutations in complex I subunits are markers of oncocytic phenotype in thyroid tumors. *Proc Natl Acad Sci USA.* 2007;104(21):9001-9006.

33. Gasparre G, Bonora E, Tallini G, Romeo G. Molecular features of thyroid oncocytic tumors. *Mol Cell Endocrinol.* 2010;321(1):67-76.

34. Landa I, Ibrahimpasic T, Boucai L, et al. Genomic and transcriptomic hallmarks of poorly differentiated and anaplastic thyroid cancers. *J Clin Invest.* 2016;126(3):1052-1066.

35. Liu R, Xing M. TERT promoter mutations in thyroid cancer. *Endocr Relat Cancer.* 2016;23(3):R143.

36. Liu X, Qu S, Liu R, et al. TERT promoter mutations and their association with BRAF V600E mutation and aggressive clinicopathological characteristics of thyroid cancer. *J Clin Endocrinol Metab.* 2014;99(6):E1130-E1136.

37. Acquaviva G, Visani M, Repaci A, et al. Molecular pathology of thyroid tumours of follicular cells: a review of genetic alterations and their clinicopathological relevance. *Histopathology.* 2018;72(1):6-31.

38. Liu D, Hou P, Liu Z, Wu G, Xing M. Genetic alterations in the phosphoinositide 3-kinase/Akt signaling pathway confer sensitivity of thyroid cancer cells to therapeutic targeting of Akt and mammalian target of rapamycin. *Cancer Res.* 2009;69(18):7311-7319.

39. Wagle N, Grabiner BC, Van Allen EM, et al. Response and acquired resistance to everolimus in anaplastic thyroid cancer. *N Engl J Med.* 2014;371(15):1426-1433.

40. Wieneke JA, Smith A. Parathyroid adenoma. *Head Neck Pathol.* 2008;2(4):305-308.

41. Abele JS, Levine RA. Diagnostic criteria and risk-adapted approach to indeterminate thyroid cytodiagnosis. *Cancer Cytopathol.* 2010;118(6):415-422.

42. Sidawy MK, Costa M. The significance of paravacuolar granules of the thyroid. A histologic, cytologic and ultrastructural study. *Acta Cytol.* 1989;33(6):929-933.

43. Lim H, Devesa SS, Sosa JA, Check D, Kitahara CM. Trends in thyroid cancer incidence and mortality in the united states, 1974-2013. *JAMA.* 2017;317(13):1338-1348.

44. Guan H, VandenBussche CJ, Erozan YS, et al. Can the tall cell variant of papillary thyroid carcinoma be distinguished from the conventional type in fine needle aspirates? A cytomorphologic study with assessment of diagnostic accuracy. *Acta Cytol.* 2013;57(5):534-542.

45. Tabbara SO, Acoury N, Sidawy MK. Multinucleated giant cells in thyroid neoplasms. *Acta Cytol.* 1996;40(6):1184-1188.

46. Auger M. Hürthle cells in fine-needle aspirates of the thyroid: a review of their diagnostic criteria and significance. *Cancer Cytopathol.* 2014;122(4):241-249.

47. Geddie WR, Bedard YC, Strawbridge HT. Medullary carcinoma of the thyroid in fine-needle aspiration biopsies. *Am J Clin Pathol.* 1984;82(5):552-558.

48. Gupta S, Modi S, Gupta V, Marwah N. Hyalinizing trabecular tumor of the thyroid gland. *J Cytol.* 2010;27(2):63-65.

49. Ellison E, Lapuerta P, Martin SE. Psammoma bodies in fine-needle aspirates of the thyroid: predictive value for papillary carcinoma. *Cancer.* 1998;84(3):169-175.

50. Harvey AM, Truong LD, Mody DR. Diagnostic pitfalls of Hashimoto's/lymphocytic thyroiditis on fine-needle aspirations and strategies to avoid overdiagnosis. *Acta Cytol.* 2012;56(4):352-360.

51. Bishop JA, Ali SZ. Hyalinizing trabecular adenoma of the thyroid gland. *Diagn Cytopathol.* 2011;39(4):306-310.

52. Evenson A, Mowschenson P, Wang H, et al. Hyalinizing trabecular adenoma—an uncommon thyroid tumor frequently misdiagnosed as papillary or medullary thyroid carcinoma. *Am J Surg.* 2007;193(6):707-712.

53. Fazeli R, VandenBussche CJ, Bishop JA, Ali SZ. Cytological diagnosis of follicular variant of papillary thyroid carcinoma before and after the Bethesda system for reporting thyroid cytopathology. *Acta Cytol.* 2016;60(1):14-18.

54. Maletta F, Massa F, Torregrossa L, et al. Cytological features of "noninvasive follicular thyroid neoplasm with papillary-like nuclear features" and their correlation with tumor histology. *Hum Pathol.* 2016;54:134-142.

55. Faquin WC, Wong LQ, Afrogheh AH, et al. Impact of reclassifying noninvasive follicular variant of papillary thyroid carcinoma on the risk of malignancy in the Bethesda system for reporting thyroid cytopathology. *Cancer Cytopathol.* 2016;124(3):181-187.

56. Zhou AG, Bishop JA, Ali SZ. Non-invasive follicular thyroid neoplasm with papillary-like nuclear features (NIFTP). *JASC.* 2017;6(5):211-216.

57. Cibas ES, Ducatman BS. *Cytology: Diagnostic Principles and Clinical Correlates.* 3rd ed. Philadelphia, PA: Saunders/Elsevier; 2009.

58. Gonzalez JL, Wang HH, Ducatman BS. Fine-needle aspiration of Hurthle cell lesions. A cytomorphologic approach to diagnosis. *Am J Clin Pathol.* 1993;100(3):231-235.

59. Harach HR, Zusman SB, Saravia Day E. Nodular goiter: a histo-cytological study with some emphasis on pitfalls of fine-needle aspiration cytology. *Diagn Cytopathol.* 1992;8(4):409-419.

60. Giorgadze T, Rossi ED, Fadda G, Gupta PK, LiVolsi VA, Baloch Z. Does the fine-needle aspiration diagnosis of "Hürthle-cell neoplasm/follicular neoplasm with oncocytic features" denote increased risk of malignancy? *Diagn Cytopathol.* 2004;31(5):307-312.

61. Pu RT, Yang J, Wasserman PG, Bhuiya T, Griffith KA, Michael CW. Does Hurthle cell lesion/neoplasm predict malignancy more than follicular lesion/neoplasm on thyroid fine-needle aspiration? *Diagn Cytopathol.* 2006;34(5):330-334.

62. Gharib H, Goellner JR. Fine-needle aspiration biopsy of the thyroid: an appraisal. *Ann Intern Med.* 1993;118(4):282-289.

63. Shaha AR, Shah JP, Loree TR. Patterns of nodal and distant metastasis based on histologic varieties in differentiated carcinoma of the thyroid. *Am J.Surg.* 1996;172(6):692-694.

64. Kushchayeva Y, Duh Q-Y, Kebebew E, D'Avanzo A, Clark OH. Comparison of clinical characteristics at diagnosis and during follow-up in 118 patients with Hurthle cell or follicular thyroid cancer. *Am J Surg.* 2008;195(4):457-462.

65. Lloyd RV, Buehler D, Khanafshar E. Papillary thyroid carcinoma variants. *Head Neck Pathol.* 2011;5(1):51-56.

66. Yeo M-K, Bae JS, Lee S, et al. The warthin-like variant of papillary thyroid carcinoma: a comparison with classic type in the patients with coexisting hashimoto's thyroiditis. *Int J Endocrinol.* 2015;2015:8.

67. Berho M, Suster S. The oncocytic variant of papillary carcinoma of the thyroid: a clinicopathologic study of 15 cases. *Hum Pathol.* 1997;28(1):47-53.

68. Lee J, Hasteh F. Oncocytic variant of papillary thyroid carcinoma associated with Hashimoto's thyroiditis: a case report and review of the literature. *Diagn Cytopathol.* 2009;37(8):600-606.

69. Pedersen RK, Pedersen NT. Primary non-Hodgkin's lymphoma of the thyroid gland: a population based study. *Histopathology*. 1996;28(1):25-32.

70. Holm L-E, Blomgren H, Löwhagen T. Cancer risks in patients with chronic lymphocytic thyroiditis. *N Engl J Med*. 1985;312(10):601-604.

71. Hyjek E, Isaacson PG. Primary B cell lymphoma of the thyroid and its relationship to Hashimoto's thyroiditis. *Hum Pathol*. 1988;19(11):1315-1326.

72. Ibrahimpasic T, Ghossein R, Carlson DL, et al. Outcomes in patients with poorly differentiated thyroid carcinoma. *J Clin Endocrinol Metab*. 2014;99(4):1245-1252.

73. Volante M, Collini P, Nikiforov YE, et al. Poorly differentiated thyroid carcinoma: the Turin proposal for the use of uniform diagnostic criteria and an algorithmic diagnostic approach. *Am J Surg Pathol*. 2007;31(8):1256-1264.

74. Hossain AM, Rahman RN, Nagaiah G, Altaha R, Remick SC. Epidemiology, treatment outcome, and survival of anaplastic thyroid cancer (ATC) in the United States: a period prevalence SEER database study 1973-2006. *J Clin Oncol*. 2010;28(15 suppl):5588.

75. Bishop JA, Sharma R, Westra WH. PAX8 immunostaining of anaplastic thyroid carcinoma: a reliable means of discerning thyroid origin for undifferentiated tumors of the head and neck. *Hum Pathol*. 2011;42(12):1873-1877.

76. Roman S, Lin R, Sosa JA. Prognosis of medullary thyroid carcinoma. *Cancer*. 2006;107(9):2134-2142.

77. Figlioli G, Landi S, Romei C, Elisei R, Gemignani F. Medullary thyroid carcinoma (MTC) and RET proto-oncogene: mutation spectrum in the familial cases and a meta-analysis of studies on the sporadic form. *Mutat Res*. 2013;752(1):36-44.

78. Wells SA Jr, Asa SL, Dralle H, et al. Revised American Thyroid Association guidelines for the management of medullary thyroid carcinoma. *Thyroid*. 2015;25(6):567-610.

79. Kaushal S, Iyer VK, Mathur SR, Ray R. Fine needle aspiration cytology of medullary carcinoma of the thyroid with a focus on rare variants: a review of 78 cases. *Cytopathology*. 2011;22(2):95-105.

80. Katoh R, Miyagi E, Nakamura N, et al. Expression of thyroid transcription factor-1 (TTF-1) in human C cells and medullary thyroid carcinomas. *Hum Pathol*. 2000;31(3):386-393.

81. Ordóñez NG. Value of GATA3 immunostaining in the diagnosis of parathyroid tumors. *Appl Immunohistochem Mol Morphol*. 2014;22(10):756-761.

82. VandenBussche CJ, Ali SZ. Diagnostic challenges in thyroid cytopathology. *Diagn Histopathol*. 2016;22(5):199-205.

SALIVARY GLAND AND CERVICAL LYMPH NODES 2

CHAPTER OUTLINE

INTRODUCTION TO SALIVARY GLAND FINE-NEEDLE ASPIRATION

Salivary gland fine-needle aspiration (FNA) is a well-established and cost-effective diagnostic tool for distinguishing between nonneoplastic and neoplastic processes, as well as between low-grade and high-grade malignancies.[1-7] Importantly, these distinctions determine clinical management. In general, nonneoplastic lesions are treated medically, benign neoplasms are treated with conservative surgical excision, and high-grade malignancies are treated with aggressive surgical resection with or without lymph node dissection. Recently, the Milan System for Reporting Salivary Gland Cytopathology (MSRSGC) was published in an attempt to standardize the reporting of salivary gland lesions into diagnostic categories with associated risks of malignancies.[8] As a result, these diagnostic categories serve to improve communication between pathologists and clinicians and to more clearly inform clinical management based on the diagnosis.

THE UNREMARKABLE SALIVARY GLAND

Salivary gland FNA is typically performed to sample a mass lesion. As a result, it is imperative to note whether or not the cells sampled and visualized correlate with the targeted lesion. For example, if sampling reveals only unremarkable salivary gland components and the patient has a mass lesion, the specimen should be considered inadequate and, according to the MSRSGC, be categorized as "nondiagnostic."[8] Normal salivary gland components are often present in the background of FNA smears and should not be misinterpreted as pathologic material. As a result, it is important to have a thorough understanding of the normal components that make up major salivary glands. These normal components include serous and mucinous acinar cells, myoepithelial cells, ductal cells, and adipocytes.

SEROUS ACINAR CELLS

The acinar cells of the parotid gland are all of the serous type while those of the submandibular gland are a mix of serous and mucinous cell types. Serous acinar cells contain dense, lightly basophilic cytoplasm and small cytoplasmic vacuoles which are best appreciated on the Diff-Quik stain. The nuclei are generally basally oriented, round, uniform, and dark. Serous acinar cells can be present in grape-like clusters with interspersed salivary gland duct cells; however, the delicate nature of the cytoplasm often results in disruption during aspiration and, consequently, naked nuclei (Figures 2.1-2.6). When many serous acinar cells are present in an FNA sample, the major differential diagnosis will be between normal acinar cells and acinic cell carcinoma (ACC). The most helpful clue in recognizing unremarkable serous acinar cells is appreciating intact, clustered, grape-like configurations and associated ducts and adipocytes. ACCs are often more cellular and consist of haphazardly arranged, crowded clusters that may be associated with fibrovascular cores in a background of abundant dyshesive cells with naked nuclei.[9]

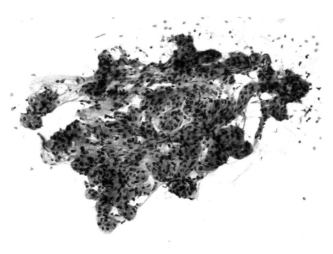

Figure 2.1. Benign salivary tissue. Lobules of benign-appearing acinar tissue form a grape-like architecture (Pap stain).

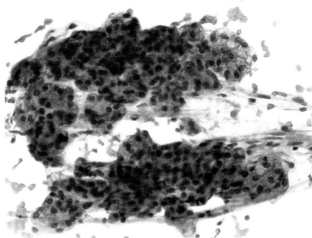

Figure 2.2. Benign salivary tissue. Clusters of serous acinar cells in the characteristic lobular configuration connected by intervening ductal type epithelium forming small tubules (Pap stain).

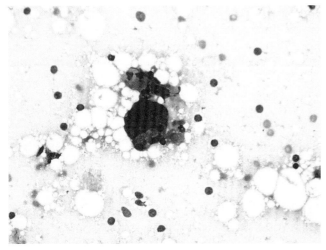

Figure 2.3. Benign salivary tissue. A high magnification view of a single lobule of unremarkable acinar cells with granular cytoplasm and eccentric, round, uniform nuclei with regular contours (Diff-Quik stain).

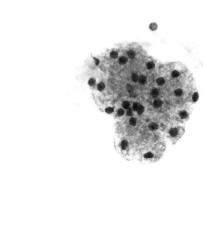

Figure 2.4. Benign salivary tissue. A high magnification view of a three-dimensional group of normal-appearing serous acinar cells with dense, granular cytoplasm and round, regular nuclei (Pap stain).

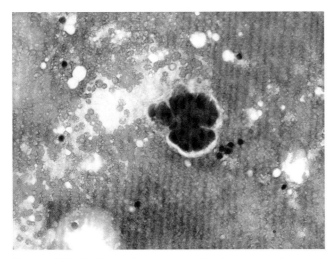

Figure 2.5. Benign salivary tissue. Single group of normal-appearing serous acinar cells with granular cytoplasm and round, regular nuclei which are 1.5-2× the size of the background lymphocytes in this field (Pap stain).

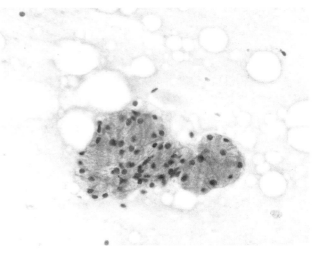

Figure 2.6. Benign salivary tissue. Unremarkable serous acinar cells displaying abundant granular cytoplasm and peripherally placed, round to oval nuclei (Pap stain).

MUCINOUS ACINAR CELLS

Mucinous acinar cells make up the majority of the acinar cells in the sublingual gland and are mixed with serous acinar cells in the submandibular gland. Mucinous acinar cells are typically larger than serous acinar cells and contain abundant, clear cytoplasm with flattened, basally oriented nuclei. The cells are typically arranged in grape-like clusters with admixed adipocytes and ductal cells. It is important to remember that mucinous cells can be seen in unremarkable submandibular and sublingual glands, as well as in malignant neoplasms, such as mucoepidermoid carcinoma (MEC). As a result, it is most important to recognize the overall grape-like structures and bland cytology of mucinous acinar cells to avoid a misdiagnosis.

MYOEPITHELIAL CELLS

Myoepithelial cells in the salivary gland surround acini and intercalated ducts, contracting and facilitating movement of salivary contents. Myoepithelial cells are often difficult to appreciate on smears of unremarkable salivary gland tissue; when present, myoepithelial cells should be seen only underlying acini and ducts and not forming a discrete cluster or a conspicuous population (Figure 2.7).

DUCTAL CELLS

The normal salivary gland contains three distinct ductal elements: 1) cuboidal, intercalated ducts, 2) columnar, striated ducts, and 3) pseudostratified, columnar excretory ducts. These ductal structures usually do not make up a large proportion of normal aspirated salivary gland tissue, but it is not uncommon to identify a few small groups of ductal cells in a honeycomb configuration with small nucleoli or small tubules in close association with normal acini (Figure 2.8). Importantly, striated ducts, which normally contain dense, abundant eosinophilic cytoplasm, can undergo squamous metaplasia—a finding that should not be confused with squamous cell carcinoma (SqCC) or mucoepidermoid carcinoma (MEC).[2]

ADIPOCYTES

FNA of unremarkable salivary gland tissue may occasionally result in a minimal amount of fibroadipose tissue on the smear. This tissue may contain small vessels and adipocytes mixed with other normal components (Figures 2.9 and 2.10). Furthermore, aging may result in fatty replacement of the parotid gland and increase the likelihood of aspirating

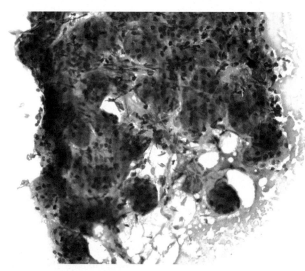

Figure 2.7. Benign salivary tissue. Normal-appearing serous acinar groups with surrounding spindle-shaped myoepithelial cells (Diff-Quik stain).

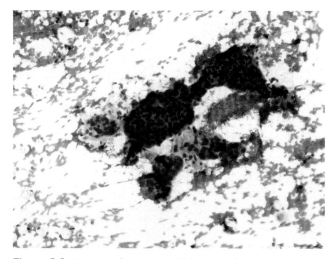

Figure 2.8. Benign salivary tissue. Thick tissue fragment consisting of ductal cells in the center of the field and serous acinar cells at the periphery. The ductal cells are well-organized within the fragment and have uniform nuclei (Pap stain).

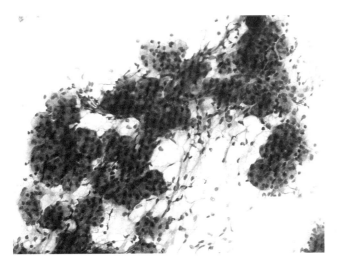

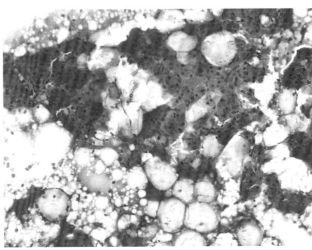

Figure 2.9. Benign salivary tissue. Bland-appearing adipocytes admixed with lobular groups of serous acinar cells (Diff-Quik stain).

Figure 2.10. Benign salivary tissue. Adipocytes of various sizes are seen surrounding and admixed within lobules of serous acinar cells (Diff-Quik stain).

this material. On rare occasions, primary salivary gland lipomas may be present and reveal a predominant population of adipocytes; however, this diagnosis requires clinical and radiographic correlation.[10]

FAQ: How can the presence of unremarkable salivary gland components be useful in an FNA of a mass lesion?

Answer: The presence of normal salivary gland components can be most helpful for two specific reasons: 1) these cell types can be directly compared with a second cell population of interest to determine whether or not cytomorphologic differences are present, and 2) it may imply that the lesion sampled is arising within the salivary gland. This latter finding may be particularly helpful when it is not entirely clear whether the lesion in question is arising from a salivary gland or from a directly adjacent focus, e.g. a dermal or subcutaneous lesion.

CYSTIC PATTERN

CHECKLIST: Etiologic Considerations for the Cystic Pattern

☐ Nonmucinous Subpattern
  ○ Epidermal Inclusion Cyst (EIC)
  ○ Lymphoepithelial Cyst
  ○ Warthin Tumor (WT)
  ○ Acinic Cell Carcinoma (ACC)
  ○ Cystic Metastatic Squamous Cell Carcinoma (SqCC)
☐ Mucinous Subpattern
  ○ Mucocele/Mucous Retention Cyst
  ○ Mucinous Metaplasia
  ○ Low-grade Mucoepidermoid Carcinoma (MEC)
  ○ Secretory Carcinoma
  ○ Salivary Duct Carcinoma (SDC)

The cystic pattern is characterized by both intrinsically cystic lesions and benign and malignant neoplasms that have undergone secondary cystic change.[11] Unfortunately, many entities fall into this pattern and at least one-third of sampled cystic salivary gland lesions are neoplastic.[12] Aspirates of cystic lesions are often paucicellular, and as a result, it is most practical to further subdivide entities based on the absence or presence of mucin. To complicate matters further, nonmucinous and mucinous cysts can undergo squamous metaplasia, which should not be interpreted as SqCC or MEC, respectively. Further diagnostic challenges include the fact that some lesions are intrinsically paucicellular while other samples will be paucicellular due to technical sampling issues. According to the MSRSGC (Table 2.1), nonmucinous cyst fluid without an epithelial component should be interpreted as "nondiagnostic" while mucinous cyst fluid without an epithelial component should be interpreted as "atypia of undermined significance (AUS)."[8] Cases with a prominent epithelial population will often be classified as "salivary gland neoplasm of uncertain malignant potential (SUMP)," unless overt malignant features are present.[8] In some instances, both benign and malignant salivary gland neoplasms are associated with characteristic cytogenetic and molecular alterations, which can be extremely helpful in making a definitive diagnosis on an FNA specimen (Table 2.2).

TABLE 2.1: Categories of the Milan System for Reporting Salivary Gland Cytopathology

Diagnostic Category	Definition and Notes	Risk of Malignancy	Clinical Management
I. *Nondiagnostic*	Insufficient cellular material for a cytologic diagnosis • Exceptions include an acellular specimen containing matrix material and mucinous cyst contents	25%	Clinical and radiologic correlation/ repeat fine-needle aspiration (FNA)
II. *Nonneoplastic*	Benign entities such as chronic sialadenitis, reactive lymph node, granulomas, and infection • Essentially includes all cases lacking cytomorphologic evidence of a neoplastic process	10%	Clinical follow-up and radiologic correlation
III. *Atypia of undetermined significance (AUS)*	Contains limited atypia and is indefinite for a neoplasm • The majority of FNAs in this category will be processes with reactive atypia or poorly sampled neoplasms	20%	Repeat FNA or surgery
IV. *Neoplasm*			
A. *Benign* *a. Epithelial origin* *b. Mesenchymal origin*	Reserved for benign neoplasms diagnosed based on established cytologic criteria • Will most often be pleomorphic adenomas and Warthin tumors	<5%	Surgery or clinical follow-up

TABLE 2.1: Categories of the Milan System for Reporting Salivary Gland Cytopathology (Continued)

Diagnostic Category	Definition and Notes	Risk of Malignancy	Clinical Management

B. Salivary *gland neoplasm of uncertain malignant potential (SUMP)*
  a. Cellular basaloid neoplasm
  b. Cellular oncocytic/oncocytoid neoplasm
  c. Cellular neoplasm with clear cell features
	Reserved for FNA samples that are diagnostic of a neoplasm but not diagnostic for a specific benign or malignant entity
	• Most cases will be cellular benign neoplasms, neoplasms with atypical features, and low-grade carcinomas
		35%	Surgery; intraoperative consultation may be helpful to determine the extent of surgery

V. *Suspicious for malignancy (SM)*	FNA samples showing features that are highly suggestive, but not definitive, for a malignant neoplasm • Report should include the suspected malignancy or the differential diagnosis	60%	Surgery; intraoperative consultation may be helpful to determine the extent of surgery
VI. *Malignant*	Features must be diagnostic of malignancy • Report should include the differential diagnosis, and there should be an attempt to grade the carcinoma as low or high grade	90%	Surgery with extent dependent on grade

Adapted from two tables in Faquin WC, Rossi ED *The Milan System for Reporting Salivary Gland Cytopathology.* New York, NY: Springer Science+Business Media; 2018 [chapter 1].

TABLE 2.2: Cytogenetic/Molecular Alterations in Primary Salivary Gland Neoplasms

Neoplasm	Chromosomal Translocation/ Molecular Alterations	Gene Fusion	Surrogate Immunomarker
Pleomorphic adenoma/ carcinoma ex pleomorphic adenoma	t(3;8)(p21;q12) t(5;8)(p12;q12)	*PLAG1*	PLAG1 antibody
	t(3;12)(p14.2;14-5) Ins(9;12)(p23;q12-15)	*HMGA2*	HMGA2 antibody
Mucoepidermoid carcinoma	t(11;19)(q21;p13)	*CRTC1-MAML2*	N/A
	t(11;15)(q21;q26)	*CRTC3-MAML2*	N/A
Adenoid cystic carcinoma	t(6;9)(q22-23;p23-24) t(8;9)	*MYB-NFIB*	MYB antibody
Secretory carcinoma	t(12;15)(p13;q12)	*ETV6-NTRK3*	N/A

(Continued)

TABLE 2.2: Cytogenetics/Molecular Alterations in Primary Salivary Gland Neoplasms (Continued)

Neoplasm	Chromosomal Translocation/ Molecular Alterations	Gene Fusion	Surrogate Immunomarker
Clear cell carcinoma and myoepithelial carcinoma, clear cell variant	t(12;22)(q13;q12)	*EWSR1-ATΓ1*	N/A
Polymorphous adenocarcinoma/cribriform adenocarcinoma of the minor salivary gland	*PRKD1* E710D activating mutations/*PRKD1* gene rearrangements	N/A	N/A
Basal cell adenoma	*CTNNB1* mutations	N/A	β-catenin

(Data adapted from Griffith CC, Schmitt AC, Little JL, Magliocca KR. New developments in salivary gland pathology: clinically useful ancillary testing and new potentially targetable molecular alterations. *Arch Pathol Lab Med.* 2017;141(3):381-395; Jo VY, Krane JF. Ancillary testing in salivary gland cytology: a practical guide. *Cancer Cytopathol.* 2018;126(S8):627-642.)

CYSTIC PATTERN: NONMUCINOUS

EPIDERMAL INCLUSION CYST

Epidermal inclusion cysts (EICs) are common lesions that often affect the skin of the face, neck, and trunk. EICs present as nodular, subcutaneous masses and, when overlying the submandibular or parotid gland, may be mistaken for a salivary gland lesion.[11,15] These cysts are unilocular, lined by squamous epithelium containing a granular layer, and are filled with laminated keratin (Figures 2.11-2.13). Furthermore, these cysts may rupture, become inflamed, and incite a granulomatous or fibrotic response; in an undersampled lesion, they may be mistaken for malignant epithelial cells and a desmoplastic stromal response. Clinical and radiographic correlation is extremely important in this setting to avoid this pitfall.

LYMPHOEPITHELIAL CYST

As the name implies, lymphoepithelial cysts are cystic lesions comprised of cyst-lining epithelial cells, a benign lymphocytic proliferation within the cyst wall, and a layer of fibrous connective tissue separating the lesion from salivary gland tissue. The epithelial component is most often made up of stratified squamous cells; however, cuboidal and columnar types may be seen. FNA most often reveals proteinaceous material with or without cholesterol crystals, vacuolated macrophages, degenerated epithelial cells, and squamous debris in a background of polymorphous lymphocytes and germinal center fragments (Figures 2.14 and 2.15). It is important to remember that the presence of lymphocytes does not automatically imply sampling of an intraparotid lymph node or a malignant lesion with tumor-associated lymphoid proliferation (TALP). The epithelial cells in lymphoepithelial cysts should be cytologically bland, although degenerative atypia is fairly common in cyst contents; as a result, a subset of these lesions are best classified as "AUS" based on the MSRSGC.[8] Most notably, however, there should be an absence of necrosis and significant cytologic atypia, which are more often present in cystic SqCCs.

WARTHIN TUMOR

Warthin tumors (WT) are benign, cystic neoplasms that occur almost exclusively in the parotid gland. WTs occur late in life, are associated with a history of smoking, and may be bilateral.[16] WTs have both epithelial and lymphocytic components, much like many other entities in the

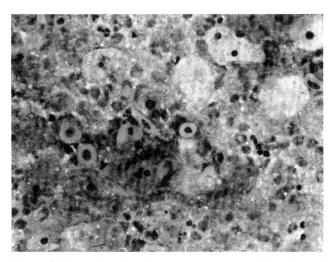

Figure 2.11. Epidermal inclusion cyst. Squamous cells with round to oval nuclei and characteristic dense blue cytoplasm are present in a background of abundant granular debris and scattered inflammatory cells. The squamous cells resemble the intermediate and superficial squamous cells seen in a cervical pap test. Additionally, note the cells with larger nuclei and a higher N/C ratio, which are reminiscent of parabasal cells. (Diff-Quik stain).

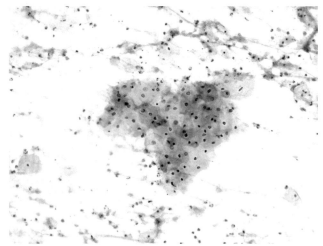

Figure 2.12. Epidermal inclusion cyst. Cyst-lining squamous cells are seen in a background of granular debris and mixed inflammatory cells. The nuclei are small and uniform with bland chromatin (Pap stain).

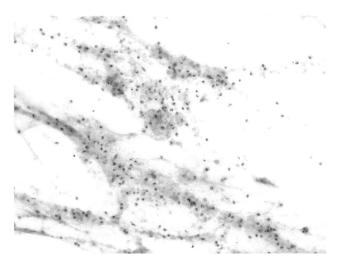

Figure 2.13. Nonmucinous cyst contents. Granular debris and mixed inflammatory cells. In the absence of a cyst-lining component, the etiology of cyst contents often cannot be definitively identified (Pap stain).

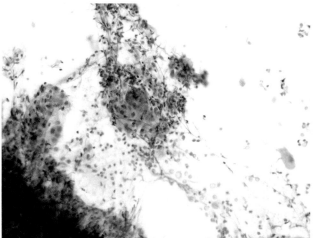

Figure 2.14. Lymphoepithelial cyst. Cyst-lining glandular epithelium is present with surrounding lymphocytes and lymphoid tangles (Pap stain).

cystic pattern. According to the MSRSGC, a definitive diagnosis of "Neoplasm: Benign" can be made if all three classic features are present: 1) sheets of oncocytes with abundant granular cytoplasm and well-defined borders in a 2) background of lymphocytes and 3) proteinaceous debris (Figures 2.16-2.19).[8] When these features are present, the diagnostic accuracy for a WT is excellent.[17] It is important to keep in mind that many entities can show oncocytic metaplasia. However, with metaplasia, the oncocytic cells are usually a minority of the epithelial component, whereas in WTs, they comprise a predominant uniform population.[17] Although extensive oncocytic metaplasia can be present in the oncocytic variant of MEC, these malignancies should contain at least rare mucinous epithelium scattered throughout.[18]

KEY FEATURES of Warthin Tumor

- The epithelial component contains cells with abundant granular cytoplasm and round nuclei with prominent nucleoli.
- The background contains abundant lymphocytes.
- Proteinaceous debris is also present in the background, and looks similar to "motor oil" when aspirated.

PEARLS & PITFALLS

It is important to remember that many entities can undergo both squamous and/ or oncocytic metaplasia. For example, the oncocytes of Warthin tumors (WT) can rarely undergo squamous metaplasia and either mimic a benign squamous-lined cyst or an invasive squamous cell carcinoma (SqCC). This latter pitfall is especially treacherous because the proteinaceous debris that is characteristically present in WTs can mimic the necrotic debris often seen in metastatic SqCC. As a result, it is important to assess whether or not a significant amount of cytologic atypia is present and to identify all the components in the specimen.

ACINIC CELL CARCINOMA

Acinic cell carcinoma (ACC) is a malignant salivary gland neoplasm which most commonly occurs in the parotid gland. The prognosis is good with the 5-year survival approaching 90%; although distant metastasis is rare, cervical lymph node involvement may occur and approximately 1/3 of cases locally recur.[19] The neoplastic cells show serous acinar

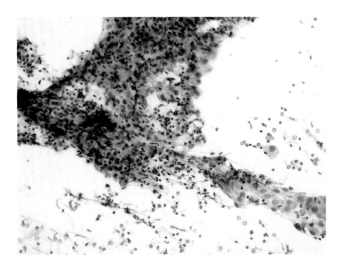

Figure 2.15. Lymphoepithelial cyst. Lymphocytes and lymphoid tangles are seen with admixed metaplastic epithelium. In the absence of cyst contents (macrophages and debris) in the background, the differential diagnosis would include sialadenitis (Pap stain).

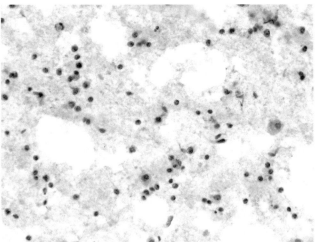

Figure 2.16. Warthin tumor. Cystic proteinaceous debris, lymphocytes, and histiocytes are present in this field and should warrant a thorough investigation for an oncocytic component to help confirm the diagnosis (Pap stain).

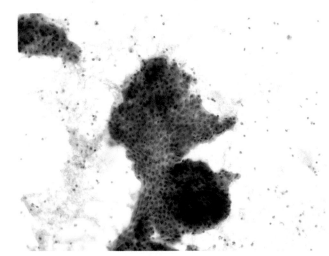

Figure 2.17. Warthin tumor. Separate field showing cohesive sheets of oncocytic epithelium in a papillary configuration with surrounding proteinaceous debris and scattered lymphocytes (Pap stain).

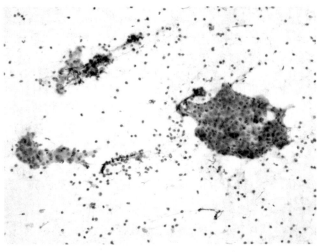

Figure 2.18. Warthin tumor with oncocytic epithelium and background lymphocytes. Note the keratinizing metaplastic squamous cell in the center of the field. This finding may occur in Warthin tumors and should not be overinterpreted as a possible squamous cell carcinoma (Pap stain).

differentiation and are most commonly solid, papillary-cystic, or microcystic in architecture. FNAs typically produce highly cellular smears comprised of large, polygonal cells with abundant, granular, and vacuolated cytoplasm and relatively bland, round nuclei with prominent nucleoli (Figures 2.20-2.23). Nuclear pleomorphism may be seen in a small subset of cases. In contrast to the lobulated architecture of ductal cells and adipocytes seen in normal salivary gland tissue, ACC is comprised of a single population of cells in three-dimensional groups, sheets, and single cells. Owing to the delicate nature of the cytoplasm, the background may be largely comprised of "naked nuclei." In papillary-cystic cases, vacuolated macrophages and proteinaceous material may be present, as well as three-dimensional groups of cells surrounding a fibrovascular core, which can mimic the lobulated architecture of normal salivary gland tissue.

PEARLS & PITFALLS

Because of the relatively bland malignant cells and their similarity to normal serous acinar cells, there is a high false-negative rate for diagnosing acinic cell carcinoma (ACC) on FNA. The most helpful clue is the lack of other salivary gland components or a cell population seen in other cystic salivary gland neoplasms, such as oncocytes from an oncocytoma or Warthin tumor, or mucocytes from a mucoepidermoid carcinoma (MEC). However, the vacuoles in cystic ACCs can be mistaken for intracytoplasmic mucin vacuoles, which may require a mucicarmine stain to rule out a MEC.[20] ACCs can also be relatively zymogen granule poor and, as a result, overlap with the cytomorphologic features of secretory carcinoma.[21] In fact, it may be nearly impossible to differentiate ACCs from secretory carcinomas without the use of immunostains. Fortunately, ACCs are positive for DOG1 while secretory carcinomas are positive for GATA3, mammaglobin, and S100 protein.

CYSTIC METASTATIC SQUAMOUS CELL CARCINOMA

Nodal metastases of squamous cell carcinoma (SqCC) in the head and neck are often cystic with a thick capsule surrounding the malignant epithelium and central, necrotic debris. Metastatic SqCC may be keratinizing or nonkeratinizing. Cutaneous primaries are by far the most common SqCCs to involve intraparotid lymph nodes, and many are keratinizing—a feature that will help rule out a MEC. On the other hand, human papillomavirus (HPV)–related oropharyngeal primaries are more likely to be nonkeratinizing, although these typically metastasize to neck lymph nodes (most notably levels II and

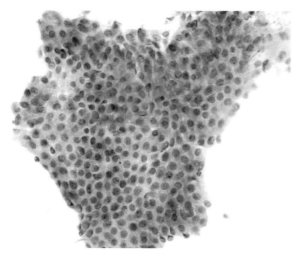

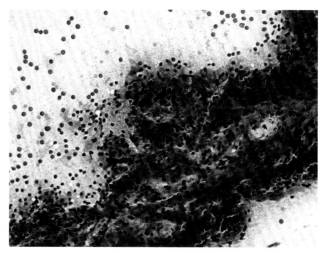

Figure 2.19. Warthin tumor. Separate case showing a large fragment of oncocytic epithelium forming a sheet. The nuclei are round and uniform and have regular contours. Note the clean background present in this SurePath preparation (Pap stain).

Figure 2.20. Acinic cell carcinoma. Disorganized sheets and single cells with a notable absence of the lobular architecture that characterizes unremarkable salivary gland tissue. The neoplasm demonstrates prominent vasculature (Diff-Quik stain).

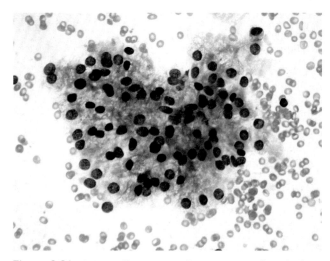

Figure 2.21. Acinic cell carcinoma. Serous acinar cells with abundant granular cytoplasm and enlarged, albeit relatively bland, nuclei. The lobular architecture of benign salivary tissue is absent; however, small fragments of finely granular/oncocytoid cells such as this may be seen in reactive processes such as sialadenitits, making a definitive diagnosis challenging (Diff-Quik stain).

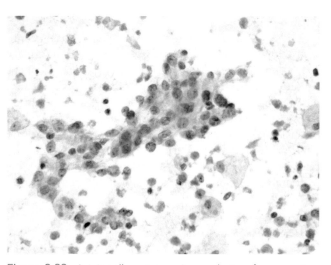

Figure 2.22. Acinic cell carcinoma. Loose cluster of serous acinar cells containing granular cytoplasm, enlarged nuclei, and distinctive nucleoli in a background of lymphocytes and cystic debris (Pap stain).

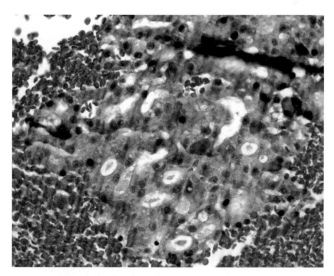

Figure 2.23. Acinic cell carcinoma. Acinar cells with basophilic, granular cytoplasm in a microcystic pattern (H&E).

III), and it would be highly unusual to see a metastasis in an intraparotid lymph node.[22] This distinction is important, however, because cutaneous HPV-negative SqCCs can be positive for p16—a screening marker for the HPV status of an SqCC.[23] Despite the cystic nature of these metastases, smears are usually cellular and comprised of fragments and isolated irregularly shaped keratinocytes with variable amounts of dense cytoplasm (Figures 2.24-2.27). The neoplastic cells generally have an increased nuclear to cytoplasmic (N/C) ratio, irregular and hyperchromatic nuclei, and mitoses. Finally, a background of necrotic tumor cells and degenerative nuclear debris can be extremely helpful in making a definitive diagnosis.

FAQ: What entities are in the differential diagnosis for an a squamous cell carcinoma (SqCC) in the parotid gland?

Answer: For scant/bland cases, an epidermal inclusion cyst may enter the differential; however, the cellular atypia and the necrotic background should point to a malignant diagnosis. For obviously malignant cases, a diagnosis of mucoepidermoid carcinoma (MEC) may be entertained due to the epidermoid cells (squamous cells resembling those seen in the epidermis); however, the absence of mucin and presence of keratinization will point toward a diagnosis of SqCC. Immunostains should be interpreted with caution because p63/p40, which are often used to confirm squamous differentiation, will stain the basal cells of salivary gland lesions and the intermediate (neither fully mucous or epidermoid in differentiation) and epidermoid cells of MECs.

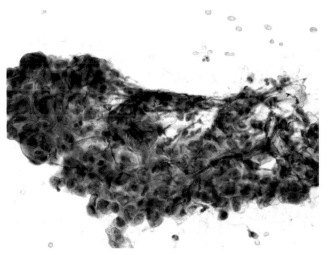

Figure 2.24. Squamous cell carcinoma. Fragment of markedly atypical cohesive cells with enlarged, pleomorphic nuclei and prominent nucleoli. Note the keratin pearls (Pap stain).

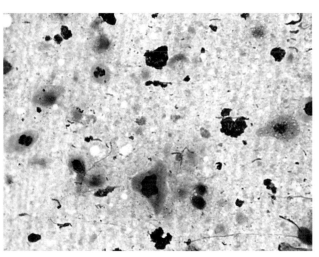

Figure 2.25. Squamous cell carcinoma. Large, polygonal cells with abundant, dense, "Robin egg" blue cytoplasm and hyperchromatic, enlarged, irregular nuclei in a background of cystic debris. The cells are too atypical to represent a benign squamous-lined cyst (Diff-Quik stain).

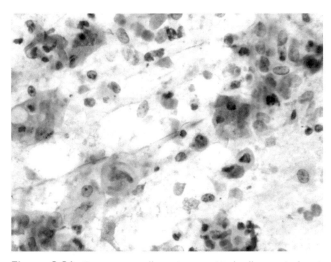

Figure 2.26. Squamous cell carcinoma. Markedly atypical epithelial cells with abnormal keratinization in a background of cystic debris (Pap stain).

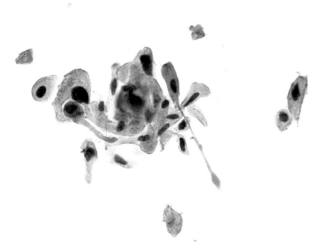

Figure 2.27. Squamous cell carcinoma. Malignant squamous cells showing markedly irregular cytoplasmic extensions, characteristic of tadpole cells, as well as nuclear hyperchromasia and pleomorphism (Pap stain).

CYSTIC PATTERN: MUCINOUS

MUCOCELE/MUCOUS RETENTION CYST

Mucoceles are relatively common lesions that most often arise in the minor salivary glands of the oral cavity, especially those of the lower lip. These lesions are pseudocysts that result from the extravasation of mucin from the salivary excretory ducts due to trauma or obstruction with a sialolith.[24] As a result, there may be an inflammatory component (Figures 2.28-2.31). Mucous retention cysts, on the other hand, are true cysts that occur when an excretory duct dilates. The epithelium will, therefore, be comprised of whatever cell type is lining that particular portion of the duct: cuboidal, columnar, oncocytic, or squamous epithelium.[24] In the parotid gland, these are more commonly referred to as salivary duct cysts; however, as the parotid gland is primarily composed of serous epithelium, the contents tend to be watery as opposed to mucinous.[24] Therefore, in the parotid gland, the presence of mucin (even acellular mucin) is an ominous finding and will trigger a diagnosis of "AUS" based on the MSRSGC due to the possibility of an undersampled MEC.[8] When mucin and an epithelial component are present, it is crucial to look for the presence of epidermoid or intermediate cells, which would be indicative of a MEC.

SAMPLE NOTE: MUCINOUS CYSTIC CONTENTS WITHOUT AN EPITHELIAL COMPONENT

Atypia of undetermined significance:
Acellular mucin, vacuolated macrophages, and mixed inflammation. Evaluation limited by scant cellularity. See note.

Note: Cyst-lining epithelial cells are not definitively identified. Therefore, this FNA may not be representative of the entire lesion. Although these findings may be consistent with a mucocele, the absence of an epithelial component from an undersampled low-grade mucoepidermoid carcinoma cannot be ruled out. Recommend clinical and radiographic correlation, as well as repeat FNA in a persistent or expanding mass lesion.

MUCINOUS METAPLASIA

Many secondary changes, including both squamous and mucinous metaplasia, are not uncommon in primary salivary gland neoplasms. As a result, the presence of mucin should warrant a thorough evaluation of all the material to rule out the presence of epidermoid and intermediate cells from a MEC or diagnostic features of a separate diagnosis. Most notably, WTs and pleomorphic adenomas (PAs) may contain metaplastic, mucin-producing cells

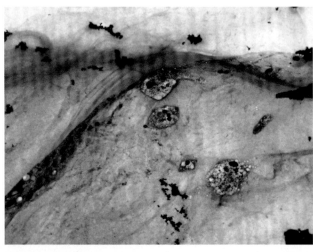

Figure 2.28. Mucocele. Thick, acellular mucin and multiple vacuolated macrophages (Diff-Quik stain).

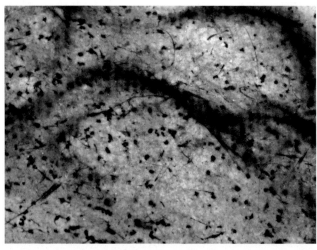

Figure 2.29. Mucocele. Acellular mucin with macrophages and granular debris (Diff-Quik stain).

(Figures 2.32 and 2.33).[25] However, for most cases of WTs, the classic cytomorphologic features of oncocytic epithelium, lymphocytes, and granular debris predominate.[24] For PAs, the presence of the metachromatic, fibrillary matrix material and myoepithelial cells will clinch the diagnosis and prevent a misdiagnosis.[26]

LOW-GRADE MUCOEPIDERMOID CARCINOMA

Mucoepidermoid carcinoma (MEC) is the most common malignant tumor of the major salivary glands and affects a wide range of patient ages with a slight female predominance. MECs are comprised of varying amounts of epidermoid (resemble squamous cells of the epidermis), mucinous epithelial cells, and intermediate cells (contain clear cytoplasm without obvious squamoid or mucinous differentiation) and are variably solid and cystic (Figures 2.34-2.38). The grade of MEC is the most important predictor for patient survival and is classified as either low-, intermediate-, or high-grade. Low-grade MECs tend to be largely cystic and less cellular, resulting in FNAs that often reveal acellular mucin and macrophages only.[27] Unlike nonmucinous cystic contents, the mere presence of mucin on FNA, even in the absence of an epithelial component (or scant epithelial component), should trigger a diagnosis of "AUS" based on the MSRSGC due to the possibility of an undersampled

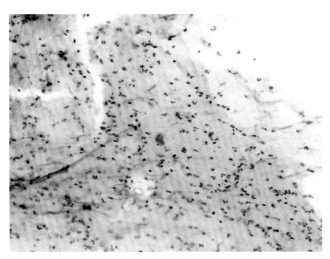

Figure 2.30. Mucocele. Acellular mucin admixed with predominantly neutrophils (Pap stain).

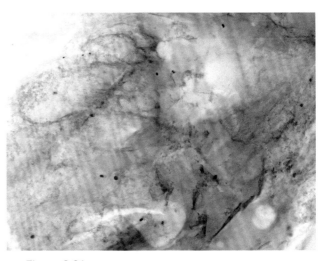

Figure 2.31. Mucocele. Thick, acellular mucin (Pap stain).

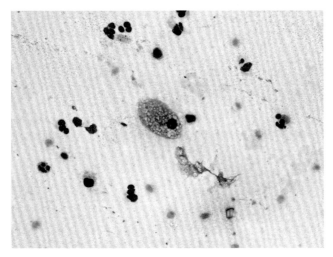

Figure 2.32. Mucinous metaplasia. Macrophages filled with mucin-containing vacuoles and surrounding inflammatory cells. Other fields contained oncocytic epithelium diagnostic for a Warthin tumor, as well as squamous metaplasia (Diff-Quik stain).

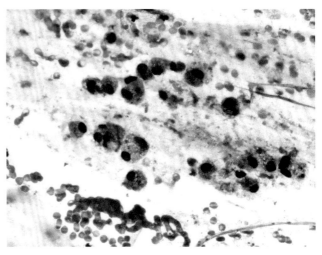

Figure 2.33. Mucinous metaplasia. Macrophages with mucin-filled vacuoles from the same Warthin tumor with mucinous metaplasia (Diff-Quik stain).

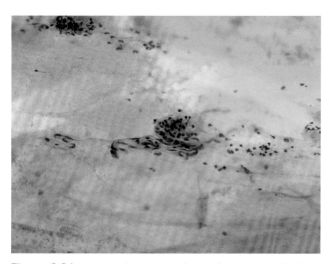

Figure 2.34. Low-grade mucoepidermoid carcinoma. Crushed epithelial cells in a background of abundant, thick mucin (Pap stain).

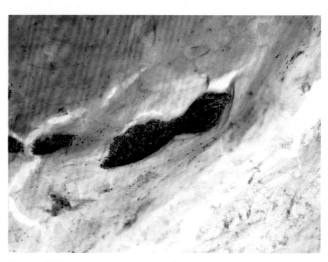

Figure 2.35. Low-grade mucoepidermoid carcinoma. A low magnification view showing abundant mucin and an epithelial tissue fragment, which should raise the possibility of a low-grade mucoepidermoid carcinoma (Pap stain).

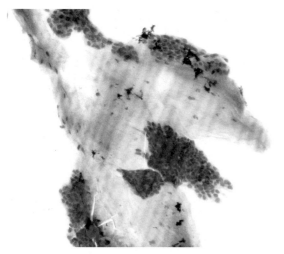

Figure 2.36. Low-grade mucoepidermoid carcinoma. Sheets of epithelial cells in a background of mucin (Diff-Quik stain).

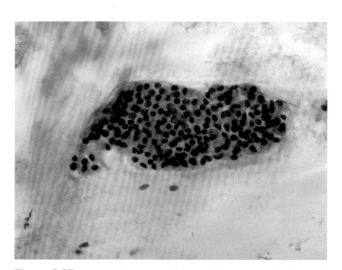

Figure 2.37. Low-grade mucoepidermoid carcinoma. A cluster of intermediate cells without obvious squamous or glandular differentiation is seen floating in a background of abundant clean mucin (Pap stain).

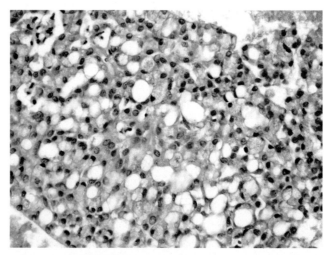

Figure 2.38. Low-grade mucoepidermoid carcinoma. Vacuolated cells with intracytoplasmic mucin can be seen admixed with intermediate cells (H&E).

MEC.[8] In contrast, high-grade MECs are highly cellular and composed predominantly of epidermoid cells with significant nuclear pleomorphism and mitoses, with or without a necrotic background.[28]

KEY FEATURES of Low-Grade Mucoepidermoid Carcinoma

- Low-grade MEC is a cystic lesion and yields a mucinous background.
- Epithelium with intracytoplasmic mucin may be present.
- Intermediate cells contain variable amounts of cytoplasmic clearing without obvious squamous or mucinous differentiation.
- Epidermoid cells have dense, nonkeratinizing cytoplasm that resemble squamous cells of the epidermis.

SECRETORY CARCINOMA

Secretory carcinoma, previously known as mammary analogue secretory carcinoma (MASC), is a low-grade malignant neoplasm of the salivary gland characterized most commonly by the *ETV6-NTRK3* gene fusion product from the t(12;15)(p13;q25) translocation; however, additional translocation partners have been identified.[29] Like ACCs, the architecture of secretory carcinomas is variable and may be solid, cystic, microcystic, papillary-cystic, tubular, or microfollicular. On FNA, smears are usually highly cellular and composed of small groups with or without papillary fragments as well as single cells, including "naked nuclei." The background often shows eosinophilic, colloid-like mucoproteinaceous secretory material and abundant vacuolated/foamy macrophages (Figures 2.39-2.41). Overall, the malignant cells are relatively bland with abundant, eosinophilic cytoplasm containing micro- or macrovesicles that stain positively with mucicarmine. Of note, there is a conspicuous lack of cytoplasmic zymogen granules, which may aid in the distinction from ACC. The nuclei are typically uniform and round with vesicular chromatin and prominent nucleoli, which help distinguish it from the high-grade malignant neoplasms. The malignant cells share many overlapping cytomorphologic features with ACC, particularly those that are zymogen granule poor. As discussed above in the "Acinic Cell Carcinoma" section, immunochemistry or molecular studies may be necessary to differentiate between these two entities: secretory carcinomas are positive for S100 protein, mammaglobin, and GATA3 while ACCs are positive for DOG1.[14] Additionally, the presence of mucin-containing epithelium may bring MEC into the differential; however, the lack of intermediate and epidermoid cells would not support this diagnosis.

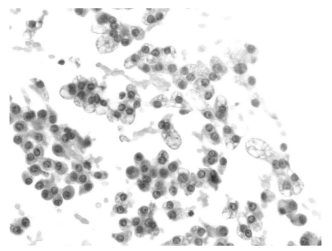

Figure 2.39. Secretory carcinoma. Many "histiocytoid" cells are present with round nuclei and abundant cytoplasm containing small and large clear vacuoles (Pap stain).

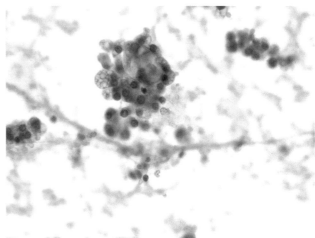

Figure 2.40. Secretory carcinoma. Neoplastic cells with abundant and large cytoplasmic vacuoles with a bubbly appearance are present. Note the small, round, and often eccentric nuclei giving the cells a "histiocytoid" appearance (Pap stain).

SALIVARY DUCT CARCINOMA

Salivary duct carcinoma (SDC) is a high-grade malignancy that most commonly arises in the parotid gland. SDC most commonly occurs in older, male patients and accounts for approximately 10% of all primary salivary gland malignancies. Unfortunately, SDC is aggressive with frequent recurrences and a propensity for regional and distant metastases, with a 5-year disease-specific survival ranging from 55-65%.[30] Not infrequently, SDC may form microcystic spaces or have larger, degenerative cystic spaces secondary to tumor necrosis. Mucin may be present, especially in the mucin-rich variant, which is characterized by islands of high-grade mucin-producing epithelium in a background of abundant extracellular mucin. SDC is cytomorphologically similar to high-grade ductal carcinoma of the breast; the neoplastic cells may have abundant oncocytic cytoplasm and large, pleomorphic nuclei with prominent nucleoli and frequent mitotic figures (Figures 2.42 and 2.43). The differential may include an oncocytic carcinoma, high-grade MEC, or adenocarcinoma not otherwise specified; however, on a well-sampled FNA, any high-grade malignant features will warrant categorization as "malignant" according to on the MSRSGC.[8] For a more definitive diagnosis, the majority of SDCs are positive for androgen receptor (AR) and approximately 30% of cases show HER2 amplification, both of which have therapeutic implications.[31,32]

> **FAQ:** What are the surgical options for treating benign and malignant salivary glands neoplasms?
>
> **Answer:** There are three main surgical procedures for the parotid gland: superficial, total, or radical parotidectomy. Most benign neoplasms can be treated with the superficial procedure where the neoplasm is narrowly excised with clean margins. The total procedure is required if the neoplasm is located in the deep portion of the parotid gland; however, this procedure is more risky because it requires dissecting the gland off the facial nerve. As a result, it is more often performed for malignant lesions that cannot be conservatively managed. For malignancies that are impinging upon the facial nerve, the radical procedure is most often performed, which involves removing the entire parotid gland and excising a portion of the facial nerve.

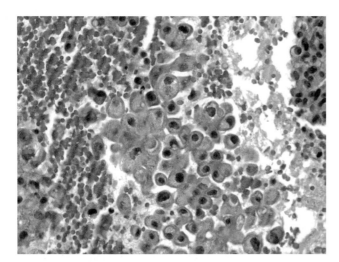

Figure 2.41. Secretory carcinoma. Cell block material comprised of neoplastic cells with abundant eosinophilic cytoplasm with small vacuoles, creating a clearing appearance. Nuclei are relatively bland and predominantly round to oval with smooth nuclear contours and occasional nucleoli (H&E).

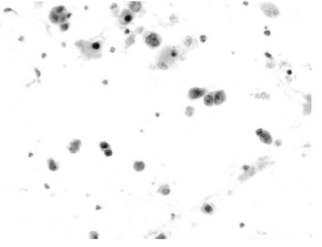

Figure 2.42. Salivary duct carcinoma. Scattered single cells are present in a background of necrotic material and inflammatory debris (Pap stain).

LYMPHOCYTE-RICH PATTERN

CHECKLIST: Etiologic Considerations for the Lymphocyte-Rich Pattern

- ☐ Sialadenitis
- ☐ Lymphoepithelial Cyst
- ☐ Warthin Tumor (WT)
- ☐ Mucoepidermoid Carcinoma (MEC)
- ☐ Acinic Cell Carcinoma (ACC)
- ☐ Intraparotid Lymph Node
- ☐ Lymphoma

The lymphocyte-rich pattern is characteristic of many processes in the salivary gland, including infectious and noninfectious inflammatory diseases, nonneoplastic cysts, and benign and malignant neoplasms. An interesting phenomenon called tumor associated lymphoid proliferation (TALP), which consists of a prominent population of reactive lymphocytes with or without germinal centers, can occur as a response to several salivary gland neoplasms. The presence of TALP is known to mimic the appearance of a lymph node and should not be confused with a metastasis. This point is particularly important given the fact that the parotid gland often contains multiple lymph nodes, which can be sites of metastasis or lymphoma. This section will provide a practical overview of the lymphocyte-rich pattern with a focus on practical diagnostic issues.

SIALADENITIS

Sialadenitis can present as acute, chronic, or lymphoepithelial types. According to the MSRSGC, each case should be diagnosed as "nonneoplastic," followed by a brief description of the findings and a note suggesting clinical, imaging, and/or microbiology correlation as appropriate.[8]

Acute sialadenitis can be suppurative (caused by bacterial infections in adults) or nonsuppurative (caused by viral infections in children). These lesions do not typically warrant FNA; however, unusual cases or those refractory to standard therapy may be aspirated to exclude a neoplasm. On FNA, numerous neutrophils may indicate a bacterial infection

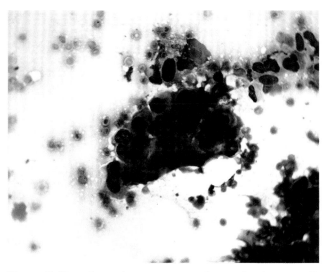

Figure 2.43. Salivary duct carcinoma. Cluster of malignant cells showing high-grade nuclear features and dense blue cytoplasm with occasional vacuoles (Diff-Quik stain).

while granulomatous inflammation may be indicative of a fungal or acid-fast bacilli infection (Figures 2.44-2.46). For a suppurative infection, there may be abundant necroinflammatory debris. It is important, however, not to interpret this finding as tumor diathesis or to overinterpret reactive atypia as a sign of malignancy.

Chronic sialadenitis most commonly affects the submandibular gland and is typically the result of salivary duct obstruction secondary to sialolithiasis. A chronic sclerosing form, which is likely an IgG4-related disease, can result in the formation of a mass, historically known as Küttner tumor.[33] FNAs should be hypocellular and composed of lymphocytes, plasma cells, and small, cohesive basaloid or metaplastic ductal cells with or without amylase crystalloids (Figure 2.47). Acinar cells should be scant, and fibrotic stromal elements may or may not be aspirated.

Lymphoepithelial sialadenitis (LESA) is an autoimmune process that afflicts patients with Sjogren syndrome and other connective tissue disorders and carries an increased risk for extranodal marginal zone lymphoma.[34] FNAs show lymphoepithelial complexes composed of sheets of ductal cells with infiltrating lymphocytes present in a cellular background of polymorphous lymphocytes and tingible body macrophages, which reflect the presence of germinal centers. Squamous metaplasia of the ductal epithelium is common and should lack cytologic atypia, precluding misinterpretation as SqCC arising in an intraparotid lymph node.

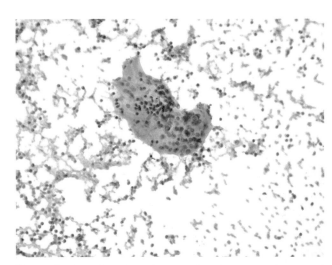

Figure 2.44. Multinucleated giant cell with a surrounding mixed inflammatory component (Pap stain).

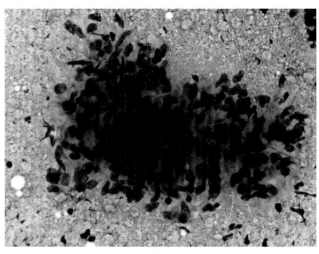

Figure 2.45. Granulomatous inflammation. Aggregate of epithelioid histiocytes with elongated nuclei, occasional nucleoli, and syncytial cytoplasm, characteristic of a granuloma (Diff-Quik stain).

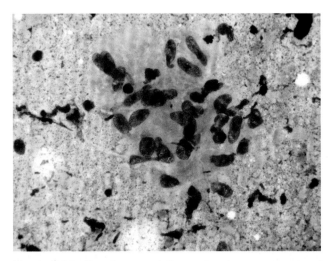

Figure 2.46. Granulomatous inflammation. Loose aggregate of epithelioid histiocytes forming a granuloma (Diff-Quik stain).

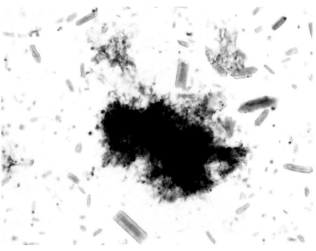

Figure 2.47. Chronic sialadenitis with amylase crystalloids, cystic debris, and lymphocytes (Pap stain).

LYMPHOEPITHELIAL CYSTS

Lymphoepithelial cysts, including human immunodeficiency virus (HIV)–associated cystic lesions, contain a thick wall composed of a dense lymphoid proliferation with germinal centers; the cysts are lined by a thin layer of epithelium, most often squamous and less often cuboidal or columnar epithelium with or without cilia. The aspirate often contains proteinaceous material with or without cholesterol crystals, vacuolated macrophages, degenerated epithelial cells, and squamous debris in a background of polymorphous lymphocytes and germinal center components (Figures 2.48 and 2.49). Most notably, lymphoepithelial cysts lack the sheets of ductal cells that are characteristic of LESA. See the "Lymphoepithelial Cyst" section in the "Cystic Pattern" for further discussion.

WARTHIN TUMOR

As previously discussed under the "Warthin Tumor" section in the "Cystic Pattern", Warthin tumors (WTs) are composed of an epithelioid and a lymphoid component (Figures 2.50-2.52). Lymphocytes may be intimately associated with the oncocytic cells and germinal center fragments containing tingible body macrophages. Most of the lymphocytes, however, should

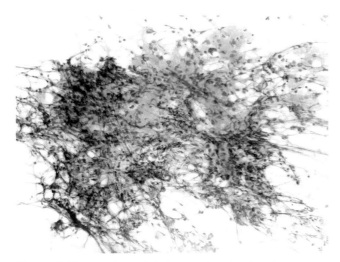

Figure 2.48. Lymphoepithelial cyst. Abundant lymphocytes are seen in this field with crush artifact, forming what is referred to as "lymphoid tangles" (Pap stain).

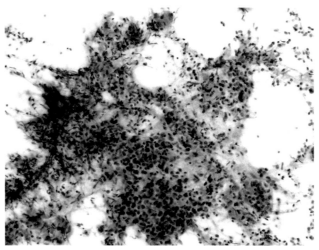

Figure 2.49. Lymphoepithelial cyst. Occasional columnar epithelial cells are present in an inflammatory background comprised of germinal centers, lymphocytes, histiocytes, and debris (Pap stain).

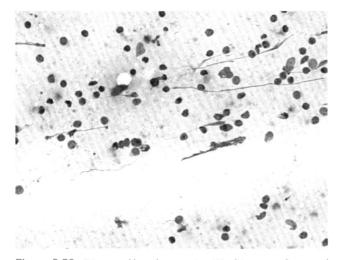

Figure 2.50. Dispersed lymphocytes in a Warthin tumor. Scattered lymphocytes with occasional crush artifact (Diff-Quik stain).

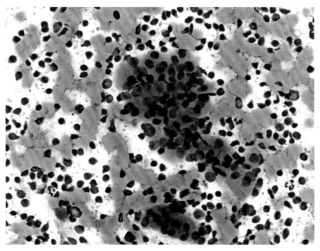

Figure 2.51. Warthin tumor. An aggregate of oncocytic epithelium is present in a background of lymphocytes and debris (Diff-Quik stain).

be small and mature in appearance. The presence of the oncocytic cell population should exclude other diagnoses such as LESA, lymphoepithelial cysts, and lymphoma, while the lymphocytic background and proteinaceous debris should favor against an oncocytoma.

MUCOEPIDERMOID CARCINOMA

Mucoepidermoid carcinoma (MEC) is the most common primary salivary gland malignancy and most often occurs in the parotid gland, followed by the minor salivary glands of the palate. MEC may be low-, intermediate-, or high-grade with increasingly atypical features and aggressive clinical outcomes. Approximately 20% of cases contain a significant amount of tumor associated lymphoid proliferation (TALP), consisting of a mixed lymphocytic response to neoplastic cells with or without germinal centers. In these cases, it is important to recognize the tripartite malignant population of epithelial cells, consisting of mucinous, intermediate (clear), and epidermoid (squamoid) cells (Figure 2.53). Furthermore, it is important not to mistake the lymphocytic population as evidence of involvement in an intraparotid lymph node. Low-grade tumors are typically cystic with abundant mucin (see discussion under the "Low-Grade Mucoepidermoid Carcinoma" in the "Cystic Pattern") while intermediate-grade tumors are more solid. High-grade tumors typically have scant mucin and may require special staining with mucicarmine if cell block material is available. Occasionally, oncocytic differentiation may be present and mimic a WT. In these cases, the presence of cells with intracytoplasmic mucin will support a diagnosis of MEC. Additionally, acinic cell carcinoma (ACC) can be associated with TALP; however, the malignant cells of ACC should have vacuolated, granular cytoplasm with many background naked nuclei and should lack the mucinous, intermediate, and epidermoid components.

ACINIC CELL CARCINOMA

Acinic cell carcinoma (ACC) is the second most common malignant primary salivary gland tumor and is considered to be a low-grade carcinoma (see the "Acinic Cell Carcinoma" under the "Cystic Pattern" for further discussion). In a subset of cases, there is a significant amount of TALP. As seen in MEC, TALP consists of a mixed lymphocytic population with or without the presence of germinal center fragments. In these cases, it is important to identify the neoplastic epithelial component, which is composed of large, dyshesive cells or loosely cohesive groups with varying amounts of delicate, vacuolated cytoplasm containing zymogen granules (Figures 2.54-2.57). The background may contain many nuclei stripped of their cytoplasm, which should be distinguished from lymphocytes. The nuclei are typically round and uniform, are eccentrically placed, and contain conspicuous nucleoli. Nuclear atypia, mitotic activity, and necrosis should be absent. It is important not to confuse the

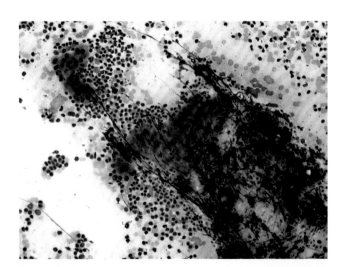

Figure 2.52. Warthin tumor. Oncocytic epithelium is present at the top left corner in a background of abundant lymphocytes and lymphoid tangles (Diff-Quik stain).

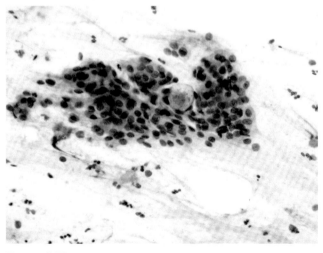

Figure 2.53. Low-grade mucoepidermoid carcinoma. A central mucocyte is seen with surrounding intermediate-type epithelium in a background of mucin and lymphocytes (Pap stain).

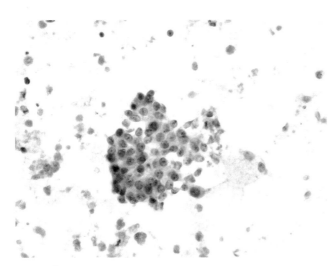

Figure 2.54. Acinic cell carcinoma. An aggregate of malignant acinar cells is seen in the center with surrounding debris and occasional lymphocytes (Pap stain).

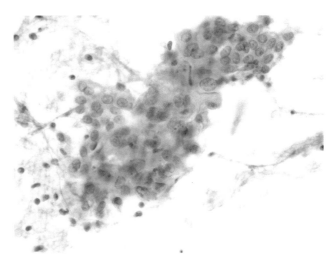

Figure 2.55. Acinic cell carcinoma. Malignant cells are seen in a lymphocytic background. Note the size of the lymphocytes compared with the malignant acinar cells (Pap stain).

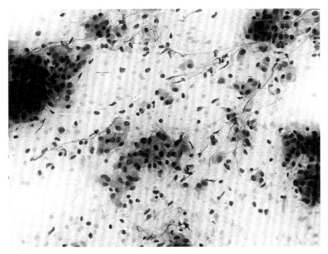

Figure 2.56. Acinic cell carcinoma. Malignant cells with "oncocytoid" cytoplasm are present in a background of intact lymphocytes and lymphoid tangles (Diff-Quik stain).

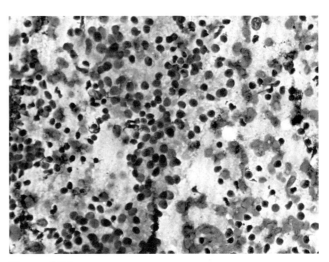

Figure 2.57. Acinic cell carcinoma. Loose clusters of malignant acinar cells are seen with numerous, admixed small lymphocytes (Diff-Quik stain).

presence of TALP for ACC involvement in an intraparotid lymph node. Furthermore, ACCs may have granular cytoplasm with an "oncocytoid" appearance, bringing WT into the differential diagnosis; however, the oncocytes of WT have denser cytoplasm and lack vacuoles and naked nuclei. The acinar cells in nonneoplastic entities, such as sialadenitis, may show grape-like clusters—a finding that should be absent in ACC.

INTRAPAROTID LYMPH NODE

The parotid gland often contains several intraparotid lymph nodes that are usually located in the preauricular area or the apex of the superficial lobe. On occasion, these lymph nodes may become enlarged and present as a parotid gland mass. Aspirates from these lymph nodes will reveal polymorphous lymphocytes and tingible body macrophages (Figures 2.58-2.60). It is important to search for an epithelial component to rule out a salivary gland malignancy with TALP or a metastatic carcinoma, oftentimes from a cutaneous SqCC. If there is a clinical suspicion for lymphoma, additional material for flow cytometry should be obtained if possible.

FAQ: Can radiologic imaging accurately identify an intraparotid lymph node?

Answer: The short answer is yes, but the long answer is more complicated. Briefly, intraparotid lymph nodes display the same imaging characteristics as lymph nodes of any location. On ultrasound, intraparotid lymph nodes are round to oval and contain a central echogenic hilum, as well as central hypervascularity on Doppler flow studies. Deep lesions, however, are not adequately assessed on ultrasound because the mandibular ramus obstructs the signal. On contrast-enhanced computed tomography (CT), intraparotid lymph nodes are well-circumscribed nodular structures with homogenous enhancement. Additional pertinent imaging features are generally not present. In contrast, the presence of calcifications may favor a pleomorphic adenoma, the presence of anechoic areas may favor a WT, and the presence of an irregularly shaped, heterogeneous mass may favor a malignant neoplasm. In a subset of cases, there may be overlap in the observed features, and the radiologist will rely on the cytopathologist to determine what is sampled.

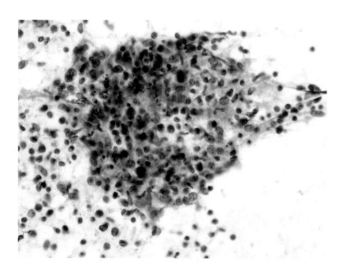

Figure 2.58. Intraparotid lymph node. This germinal center shows a heterogeneous population of lymphocytes and dendritic cells from an intraparotid lymph node (Pap stain).

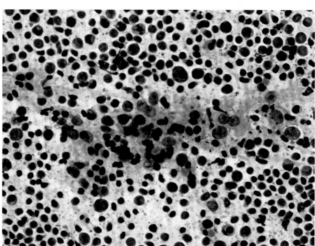

Figure 2.59. Intraparotid lymph node. Germinal center composed of a polymorphous population of lymphocytes, centrocytes, centroblasts, and tingible body macrophages (Diff-Quik stain).

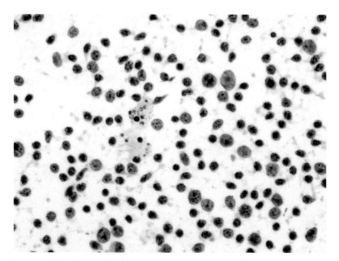

Figure 2.60. Intraparotid lymph node. Germinal center components, including tingible body macrophages (Pap stain).

LYMPHOMA

Primary salivary gland lymphoma is rare, representing only 2% of all salivary gland neoplasms. Patients often have a history of LESA (Sjogren syndrome), and as a result, extranodal marginal zone lymphomas of mucosa-associated lymphoid tissue (MALT) represent most primary lymphoma cases, followed by diffuse large B-cell lymphoma (DLBCL) in a minority. FNA is, therefore, useful for obtaining material for immunophenotyping by flow cytometry and/or mmunostains if lymphoma is suspected. MALT lymphoma is a low-grade B-cell lymphoma and is nearly indistinguishable from a reactive lymph node. FNA produces a cellular smear with an increase in small- to intermediate-sized lymphocytes with pale cytoplasm, condensed chromatin, and indistinct nucleoli (referred to as monocytoid B-cells) (Figure 2.61). Germinal center fragments, plasma cells, and immunoblasts may also be present, adding to the difficulty in distinguishing this entity from a reactive lymphocytic process. On the other hand, DLBCL is usually recognized as a malignant neoplasm on FNA. Aspirates contain sheets of large, atypical dispersed lymphocytes with round nuclei and often distinct nucleoli (Figure 2.62). The differential diagnosis based on cytomorphologic features alone is broad and includes other high-grade B-cell lymphomas, as well as nonhematologic malignancies such as melanoma and poorly differentiated carcinoma.

FAQ: When performing rapid on-site evaluation, when should flow cytometry be considered?

Answer: On FNA, it can be very difficult to distinguish several of the entities in the lymphocyte-rich pattern. As a result, there should be a low threshold for performing flow cytometry on a lymphocyte-rich specimen, especially in a patient with Sjogren syndrome. Flow cytometry is considerably more helpful than immunostains in this setting because it can demonstrate B-cell clonality, which is critical for distinguishing MALT lymphomas from reactive lymphoid processes. However, if the lymphocyte-rich specimen looks concerning for a large cell lymphoma like DLBCL, flow cytometry may or may not be helpful because DLBCL cells often do not survive the processing steps of flow cytometry and may be negative in up to 25% of large cell lymphomas.[35] In this setting, obtaining adequate cell block and/ or tissue core biopsy material is important so that the appropriate immunostains can be performed to: 1) distinguish a B-cell lymphoid malignancy (e.g. CD20 and PAX5 positive) from a carcinoma or melanoma and 2) to demonstrate an abnormal phenotype and further subclassify the DLBCL.

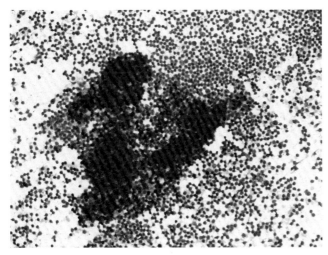

Figure 2.61. Extranodal marginal zone lymphoma of mucosa-associated lymphoid tissue (MALT). Sheets of intermediate sized, relatively monomorphic lymphocytes with a notable lack of interspersed tingible body macrophages (Pap stain).

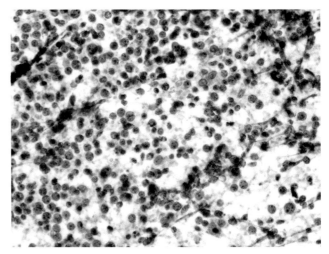

Figure 2.62. Diffuse large B-cell lymphoma. Sheets of large lymphocytes with clumped chromatin and prominent nucleoli are seen (Pap stain).

DISPERSED PATTERN

CHECKLIST: Etiologic Considerations for the Dispersed Pattern

☐ Myoepithelioma/Myoepithelial Carcinoma

☐ Acinic Cell Carcinoma (ACC)

☐ Poorly Differentiated Carcinoma

☐ Melanoma

The dispersed pattern is characterized by smears composed of predominantly scattered, dyshesive cells. The lymphocyte-rich pattern is typically also dyshesive; however, for the purposes of making these patterns more manageable, the dispersed pattern consists of dyshesive, nonlymphoid cells. The differential diagnosis for this pattern is long, as many nonneoplastic, benign neoplastic, and malignant neoplastic entities can show these features. As a result, a specific focus on the cell type and any background material will help to narrow the differential diagnosis.

MYOEPITHELIOMA/MYOEPITHELIAL CARCINOMA

Myoepithelioma is a rare, benign neoplasm most often present in the parotid but also commonly found in the minor salivary glands of the hard palate. FNA typically yields cellular smears composed of epithelioid, spindled, or plasmacytoid cells with a notable absence of chondromyxoid and mucoid stroma; however, some degree of myxoid or basement membrane material may be seen (Figures 2.63 and 2.64). Although the myoepithelial cells are often present in sheets and clusters, a dispersed pattern may be seen in a minority of cases, particularly when the plasmacytoid morphology predominates. Nuclei are bland with even chromatin and a lack of mitotic activity. Dispersed, plasmacytoid myoepitheliomas may mimic a plasmacytoma; however, plasma cells have the characteristic "clockface" chromatin and a perinuclear hof. Myoepitheliomas can be distinguished from pleomorphic adenomas (PAs) by the lack of ductal epithelial cells and fibrillary, chondromyxoid stroma.[36] Another entity that may arise in the differential diagnosis is basal cell adenoma (BCA), which typically consists of sheets and clusters; however, the basal cells may occasionally be dispersed. These cells can be distinguished from myoepithelial cells by their smaller size, less abundant cytoplasm, and darker nuclei.[36]

Myoepithelial carcinoma is a rare malignant salivary gland neoplasm that can involve major or minor salivary glands. FNA will result in a cellular smear with irregular clusters of neoplastic myoepithelial cells, often in a background of numerous dispersed myoepithelial

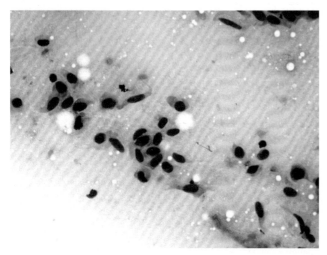

Figure 2.63. Myoepithelial neoplasm. Dispersed spindled myoepithelial cells with elongated nuclei and bipolar cytoplasmic processes (Diff-Quik stain).

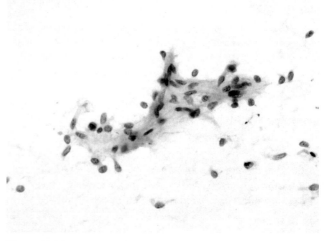

Figure 2.64. Myoepithelial neoplasm. Spindled myoepithelial cells embedded in a basement membrane–like material (Pap stain).

cells with variably epithelioid, plasmacytoid, and/or spindled morphology. Myxoid or hyaline stroma may be present. The nuclei are relatively bland for a malignant neoplasm: they are round with coarse chromatin, occasional intranuclear inclusions, and inconspicuous nucleoli. A subset of cases, however, may show a significant degree of nuclear atypia. Unlike myoepitheliomas, necrosis and mitotic activity may be present. However, in the absence of overt nuclear atypia, mitotic activity, and necrosis, myoepitheliomas and myoepithelial carcinomas are virtually cytomorphologically identical.[37,38] As a result, both myoepitheliomas and myoepithelial carcinomas lacking necrosis and mitosis on FNA should be classified as "salivary gland neoplasm of uncertain malignant potential (SUMP)."[8] Myoepithelial carcinomas and myoepithelial-rich PAs can be virtually indistinguishable if ductal cells are not present in the aspirated sample.[38] If cell block material is available, using c-kit (CD117) and EMA immunostains may help highlight a ductal component in a PA.

ACINIC CELL CARCINOMA

Acinic cell carcinoma (ACC) has been previously discussed in the "Cystic Pattern" and "Lymphocyte-Rich Pattern". Although the malignant epithelial cells in ACC are most often present in cohesive clusters and sheets, the delicate cytoplasm frequently becomes disrupted, resulting in single cell dispersion (Figures 2.65-2.67). These single cells are often stripped of cytoplasm and appear as "naked nuclei." They can be distinguished from lymphocytes by

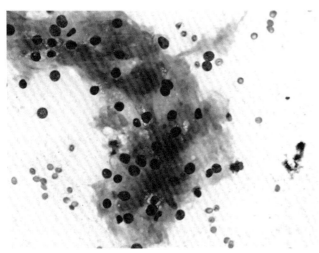

Figure 2.65. Acinic cell carcinoma. Loosely cohesive malignant cells are seen with dispersed and isolated round nuclei at the periphery (Diff-Quik stain).

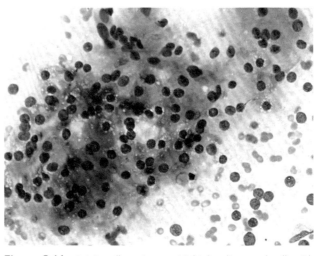

Figure 2.66. Acinic cell carcinoma. Multiple, dispersed cells with syncytial cytoplasm and naked, round nuclei are present in this field. (Diff-Quik stain).

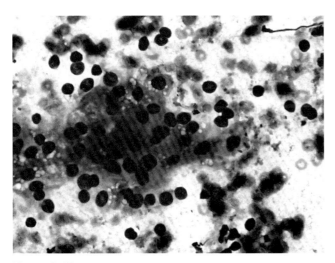

Figure 2.67. Acinic cell carcinoma. Cluster of malignant cells are present in the center with multiple surrounding dispersed naked nuclei (Diff-Quik stain).

comparison to the nuclei of intact malignant cells, which should appear identical. Because intact cells may have granular "oncocytoid" cytoplasm and the "naked nuclei" may mimic lymphocytes, a diagnosis of a WT may be entertained. Additionally, lymphoma and melanoma, which could also be on the differential, will lack the clustered epithelial components of ACC.

KEY FEATURES of Acinic Cell Carcinoma

- The specimen contains sheets of large, polygonal cells with vacuolated, basophilic granular cytoplasm
- The carcinoma cells have large, round, and eccentric nuclei with prominent nucleoli
- Numerous scattered, single malignant cells that have lost their delicate cytoplasm—referred to as naked nuclei—are often seen.
- The presence of TALP often results in a smear with a lymphocytic background.

POORLY DIFFERENTIATED CARCINOMA

Poorly differentiated carcinoma refers to primary small cell, large cell, or undifferentiated carcinomas of the salivary gland, primarily the parotid gland. The cytomorphologic features of these subtypes are identical to those seen in other primary locations (Figures 2.68-2.70). For example, FNA of small cell carcinoma typically produces a cellular smear in a background of necrotic debris. The malignant cells are large with an increased N/C ratio and have "salt-and-pepper" chromatin, frequent mitoses and apoptosis, and nuclear molding. In contrast, large cell carcinoma has more cytoplasm and prominent nucleoli. In addition to forming small clusters, poorly differentiated carcinomas may be highly cellular with many single, dispersed cells comprising the background. As a result, a high-grade lymphoma should be considered in certain cases, especially undifferentiated carcinomas which lack neuroendocrine nuclear features. In addition, the small cell variant of poorly differentiated carcinoma should be distinguished from Merkel cell carcinoma and small round blue cell tumors, including Ewing sarcoma, metastatic melanoma, and neuroblastoma.[39]

MELANOMA

Melanoma is the second most common metastatic tumor to the parotid gland after SqCC.[40-42] On FNA, smears may be variably cellular depending on the disease burden with variable morphology depending on the subtype. In most instances, melanoma is dyshesive with hyperchromatic, pleomorphic nuclei, irregular nuclear membranes, and prominent eosinophilic nucleoli (Figures 2.71-2.74). Because these cells may be small, large, epithelioid, signet ring–like, rhabdoid, plasmacytoid, or spindled, melanoma should be included in

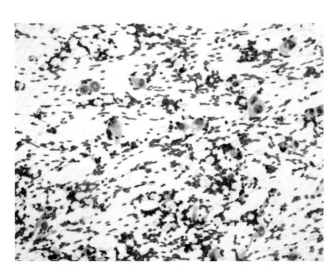

Figure 2.68. Poorly differentiated carcinoma. This field is comprised of scattered, dispersed single cells with variable amounts of cytoplasm, large nuclei, and prominent nucleoli (Pap stain).

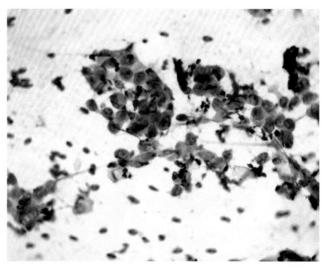

Figure 2.69. Poorly differentiated carcinoma. Loose aggregates and single cells with enlarged nuclei and prominent nucleoli are present (Pap stain).

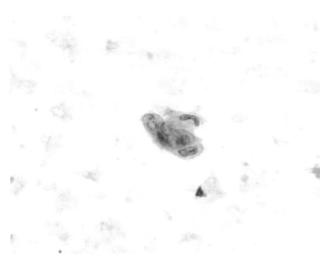

Figure 2.70. Poorly differentiated carcinoma. Scattered small aggregates of pleomorphic cells with enlarged nuclei and irregular nuclear membranes are seen (Pap stain).

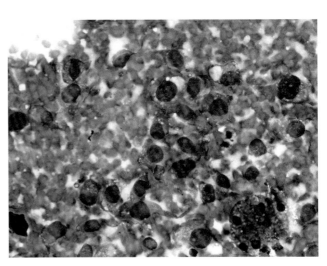

Figure 2.71. Melanoma. Dispersed cells with abundant vacuolated cytoplasm and enlarged nuclei with prominent nucleoli are suggestive of melanoma. Note the small acinar lobule at the bottom right portion of the image, suggesting parenchymal involvement of the parotid gland (Diff-Quik stain).

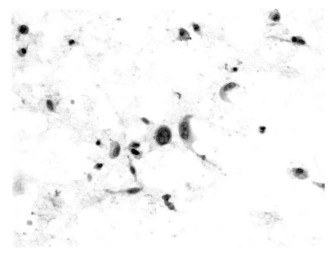

Figure 2.72. Melanoma. Dispersed pleomorphic cells with variable amounts of cytoplasm and large nuclei with prominent nucleoli are present in this case of metastatic melanoma (Pap stain).

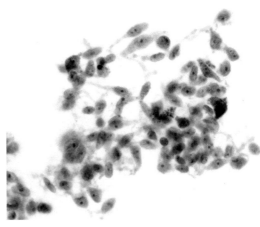

Figure 2.73. Melanoma. Malignant spindle and epithelioid cells are seen with cytoplasmic melanin pigment, elongated nuclei, and prominent nucleoli. The presence of brown to black pigment is present in clearly malignant cells (i.e., not histiocytes) is highly suggestive of melanoma (Pap stain).

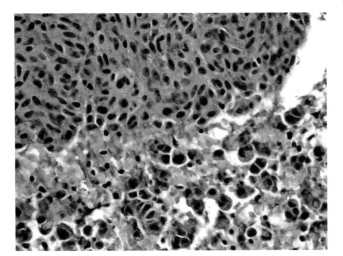

Figure 2.74. Melanoma. Cell block shows an aggregate, as well as dispersed cells, in a case of melanoma with pleomorphic features (H&E).

many differential diagnoses. Occasionally, cytoplasmic melanin pigment may be present, suggesting melanoma. In most cases, however, a panel of immunostains including multiple melanocytic markers such as S100 protein, SOX10, and HMB-45 are necessary for a definitive diagnosis, which should differentiate between other entities on the differential such as lymphoma and poorly differentiated carcinoma.

BASALOID PATTERN

CHECKLIST: Etiologic Considerations for the Basaloid Pattern

☐ Basal Cell Adenoma (BCA)/Basal Cell Adenocarcinoma (BAC)

☐ Myoepithelioma/Myoepithelial Carcinoma

☐ Myoepithelial-Rich Pleomorphic Adenoma

☐ Adenoid Cystic Carcinoma (AdCC), Solid Variant

☐ Polymorphous Adenocarcinoma

The basaloid pattern is characterized by the presence of epithelial/myoepithelial cells with scant cytoplasm and dark nuclei. The differential for this pattern is broad and contains a number of benign and malignant neoplasms. Diagnostically, these entities can be broken down into those with matrix material—such as AdCC, PA, or polymorphous adenocarcinoma—and those lacking this component—such as BCA/BAC, myoepithelioma/myoepithelial carcinoma, sialoblastoma, a metastasis from a basaloid SqCC, or direct extension from a cutaneous basal cell carcinoma. If sampling is limited, matrix material may not be present, especially in the solid variant of AdCC and in a myoepithelial-rich PA which may have very limited amounts of the characteristic fibrillary chondromyxoid matrix material. Furthermore, invasion is required to make the diagnosis of both BAC and myoepithelial carcinoma. As a result, many FNAs with a basaloid pattern will be classified as "SUMP" with a subcategory of "cellular basaloid neoplasm" according to the MSRSGC.[8] Thankfully, there are a few immunostains that may allow for a more definitive diagnosis.

BASAL CELL ADENOMA/ADENOCARCINOMA

Basal cell adenoma (BCA) and basal cell adenocarcinoma (BAC) are the prototypical primary salivary gland neoplasms that exemplify the basaloid pattern. BCAs are rare and comprise <5% of all salivary gland neoplasms, while BACs are even rarer. Both entities are more common in elderly patients, and the overwhelming majority arises from the major salivary glands, most notably the parotid gland.[43] These benign and malignant counterparts are slow growing and portend an excellent prognosis. Recurrence is rare with BCAs with the exception being the membranous type, which recurs locally in up to a quarter of cases.[44] Approximately 1/3 of BACs recur locally, but reports of regional and distant metastases are extremely rare, resulting in a low disease specific mortality rate.[45] On FNA, the cytomorphologic features of BCA and BAC are essentially indistinguishable. Smears are typically cellular and comprised of clusters and single cells with uniform, dark, round to oval nuclei and scant cytoplasm (Figures 2.75-2.77). Small clusters may show peripheral palisading, and a second cell population of larger cells with pale nuclei may be present in the center of the clusters. Additionally, tubular, trabecular, solid, and membranous patterns may be intermixed. With the exception of the membranous type—which contains hyaline matrix that may be strand-like or droplet-like within nests—stromal/matrix material should be absent. In all cases, however, the fibrillary, chondromyxoid matrix characteristic of PAs should be absent. Cytologic atypia is generally absent in both BCAs and BACs; however, BACs may show increased mitoses or tumor necrosis (Figures 2.78 and 2.79).[43] These features, if present, may warrant classification as "suspicious for malignancy" according to the MSRSGC.[8] Otherwise, many of these neoplasms will be classified as "SUMP" with the subcategory of "cellular basaloid neoplasm" according to the MSRSGC.[8] Immunostains may help further narrow the differential diagnosis in some cases. For example, the

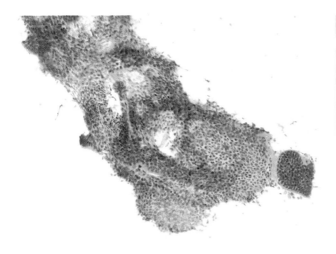

Figure 2.75. Basal cell adenoma. Sheet of monomorphic basaloid cells with scant cytoplasm (Pap stain).

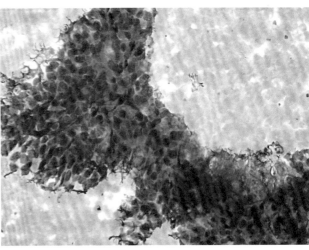

Figure 2.76. Basal cell adenoma. Cohesive cluster of basaloid cells containing scant cytoplasm and hyperchromatic, oval nuclei (Diff-Quik stain).

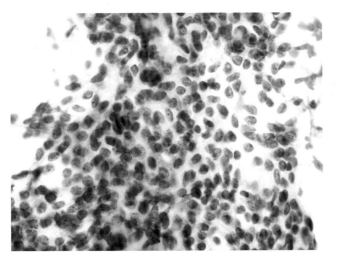

Figure 2.77. Basal cell adenoma. A high magnification view of a cluster of haphazardly arranged basaloid cells with scant cytoplasm and round to oval nuclei with coarse chromatin (Pap stain).

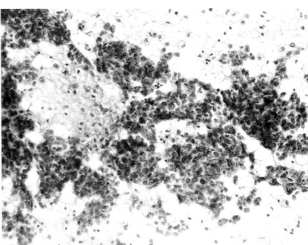

Figure 2.78. Basal cell adenocarcinoma. A low magnification view showing irregular clusters of basaloid cells in a background of necrosis (Pap stain).

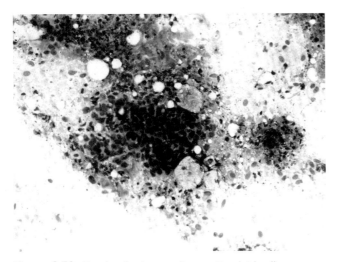

Figure 2.79. Basal cell adenocarcinoma. Basaloid cells are present and admixed with a hyaline basement membrane material and necrosis (Diff-Quik stain).

majority of PAs are positive for PLAG1 or HMGA2 while the majority of AdCCs are positive for MYB and CD117 (c-kit).[46] In contrast, nuclear β-catenin expression, corresponding to *CTNNB1* mutations, is fairly sensitive and highly specific for BCA/BAC.[47]

MYOEPITHELIOMA/MYOEPITHELIAL CARCINOMA

Myoepitheliomas and myoepithelial carcinomas are benign and malignant counterparts of one another with otherwise relatively indistinguishable benign-appearing cytomorphologic features, previously discussed under the "Dispersed Pattern". FNA typically produces cellular smears comprised of small groups and single cells with variable cytomorphologic features, including spindled, epithelioid, plasmacytoid, and clear cell populations; myxoid matrix material is scant, if present.[48] Nuclei are typically round to oval and bland in both the benign and carcinomatous counterparts. When the cytoplasm is scant, it can take the appearance of a basaloid pattern (Figure 2.80). Immunostains are is not always helpful with the differential diagnosis because any biphasic tumor with a myoepithelial component can have a similar staining pattern. Furthermore, expression of markers such as p63/p40, smooth muscle actin, S100 protein, and cytokeratins in cells with myoepithelial differentiation shows variability in the staining pattern, even within the same tumor. As a result, this diagnosis and differential is extremely challenging on FNA. Fortunately, recognizing that the tumor is neoplastic based on the cellularity should trigger the appropriate clinical management in most instances.

MYOEPITHELIAL-RICH PLEOMORPHIC ADENOMA

Pleomorphic adenoma (PA) is the most common primary salivary gland neoplasm, occurs in both children and adults, and originates from both major and minor salivary glands. PAs are the prototypical biphenotypic neoplasms comprised of varying proportions of ductal epithelial cells, myoepithelial cells, and a characteristic fibrillary chondromyxoid matrix material—an essential feature for diagnosis on FNA (Figures 2.81-2.84). A subset of PAs are myoepithelial-rich and tend to be very cellular (also referred to as "cellular PA") with a scant stromal component. Just like myoepithelioma/myoepithelial carcinoma, the myoepithelial cells in a myoepithelial-rich PA can have spindled, epithelioid, plasmacytoid, or clear cell appearances. When the population is predominantly comprised of epithelioid cells with scant cytoplasm, the tumor has a basaloid appearance (Figures 2.85-2.87). In these cases, distinguishing this tumor from others with a basaloid pattern, such as BCA/BAC, myoepithelioma/myoepithelial carcinoma, solid ACC, and polymorphous adenocarcinoma can be nearly impossible on cytomorphologic features alone. Fortunately, the majority of PAs are positive for PLAG1 or HMGA2 immunostains while most AdCCs are positive for MYB and c-kit (CD117), and BCA/BACs are positive for nuclear β-catenin.[47] Finally, polymorphous

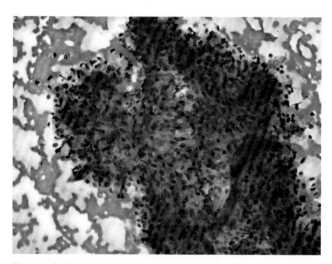

Figure 2.80. Myoepithelioma. Cluster of oval to spindled cells embedded in a scant stromal substance, with a basaloid appearance (Diff-Quik stain).

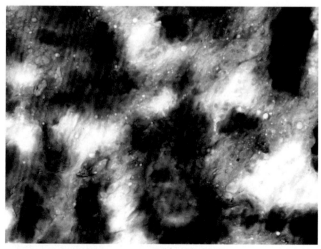

Figure 2.81. Pleomorphic adenoma. In contrast to the myoepithelial-rich variant, the classic appearance of pleomorphic adenoma has an abundance of the characteristic fibrillary chondromyxoid matrix material (Diff-Quik stain).

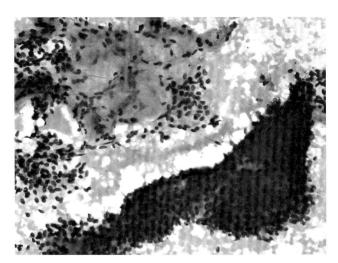

Figure 2.82. Pleomorphic adenoma. Note the basaloid population of myoepithelial cells adjacent to the magenta chondroid material, which also contains embedded myoepithelial cells (Diff-Quik stain).

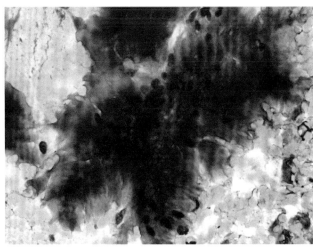

Figure 2.83. Pleomorphic adenoma. Basaloid cells are embedded in the fibrillary chondromyxoid matrix material (Diff-Quik stain).

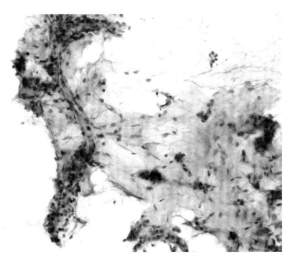

Figure 2.84. Pleomorphic adenoma. Single cells and clusters of basaloid cells are present in a background of chondroid matrix (Pap stain).

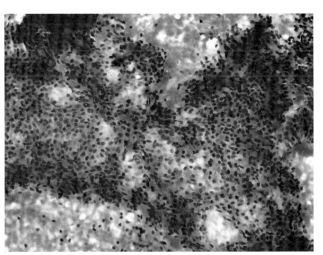

Figure 2.85. Myoepithelial-rich pleomorphic adenoma. This field shows a predominance of epithelioid and spindled myoepithelial cells with a conspicuous lack of fibrillary chondromyxoid matrix material (Diff-Quik stain).

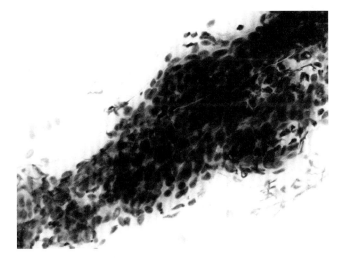

Figure 2.86. Myoepithelial-rich pleomorphic adenoma. This specimen was composed of predominantly spindle-shaped myoepithelial cells with scant cytoplasm, giving the cells a basaloid appearance (Diff-Quik stain).

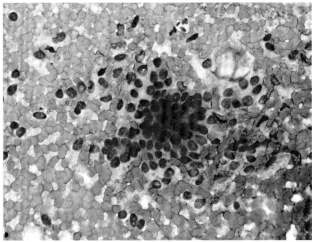

Figure 2.87. Myoepithelial-rich pleomorphic adenoma. Cluster and single round to oval myoepithelial cells with scant cytoplasm (Diff-Quik stain).

adenocarcinomas have a characteristic p63-positive, p40-negative phenotype, which is highly specific for the diagnosis in this setting.[49] When immunostains cannot be used, most myoepithelial-rich PAs may be categorized in the "benign" category when some amount of characteristic matrix material is present or as "SUMP" and subcategorized as "cellular basaloid neoplasm" when the matrix is not appreciated.[8]

KEY FEATURES of Pleomorphic Adenoma

- A variable amount of characteristic fibrillary metachromatic chondromyxoid matrix material is usually seen.
- Bland, cuboidal ductal epithelial cells form cohesive groups.
- Single cells and clusters of bland myoepithelial cells can demonstrate spindled, epithelioid, plasmacytoid, and/or clear cells features.

ADENOID CYSTIC CARCINOMA, SOLID VARIANT

Adenoid cystic carcinoma (AdCC) is a malignant primary major and minor salivary gland neoplasm with a variable recurrence rate and a propensity for distant metastases in over half of cases.[50] Like many salivary gland neoplasms, AdCC can have various architectural features and variations in the cellular components, being comprised of both epithelial ductal cells and abluminal cells with myoepithelial differentiation. In fact, the predominant architecture may be tubular, cribriform, or cellular and comprised of nodules of myoepithelial cells with only occasional ductal epithelium forming the "punched-out" spaces that are filled with a myxoid ground substance. Like other basaloid neoplasms, these cells typically have scant cytoplasm, dark nuclei, and a lack of overt malignant cytologic features (Figures 2.88-2.91). As a result, it may be extremely difficult to further classify these solid AdCCs as something other than "SUMP" and subcategorized as "cellular basaloid neoplasm" according to the MSRSGC.[8] Fortunately, the combination of strong and diffuse expression of MYB and c-kit (CD117) immunostains has been shown to be highly sensitive for the diagnosis of AdCC.[46] Furthermore, half of cases show a characteristic t(6;9) translocation involving the *MYB* proto-oncogene with the *NFIB* transcription factor gene (Table 2.2).[51-53] If used, these ancillary studies may provide support for a "malignant" diagnosis and appropriately trigger a broader preoperative workup.

KEY FEATURES of Adenoid Cystic Carcinoma

- Metachromatic matrix material forms spheres and/or tubules.
- Bland basaloid neoplastic cells have faint pale cytoplasm and dark, angulated nuclei line the matrix material.
- The solid variant contains less matrix material and more basaloid cells in clusters and groups.

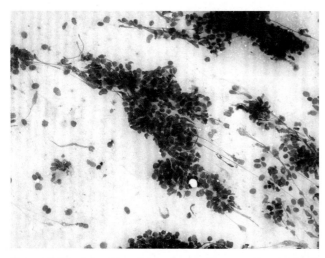

Figure 2.88. Adenoid cystic carcinoma. Clusters of basaloid cells with no appreciable matrix component (Diff-Quik stain).

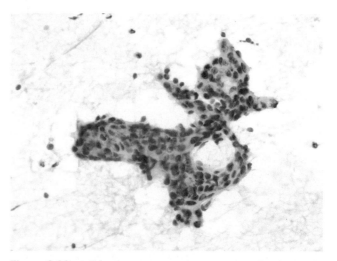

Figure 2.89. Adenoid cystic carcinoma. Fragment of basaloid cells with elongated and angulated nuclei and virtually no matrix material (Pap stain).

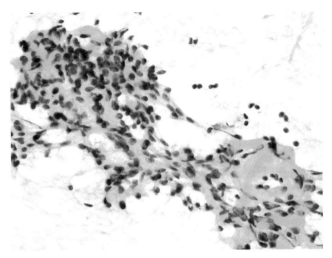

Figure 2.90. Adenoid cystic carcinoma. Elongated basaloid cells are present with the characteristic light green, dense mucopolysaccharide material of adenoid cystic carcinoma (Pap stain).

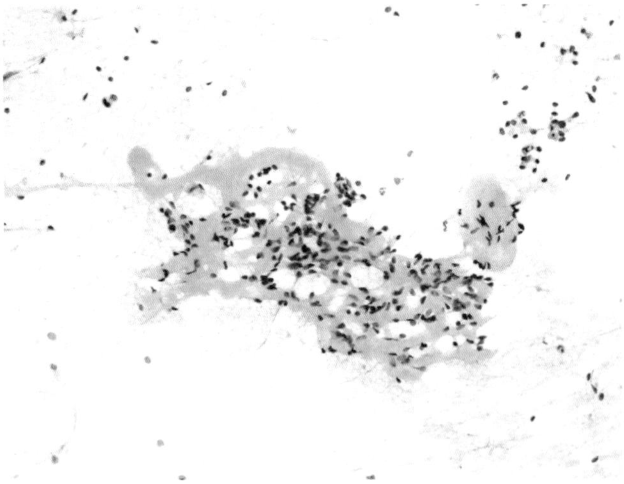

Figure 2.91. Adenoid cystic carcinoma. Basaloid cells are present and intimately associated with an abundant amount of the characteristic acellular mucopolysaccharide material (Pap stain).

POLYMORPHOUS ADENOCARCINOMA

Polymorphous adenocarcinoma, previously known as polymorphous low-grade adenocarcinoma (PLGA), is the second most common malignant salivary gland neoplasm of the oral cavity, most commonly occurring in the hard palate, followed by the soft palate.[54,55] Polymorphous adenocarcinoma occurs in the major salivary glands in <10% of cases; as a result, it is an entity that is rarely encountered on FNA.[55,56] When encountered, the cytomorphologic characteristics are fairly nonspecific. Smears are cellular and contain sheets, three-dimensional clusters, or papillary fragments comprised of uniform epithelial cells with scant cytoplasm and bland, slightly hyperchromatic, oval nuclei with rare, if any, mitotic figures. Despite the uniform cytomorphology, the histologic architecture may be diverse—hence the term "polymorphous." On FNA, the bland cytologic features will make an outright malignant diagnosis impossible on cytomorphology alone. Therefore, many of these entities will be classified as "SUMP" and may be subclassified as "cellular basaloid neoplasm."[8] The differential diagnosis will include the other basaloid neoplasms; however, the epithelium in polymorphous adenocarcinoma is not myoepithelial in differentiation. Thus, these tumors are characteristically positive for p63 while negative for p40—a specific myoepithelial marker.[49] This immunophenotype in this setting is fairly sensitive and specific for polymorphous adenocarcinoma. Additionally, polymorphous adenocarcinoma is recognized as "carcinoma" due to its infiltrative growth pattern with a predilection for perineural invasion, as well as invasion into bone. Despite invasion, the prognosis is generally good with surgical resection. Only about 20% of cases recur locally and distant metastases are extremely rare.[55] Surgical resection is important to prevent destructive invasion and high-grade transformation.[54-56]

FAQ: Why is it necessary to distinguish between a benign and malignant neoplasm when both diagnoses typically warrant surgical excision?

Answer: Most surgeons will choose to perform a total parotidectomy (versus a superficial parotidectomy) for malignant neoplasms, regardless of the location of the lesion, to ensure complete resection and negative margins. Furthermore, for malignant neoplasms, particularly high-grade lesions with a propensity to involve regional lymph nodes, an elective neck dissection may be performed at the time of parotidectomy, precluding the need for an additional surgical procedure.

ONCOCYTIC PATTERN

CHECKLIST: Etiologic Considerations for the Oncocytic Pattern

☐ Nodular Oncocytic Hyperplasia
☐ Oncocytoma/Oncocytic Carcinoma
☐ Warthin Tumor (WT)
☐ Mucoepidermoid Carcinoma (MEC)
☐ Acinic Cell Carcinoma (ACC)
☐ Salivary Duct Carcinoma (SDC)

The oncocytic pattern is characterized by a wide range of, benign and malignant neoplastic entities. "Oncocytic" refers to a cellular morphologic pattern characterized by epithelial cells with abundant, dense, granular cytoplasm and large, round nuclei with prominent nucleoli. The characteristic cytoplasm is the result of numerous metabolically active mitochondria, which may be incidentally detected on staging radiologic imaging. Lesions in this pattern may be comprised of purely oncocytic epithelium (oncocytoma and oncocytic carcinoma), a mixed population of oncocytic epithelium and a lymphoid population (WT), oncocytic/oncocytoid metaplasia involving benign glands (nodular oncocytic hyperplasia), or a neoplastic process (MEC, ACC, and SDC). In fact, oncocytoid metaplasia can be seen in nearly every entity involving a major salivary gland. As a result, this pattern is particularly challenging on FNA when tumor heterogeneity may greatly affect evaluation.

NODULAR ONCOCYTIC HYPERPLASIA

Nodular oncocytic hyperplasia (NOH) is a rare, nonneoplastic, multifocal, nodular proliferation of oncocytic epithelial cells. NOH is more common in women, occurs exclusively in the parotid gland, and is often bilateral. Histologically, NOH can be distinguished from an oncocytoma by the lack of a capsule and by the presence of entrapped normal salivary gland tissue within the oncocytic nodules. On FNA, however, this distinction is not possible, as both lesions are comprised of sheets and clusters of polygonal cells with abundant, densely granular cytoplasm and large, round nuclei with prominent nucleoli, and no cytologic atypia (Figure 2.92).[57] In fact, it can even be extremely difficult to distinguish NOH or oncocytoma from an oncocytic carcinoma by cytomorphologic features alone; however, the cells of an oncocytic carcinoma show more pleomorphism, mitoses, and occasionally necrosis.

PEARLS & PITFALLS

Owing to the morphologic overlap between nodular oncocytic hyperplasia, oncocytoma, and oncocytic carcinoma, these specimens will most often require a descriptive diagnosis with a differential listing these entities. As a result, these purely oncocytic lesions are best classified as "SUMP" according to the MSRSGC, despite the fact that a nonneoplastic entity is in the differential diagnosis.[8] If, however, the sample shows a mixed population of unremarkable salivary gland tissue and is only focally oncocytic, categorization as "AUS" is most often applied.[8]

ONCOCYTOMA/ONCOCYTIC CARCINOMA

Oncocytomas and oncocytic carcinomas are the prototypical lesions of the "oncocytic pattern." Oncocytomas and oncocytic carcinomas are rare and occur predominantly in the parotid gland. Both neoplasms are composed of a pure population of oncocytic

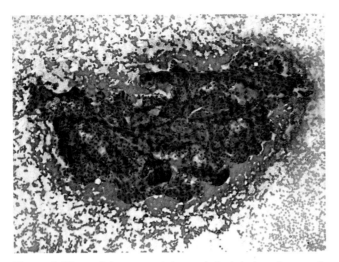

Figure 2.92. Nodular oncocytic hyperplasia. Lobules of oncocytic epithelium (Diff-Quik stain).

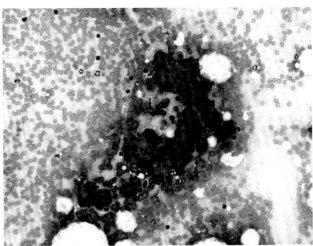

Figure 2.93. Oncocytoma. Clusters of oncocytic epithelium with abundant granular cytoplasm and round, regular nuclei (Diff-Quik stain).

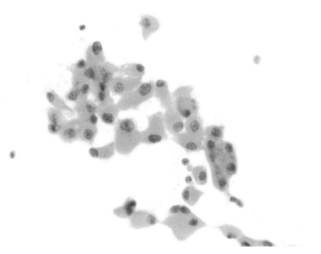

Figure 2.94. Oncocytoma. Oncocytic epithelium with the characteristic abundant cytoplasm, round nuclei, and prominent nucleoli (Pap stain).

epithelial cells with abundant, densely granular cytoplasm, enlarged round nuclei, and prominent nucleoli (Figures 2.93 and 2.94). Oncocytic carcinoma is the malignant counterpart of oncocytoma and can be most easily distinguished by the presence of invasion on resection and by its moderate nuclear pleomorphism, increased mitotic activity, and occasional necrotic debris on FNA. However, these features can be subtle, and as a result, most of these neoplasms will be classified as "SUMP" and subcategorized as "cellular oncocytic/oncocytoid neoplasm" according to the MSRSGC.[8] The differential diagnosis is broad and includes all of the entities that make up the "oncocytic pattern." The key feature for both oncocytomas and oncocytic carcinomas is the lack of additional neoplastic components, such as the lymphoid stroma and cystic contents of a WT, the mucocytes of a MEC, or the cytoplasmic vacuoles and basophilic zymogen granules of an ACC.

SAMPLE NOTE: PURELY ONCOCYTIC LESION

Salivary gland neoplasm of uncertain malignant potential:
Proliferation of purely oncocytic-type epithelium. Overt atypia, lymphocytes, and otherwise diagnostic features are notably absent. See note.

Note: The differential diagnosis for a purely oncocytic/oncocytoid lesion includes nodular oncocytic hyperplasia, oncocytoma, oncocytic carcinoma, acinic cell carcinoma, and oncocytic mucoepidermoid carcinoma. Owing to the morphologic overlap between these entities and a lack of overt cytomorphologic atypia, mucocytes, and cytoplasmic vacuoles, a definitive diagnosis cannot be made on FNA samples alone. Clinical and radiographic correlation is recommended.

Reference:
Faquin WC, Rossi ED. *The Milan System for Reporting Salivary Gland Cytopathology.* New York, NY: Springer Science+Business Media; 2018:75-77.

WARTHIN TUMOR

Warthin tumors (WTs) typically occur in the parotid gland of older patients and are often associated a history of smoking (see additional discussion under the "Cystic Pattern" and the "Lymphocyte-rich Pattern"). WTs are benign, neoplastic, cystic lesions composed of oncocytic epithelium, lymphocytes, and proteinaceous background material (Figures 2.95-2.99). The oncocytes contain abundant granular cytoplasm, well-defined cell borders, and round nuclei with prominent nucleoli, not unlike the oncocytes of oncocytomas/oncocytic carcinoma. However, when all three components are present, a definitive diagnosis of WT can be made with categorization as "neoplasm: benign" according to the MSRSGC.[8]

MUCOEPIDERMOID CARCINOMA

Mucoepidermoid carcinoma (MEC) is composed of mucinous, intermediate, and squamoid cells and can be cystic or solid (see additional discussion under the "Cystic Pattern" and "Lymphocyte-rich Pattern"). Furthermore, there are three main variants: oncocytic, clear cell, and sclerosing variants. The oncocytic variant is characterized by a nodular proliferation of predominantly large, polygonal oncocytic epithelial cells with abundant eosinophilic, granular cytoplasm, and small nuclei with prominent nucleoli; mucocytes are scattered throughout, although squamoid cells are rare (Figure 2.100).[58] For cases that are cystic and have tumor associated lymphoid proliferation (TALP),

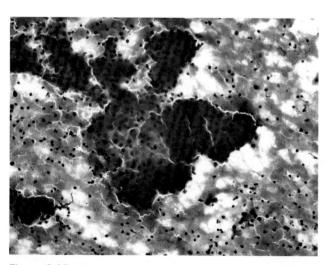

Figure 2.95. Warthin tumor. Fragments of oncocytic epithelium in a background of scattered small lymphocytes (Diff-Quik stain).

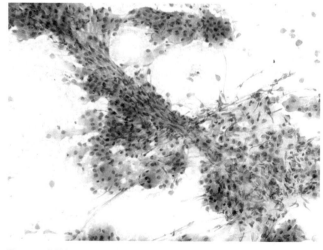

Figure 2.96. Warthin tumor. Oncocytic epithelium and adjacent lymphoid tangles (Pap stain).

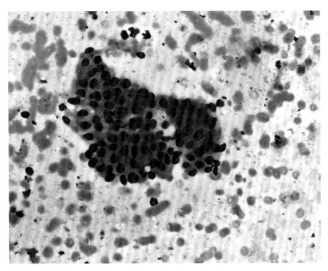

Figure 2.97. Warthin tumor. Oncocytic epithelial component of a Warthin tumor (Diff-Quik stain).

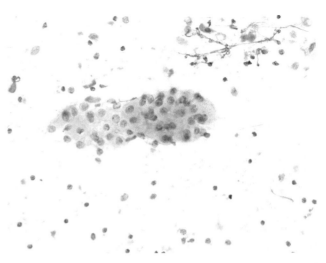

Figure 2.98. Warthin tumor. Oncocytic epithelium with scattered small lymphocytes and lymphoid tangles in the background (Pap stain).

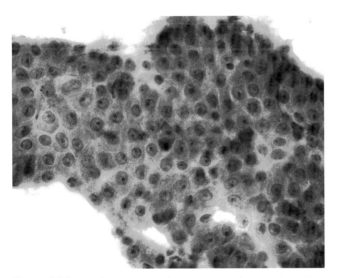

Figure 2.99. Warthin tumor. High-power view of oncocytic epithelium with abundant granular cytoplasm, round nuclei, and prominent nucleoli (Pap stain).

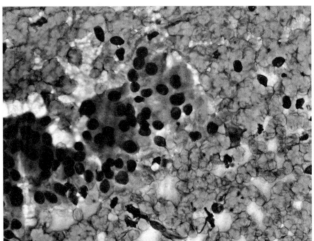

Figure 2.100. Mucoepidermoid carcinoma. Oncocytic epithelium in a lesion that proved to be a mucoepidermoid carcinoma, oncocytic type, on follow-up (Diff-Quik stain).

oncocytic MECs may appear similar to WTs. Fortunately, the presence of mucocytes will point to the correct diagnosis. In some cases, confirmatory staining with mucicarmine and periodic acid-Schiff (PAS) with diastase is warranted.

ACINIC CELL CARCINOMA

Acinic cell carcinoma (ACC) is usually a low-grade malignant neoplasm which most often occurs in the parotid gland (see additional discussion under the "Cystic Pattern", the "Lymphocyte-Rich Pattern", and the "Dispersed Pattern"). ACCs are characterized by at least focal serous acinar differentiation. The epithelial cells are large and polygonal with abundant granular, vacuolated cytoplasm and bland, eccentric nuclei with prominent nucleoli (Figures 2.101-2.103). The cytoplasm often appears eosinophilic and can look "oncocytoid." Fortunately, ACC is the only primary salivary gland neoplasm in the oncocytic pattern that contains cytoplasmic vacuoles, which are most easily appreciated on the Diff-Quik stain.

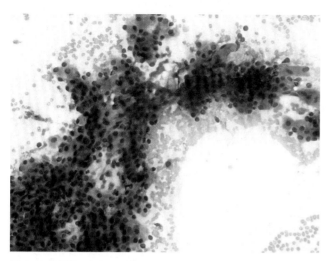

Figure 2.101. Acinic cell carcinoma. Malignant acinar cells with abundant granular cytoplasm, resulting in an oncocytoid appearance (Diff-Quik stain).

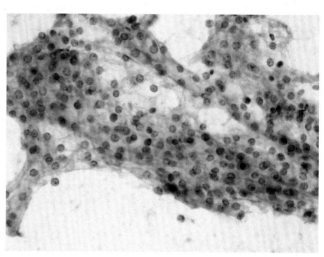

Figure 2.102. Acinic cell carcinoma. Malignant acinar cells with round, regular nuclei, punctate nucleoli, and granular cytoplasm, creating an appearance that is somewhat oncocytoid (Pap stain).

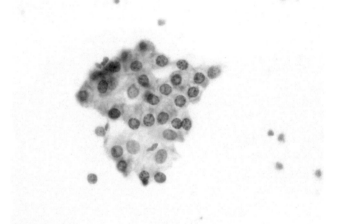

Figure 2.103. Acinic cell carcinoma. High-power view of malignant acinar cells showing oncocytoid features (Pap stain).

SALIVARY DUCT CARCINOMA

Salivary duct carcinoma (SDC) is one of the most aggressive malignant salivary gland neoplasms and most frequently arises in the parotid gland (see additional discussion under the Cystic Pattern). Interestingly, SDC somewhat resembles high-grade ductal carcinoma of the breast: ER and PR are negative, AR is positive in 70% of cases, and a high HER2 expression is seen in >25% of cases.[59-61] FNAs are cellular with sheets and clusters of epithelial cells in a background of necrotic debris. The epithelial cells contain abundant oncocytic cytoplasm, large pleomorphic nuclei, prominent nucleoli, and frequent mitoses (Figures 2.104 and 2.105). The presence of highly atypical nuclei, frequent mitoses, and necrosis, in addition to immunostains, are the most helpful clues for making an accurate diagnosis.

CLEAR CELL PATTERN

CHECKLIST: Etiologic Considerations for the Clear Cell Pattern

☐ Myoepithelioma/Myoepithelial Carcinoma

☐ Epithelial-Myoepithelial Carcinoma (EMC)

☐ Mucoepidermoid Carcinoma (MEC)

The clear cell pattern is characterized by cells containing abundant, clear cytoplasm. Although this is a relatively simple feature to recognize, making a specific diagnosis based on the presence of clear cells alone is often not justified. Recognizing clear cells on FNA is the first step to formulating a differential diagnosis that triggers a search for additional cytomorphologic features characteristic of a specific entity. Although clear cell carcinoma is arguably the purest example of this pattern, it predominantly arises from intraoral minor salivary glands, is rarely sampled on FNA, and is a diagnosis of exclusion due to its lack of additional cytomorphologic features. Interestingly, many of the lesions that populate this pattern are actually myoepithelial in origin, owing to the fact that myoepithelial cells can have a number of cytomorphologic characteristics, including abundant, clear cytoplasm.

MYOEPITHELIOMA/MYOEPITHELIAL CARCINOMA

Both myoepitheliomas and myoepithelial carcinomas are composed entirely of myoepithelial cells, which can have various cytomorphologic characteristics, including abundant clear cytoplasm (Figure 2.106). The major diagnostic distinction between these two entities is the presence of invasion that is determined at the time of resection; in most cases, the cytomorphology is indistinguishable. Interestingly, clear cell myoepithelial carcinoma may be a distinct subtype of myoepithelial carcinoma that is frequently associated with necrosis, poor outcomes, and an *EWSR1* gene rearrangement—the same *EWSR1-ATF1* translocation characteristic of clear cell carcinoma of the salivary gland and at other locations.[62] As a result, most clear cell

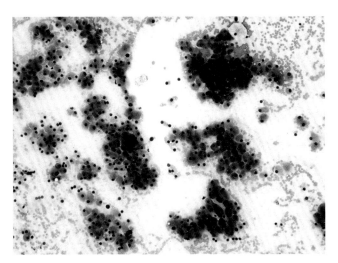

Figure 2.104. Salivary duct carcinoma. Cellular smear comprised of loosely cohesive fragments of oncocytic epithelium (Diff-Quik stain).

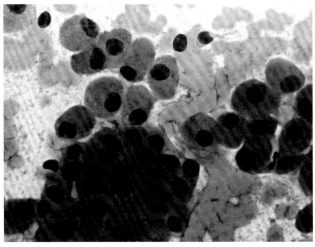

Figure 2.105. Salivary duct carcinoma. High-power view of clustered and dispersed epithelial cells with oncocytic features (Diff-Quik stain).

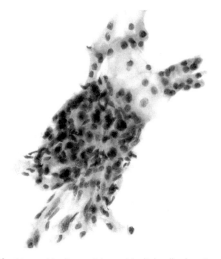

Figure 2.106. Myoepithelioma. Myoepithelial cells showing varying morphologies, including spindled and clear cell features (Pap stain).

myoepitheliomas/myoepithelial carcinomas will be categorized as "SUMP" and further subcategorized as "cellular neoplasm with clear cell features." For further information, please see the "Myoepithelioma/Myoepithelial Carcinoma" section under the "Dispersed Pattern" and the "Basaloid Pattern".

EPITHELIAL-MYOEPITHELIAL CARCINOMA

Epithelial-myoepithelial carcinoma (EMC) is an uncommon low-grade malignant salivary gland neoplasm most commonly arising in the parotid and submandibular glands.[63,64] As the name implies, EMC is biphasic neoplasm composed of gland-forming ductal epithelium with an abluminal myoepithelial population. On FNA, EMC usually produces hypercellular smears composed of scattered, large three-dimensional groups and sheets containing polygonal myoepithelial cells and cuboidal ductal cells (Figure 2.107). Most of the myoepithelial cells have abundant, clear cytoplasm and oval nuclei with open chromatin and prominent nucleoli while the cuboidal ductal epithelial cells have finely granular cytoplasm, high N/C ratios, oval nuclei, and prominent nucleoli. Overall, the nuclear atypia is mild, and mitoses and necrosis are rarely encountered on FNA.

PEARLS & PITFALLS

Not all lesions with myoepithelial cells and matrix material are pleomorphic adenomas (PA). The background material from smearing epithelial-myoepithelial carcinomas (EMC) often largely consists of single myoepithelial cells that have been stripped of their cytoplasm ("naked nuclei") and secreted, concentrically laminated hyaline material. In fact, this secreted material may mimic the myxoid ground substance characteristic of adenoid cystic carcinoma. Furthermore, depending on the paucity of the glandular epithelial component, the clear cell myoepithelial population may dominate and lead to diagnostic consideration for a myoepithelioma/myoepithelial carcinoma. Finally, it is important to realize that the presence of both a myoepithelial and an epithelial population does not automatically lead to a diagnosis of PA. When the myoepithelial population is predominantly of a clear cell type, EMC should be considered in the differential on FNA.

MUCOEPIDERMOID CARCINOMA

Mucoepidermoid carcinoma (MEC) is composed of mucinous, intermediate, and squamous/epidermoid cells. The intermediate population can, in some cases, undergo clear cell change and result in a prominent population of cells with abundantly clear, glycogenated cytoplasm (Figures 2.108 and 2.109). In fact, clear cell is one of three major

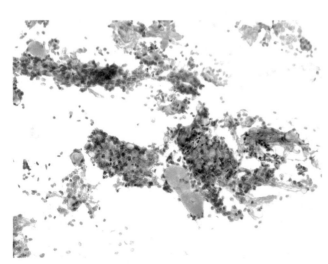

Figure 2.107. Epithelial-myoepithelial carcinoma. Cellular smear comprised of ductal epithelium and larger myoepithelial cells with clear cytoplasm, along with scattered concentrically laminated hyaline material (Pap stain).

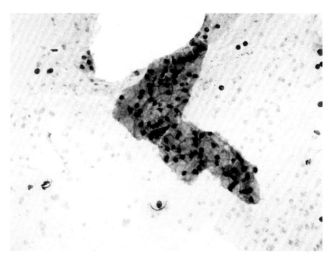

Figure 2.108. Mucoepidermoid carcinoma. A population of cells containing abundant, clear cytoplasm can occasionally be seen in cases of mucoepidermoid carcinoma (Diff-Quik stain).

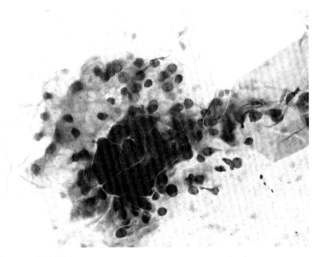

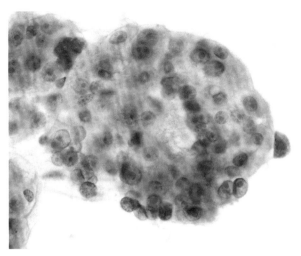

Figure 2.109. Mucoepidermoid carcinoma. A high-power view highlighting the clear, glycogenated cells that can be seen in mucoepidermoid carcinomas (Diff-Quik stain).

Figure 2.110. Metastatic clear cell renal cell carcinoma. A disorganized cluster of epithelial cells with clear cytoplasm, round nuclei, and prominent nucleoli are characteristic of this entity regardless of the site of involvement (Pap stain).

variants of MEC, along with the oncocytic and sclerosing variants. The key to making the correct diagnosis is to recognize the presence of cells with intracytoplasmic mucin vacuoles. For additional details, please refer to the "Mucoepidermoid Carcinoma" sections in the "Cystic Pattern", the "Lymphocyte-Rich Pattern", and the "Oncocytic Pattern". Furthermore, it is important to keep in mind that a metastasis, such as a clear cell renal cell carcinoma (CC-RCC), can rarely occur; however, CC-RCCs should lack a mucinous component (Figure 2.110).

SPINDLE CELL PATTERN

CHECKLIST: Etiologic Considerations for the Spindle Cell Pattern

☐ Myoepithelioma/Myoepithelial-rich Pleomorphic Adenoma

☐ Schwannoma

☐ Nodular Fasciitis (NF)

The spindle cell pattern is comprised of reactive, benign, and malignant lesions. Although a long list of diagnoses could fall into this category, only a few are encountered in routine practice. The majority of the lesions with a pure spindle cell pattern are myoepithelial in origin, including myoepithelioma (much less commonly myoepithelial carcinoma) and myoepithelial-rich pleomorphic adenoma (PA). Other rare entities worth mentioning include NF and schwannoma, as well as melanoma and sarcomatoid carcinoma.

MYOEPITHELIOMA/MYOEPITHELIAL-RICH PLEOMORPHIC ADENOMA

Myoepithelial cells—and as a result, myoepithelial neoplasms—can be spindled, epithelioid, or plasmacytoid in appearance. Although myoepitheliomas are extremely rare and represents approximately 1% of salivary gland neoplasms, the spindle cell subtype is the most common overall (Figures 2.111 and 2.112).[65] Furthermore, the spindle cell subtype is more commonly seen in the major salivary glands and can be easily confused with schwannoma in this location. Myoepithelial-rich PAs are essentially indistinguishable from myoepitheliomas in most

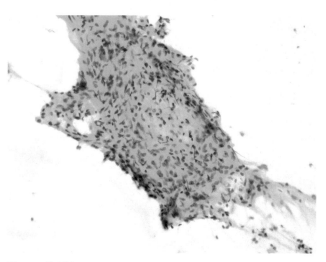

Figure 2.111. Myoepithelioma. Fragment of monotonous spindled cells with a notable absence of fibrillary myxoid matrix (Pap stain).

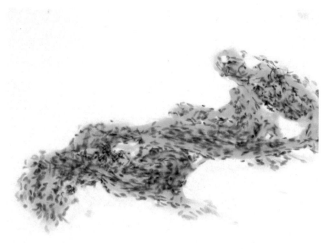

Figure 2.112. Myoepithelioma. Streaming fragments of spindled myoepithelial cells embedded in a collagenized stroma. (Pap stain).

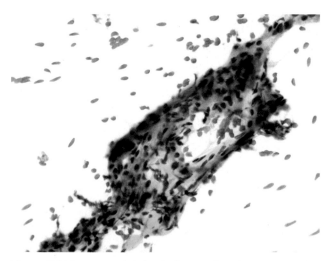

Figure 2.113. Myoepithelial-rich pleomorphic adenoma. Spindled cells with dark nuclei in a clean background (Pap stain).

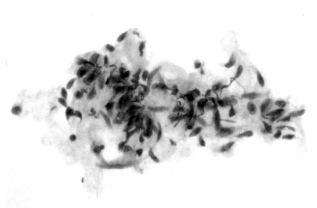

Figure 2.114. Myoepithelial-rich pleomorphic adenoma. High-power view of loosely cohesive spindled myoepithelial cells from a myoepithelial-rich pleomorphic adenoma (Pap stain).

cases. On FNA, the smears are cellular and comprised of clusters and single cells that are bland with fusiform nuclei, fine to coarse chromatin, and scant, pale cytoplasm (Figures 2.113 and 2.114). Fascicular growth or cellular swirling may be seen in small groups. Importantly, myoepitheliomas lack atypical mitoses and necrosis and should not be mistaken for a malignant neoplasm. The only distinguishing cytomorphologic feature seen in myoepithelial-rich PAs is the presence of ductal or fibrillary myxoid material; however, this might not be present on a limited specimen. Importantly, the management is identical and most cases will be categorized as either "benign" or "SUMP" when the specimen is particularly cellular.[8] See the "Dispersed Pattern", the "Basaloid Pattern", and the "Clear Cell Pattern" for further discussion.

FAQ: How do you distinguish a spindled myoepithelial neoplasm from a schwannoma?

Answer: To distinguish a myoepithelial neoplasm from a schwannoma, p40 can be a helpful stain to support myoepithelial differentiation.[66,67] This finding is particularly useful because both entities are positive for S100 and can be positive for cytokeratin stains.[68]

SCHWANNOMA

Schwannoma is a benign peripheral nerve sheath tumor that rarely arises within the parotid gland. There is a considerable amount of overlap between schwannomas and myoepitheliomas/myoepithelial-rich PAs. FNAs tend to be less cellular and comprised of clusters and groups of spindle cells with pale, wispy cytoplasm and hyperchromatic, elongated nuclei that are typically wavy or bent (Figures 2.115-2.118). If present, the most important but rarely seen clue favoring a diagnosis of schwannoma is the presence of Verocay bodies—nuclear palisading within an Antoni A (cellular) area.[69] Although "ancient change," also known as degenerative atypia, may be present in long-standing lesions, increased mitoses, atypical mitoses, and necrosis should not be present. Positive expression for S100 protein and SOX10, and lack of myoepithelial markers such as p40, will strongly favor a schwannoma; this setting may allow a categorization as "benign" with subcategorization as "mesenchymal origin" according to the MSRSGC.[8]

NODULAR FASCIITIS

Nodular fasciitis (NF) is a rare, clonal, benign fibroblastic/myofibroblastic proliferation that grows quickly along muscular fascial planes and is a well-established mimic of malignancy. The lesion occurs across a wide range of ages and has no clear sex

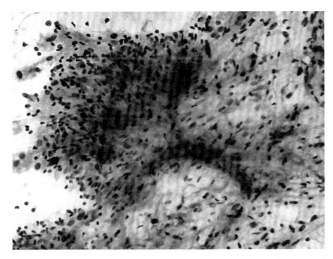

Figure 2.115. Schwannoma. Variably cellular areas of spindled cells in a magenta, fibrillary stroma that can easily be mistaken for the matrix material in a pleomorphic adenoma (Diff-Quik stain).

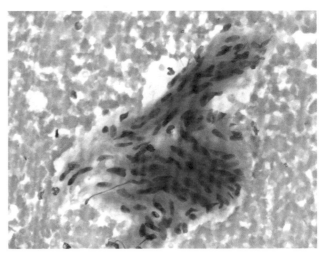

Figure 2.116. Schwannoma. Cluster of closely packed spindled cells, as seen from an Antoni A area (Diff-Quik stain).

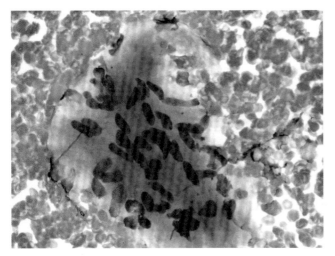

Figure 2.117. Schwannoma. Spindled cells with elongated, fusiform nuclei embedded within a magenta, fibrillary stroma (Diff-Quik stain).

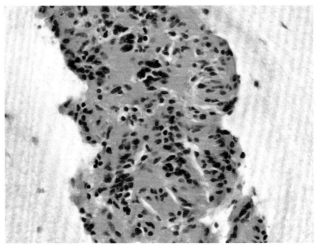

Figure 2.118. Schwannoma. Cell block showing Antoni A areas with nuclear palisading (H&E).

predilection. Fortunately, NF is self-limited and resolves without the need for surgery. As a result, it is important to keep this entity in the differential to avoid unnecessary surgery to the patient. Unfortunately, NF is a challenging diagnosis to make on FNA.[70] Furthermore, NF is an extremely rare entity to arise within or indistinguishably from the parotid gland.[71] On FNA, NF tends to produce smears composed of predominantly single, uniform, spindled cells in a tissue-culture appearance within myxoid to collagenous stroma. The spindled cells contain short, unipolar or bipolar cytoplasmic processes and have round to elongated, hypochromatic nuclei without readily identifiable nucleoli (Figures 2.119-2.121).[70,71] Importantly, overt cytologic atypia, atypical mitoses, and necrosis should be absent, as well as any other feature characteristic of another entity. NF shows variable labeling with SMA and calponin but should generally be negative with other immunostains of myoepithelial neoplasms, schwannomas, and melanoma—which can be spindled and have some cytomorphologic overlap with many of the entities in this pattern (Figures 2.122-2.124). Additionally, NF has recently been shown to be characterized by a *MYH9-USP6* gene fusion, which can be detected on FNA material by fluorescence in situ hybridization (FISH).[72,73]

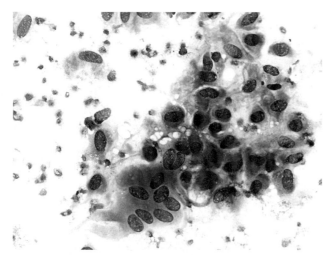

Figure 2.119. Nodular fasciitis. This field is composed of predominately single spindled cells with short, blue cytoplasmic processes embedded in a magenta myxoid stroma (Diff-Quik stain).

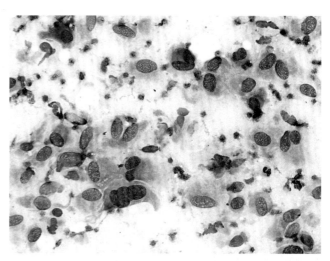

Figure 2.120. Nodular fasciitis. A different field from the same case showing single spindled cells, as well as multinucleated cells, with occasional small nucleoli (Diff-Quik stain).

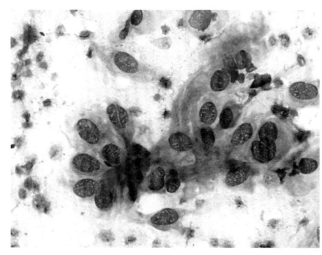

Figure 2.121. Nodular fasciitis. Spindled cells with abundant blue cytoplasm and a magenta myxoid stroma. Notice the bland cytomorphologic features of the nuclei (Diff-Quik stain).

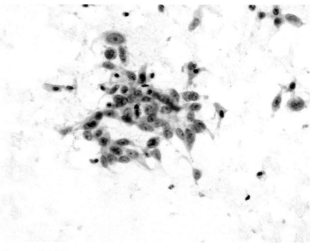

Figure 2.122. Metastatic melanoma. Loose cluster of spindled cells with enlarged nuclei and prominent nucleoli (Pap stain).

PLEOMORPHIC PATTERN

CHECKLIST: Etiologic Considerations for the Pleomorphic Pattern

☐ Salivary Duct Carcinoma (SDC)

☐ High-grade Mucoepidermoid Carcinoma (MEC)

☐ Carcinoma ex Pleomorphic Adenoma (PA)

☐ Metastases

The pleomorphic pattern is characterized by the presence of high-grade malignant nuclear features—mainly nuclear pleomorphism, coarse chromatin, and frequent and/or atypical mitotic figures. There is a considerable amount of overlap between several of the entities in this differential diagnosis, only some of which can be addressed with immunostains. Fortunately, high-grade malignant salivary gland neoplasms on FNA will most immediately managed similarly with aggressive surgical excision with or without lymph node dissection depending on additional radiologic features. Thus, specifically differentiating these entities is not necessary on FNA; rather, it is more important to categorize them as "malignant" according to the MSRSGC.[8] However, it may be important to distinguish a primary salivary gland malignancy from a metastatic lesion because metastases are more likely to necessitate systemic treatment versus locoregional surgical intervention.

SALIVARY DUCT CARCINOMA

Salivary duct carcinoma (SDC) is the prototypical salivary gland entity with a pleomorphic pattern. SDC is rapidly growing and can occur as a primary lesion or arise secondarily from a carcinoma ex PA. FNA reveals cellular smears comprised of three-dimensional clusters and sheets of large, polygonal cells with abundant granular/oncocytic cytoplasm and large, pleomorphic nuclei with coarse chromatin, prominent nucleoli, and frequent mitoses in a background of necrosis (Figures 2.125-2.127). Fortunately, SDCs typically yield diagnostic samples, and these features are not difficult to recognize as malignant. If cell block material is available and a definitive diagnosis is sought, positive AR and HER2 expression can be helpful in making the diagnosis and inform important therapeutic decisions.[60] For further information, see the "Salivary Duct Carcinoma" section under the "Cystic Pattern" and the "Oncocytic Pattern".

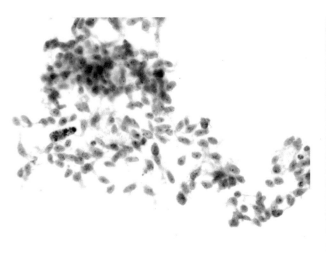

Figure 2.123. Metastatic melanoma. Dispersed spindled cells containing melanin pigment and enlarged nuclei with prominent nucleoli. These findings are virtually diagnostic for melanoma (Pap stain).

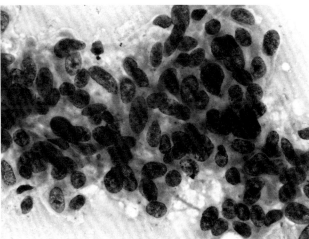

Figure 2.124. Metastatic melanoma. High-power view showing enlarged oval to spindled nuclei with prominent nucleoli (Diff-Quik stain).

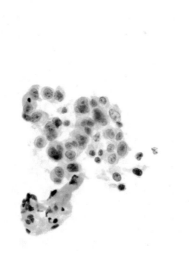

Figure 2.125. Salivary duct carcinoma. Note the large, polygonal cells with abundant granular cytoplasm and large nuclei with coarse chromatin and prominent nucleoli (Pap stain).

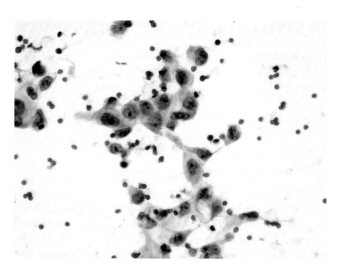

Figure 2.126. Salivary duct carcinoma. This field shows malignant cells with abundant cytoplasm and pleomorphic nuclei with coarse chromatin and prominent nucleoli (Pap stain).

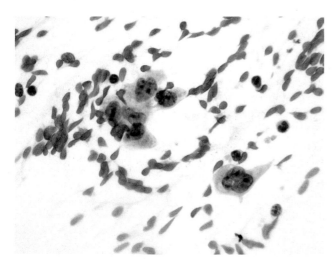

Figure 2.127. Salivary duct carcinoma. Same case showing large, highly atypical cells with irregular nuclear borders and clumped chromatin (Pap stain).

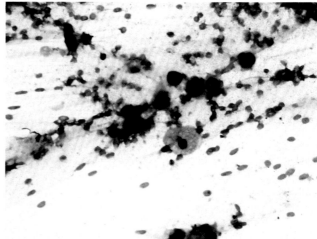

Figure 2.128. High-grade mucoepidermoid carcinoma. A mucocyte can be seen adjacent to pleomorphic cells with enlarged nuclei, high nuclear to cytoplasmic (N/C) ratios, and prominent nucleoli (Diff-Quik stain).

HIGH-GRADE MUCOEPIDERMOID CARCINOMA

High-grade mucoepidermoid carcinomas (MECs) are less common than low- and intermediate-grade MECs, which are further discussed in previous "Mucoepidermoid Carcinoma" sections. High-grade MECs are usually solid masses that produce cellular smears of groups and sheets of large neoplastic cells that are predominantly squamoid in appearance with much rarer intermediate and mucin-containing cells. The epidermoid cells have a moderate amount of dense cytoplasm, which may also be vacuolated, and contain large, pleomorphic nuclei with hyperchromatic chromatin, prominent nucleoli, and brisk mitotic activity (Figures 2.128-2.130). The key to making a specific diagnosis, however, relies on the identification of cells with intracytoplasmic mucin—a finding that can be confirmed with positive mucicarmine or PAS with diastase staining. A pitfall is to interpret the squamoid cells as part of a SqCC. In fact, if keratin pearls or overt keratinization is present, a high-grade MEC is unlikely.

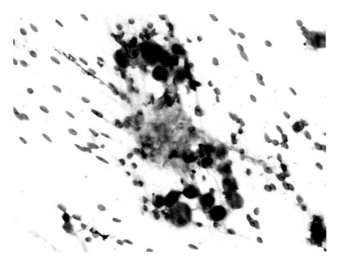

Figure 2.129. High-grade mucoepidermoid carcinoma. Atypical cells with large nuclei, high nuclear to cytoplasmic (N/C) ratios, and prominent nucleoli are present (Diff-Quik stain).

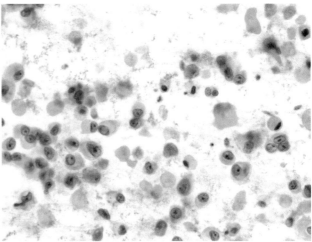

Figure 2.130. High-grade mucoepidermoid carcinoma. Dispersed, pleomorphic single cells, as well orangeophilic cells showing squamous metaplasia are present (Pap stain).

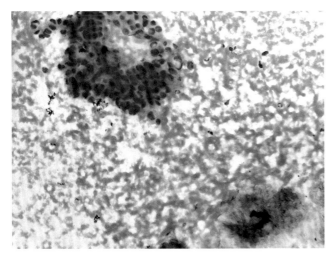

Figure 2.131. Carcinoma ex pleomorphic adenoma. A poorly differentiated carcinomatous component can be seen at the upper left-hand corner with some magenta-colored, fibrillary chondromyxoid material in the bottom right corner, supporting a diagnosis of carcinoma ex pleomorphic adenoma (Diff-Quik stain).

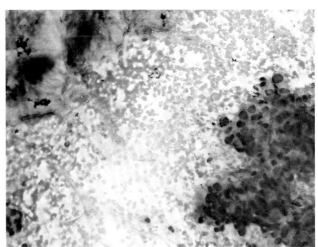

Figure 2.132. Carcinoma ex pleomorphic adenoma. Fibrillary chondromyxoid material is present alongside a poorly differentiated carcinoma, providing a clue that this carcinoma arose from a pleomorphic adenoma (Diff-Quik stain).

CARCINOMA EX PLEOMORPHIC ADENOMA

Carcinoma ex PA is essentially carcinomatous transformation of a PA. Although rare, it is an aggressive malignancy, and local and distant metastases are common. The malignant component is most commonly SDC; however, any other primary salivary gland neoplasm of epithelial or myoepithelial origin can arise from a PA. As a result, the cytomorphologic features will be characteristic of the malignant entity to which it has transformed. The most helpful clue, besides patient history and clinical presentation, will be the presence of background metachromatic fibrillary chondromyxoid material, which, unfortunately, may or may not be present in the aspirated material (Figures 2.131 and 2.132). Carcinoma ex PAs also retain the *PLAG1* or *HMGA2* gene fusions characteristic of the benign counterpart; however, this finding has little clinical utility in this setting. The most important goal is identification of malignant transformation on aspirated material, which will result in aggressive surgical management.

METASTASES

The parotid gland may contain both intraparotid and periparotid lymph nodes. As a result, metastases to these lymph nodes, particularly from a cutaneous lesion of the face or scalp, are not uncommon. SqCC is the most common primary malignancy to metastasize to the parotid gland and is discussed above in the "Cystic Pattern"; melanoma is the second most common and is discussed above in the "Dispersed Pattern" (Figure 2.133). On FNA, SqCC will often result in a cellular smear in a background of necrotic debris. The malignant cells are highly variable in size, shape, and appearance. Nuclei are usually enlarged and hyperchromatic, but some cells may contain smaller, pyknotic nuclei—especially keratinizing cells. As a result, some cells have a high N/C ratio while others have abundant dense/"hard" cytoplasm. The cytoplasm may or may not appear orangeophilic, like that which is seen in dyskeratotic cells. One of the most specific features for SqCC is the presence of tadpole cells, which are characterized by elongated, orangeophilic cytoplasmic tails (Figure 2.134). Fortunately, the majority of patients have a known history of a cutaneous primary, which is most often keratinizing. In fact, if a patient lacks a history and a primary SqCC is a diagnostic consideration, it is more likely to represent squamous differentiation of another high-grade malignant salivary gland neoplasm or a metastasis from an unknown primary cutaneous lesion.[74]

NEAR MISSES

PROTEINACEOUS DEBRIS OF A WARTHIN TUMOR MISTAKEN FOR NECROSIS

Many salivary gland lesions are either intrinsically cystic or can undergo secondary cystic degenerative changes. These contents may be predominantly mucinous, as in a mucocele or low-grade mucoepidermoid carcinoma, or predominantly proteinaceous, as classically seen in a Warthin tumor (WT). The proteinaceous debris of WTs gives the aspirated fluid a macroscopic "motor oil" greenish-brown appearance and microscopically consists of granular, dirty debris with scattered lymphocytes and histiocytes (Figures 2.135-2.138). These findings are not too dissimilar from the tumor necrosis (coagulative necrosis) seen in high-grade salivary gland malignancies and metastatic squamous cell carcinomas. The most helpful distinguishing features favoring tumor necrosis include the following: the presence of dying, degenerating, and fragmented nuclear material and the presence of an intact morphologically atypical component. The latter feature is particularly helpful when differentiating between WTs that contain mucinous or squamous metaplasia.

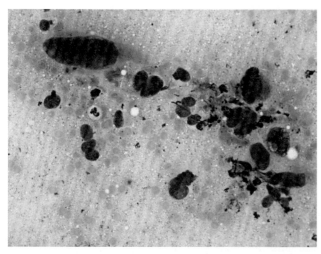

Figure 2.133. Metastatic melanoma. Highly pleomorphic cells with enlarged and irregular nuclei from a metastatic melanoma involving the parotid gland (Diff-Quik stain).

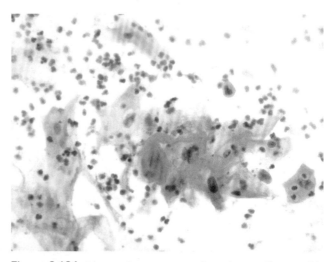

Figure 2.134. Metastatic squamous cell carcinoma. Pleomorphic cells are present with elongated orangeophilic cytoplasmic processes, a finding that suggests abnormal keratinization (Pap stain).

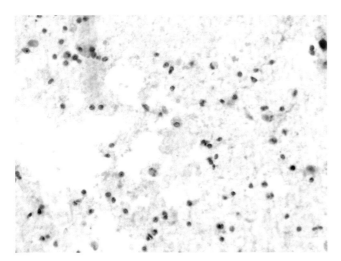

Figure 2.135. Warthin tumor. Abundant proteinaceous debris, lymphocytes, and macrophages which should not be overinterpreted as tumor necrosis (Pap stain).

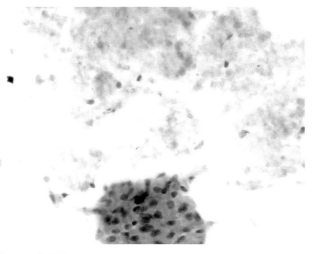

Figure 2.136. Warthin tumor. Note the oncocytic epithelium and adjacent proteinaceous debris, not to be confused with tumor necrosis (Pap stain).

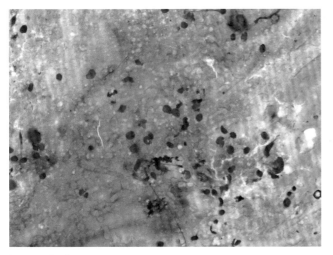

Figure 2.137. Warthin tumor. Thick protein-rich fluid and mixed inflammatory cells that could easily be mistaken for mucin or necrotic debris (Diff-Quik stain).

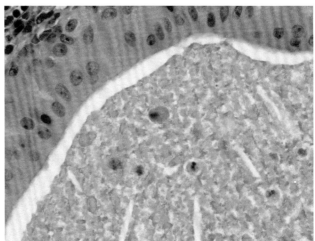

Figure 2.138. Warthin tumor. High magnification field showing the characteristic bilayer of oncocytic epithelium and central proteinaceous material (H&E).

AN EPITHELIOID, PLASMACYTOID, OR SPINDLED NEOPLASM POSITIVE FOR "MELANOMA MARKERS" IN THE SALIVARY GLAND MISTAKEN FOR MELANOMA

Both melanoma and myoepithelial-rich neoplasms may be characterized by epithelioid, plasmacytoid, or spindled cell populations (Figures 2.139 and 2.140). Additionally, there is considerable overlap of the immunoprofiles between melanoma and myoepithelial cells. Given its high sensitivity, S100 protein has historically been considered the gold standard to screen for melanoma; however, more recently, SOX10 has been shown to be more sensitive and specific than S100 protein. Furthermore, a number of additional melanoma markers, such as HMB-45, MelanA, Mart-1, and MITF may be employed. In fact, multiple melanocytic markers should be used in such cases, and the combination of morphology and positive immunostaining for more than one of these markers is often sufficient to make a correct diagnosis. However, for example, PAs can be positive for S100 protein and SOX10, as well as focally positive for MelanA. In the salivary gland, it is important to perform additional markers, such as p63/p40, high-molecular-weight cytokeratin, smooth muscle actin, or calponin. Positivity with one or more of these markers in this setting would favor a myoepithelial-rich neoplasm over a melanoma.

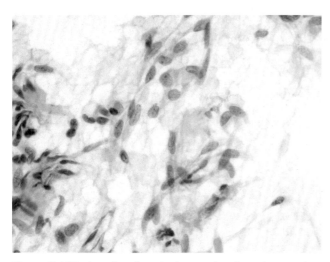

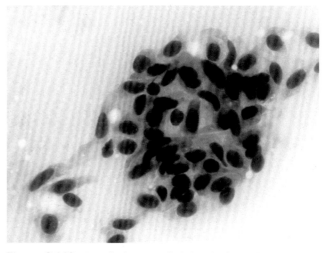

Figure 2.139. Spindle cells with elongated nuclei with open chromatin and wispy bipolar cytoplasmic processes, consistent with myoepithelial cells. The presence of a prominent spindle cell population positive for S100 protein may initially cause concern for a metastatic melanoma (Pap stain).

Figure 2.140. Spindled myoepithelial cells that lack the nuclear irregularity, hyperchromasia, and nucleoli typically seen in melanoma (Diff-Quik stain).

INTRODUCTION TO CERVICAL LYMPH NODES

Cervical lymph nodes are anatomically divided into eight unique, clinically relevant regions, also known as levels: Ia (submental triangle), Ib (submandibular triangle), IIa (anterior-inferior to spinal accessory), IIb (posterior-superior to spinal accessory), III (middle 1/3 of internal jugular vein), IV (lower 1/3 of internal jugular vein), V (posterior triangle), and VI (anterior central compartment). These lymph nodes can be involved by reactive or malignant processes including infections, metastases, and lymphoma. Furthermore, certain primary anatomic sites have a proclivity to drain to certain lymph node levels, which can be specifically assessed for metastatic involvement or, conversely, used to help localize a carcinoma of unknown primary. The most common malignances that involve cervical lymph nodes are metastatic carcinomas from the head and neck (SqCC), papillary thyroid carcinoma (PTC), and metastatic melanoma. The evaluation of cervical lymph node involvement is extremely important for both prognosis and treatment planning. Given the anatomic proximity to vital neck structures, minimally invasive sampling with FNA is the most common method of assessing lymph node status.

METASTATIC CARCINOMA PATTERN

CHECKLIST: Etiologic Considerations for the Metastatic Carcinoma Pattern

☐ Metastatic HPV-positive Squamous Cell Carcinoma (SqCC)

☐ Metastatic HPV-negative Squamous Cell Carcinoma (SqCC)

☐ Metastatic Nasopharyngeal Carcinoma (NPC)

☐ Metastatic Papillary Thyroid Carcinoma (PTC)

The metastatic carcinoma pattern is characterized by the presence of malignant, epithelial cells in an aspirated lymph node. The only difference between metastatic carcinomas in the cervical lymph nodes versus a separate region (e.g., mediastinal lymph nodes) is the primary malignancies that tend to involve these nodes. The majority of cervical lymph node metastases come from head and neck SqCCs. In fact, as many as 50% of patients with head and neck SqCC present with a neck mass as their first clinical symptom.[75] As a result, a patient may or may not have a history of malignancy, and the cytopathologist may be able to both diagnose a malignancy and suggest the primary site of origin.

HPV-negative SqCC primaries are more likely to be overtly keratinizing than HPV-positive SqCCs. To determine the HPV status of SqCC, p16 can be used as a screening marker (all lymph node levels) or as a surrogate marker (levels II/III) for HPV.[22] When confirmatory testing is required, an HPV-specific test, such as high-risk HPV RNA in situ hybridization (HR-HPV ISH), can be used. The overwhelming majority of these HPV-related SqCCs will be from an oropharyngeal primary lesion. The most common nonsquamous epithelial carcinoma will be PTC, which have the classic nuclear features, follicles and papillary structures, and may contain abundant psammoma bodies. Confirmatory immunostaining with PAX-8 and TTF-1 may be helpful but is typically not required.

METASTATIC HPV-POSITIVE SQUAMOUS CELL CARCINOMA

HPV-positive SqCC is a distinct epidemiologic, clinical, and pathologic malignancy that most often arises from the palatine and lingual tonsils of the oropharynx.[76] Because of the unique anatomy of these tonsils, malignant cells have immediate access to the lymphatics. As a result, patients frequently present at advanced clinical stage with cervical lymph node involvement, most commonly levels II and III, without an obvious oropharyngeal mass.[77] Despite the frequency of regional lymph node involvement, HPV is associated with an improved prognosis and response to chemotherapy and radiation therapy versus conventional, HPV-negative SqCC. Furthermore, the HPV status is required for enrollment in clinical trials and possible de-escalation of therapy. Therefore, determining the HPV status is important. HPV-positive SqCC tends to produce cellular smears consisting of cohesive fragments of minimally keratinizing, basaloid squamous cells with scant but dense cytoplasm and enlarged, hyperchromatic nuclei (Figures 2.141-2.144).[78] Necrosis is common, resulting in secondary cystic change in lymph node metastases. When overt squamous differentiation is not present, a p40 immunostain is the single most helpful marker; however, it is important to note that other entities in the differential diagnosis, such as NPC, are also p40 positive (Figure 2.145). According to the most recent guidelines from the College of American Pathologists (CAP), high-risk HPV testing is recommended for all patients with SqCC cervical lymph node metastases with either an oropharyngeal mass or carcinoma of unknown primary (Figures 2.146 and 2.147).[22] Importantly, this testing can be reliably performed on cell block material.[79-81]

SAMPLE NOTE: HPV-POSITIVE SQUAMOUS CELL CARCINOMA

Metastatic HPV-positive squamous cell carcinoma. See note.

Note: Ancillary studies were performed on the cell block with the following expression patterns: p16 positive and HR-HPV RNA ISH positive. HPV-positive SqCCs are most likely to arise from the palatine and lingual (base of tongue) tonsils, although other primary sites, such as the nasopharynx, have also been documented. Based on the literature, HR-HPV positivity is associated with an improved prognosis and clinical response to chemotherapy and radiation therapy when compared with HPV-negative, conventional squamous cell carcinoma.

METASTATIC HPV-NEGATIVE SQUAMOUS CELL CARCINOMA

Despite the increasing incidence of HPV-positive SqCC, the majority of head and neck SqCCs are HPV negative (conventional), most often arising from the larynx and the oral cavity.[82,83] As a result, it is not uncommon for an HPV-negative SqCC to metastasize to

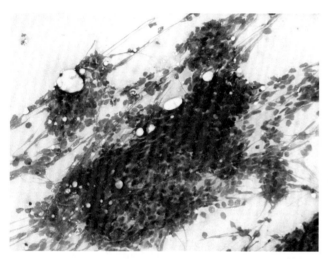

Figure 2.141. Metastatic HPV-positive squamous cell carcinoma. Cellular proliferation of large cells showing crush artifact (Diff-Quik stain).

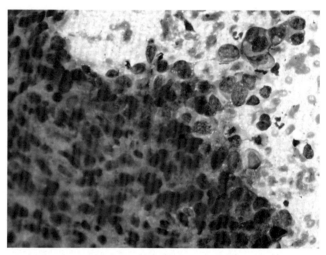

Figure 2.142. Metastatic HPV-positive squamous cell carcinoma. This field is comprised of large, basaloid cells with a high nuclear to cytoplasmic ratio and a lack of keratinization (Diff-Quik stain).

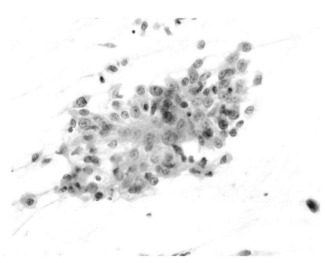

Figure 2.143. Metastatic HPV-positive squamous cell carcinoma. Cluster of malignant cells with large nuclei, abundant blue cytoplasm, and small nucleoli (Pap stain).

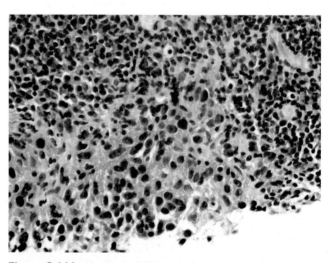

Figure 2.144. Metastatic HPV-positive squamous cell carcinoma. Core biopsy showing non-keratinizing squamous cell carcinoma colonizing a lymph node (H&E).

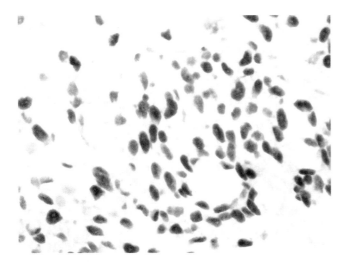

Figure 2.145. Metastatic HPV-positive squamous cell carcinoma. Diffuse p40 positivity seen on cell block material, supporting squamous differentiation (p40 immunostain).

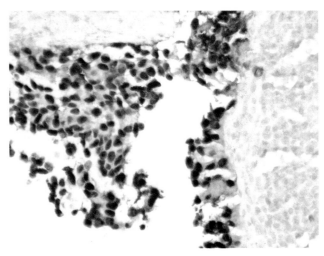

Figure 2.146. Metastatic HPV-positive squamous cell carcinoma. Diffuse p16 positivity seen on cell block material, which is often used as a screening marker for the HPV status of a tumor (p16 immunostain).

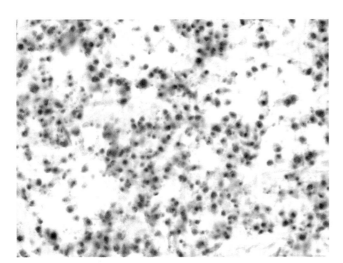

Figure 2.147. Metastatic HPV-positive squamous cell carcinoma. Punctate nuclear and cytoplasmic staining by HPV high-risk in situ hybridization on cell block material (HPV-HR ISH stain).

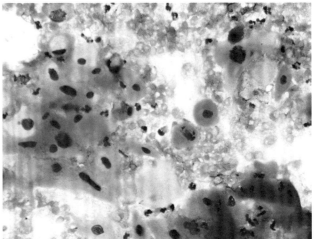

Figure 2.148. Metastatic HPV-negative squamous cell carcinoma. Malignant cells with abundant amounts of the characteristic Robin egg blue cytoplasm seen in keratinizing squamous cell carcinoma (Diff-Quik stain).

a cervical lymph node. Conventional SqCCs may be keratinizing, nonkeratinizing, or poorly differentiated with no specific morphologic or immunophenotype suggesting a primary site of origin. As a result, once HPV-association is ruled out by a lack of p16 immunolabeling, no additional workup is required. Like metastases to other lymph node regions, HPV-negative SqCCs are often cystic with central, necrotic debris. FNA, however, most often produces cellular smears of variably keratinizing squamous cells with dense cytoplasm, enlarged and hyperchromatic nuclei with irregular nuclear membranes, and frequent mitotic figures (Figures 2.148-2.152). For additional discussion and figures, see the "Metastatic Squamous Cell Carcinoma" section under the "Cystic Pattern".

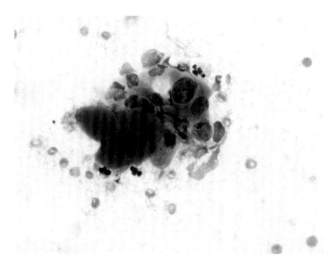

Figure 2.149. Metastatic HPV-negative squamous cell carcinoma. Thick, glassy blue keratin material is seen extruding from large cells with pleomorphic nuclei (Diff-Quik stain).

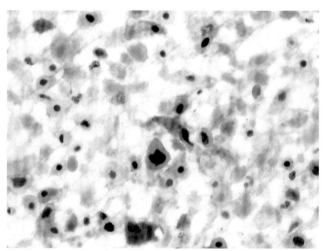

Figure 2.150. Metastatic HPV-negative squamous cell carcinoma. Single malignant cells with abundant, orangeophilic cytoplasm and complex, hyperchromatic nuclei from a metastatic keratinizing squamous cell carcinoma (Pap stain).

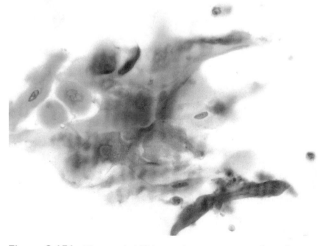

Figure 2.151. Metastatic HPV-negative squamous cell carcinoma. Malignant squamous cells with dense, hard cytoplasm and atypical keratinizing cytoplasmic extensions (Pap stain).

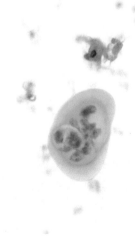

Figure 2.152. Metastatic HPV-negative squamous cell carcinoma. A single, bizarre malignant cell with dense, hard cytoplasm is present in a background of smaller keratinizing cells (Pap stain).

METASTATIC NASOPHARYNGEAL CARCINOMA

Nasopharyngeal carcinoma (NPC) is a rare carcinoma with squamous differentiation arising from the nasopharynx. NPC can be of two main subtypes that have distinct epidemiology and morphology: keratinizing (K-NPC), which is associated with tobacco and alcohol consumption, and nonkeratinizing (NK-NPC), which is strongly associated with EBV. Additionally, NK-NPC can be differentiated or undifferentiated depending on the degree of overt squamous differentiation. Although NPC is rare, these malignancies frequently exhibit locoregional metastasis; as many as 42% of patients present with a neck mass, and as many as 72% have enlarged lymph nodes on physical examination.[16] NPC most commonly metastasizes to the retropharyngeal lymph nodes and cervical lymph node levels II and V. On FNA, K-NPC is indistinguishable from a keratinizing SqCC. The NK-NPC differentiated type is often cystic due to necrosis and consists of clusters of cells with pleomorphic nuclei and well-defined cytoplasmic borders and intercellular bridges (Figures 2.153-2.155). In contrast, NK-NPC undifferentiated type consists of sheets, irregular groups, and dispersed large, atypical cells with vesicular chromatin and prominent nucleoli in a lymphocyte-rich background. NPCs are positive for markers of squamous differentiation, such as

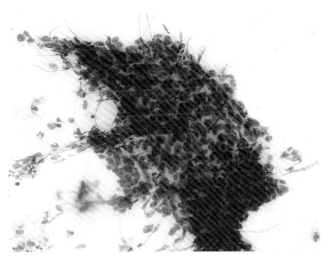

Figure 2.153. Metastatic nasopharyngeal carcinoma, nonkeratinizing type. Cluster of haphazardly arranged malignant cells with crush artifact, high nuclear to cytoplasmic ratios and vesicular chromatin (Diff-Quik stain).

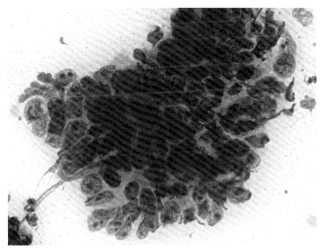

Figure 2.154. Metastatic nasopharyngeal carcinoma, nonkeratinizing type. High-power view from the same case highlighting enlarged nuclei with irregular nuclear borders, vesicular chromatin, and prominent nucleoli (Diff-Quik stain).

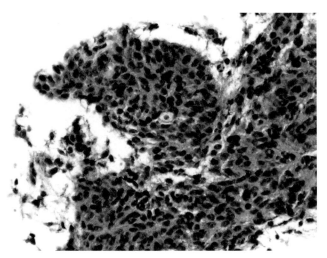

Figure 2.155. Metastatic nasopharyngeal carcinoma, nonkeratinizing type. Syncytial group of malignant cells with enlarged and hyperchromatic nuclei containing frequent apoptotic bodies and mitoses (H&E).

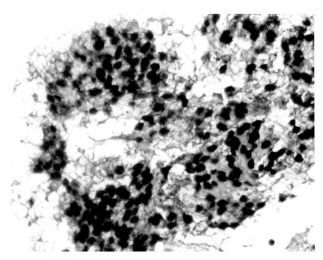

Figure 2.156. Metastatic nasopharyngeal carcinoma, nonkeratinizing type. Strong and diffuse staining with in situ hybridization for Epstein-Barr encoded RNA (EBER) studies confirms the diagnosis (EBER stain).

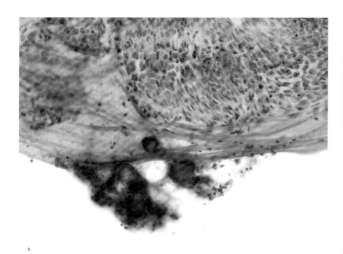

Figure 2.157. Metastatic papillary thyroid carcinoma. Sheets of malignant cells with adjacent psammoma bodies, an extremely helpful features that can clinch the diagnosis at a metastatic site (Pap stain).

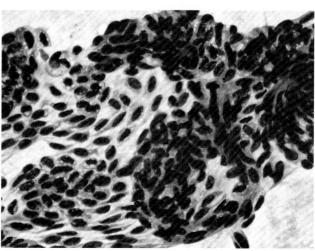

Figure 2.158. Metastatic papillary thyroid carcinoma. Streaming sheets and clusters of epithelial cells showing nuclear enlargement, elongation, and overlap (Diff-Quik stain).

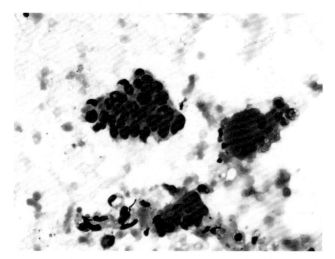

Figure 2.159. Metastatic papillary thyroid carcinoma. Clusters of epithelial cells with cytoplasmic vacuolizationand nuclear enlargement in a background of colloid (Diff-Quik stain).

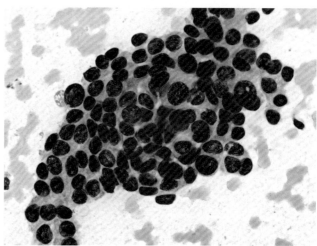

Figure 2.160. Metastatic papillary thyroid carcinoma. Cluster of disorganized epithelial cells showing the nuclear enlargement, elongation, overlap, and grooves (Diff-Quik stain).

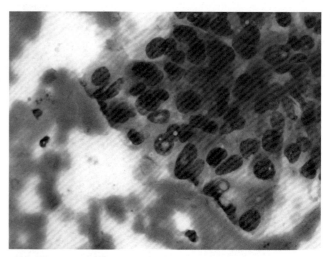

Figure 2.161. Metastatic papillary thyroid carcinoma. High-power view of a cluster of disorganized epithelial cells showing characteristic nuclear features, including classic nuclear pseudoinclusions, which resemble the cytoplasm of the malignant cells (Diff-Quik stain).

p63/p40, and the NK-NPCs are most often positive for EBV ISH (Figure 2.156). Notably, a subset of NK-NPCs that are EBV negative may be p16 positive and associated with HR-HPV. Correlation with clinical and radiographic studies will be the most helpful in localizing a cervical lymph node metastasis of unknown origin.

METASTATIC PAPILLARY THYROID CARCINOMA

Papillary thyroid carcinoma (PTC) frequently metastasizes to regional lymph nodes. Most notably, the central neck (level VI) is often the first site of metastatic involvement, followed by involvement of the lateral neck (levels III and IV). The diagnostic features of metastatic PTC are identical to those seen in primary thyroid FNA: enlarged and overlapping follicular cells with an increased N/C ratio and large nuclei with irregular nuclear contours, nuclear grooves, intranuclear pseudoinclusions, and pale chromatin (Figures 2.157-2.161). Like primary thyroid PTCs, psammoma bodies are rarely identified by FNA, most likely due to the size of the procedure needles and mechanics of aspiration. The most helpful immunochemical stains to prove a thyroid origin are TTF-1, PAX-8, and thyroglobulin.

LYMPHOID PATTERN

CHECKLIST: Etiologic Considerations for the Lymphoid pattern

☐ Reactive Lymphoid Hyperplasia

☐ Low-grade B-cell Lymphomas

☐ High-grade B-cell Lymphomas (Diffuse Large B-Cell Lymphoma and Burkitt Lymphoma)

☐ Hodgkin Lymphoma

The lymphoid pattern consists of both reactive and neoplastic lymphocytic lesions. FNA is often considered to be the first-line diagnostic method for evaluating lymphadenopathy, especially when lymph nodes are near vital structures (such as cervical lymph nodes). FNA may be used to triage the diagnostic workup for cases with a lymphocytic pattern by diverting material for culture, flow cytometry, cell block preparation, and/or core biopsy when appropriate. Most cases can be divided into one of four categories: reactive (including infectious etiologies), low-grade non-Hodgkin lymphomas, high-grade non-Hodgkin lymphomas, and Hodgkin lymphomas.

REACTIVE LYMPHOID HYPERPLASIA

Reactive lymphoid hyperplasia (RLH) is a nonspecific finding which can occur due to a variety of etiologies. Although not as easily appreciated on FNA specimens, RLH can be due to the proliferation of the follicular centers or to the expansion of the paracortical space. In both cases, however, the unifying theme is that the sample is polymorphous in nature (Figures 2.162-2.164). A variety of lymphoid cell types should be present, including small lymphocytes and plasma cells, as well as germinal center cells (centrocytes, centroblasts, tingible body macrophages). The germinal center cells may cluster together to form aggregates, which are very reassuring of a reactive lesion. For RLH, the lack of a monotonous population and the presence of tingible body macrophages favor against a low-grade B-cell lymphoma, while the lack of an atypical, pleomorphic population favors against a high-grade lymphoma, such as DLBCL or Burkitt lymphoma. Like lymph nodes from all other sites, granulomatous inflammation may involve the cervical lymph nodes (Figures 2.165-2.167). The differential diagnosis for granulomatous inflammation is broad and includes foreign-body giant cell reaction, fungal and acid-fast bacilli infections, sarcoidosis, or malignancy, to name a few.

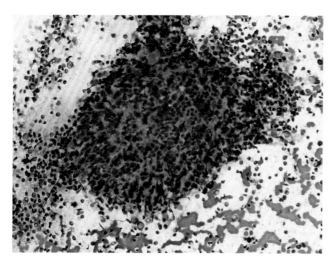

Figure 2.162. Reactive lymphoid hyperplasia. Low-power view of an aggregate of lymphocytes and histiocytes, consistent with an enlarged germinal center (Diff-Quik stain).

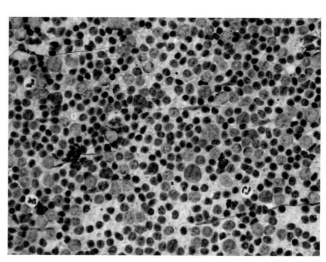

Figure 2.163. Reactive lymphoid hyperplasia. A polymorphous population of lymphocytes, including small lymphocytes, centrocytes, and centroblasts (Diff-Quik stain).

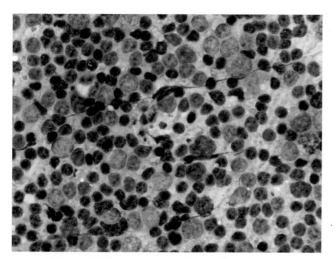

Figure 2.164. Reactive lymphoid hyperplasia. High-power view of a germinal center containing a tingible body macrophage (center), a finding that almost always suggests sampling of a benign process (Diff-Quik stain).

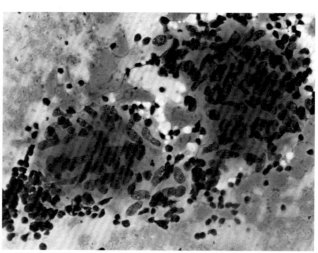

Figure 2.165. Granulomatous inflammation. Two nonnecrotizing granulomas are present with epithelioid histiocytes and surrounding small lymphocytes (Diff-Quik stain).

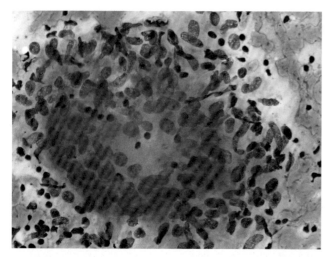

Figure 2.166. Granulomatous inflammation. This granuloma consists of epithelioid histiocytes and admixed lymphocytes (Diff-Quik stain).

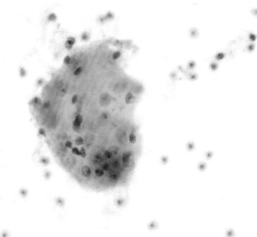

Figure 2.167. Granulomatous inflammation. A multinucleated giant cell is present with small, round nuclei (Pap stain).

LOW-GRADE B-CELL LYMPHOMAS

Low-grade B-cell lymphomas include a variety of entities, such as follicular lymphoma (WHO grades I/II), chronic lymphocytic leukemia/small lymphocytic lymphoma (CLL/SLL), lymphoplasmacytic lymphoma, and nodal marginal zone lymphoma, to name a few. For the most part, these entities are largely indistinguishable on cytomorphologic smears alone and are comprised of predominantly small- to medium-sized, monotonous lymphocytes with scant to moderate amounts of cytoplasm and variably irregular nuclear contours (Figures 2.168-2.170). Lymphoplasmacytic lymphoma, however, will be comprised of lymphocytes with variable plasmacytoid features. The most helpful diagnostic clue to suggest the possibility of a low-grade B-cell lymphoma is the presence of a monotonous population of lymphocytes with a notable lack of tingible body macrophages or other normal lymph node components. This smear appearance should trigger dedicated passes for flow cytometry (most importantly) and core biopsy, if amenable.

HIGH-GRADE B-CELL LYMPHOMAS

The two most notable high-grade B-cell lymphomas are DLBCL and Burkitt lymphoma. DLBCL tends to occur in older patients and is the most common subtype of non-Hodgkin lymphoma overall. DLBCL most often consists of sheets of dyshesive, large, atypical

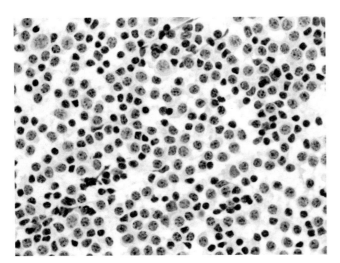

Figure 2.168. Small lymphocytic lymphoma. Monomorphic population of small lymphocytes with smooth nuclear contours and clumped chromatin (Pap stain).

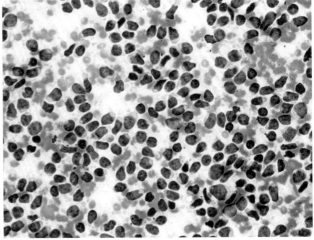

Figure 2.169. Mantle cell lymphoma. Sheets of monomorphic, medium-sized lymphocytes with irregular nuclear contours. Cytogenetic studies detected a t(11;14) translocation, confirming a diagnosis of mantle cell lymphoma (Diff-Quik stain).

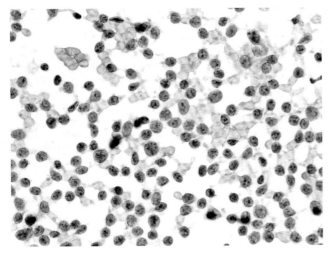

Figure 2.170. Mantle cell lymphoma. Pap stain from the same case of mantle cell lymphoma, highlighting the fine nuclear chromatin present in these cells (Pap stain).

lymphocytes with scant cytoplasm and round, noncleaved nuclei with prominent nucleoli (Figures 2.171 and 2.172). DLBCL cells may not survive the processing steps required for flow cytometry; as a result, obtaining a dedicated pass for cell block preparation or for a core biopsy is important. DLBCL is positive for B-cell markers, such as CD20 and Pax5, which can help to distinguish it from other non–B-cell high-grade malignancies.

Burkitt lymphoma has three epidemiological variants: 1) endemic type (EBV-related), most commonly arising in the jaws and facial bones of children, 2) sporadic type, most commonly involving the ileocecal region with rare lymph node involvement, and 3) immunodeficiency-associated type, most commonly seen in the setting of HIV infection.[84] Burkitt lymphoma smears consist of sheets of monotonous, medium-sized lymphocytes in a background of necrosis, apoptosis, and tingible body macrophages (which impart the classic "starry sky" appearance on histology) (Figures 2.173 and 2.174). The lymphocytes contain a moderate amount of basophilic cytoplasm that often contains vacuoles, which can be a helpful diagnostic clue. The nuclei are round to oval with chunky, coarse chromatin and several nucleoli. Like DLBCL, Burkitt lymphoma is positive for B-cell markers. In addition, almost all cases of Burkitt lymphoma are positive for nuclear MYC expression by on immunostaining, most commonly reflecting a t(8;14) *IGH-MYC* rearrangement, and have a Ki-67 proliferation index of >99%.

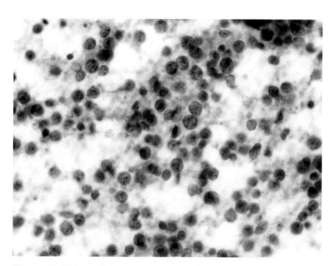

Figure 2.171. Diffuse large B-cell lymphoma, confirmed by ancillary studies. Dispersed large lymphocytes with coarse chromatin and a background of necrotic debris (Pap stain).

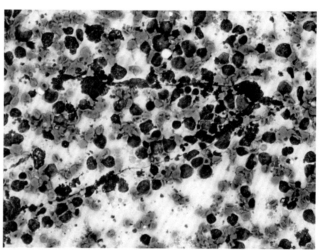

Figure 2.172. Diffuse large B-cell lymphoma. Single, large lymphocytes in a background of lymphoglandular bodies and necrotic debris (Diff-Quik stain).

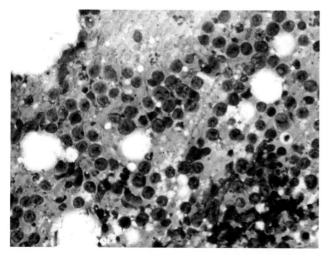

Figure 2.173. Burkitt lymphoma, confirmed by ancillary studies. Single, high-grade malignant cells with prominent nucleoli, apoptotic bodies, and necrotic debris. (Diff-Quik stain).

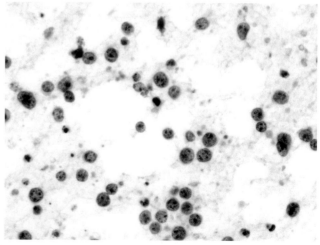

Figure 2.174. Burkitt lymphoma. Medium- and large-sized scattered lymphocytes with round nuclei, coarse chromatin, and prominent nucleoli in a background of necrotic debris (Pap stain).

HODGKIN LYMPHOMA

Hodgkin lymphomas (HL) include both the classical (nodular sclerosing, lymphocyte-rich, mixed cellularity, and lymphocyte-depleted types) and nonclassical (nodular lymphocyte–predominant) types of lymphomas. Both main categories of HL are characterized by scattered, large and atypical cells in a mixed inflammatory and/or sclerotic background. The main difference between classical and nonclassical types is the presence of Reed-Sternberg (RS)/RS-like cells (CD15, CD30, PAX-5 positive) versus multilobulated "popcorn" cells (CD20 positive), respectively. The main difference between the subtypes of classical HL is the inflammatory background within which the RS/RS-like cells are present. Briefly, RS cells are large, binucleated cells with prominent "owl eye" nucleoli while RS-like cells are similarly atypical with a single nucleus containing a prominent nucleolus (Figures 2.175-2.178). Owing to the rarity of these malignant cells within the inflammatory background, it is often necessary to obtain a dedicated pass for cell block preparation or a core needle biopsy for immunophenotypic characterization.

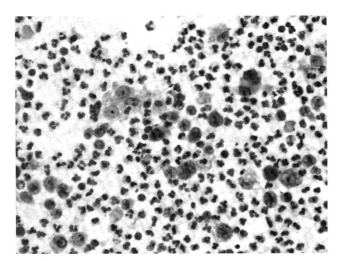

Figure 2.175. Hodgkin lymphoma. Note the binucleated Reed-Sternberg (RS) cells and mononuclear RS-like cells in a background of mixed inflammation (Diff-Quik stain).

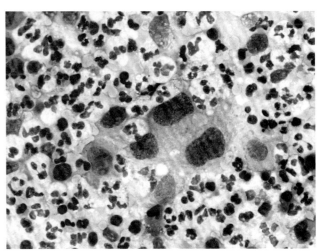

Figure 2.176. Hodgkin lymphoma. High-power view of Reed-Sternberg/Reed Sternberg-like cells from the same case of Hodgkin lymphoma (Diff-Quik stain).

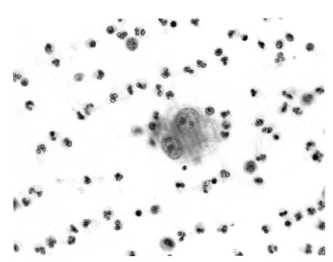

Figure 2.177. Hodgkin lymphoma. Classical binucleated Reed-Sternberg cell with prominent nucleoli (Pap stain).

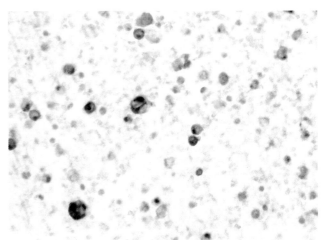

Figure 2.178. Hodgkin lymphoma. The Reed-Sternberg cells stain positivity with CD30 (CD30 immunostain).

PEARLS & PITFALLS

Unfortunately, some lymphomas, such as Hodgkin lymphoma (HL), are comprised of predominantly reactive inflammatory cells with only rare neoplastic cells. Fortunately, several clues, such as the presence of RS/RS-like cells or the presence of an unexpected cell population, such as eosinophils, can be extremely helpful. Most cases, however, reveal reactive lymphoid hyperplasia (RLH) and will not require an ancillary workup. In cases of RLH versus low-grade B-cell lymphoma, flow cytometry can be extremely helpful in confirming a polymorphous (polyclonal) population without an aberrant or abnormal phenotype. It is important to note that not all lymphomas are readily identifiable by flow cytometry; in particular, flow cytometry is insensitive to HL and large cell lymphomas, and immunostains may be the more helpful ancillary tests for these cases.

OTHER

MELANOMA

The majority of the melanomas that metastasize to the cervical lymph nodes are cutaneous in origin, and most patients will have a prior diagnosis. Melanoma can show many different morphologic features; most classically, the nuclei are eccentric, occasionally binucleated, and enlarged with prominent nucleoli (Figure 2.179). Alternatively, melanoma may be spindled, epithelioid, or pleomorphic. Unfortunately, melanin pigment is often absent, and the cytomorphology is typically not specific enough to make a definitive diagnosis, unless there is prior material from a known diagnosis to which the current sample can be compared. As a result, a dedicated pass for cell block/core biopsy should be attempted to facilitate a workup with melanocytic immuno markers such as S100 protein, SOX10, HMB-45, MITF, Mart-1, and/or MelanA. For additional discussion, see the "Melanoma" section in the "Dispersed Pattern."

ADENOCARCINOMA

Occasionally, primary malignancies—many of which are adenocarcinomas—metastasize to a cervical lymph node from the major salivary glands, oral cavity, lung, breast, or kidneys (Figures 2.180-2.190). These include SDC, high-grade MEC, lung adenocarcinoma, and ductal carcinoma of the breast, to name a few. Most of these patients will have a known primary diagnosis, which makes either cytomorphologic comparison or confirmation with immunostains the most effective way to make the diagnosis.

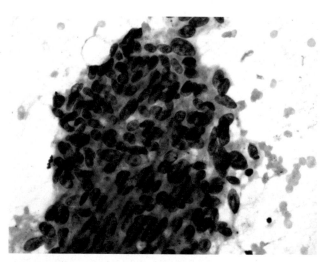

Figure 2.179. Metastatic melanoma. Cluster of malignant cells containing enlarged, elongated nuclei with prominent nucleoli (Diff-Quik stain).

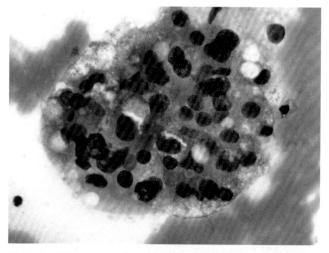

Figure 2.180. Metastatic clear cell renal cell carcinoma. Cohesive cluster of malignant epithelial cells with abundant, vacuolated cytoplasm and prominent nucleoli (Diff-Quik stain).

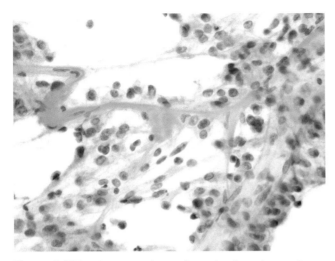

Figure 2.181. Metastatic clear cell renal cell carcinoma. Loose fragments of malignant epithelial cells are associated with prominent vessels (Pap stain).

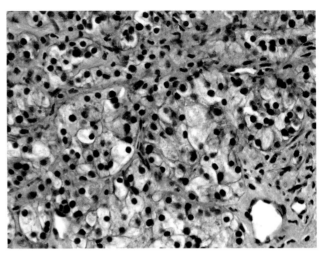

Figure 2.182. Metastatic clear cell renal cell carcinoma. Core biopsy showing the nested nature of this cell population and the prominent, vacuolated cytoplasm (H&E).

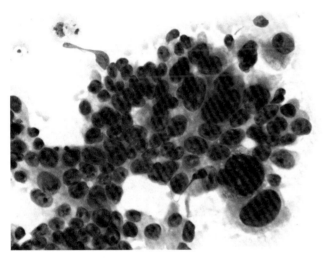

Figure 2.183. Metastatic adenocarcinoma of the lung. Cluster of disorganized malignant cells with enlarged, irregular nuclei and prominent nucleoli (Diff-Quik stain).

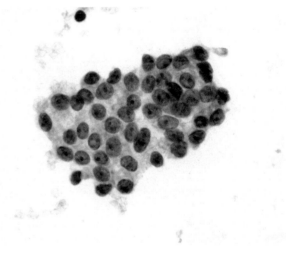

Figure 2.184. Metastatic adenocarcinoma of the lung. Cohesive cluster of epithelial cells showing a loss of the normal honeycomb architecture, as well as enlarged nuclei with prominent nucleoli (Pap stain).

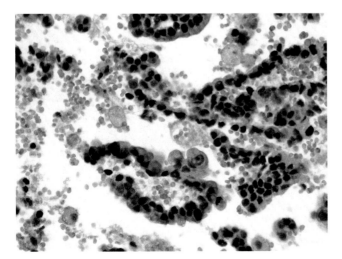

Figure 2.185. Metastatic adenocarcinoma of the lung. Cell block material showing rudimentary gland formation, cytoplasmic mucin, and nuclear atypia (H&E).

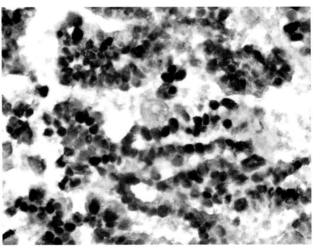

Figure 2.186. Metastatic adenocarcinoma of the lung. Diffuse nuclear TTF-1 staining, which, in this context, supports a diagnosis of a primary adenocarcinoma of the lung. Notably, a Pax-8 stain was also negative, which excluded a thyroid origin (TTF-1 immuno stain).

NEAR MISSES

THYROID TISSUE REMNANT

Although many patients with PTC receive radioactive iodine treatment after a total thyroidectomy, there is no proven benefit to administering this therapy for patients who have PTCs that are <1 cm.[85] As a result, some patients with a history of low-risk PTC may have thyroidal remnants left after thyroidectomy. It is important to keep the anatomy of the cervical lymph nodes in mind when interpreting the FNA material. Level VI is located in the central neck, and many lymph nodes are essentially at the site of the peripheral thyroidectomy surgical bed. If incompletely resected, a portion of the thyroid may be left behind and interpreted as lymphadenopathy on examination. In a patient with a history of lymphocytic thyroiditis, the remnant thyroidal tissue may even mimic a lymph node, owing to the presence of many lymphocytes and germinal centers (Figures 2.191-2.193). Furthermore, there may be reactive atypia secondary to the lymphocytic thyroiditis that is interpreted to be in keeping with PTC. The most important clue is the absence of diagnostic atypical nuclear features; however, many metastatic PTCs are deceptively bland. As a result, it is recommended to exercise caution when interpreting a level VI lymph node in a postthyroidectomy patient who has not received thyroid ablation therapy.

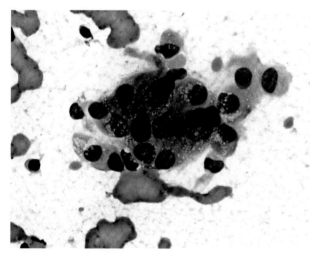

Figure 2.187. Metastatic adenocarcinoma of the breast. Small cluster of atypical epithelial cells with abundant oncocytic cytoplasm and prominent nucleoli (Diff-Quik stain).

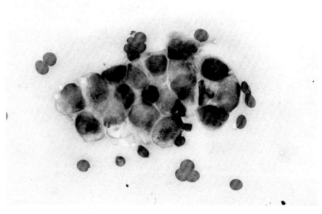

Figure 2.188. Metastatic adenocarcinoma of the breast. Small, cohesive cluster of malignant epithelial cells with large eccentric nuclei and small cytoplasmic mucin vacuoles (Pap stain).

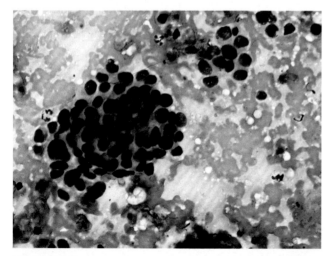

Figure 2.189. Metastatic medullary thyroid carcinoma, confirmed by a positive calcitonin immunostain. Cluster of malignant cells with scant cytoplasm and round to oval, enlarged and hyperchromatic nuclei (Diff-Quik stain).

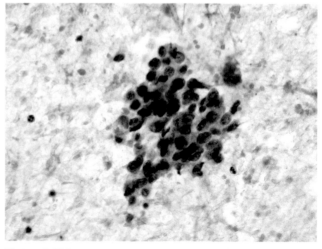

Figure 2.190. Metastatic medullary thyroid carcinoma. Cluster of malignant epithelial cells with salt-and-pepper chromatin (Pap stain).

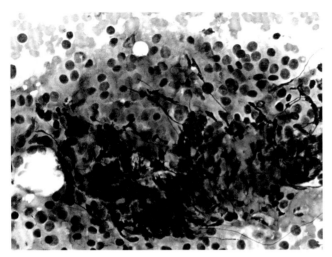

Figure 2.191. Lymphocytic thyroiditis in a thyroid remnant. Follicular epithelium showing Hurthle cell changes adjacent to a lymphoid tangle. Such atypical findings on the aspiration of a suspected lymph node may result in an incorrect diagnosis of metastatic papillary thyroid carcinoma (Diff-Quik stain).

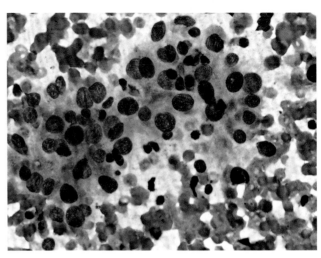

Figure 2.192. Lymphocytic thyroiditis in a thyroid remnant. Follicular epithelium showing Hurthle cell changes/atypia (Diff-Quik stain).

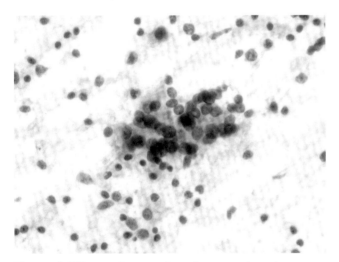

Figure 2.193. Lymphocytic thyroiditis in a thyroid remnant. Follicular epithelium with Hurthle cell changes in a background of lymphocytes (Pap stain).

References

1. Colella G, Cannavale R, Flamminio F, Foschini MP. Fine-needle aspiration cytology of salivary gland lesions: a systematic review. *J Oral Maxillofac Surg*. 2010;68(9):2146-2153.

2. Faquin WC, Powers C. Salivary gland cytopathology. In: Rosenthal DL, ed. *Essentials in Cytopathology*. Vol 5. New York: Springer; 2008.

3. Layfield LJ, Gopez E, Hirschowitz S. Cost efficiency analysis for fine-needle aspiration in the workup of parotid and submandibular gland nodules. *Diagn Cytopathol*. 2006;34(11):734-738.

4. Novoa E, Gurtler N, Arnoux A, Kraft M. Diagnostic value of core needle biopsy and fine-needle aspiration in salivary gland lesions. *Head Neck*. 2016;38(suppl 1):E346-E352.

5. Schmidt RL, Hall BJ, Wilson AR, Layfield LJ. A systematic review and meta-analysis of the diagnostic accuracy of fine-needle aspiration cytology for parotid gland lesions. *Am J Clin Pathol*. 2011;136(1):45-59.

6. Song IH, Song JS, Sung CO, et al. Accuracy of core needle biopsy versus fine needle aspiration cytology for diagnosing salivary gland tumors. *J Pathol Transl Med*. 2015;49(2):136-143.

7. Wei S, Layfield LJ, LiVolsi VA, Montone KT, Baloch ZW. Reporting of fine needle aspiration (FNA) specimens of salivary gland lesions: a comprehensive review. *Diagn Cytopathol*. 2017;45(9):820-827.

8. Faquin WC, Rossi ED. *The Milan System for Reporting Salivary Gland Cytopathology*. New York, NY: Springer Science+Business Media; 2018.

9. Nagel H, Laskawi R, Büter Johann J, Schröder M, Chilla R, Droese M. Cytologic diagnosis of acinic-cell carcinoma of salivary glands. *Diagn Cytopathol*. 1998;16(5):402-412.

10. VandenBussche CJ, Ali SZ, Faquin WC, Maleki Z, Bishop JA. *Atlas of Salivary Gland Cytopathology With Histopathologic Correlations*. New York: Demos; 2018.

11. Hegde PN, Prasad HLK, Kumar YS, et al. A rare case of an epidermoid cyst in the parotid gland – which was diagnosed by fine needle aspiration cytology. *J Clin Diagn Res*. 2013;7(3):550-552.

12. Allison Derek B, McCuiston Austin M, Kawamoto S, Eisele David W, Bishop Justin A, Maleki Z. Cystic major salivary gland lesions: utilizing fine needle aspiration to optimize the clinical management of a broad and diverse differential diagnosis. *Diagn Cytopathol*. 2017;45(9):800-807.

13. Griffith CC, Schmitt AC, Little JL, Magliocca KR. New developments in salivary gland pathology: clinically useful ancillary testing and new potentially targetable molecular alterations. *Arch Pathol Lab Med*. 2017;141(3):381-395.

14. Jo VY, Krane JF. Ancillary testing in salivary gland cytology: a practical guide. *Cancer Cytopathol*. 2018;126(S8):627-642.

15. Ganesan A, Nandakumar GK. Epidermal cyst of parotid gland: a rarity and a diagnostic dilemma. *Case Rep Dent*. 2015;2015:3.

16. El-Naggar AK, Chan JK, Grandis JR, et al. *World Health Organization (WHO) Classification of Head and Neck Tumours*. Lyon, France: IARC Press; 2017.

17. Veder LL, Kerrebijn JDF, Smedts FM, den Bakker MA. Diagnostic accuracy of fine-needle aspiration cytology in Warthin tumors. *Head Neck*. 2010;32(12):1635-1640.

18. Liao X, Haghighi P, Coffey CS, Xu X. A rare case of exclusively oncocytic mucoepidermoid carcinoma with MAML2 translocation. *Rare Tumors*. 2016;8(2):6166.

19. Patel NR, Sanghvi S, Khan MN, Husain Q, Baredes S, Eloy JA. Demographic trends and disease-specific survival in salivary acinic cell carcinoma: an analysis of 1129 cases. *Laryngoscope*. 2014;124(1):172-178.

20. Ali SZ. Acinic-cell carcinoma, papillary-cystic variant: a diagnostic dilemma in salivary gland aspiration. *Diagn Cytopathol*. 2002;27(4):244-250.

21. Inaba T, Fukumura Y, Saito T, et al. Cytological features of mammary analogue secretory carcinoma of the parotid gland in a 15-year-old girl: a case report with review of the literature. *Case Rep Pathol*. 2015;2015:656107.

22. Lewis JS, Beadle B, Bishop JA, et al. Human papillomavirus testing in head and neck carcinomas: guideline from the College of American Pathologists. *Arch Pathol Lab Med*. 2017;142(5):559-597.

23. McDowell LJ, Young RJ, Johnston ML, et al. p16-positive lymph node metastases from cutaneous head and neck squamous cell carcinoma: No association with high-risk human papillomavirus or prognosis and implications for the workup of the unknown primary. *Cancer*. 2016;122(8):1201-1208.

24. Faquin WC, Powers CN. Cystic and mucinous lesions: mucocele and low-grade mucoepidermoid carcinoma. In: Faquin WC, Powers CN, eds. *Salivary Gland Cytopathology*. Boston, MA: Springer US; 2008:159-181.

25. Taxy JB. Necrotizing squamous/mucinous metaplasia in oncocytic salivary gland tumors. A potential diagnostic problem. *Am J Clin Pathol*. 1992;97(1):40-45.

26. Guo SP, Cheuk W, Chan JKC. Pleomorphic adenoma with mucinous and squamous differentiation: a mimicker of mucoepidermoid carcinoma. *Int J Surg Pathol*. 2009;17(4):335-337.

27. Rupani A, Kavishwar V, Achinmane V, Puranik G. Fine needle aspiration cytology of low-grade mucoepidermoid carcinoma of the parotid gland: a diagnostic challenge. *J Cytol*. 2008;25(3):115-116.

28. Klijanienko J, Vielh P. Fine-needle sampling of salivary gland lesions IV. Review of 50 cases of mucoepidermoid carcinoma with histologic correlation. *Diagn Cytopathol*. 1997;17(2):92-98.

29. Skálová A, Vanecek T, Sima R, et al. Mammary analogue secretory carcinoma of salivary glands, containing the ETV6-NTRK3 fusion gene: a hitherto undescribed salivary gland tumor entity. *Am J Surg Pathol*. 2010;34(5):599-608.

30. Jayaprakash V, Merzianu M, Warren GW, et al. Survival rates and prognostic factors for infiltrating salivary duct carcinoma: analysis of 228 cases from the surveillance, epidemiology, and end results database. *Head Neck*. 2014;36(5):694-701.

31. Williams L, Thompson LDR, Seethala RR, et al. Salivary duct carcinoma: the predominance of apocrine morphology, prevalence of histologic variants, and androgen receptor expression. *Am J Surg Pathol.* 2015;39(5):705-713.

32. Masubuchi T, Tada Y, Maruya S, et al. Clinicopathological significance of androgen receptor, HER2, Ki-67 and EGFR expressions in salivary duct carcinoma. *Int J Clin Oncol.* 2015;20(1): 35-44.

33. Geyer JT, Ferry JA, Harris NL, et al. Chronic sclerosing sialadenitis (Küttner tumor) is an IgG4-associated disease. *Am J Surg Pathol.* 2010;34(2):202-210.

34. Carbone A, Gloghini A, Ferlito A. Pathological features of lymphoid proliferations of the salivary glands: lymphoepithelial sialadenitis versus low-grade B-cell lymphoma of the malt type. *Ann Otol Rhinol Laryngol.* 2000;109(12):1170-1175.

35. Bertram HC, Check IJ, Milano MA. Immunophenotyping large B-cell lymphomas. Flow cytometric pitfalls and pathologic correlation. *Am J Clin Pathol.* 2001;116(2):191-203.

36. Chen L, Ray N, He H, Hoschar A. Cytopathologic analysis of stroma-poor salivary gland epithelial/myoepithelial neoplasms on fine needle aspiration. *Acta Cytol.* 2012;56(1):25-33.

37. Savera AT, Sloman A, Huvos AG, Klimstra DS. Myoepithelial carcinoma of the salivary glands: a clinicopathologic study of 25 patients. *Am J Surg Pathol.* 2000;24(6):761-774.

38. Ahn S, Kim Y, Oh YL. Fine needle aspiration cytology of benign salivary gland tumors with myoepithelial cell participation: an institutional experience of 575 cases. *Acta Cytol.* 2013;57(6):567-574.

39. Allison DB, McCuiston A, VandenBussche CJ. The presence of neuroendocrine features generates a broad differential diagnosis in the fine-needle aspiration of bone and soft tissue neoplasms. *J Am Soc Cytopathol.* 2017;6(5):185-193.

40. Prayson RA, Sebek BA. Parotid gland malignant melanomas. *Arch Pathol Lab Med.* 2000;124(12):1780-1784.

41. Mesa M, Quesada JL, Piñas J. Metastasis of amelanotic melanoma of unknown origin in the parotid gland. *Br J Oral Maxillofac Surg.* 2009;47(7):569-571.

42. Wang BY, Lawson W, Robinson RA, Perez-Ordonez B, Brandwein M. Malignant melanomas of the parotid: comparison of survival for patients with metastases from known vs unknown primary tumor sites. *Arch Otolaryngol Head Neck Surg.* 1999;125(6):635-639.

43. Wilson TC, Robinson RA. Basal cell adenocarcinoma and basal cell adenoma of the salivary glands: a clinicopathological review of seventy tumors with comparison of morphologic features and growth control indices. *Head Neck Pathol.* 2015;9(2):205-213.

44. Luna MA, Batsakis JG, El-Naggar AK. Basaloid monomorphic adenomas. *Ann Otol Rhinol Laryngol.* 1991;100(8):687-690.

45. Muller S, Barnes L. Basal cell adenocarcinoma of the salivary glands: report of seven cases and review of the literature. *Cancer.* 1996;78(12):2471-2477.

46. Aisagbonhi OA, Tulecke MA, Wilbur DC, et al. Fine-needle aspiration of epithelial-myoepithelial carcinoma of the parotid gland with prominent adenoid cystic carcinoma–like cribriform features: avoiding a diagnostic pitfall. *Am J Clin Pathol.* 2016;146(6):741-746.

47. Jo VY, Sholl LM, Krane JF. Distinctive patterns of CTNNB1 (β-catenin) alterations in salivary gland basal cell adenoma and basal cell adenocarcinoma. *Am J Surg Pathol.* 2016;40(8):1143-1150.

48. Das DK, Haji BE, Ahmed MS, Riyad Hossain MN. Myoepithelioma of the parotid gland initially diagnosed by fine needle aspiration cytology and immunocytochemistry. *Acta Cytol.* 2005;49(1):65-70.

49. Rooper L, Sharma R, Bishop JA. Polymorphous low grade adenocarcinoma has a consistent p63+/p40− immunophenotype that helps distinguish it from adenoid cystic carcinoma and cellular pleomorphic adenoma. *Head Neck Pathol.* 2015;9(1):79-84.

50. Singh FM, Mak SY, Bonington SC. Patterns of spread of head and neck adenoid cystic carcinoma. *Clin Radiol.* 2015;70(6):644-653.

51. West RB, Kong C, Clarke N, et al. MYB expression and translocation in adenoid cystic carcinomas and other salivary gland tumors with clinicopathologic correlation. *Am J Surg Pathol.* 2011;35(1):92-99.

52. Brill Ii LB, Kanner WA, Fehr A, et al. Analysis of MYB expression and MYB-NFIB gene fusions in adenoid cystic carcinoma and other salivary neoplasms. *Mod Pathol.* 2011;24:1169.

53. Persson M, Andrén Y, Mark J, Horlings HM, Persson F, Stenman G. Recurrent fusion of MYB and NFIB transcription factor genes in carcinomas of the breast and head and neck. *Proc Natl Acad Sci USA.* 2009;106(44):18740-18744.

54. Kimple AJ, Austin GK, Shah RN, et al. Polymorphous low-grade adenocarcinoma: a case series and determination of recurrence. *Laryngoscope*. 2014;124(12):2714-2719.

55. Patel TD, Vazquez A, Marchiano E, Park RC, Baredes S, Eloy JA. Polymorphous low-grade adenocarcinoma of the head and neck: a population-based study of 460 cases. *Laryngoscope*. 2015;125(7):1644-1649.

56. Klijanienko J, Vielh P. Salivary carcinomas with papillae: cytology and histology analysis of polymorphous low-grade adenocarcinoma and papillary cystadenocarcinoma. *Diagn Cytopathol*. 1998;19(4):244-249.

57. Rooper LM, Onenerk M, Siddiqui MT, Faquin WC, Bishop JA, Ali SZ. Nodular oncocytic hyperplasia: can cytomorphology allow for the preoperative diagnosis of a nonneoplastic salivary disease? *Cancer Cytopathol*. 2017;125(8):627-634.

58. Fujimaki M, Fukumura Y, Saito T, et al. Oncocytic mucoepidermoid carcinoma of the parotid gland with CRTC1-MAML2 fusion transcript: report of a case with review of literature. *Hum Pathol*. 2011;42(12):2052-2055.

59. Di Palma S, Simpson RHW, Marchiò C, et al. Salivary duct carcinomas can be classified into luminal androgen receptor-positive, HER2 and basal-like phenotypes*. *Histopathology*. 2012;61(4):629-643.

60. Locati LD, Perrone F, Cortelazzi B, et al. Clinical activity of androgen deprivation therapy in patients with metastatic/relapsed androgen receptor–positive salivary gland cancers. *Head Neck*. 2016;38(5):724-731.

61. Kapadia SB, Barnes L. Expression of androgen receptor, gross cystic disease fluid protein, and CD44 in salivary duct carcinoma. *Mod Pathol*. 1998;11(11):1033-1038.

62. Skalova A, Weinreb I, Hyrcza M, et al. Clear cell myoepithelial carcinoma of salivary glands showing EWSR1 rearrangement: molecular analysis of 94 salivary gland carcinomas with prominent clear cell component. *Am J Surg Pathol*. 2015;39(3):338-348.

63. Seethala RR, Barnes EL, Hunt JL. Epithelial-myoepithelial carcinoma: a review of the clinicopathologic spectrum and immunophenotypic characteristics in 61 tumors of the salivary glands and upper aerodigestive tract. *Am J Surg Pathol*. 2007;31(1):44-57.

64. Vazquez A, Patel TD, D'Aguillo CM, et al. Epithelial-myoepithelial carcinoma of the salivary glands: an analysis of 246 cases. *Otolaryngol Head Neck Surg*. 2015;153(4):569-574.

65. Testa D, Galera F, Insabato L, Vassallo A, Mesolella M, Galli V. Submandibular gland myoepithelioma. *Acta Otolaryngol*. 2005;125(6):664-666.

66. Owosho AA, Aguilar CE, Seethala RR. Comparison of p63 and p40 (ΔNp63) as basal, squamoid, and myoepithelial markers in salivary gland tumors. *Appl Immunohistochem Mol Morphol*. 2016;24(7):501-508.

67. Bishop JA, Montgomery EA, Westra WH. Use of p40 and p63 immunohistochemistry and human papillomavirus testing as ancillary tools for the recognition of head and neck sarcomatoid carcinoma and its distinction from benign and malignant mesenchymal processes. *Am J Surg Pathol*. 2014;38(2):257-264.

68. Fanburg-Smith JC, Majidi M, Miettinen M. Keratin expression in schwannoma; a study of 115 retroperitoneal and 22 peripheral schwannomas. *Mod Pathol*. 2005;19:115.

69. Faquin WC, Powers CN. Spindle cell tumors: spindled myoepithelioma, myoepithelial-predominant pleomorphic adenoma, and schwannoma. In: Faquin WC, Powers CN, eds. *Salivary Gland Cytopathology*. Boston, MA: Springer US; 2008:203-231.

70. Allison DB, Wakely PE Jr, Siddiqui MT, Ali SZ. Nodular fasciitis: a frequent diagnostic pitfall on fine-needle aspiration. *Cancer Cytopathol*. 2017;125(1):20-29.

71. Allison DB, VandenBussche CJ, Rooper LM, et al. Nodular fasciitis of the parotid gland: a challenging diagnosis on FNA. *Cancer Cytopathol*. 2018;126(10):872-880.

72. Erickson-Johnson MR, Chou MM, Evers BR, et al. Nodular fasciitis: a novel model of transient neoplasia induced by MYH9-USP6 gene fusion. *Lab Invest*. 2011;91:1427.

73. Oliveira AM, Chou MM. USP6-induced neoplasms: the biologic spectrum of aneurysmal bone cyst and nodular fasciitis. *Hum Pathol*. 2014;45(1):1-11.

74. Chen MM, Roman SA, Sosa JA, Judson BL. Prognostic factors for squamous cell cancer of the parotid gland: an analysis of 2104 patients. *Head Neck*. 2015;37(1):1-7.

75. McIlwain WR, Sood AJ, Nguyen SA, Day TA. Initial symptoms in patients with HPV-positive and HPV-negative oropharyngeal cancer. *JAMA Otolaryngol Head Neck Surg*. 2014;140(5):441-447.

76. Begum S, Cao D, Gillison M, Zahurak M, Westra WH. Tissue distribution of human papillomavirus 16 DNA integration in patients with tonsillar carcinoma. *Clin Cancer Res.* 2005;11(16):5694-5699.

77. Gillison ML. Current topics in the epidemiology of oral cavity and oropharyngeal cancers. *Head Neck.* 2007;29(8):779-792.

78. Allison DB, Maleki Z. HPV-related head and neck squamous cell carcinoma: an update and review. *J Am Soc Cytopathol.* 2016;5(4):203-215.

79. Allison DB, Miller JA, Coquia SF, Maleki Z. Ultrasonography-guided fine-needle aspiration with concurrent small core biopsy of neck masses and lymph nodes yields adequate material for HPV testing in head and neck squamous cell carcinomas. *J Am Soc Cytopathol.* 2016;5(1):22-30.

80. Miller JA, Allison DB, Maleki Z. Interpretation of HPV DNA in situ hybridization in HPV-related head and neck squamous cell carcinoma: an achievable task in cell block and small biopsy material. *J Am Soc Cytopathol.* 2017;6(3):89-95.

81. Jalaly JB, Lewis JS, Collins BT, et al. Correlation of p16 immunohistochemistry in FNA biopsies with corresponding tissue specimens in HPV-related squamous cell carcinomas of the oropharynx. *Cancer Cytopathol.* 2015;123(12):723-731.

82. Chaturvedi AK, Anderson WF, Lortet-Tieulent J, et al. Worldwide trends in incidence rates for oral cavity and oropharyngeal cancers. *J Clin Oncol.* 2013;31(36):4550-4559.

83. Hashibe M, Brennan P, Benhamou S, et al. Alcohol drinking in never users of tobacco, cigarette smoking in never drinkers, and the risk of head and neck cancer: pooled analysis in the International Head and Neck Cancer Epidemiology Consortium. *J Natl Cancer Inst.* 2007;99(10):777-789.

84. Swerdlow SH, Campo E, Harris NL, et al, eds. *World Health Organization Classification of Tumours of Haematopoietic and Lymphoid Tissues.* 4th rev ed. Lyon: IARC Press; 2017.

85. Cooper DS, Doherty GM, Haugen BR, et al. Revised American Thyroid Association management guidelines for patients with thyroid nodules and differentiated thyroid cancer. *Thyroid.* 2009;19(11):1167-1214.

CHAPTER OUTLINE

THE UNREMARKABLE LUNG

Pulmonary cytopathology specimens are obtained through a variety of techniques, including sputum, bronchial washings/brushings, bronchoalveolar lavage (BAL), and fine-needle aspiration (FNA) with imaging guidance (computed tomography [CT] or endoscopic ultrasound). Each technique has strengths and weaknesses, and it is important to understand which technique was performed when evaluating a specimen. Pulmonary cytopathology is most often performed to evaluate a radiologic abnormality for both infectious and malignant processes. Having a solid grasp on the normal components of pulmonary cytopathology specimens is not only necessary for adequacy assessment but also serves as a benchmark for distinguishing between metaplasia, reactive atypia, and malignancy.[1] This section will provide a brief overview of the normal components of pulmonary cytology specimens.

SQUAMOUS CELLS

Squamous cells usually represent oral contamination in exfoliative cytologic specimens such as sputum, bronchial brushing, bronchial washing, and BAL specimens. These contaminating squamous cells are identical to benign squamous cells from other anatomic sites, such as those commonly seen on Pap test specimens. Most of the squamous cells are superficial and intermediate cells with small nuclei and abundant, platelike cytoplasm, although reactive and/or degenerative changes are commonly seen and should not be over-interpreted (Figure 3.1).

CILIATED BRONCHIAL COLUMNAR CELLS

These are the predominant epithelial cells that line the trachea and bronchi. At the apical surface, there are characteristic cilia attached to a terminal bar; a cytoplasmic tail may be seen at the basal surface (Figures 3.2-3.4). The nuclei are basally oriented and round to oval in shape with evenly dispersed chromatin and small nucleoli. These respiratory bronchial epithelial cells are often the most helpful normal comparator when assessing whether a separate population is malignant.

GOBLET CELLS

The bronchial epithelial lining also includes goblet cells, which are much less common than the ciliated columnar cells (1:5 ratio). Goblet cells are characterized by large, mucin-filled cytoplasmic vacuoles with oval to flattened, basally oriented nuclei (Figures 3.5-3.7).

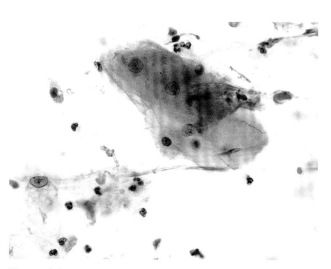

Figure 3.1. Squamous cells consistent with oral contamination. The benign squamous cells are admixed with pulmonary alveolar macrophages and inflammatory cells (Pap stain).

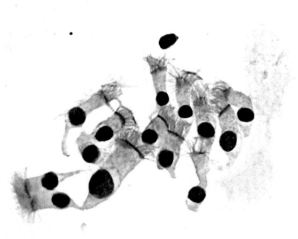

Figure 3.2. Normal ciliated bronchial columnar epithelial cells. At the apical surface, the cells have a terminal bar with attached cilia. At the basal surface, some cells have a cytoplasmic tail (Pap stain).

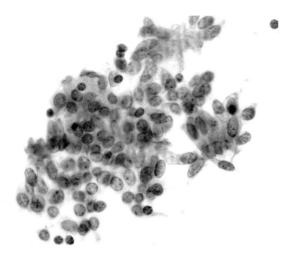

Figure 3.3. Fragment of bronchial epithelial cells. Look to the edge of clusters to find ciliated cells (Pap stain).

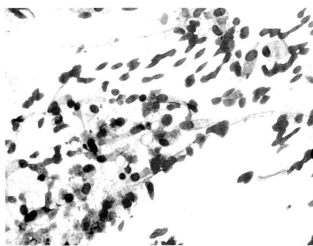

Figure 3.4. Scattered bronchial epithelial cells. Terminal bars/cilia can be seen on some cells, but all cells have basally oriented nuclei with fine, even chromatin and abundant, apical cytoplasm (Pap stain).

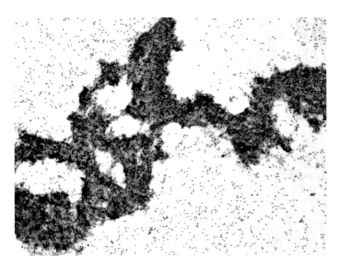

Figure 3.5. Low magnification view of a large fragment of bronchial epithelium with goblet cell hyperplasia (cells with pink vacuoles) (Pap stain).

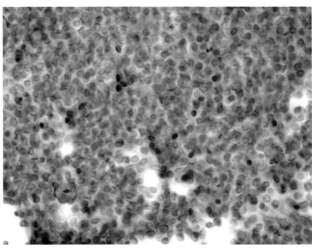

Figure 3.6. Sheet of bronchial epithelial cells with interspersed goblet cells, which are large and round and have pink-staining cytoplasmic mucin (Pap stain).

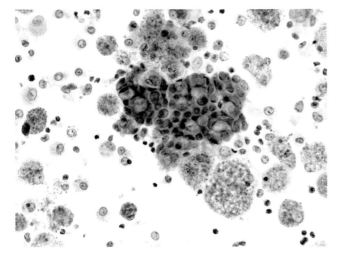

Figure 3.7. Fragment of bronchial epithelium with numerous goblet cells in a background of hemosiderin-laden macrophages. The presence of macrophages indicates adequate sampling from alveolar spaces (Pap stain).

They are more commonly seen in chronic conditions that cause goblet cell hyperplasia such as asthma, chronic bronchitis, and bronchiectasis; this finding should not be over-interpreted as a mucin-producing neoplasm.

PNEUMOCYTES

Type I alveolar pneumocytes are the flat cells that form the alveolar gas exchange surface and are not typically seen in cytologic specimens. Type II pneumocytes are responsible for secreting surfactant and are seen in cytologic specimens in reactive and pathologic states. Type II pneumocytes usually have round nuclei with regular borders and abundant cytoplasm. They can be difficult to definitively distinguish from alveolar macrophages in cytologic specimens, but this distinction is rarely, if ever, necessary.

ALVEOLAR MACROPHAGES

Alveolar macrophages float freely in the alveolar space and are required for adequacy in sputum and BAL specimens because their presence indicates that the alveolar spaces have been sampled. They appear similarly to macrophages/histiocytes seen in other locations, with variable sizes, vesicular nuclei with fine chromatin, and abundant cytoplasm. Alveolar macrophages may contain cytoplasmic pigment, including black carbon pigment (anthracosis), hemosiderin, as well as other materials ingested via phagocytosis (Figures 3.7-3.9).

EPITHELIAL PATTERN

The epithelial pattern consists of both reactive epithelial processes and malignant epithelial neoplasms comprised of cells that derive from and/or appear to recapitulate epithelial lining cells. In the lung, the most common primary carcinomas are adenocarcinomas and squamous cell carcinomas (SqCCs), which are important to distinguish from one another for treatment purposes. In addition, the lung is a common site of metastasis; thus, a common scenario involves the cytologic determination of a primary lung malignancy versus a metastasis. This section will highlight the most common entities that comprise the "Epithelial Pattern"; the presence of epithelial fragments and/or cells with squamous differentiation is additionally covered below in the "Squamous Pattern."

CHECKLIST: Etiologic Considerations for the Epithelial Pattern

☐ Reactive Bronchial Cells and Pneumocytes

☐ Adenocarcinoma

☐ Squamous Cell Carcinoma

☐ Adenosquamous Carcinoma

☐ Non–Small Cell Carcinoma

☐ Malignant Mesothelioma

☐ Metastatic Carcinoma

REACTIVE BRONCHIAL CELLS AND PNEUMOCYTES

Reactive bronchial cells can show nuclear enlargement, multinucleation, pleomorphism, hyperchromasia, coarse chromatin, and prominent nucleoli—all features that can be seen in malignant neoplasms (Figures 3.10-3.22).

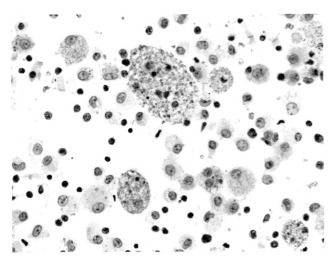

Figure 3.8. Pulmonary alveolar macrophages, some of which contain hemosiderin. There are also scattered ciliated bronchial epithelial cells in the background (Pap stain).

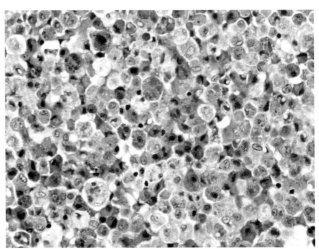

Figure 3.9. Sheet of hemosiderin-laden macrophages on cell block (H&E).

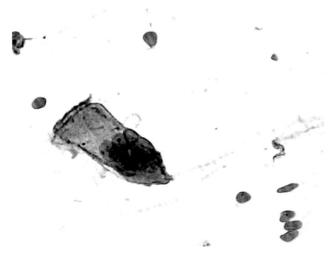

Figure 3.10. Reactive multinucleated bronchial epithelial cell. All the nuclei are still small and basally oriented, and cilia are present at the apical surface (Pap stain).

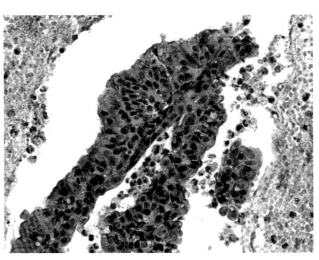

Figure 3.11. Reactive bronchial epithelium with enlarged, hyperchromatic nuclei and occasional prominent nucleoli on a cell block preparation. Although there is pseudostratification, the cells are still oriented and retain some resemblance to normal architecture. Terminal bars and cilia can also be seen (H&E).

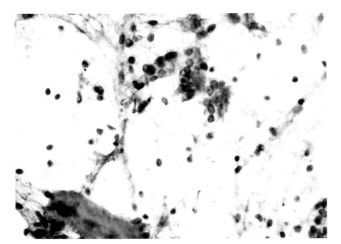

Figure 3.12. Reactive bronchial epithelial cells with enlarged nuclei and prominent nucleoli. Cilia can still be appreciated on these cells (Pap stain).

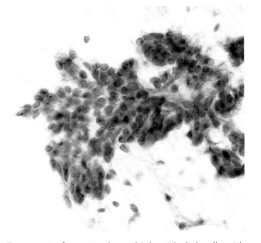

Figure 3.13. Fragment of reactive bronchial epithelial cells with enlarged, slightly overlapping, somewhat hyperchromatic nuclei with inconspicuous nucleoli. Look for cilia at the edges of fragments (Pap stain).

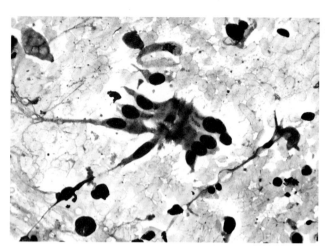

Figure 3.14. Reactive bronchial epithelial cells. Although the nuclei are enlarged, the nuclear membranes are smooth, and cilia are present at the apical surfaces (Diff-Quik stain).

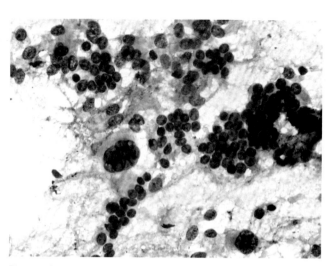

Figure 3.15. Reactive bronchial epithelial cells. They can occasionally be multinucleated, as seen scattered in this field (Diff-Quik stain).

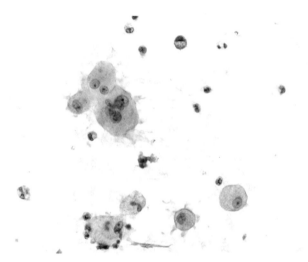

Figure 3.16. Multinucleated giant cell histiocytes and pulmonary alveolar macrophages. Note the vacuolated cytoplasm (Pap stain).

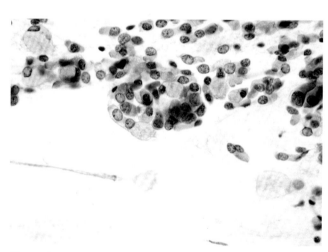

Figure 3.17. Benign bronchial epithelial cells with mucinous metaplasia (Pap stain).

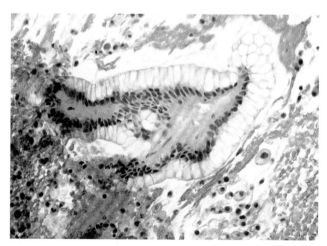

Figure 3.18. Tissue fragment of benign bronchial epithelial cells with mucinous metaplasia on a cell block preparation. The cells are uniformly polarized with small bland nuclei (H&E).

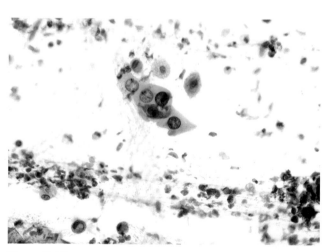

Figure 3.19. Reactive bronchial epithelial cells. In the center of the field, there are atypical epithelial cells that are favored to be reactive in origin. Although the cells are enlarged and stand out from the background inflammatory component, the nuclear contours are uniform, round, and smooth (Pap stain).

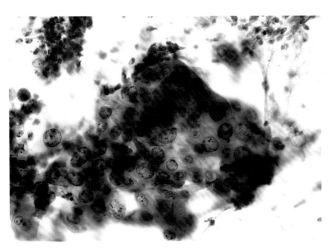

Figure 3.20. Reactive bronchial epithelial cells. This fragment of atypical cells demonstrates multinucleation and pleomorphism, but the lack of crowding, hyperchromasia, or nuclear membrane abnormalities favors these cells to be reactive in nature (Pap stain).

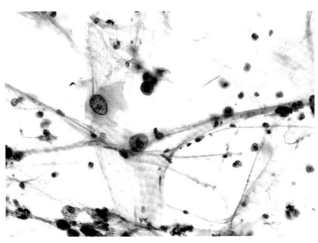

Figure 3.21. Atypical epithelial cells with degenerative changes. The nucleus of the large atypical cell is large but has smooth contours (Pap stain).

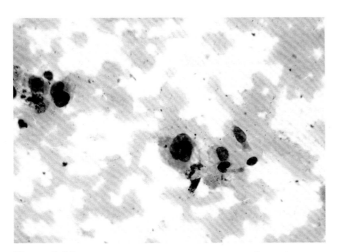

Figure 3.22. Atypical epithelial cells, suspicious for malignancy. These highly atypical cells have marked nuclear enlargement, hyperchromasia, and nuclear membrane irregularities. These single atypical cells should raise suspicion for a malignant process (Diff-Quik stain).

TABLE 3.1: Relevant Gene Biomarkers With Targeted Therapies in Non–Small Cell Lung Cancers With Adenocarcinoma Component

Gene	Frequency and Demographics	CAP/IASLC/AMP Recommendation	Testing Method
EGFR	10-20% More common in women, non smokers, and Asian patients[16]	Must be tested on all lung adenocarcinoma patients	PCR-based methods followed by multiplexed sequencing panel (e.g., next-generation sequencing)
ALK	6% Usually seen in younger patients	Must be tested on all lung adenocarcinoma patients	FISH IHC is an equivalent alternative to FISH (on FFPE samples)

TABLE 3.1: Relevant Gene Biomarkers With Targeted Therapies in Non–Small Cell Lung Cancers With Adenocarcinoma Component—Continued

Gene	Frequency and Demographics	CAP/IASLC/AMP Recommendation	Testing Method
ROS1	2% Usually seen in young non smokers	Must be tested on all lung adenocarcinoma patients	IHC can be used as a screening test; however, positive ROS1 IHC results should be confirmed by a molecular (RT-PCR) or cytogenetic (FISH) method
KRAS	30% Usually seen in smokers	Not indicated as routine stand-alone test outside the context of a clinical trial; can be included as part of larger testing panels	Multiplexed sequencing panel (e.g., next-generation sequencing)
MET, BRAF, ERBB2 (HER2), RET	6% MET 2% BRAF 2% ERBB2 (HER2) 1% RET	Not indicated as routine stand-alone test outside the context of a clinical trial; can be included as part of larger testing panels	Multiplexed sequencing panel (e.g., next-generation sequencing)

Adapted from Rodriguez EF, Monaco SE. Recent advances in the pathology and molecular genetics of lung cancer: a practical review for cytopathologists. *J Am Soc Cytopathol.* 2016;5(5):252-265 and Jain D, Roy-Chowdhuri S. Molecular pathology of lung cancer cytology specimens: a concise review. *Arch Pathol Lab Med.* 2018;142(9):1127-1133.

ALK, anaplastic lymphoma kinase; EGFR, epidermal growth factor receptor; FFPE, formalin-fixed, paraffin-embedded; FISH, fluorescence in situ hybridization; IHC, immunohistochemistry; PCR, polymerase chain reaction; RT-PCR, reverse transcriptase-polymerase chain reaction.

Reactive type II pneumocytes and alveolar macrophages can occur singly and in clusters and can appear atypical, with many of the same features seen in reactive bronchial cells. In addition, the cells can have increased nuclear to cytoplasmic (N/C) ratios and more three-dimensional clustering. In reactive conditions, they may be seen in great numbers, emulating a neoplastic process. These cells can also be mistaken for well differentiated adenocarcinoma, which is often the main differential diagnosis. Overall, the cell population of interest should be less numerous in a reactive lesion compared with a well-sampled well differentiated adenocarcinoma, especially in FNA specimens. However, exfoliative specimens can contain benign reactive cells in large numbers, and thus cellularity is not always a helpful feature in these specimen types.

ADENOCARCINOMA

Lung adenocarcinoma is the most common primary malignancy of the lung and usually arises in a peripheral location, in contrast to SqCC and small cell lung carcinoma. Invasive adenocarcinoma is classified into different subtypes based on the predominant histologic pattern: lepidic, acinar, papillary, micropapillary, and solid. The micropapillary and solid patterns portend a worse prognosis; however, invasive mucinous adenocarcinoma (a variant of lung adenocarcinoma) is also associated with a worse prognosis compared with nonmucinous adenocarcinomas.[2-4]

The cytologic features of lung adenocarcinomas vary depending on the histologic patterns.[5] Although the morphologic features of the different patterns can be seen on cytology samples, adenocarcinomas are not subclassified on cytology specimens.[6] In general, the cells resemble glandular epithelium and are cohesive with fine chromatin, large nucleoli, and thin/foamy cytoplasm (Figures 3.23-3.51). The formation of certain architectural patterns (e.g., acinar or papillary formations) or the presence of mucinous differentiation strongly suggests an adenocarcinoma.

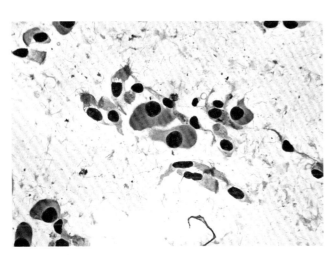

Figure 3.23. Lung adenocarcinoma. These large neoplastic epithelioid cells are admixed with benign bronchial epithelial cells (Diff-Quik stain).

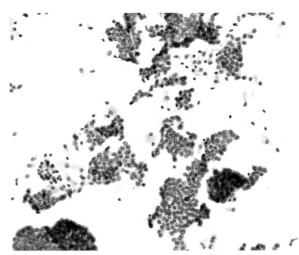

Figure 3.24. Lung adenocarcinoma. The smear is highly cellular and composed primarily glandular epithelium with nuclear enlargement and minimal overlap. The cells are monomorphic and may be difficult to distinguish from tissue fragments of benign respiratory epithelium—a challenge with many well differentiated lung adenocarcinomas (Pap stain).

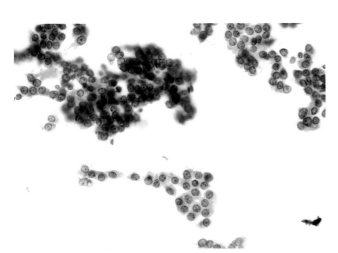

Figure 3.25. Well differentiated lung adenocarcinoma. The neoplastic cells are uniform in shape and size with minimal overlapping and inconspicuous nucleoli. The neoplastic cells are distributed in sheets and glands (Pap stain).

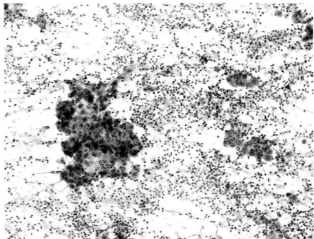

Figure 3.26. Well differentiated lung adenocarcinoma on an intraoperative smear. The fragments of neoplastic cells stand out from the background inflammation given their marked nuclear enlargement and prominent nucleoli. The neoplastic cells are monomorphic, which is a helpful distinguishing feature from reactive processes (H&E).

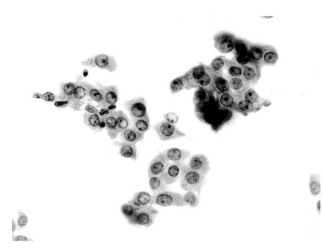

Figure 3.27. Well differentiated lung adenocarcinoma. Note the absence of a terminal bar and cilia and the presence of enlarged nuclei with prominent nucleoli (Pap stain).

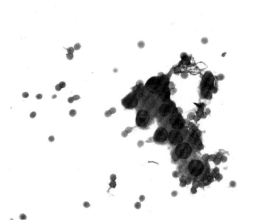

Figure 3.28. Well differentiated lung adenocarcinoma. The cells are monomorphic and have abundant cytoplasm and prominent nucleoli (Diff-Quik stain).

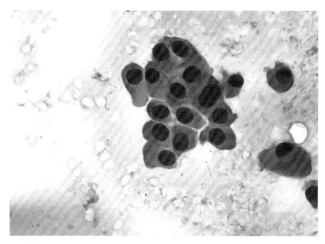

Figure 3.29. Well differentiated lung adenocarcinoma. Note the deceptively bland nuclear features (Diff-Quik stain).

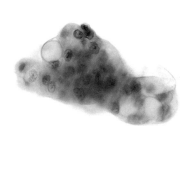

Figure 3.30. Moderately differentiated lung adenocarcinoma. Lumens are present in this three-dimensional group, indicating its glandular nature. The individual cells are notable for their marked nuclear membrane irregularities and cellular overlap (Pap stain).

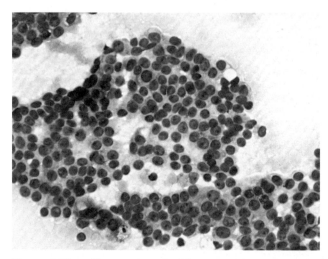

Figure 3.31. Well to moderately differentiated lung adenocarcinoma. The cells have increased N/C ratios, mild pleomorphism, and nuclear overlapping. However, the glandular architecture can still be readily appreciated (Diff-Quik stain).

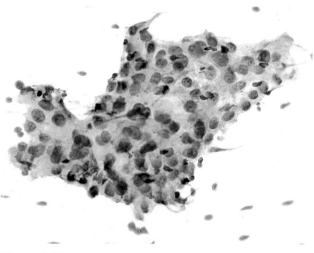

Figure 3.32. Moderately differentiated lung adenocarcinoma. Note the increased nuclear crowding and anisonucleosis. The cytoplasm is granular, and the cell borders are indistinct (Pap stain).

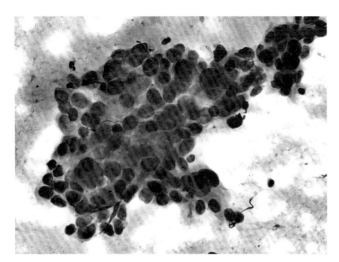

Figure 3.33. Moderately differentiated lung adenocarcinoma. The cells have a disorganized architectural arrangement (Pap stain).

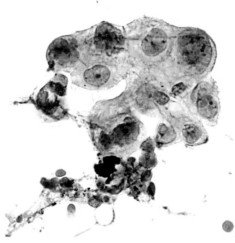

Figure 3.34. Moderately differentiated lung adenocarcinoma. There is marked nuclear enlargement, irregular chromatin, and significant pleomorphism; however, the presence of intracytoplasmic vacuoles supports a diagnosis of adenocarcinoma (Pap stain).

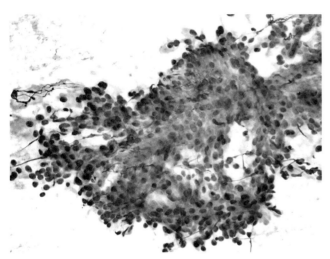

Figure 3.35. Papillary pattern of lung adenocarcinoma. Fibrovascular cores are lined by malignant glandular epithelial cells. The presence of specific patterns can aid in the diagnosis of lung adenocarcinoma (Diff-Quik stain).

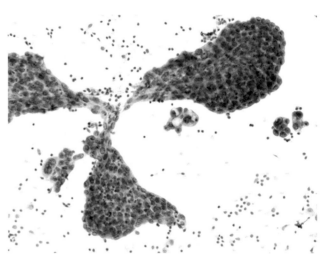

Figure 3.36. Papillary pattern of lung adenocarcinoma. The neoplastic cells are arranged in papillary fronds and in small clusters with intracytoplasmic vacuoles (Pap stain).

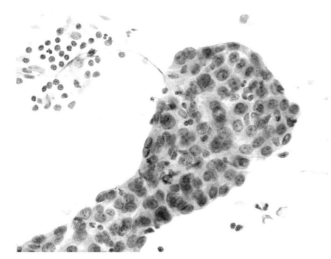

Figure 3.37. Papillary pattern of lung adenocarcinoma. Note the marked nuclear enlargement as compared with the lymphocytes present in the background (Pap stain).

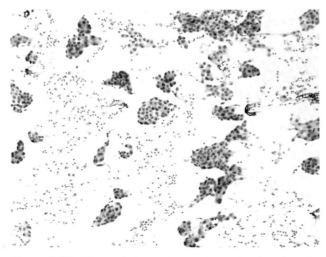

Figure 3.38. Metastatic lung adenocarcinoma in a lymph node. There are numerous cohesive fragments of malignant epithelioid cells standing out as a second population in a background of predominately lymphocytes (Pap stain).

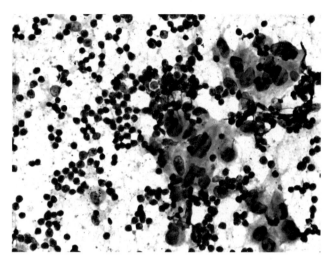

Figure 3.39. Metastatic lung adenocarcinoma in a lymph node. Note the large nuclei and abundant cytoplasm that makes the neoplastic cells easily distinguished from the background lymphoid cells (Diff-Quik stain).

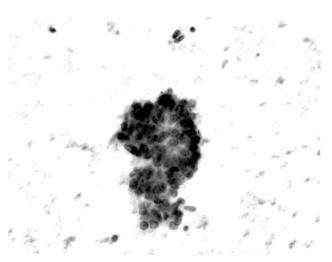

Figure 3.40. Lung adenocarcinoma. Be cautious of interpreting background blood at the periphery of atypical fragments as cilia. The cells are forming a three-dimensional structure, have high N/C ratios, and are hyperchromatic (Pap stain).

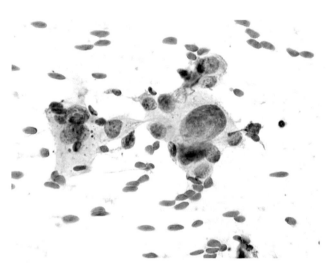

Figure 3.41. Lung adenocarcinoma with marked anisonucleosis (Pap stain).

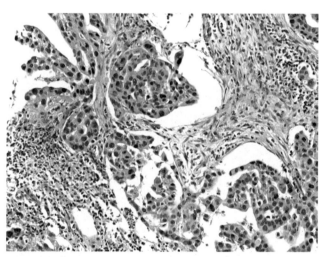

Figure 3.42. Lung adenocarcinoma on cell block with background inflammation (H&E).

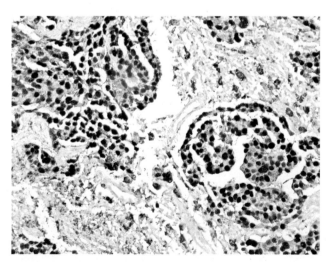

Figure 3.43. Lung adenocarcinoma with positive nuclear TTF-1 and cytoplasmic napsin A expression (brown on a TTF-1/napsin A/p40 triple immunostain).

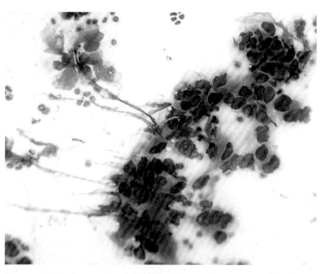

Figure 3.44. Lung adenocarcinoma smear from case with high PD-L1 expression (Diff-Quik stain).

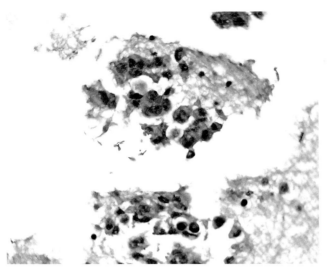

Figure 3.45. Lung adenocarcinoma cell block corresponding to the previous smear (H&E).

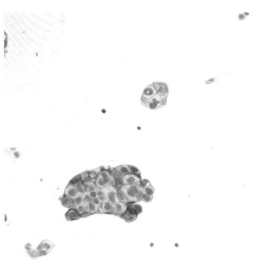

Figure 3.46. Positive membranous PD-L1 staining of lung adenocarcinoma in the previous cell block (PD-L1 immunostain).

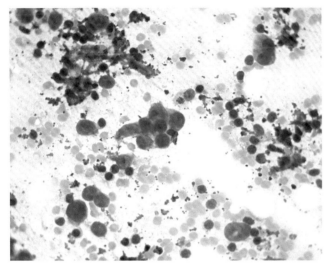

Figure 3.47. Lung adenocarcinoma smear from case with *ALK* mutation (Diff-Quik stain).

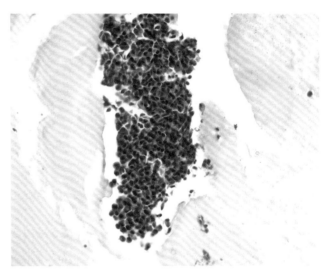

Figure 3.48. Lung adenocarcinoma cell block corresponding to the previous smear (H&E).

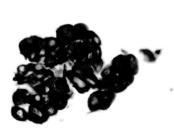

Figure 3.49. Positive cytoplasmic staining for the ALK (anaplastic lymphoma kinase) protein in lung adenocarcinoma (ALK immunostain).

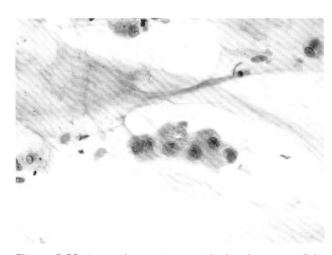

Figure 3.50. Lung adenocarcinoma with abundant extracellular mucin. The presence of only extracellular mucin without intracytoplasmic mucin is not diagnostic of mucinous adenocarcinoma (Pap stain).

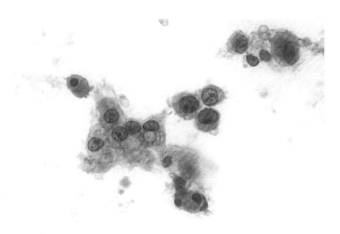

Figure 3.51. Mucinous adenocarcinoma with intracytoplasmic mucin vacuoles (Pap stain).

FAQ: What are the recommendations for molecular testing in non–small cell lung cancers?

Answer: Increasing numbers of mutations in oncogenic driver genes involved in the pathogenesis of non–small cell lung carcinomas (NSCLCs) are being identified, and approved targeted therapies are becoming increasingly available.[7-15] Thus, it has now become the standard of care to test for these molecular alterations in all NSCLCs in which an adenocarcinoma component cannot be excluded. The current basic guidelines from the College of American Pathologists/International Association for the Study of Lung Cancer/Association for Molecular Pathology (CAP/IASLC/AMP) are presented in Table 3.1.[19] Of note, programmed death-ligand 1 (PD-L1) testing using immunohistochemistry has not yet been validated on cytology specimens but has been shown to be comparable to that in histologic specimens with appropriate validation in some studies.[20,21]

SQUAMOUS CELL CARCINOMA

Squamous cell carcinoma (SqCC) accounts for around one-third of primary lung malignancies and tends to arise in a central location. The cytologic features depend on the degree of squamous differentiation: well differentiated tumors are often keratinizing while moderately to poorly differentiated tumors often do not show evidence of keratinization. Well differentiated SqCC characteristically shows abundant keratinization and markedly pleomorphic single cells (Figures 3.52-3.60). Moderately to poorly differentiated SqCC tends to be more cohesive and uniform, with individual malignant cells that have higher N/C ratios (Table 3.2). Poorly differentiated SqCC can be difficult to distinguish from adenocarcinoma. Importantly, metastatic SqCC to the lung often cannot be distinguished from a primary SqCC using morphology alone.

KEY FEATURES of Squamous Cell Carcinoma
Well differentiated SqCC

- The neoplastic cells are present in tissue fragments as well as singly dispersed.
- The neoplastic cells have diverse cell shapes: polygonal, round, tadpole/spindle, etc.
- The neoplastic cells have dense, waxy, and/or hard-appearing cytoplasm with distinct cell outlines.
- The nuclei are typically pyknotic and/or hyperchromatic, though anucleate "ghost" cells can also be seen.
- Keratinization and/or keratin pearl formation may be present and are helpful indicators of squamous differentiation.
- The background may be necrotic.

Moderately to poorly differentiated SqCC

- The neoplastic cells have large nuclei, high N/C ratios, and prominent nucleoli and/or coarse chromatin.
- There is often prominent anisonucleosis and pleomorphism of the neoplastic cells.
- There is absent to rare keratinization.

PEARLS & PITFALLS

With regard to immunostaining pattern, TTF-1 positivity carries the most weight, as it is not positive in any SqCCs. For example, if TTF-1 is positive, but p63 or p40 is also positive in some of the same cells, the favored diagnosis is still adenocarcinoma. If the staining profile is inconclusive, a diagnosis of "non–small cell carcinoma" can be rendered and molecular testing should be performed (see Non–Small Cell Carcinoma section below). Although TTF-1 is positive in most lung adenocarcinomas, a small subset can be negative; furthermore, many additional malignancies can be positive for TTF-1, including small cell lung carcinoma.[28,29] A special stain for mucin (mucicarmine) can be performed; the presence of mucinous vacuoles helps establish the diagnosis of adenocarcinoma.

PEARLS & PITFALLS

On cytology, the terminologies "adenocarcinoma in situ" and "minimally invasive adenocarcinoma" are not used. Often, such lesions are small and not targeted by FNA procedures. These entities are signed out as "adenocarcinoma," which is the goal of cytologic examination. On the other hand, it is crucial to distinguish adenocarcinoma from SqCC, as there are increasing numbers of clinically actionable molecular tests and targeted therapies for these specific carcinoma subtypes.

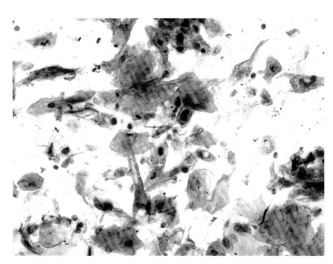

Figure 3.52. Keratinizing squamous cell carcinoma of the lung, with keratinized squamous cells staining an orangeophilic color on Pap stain (Pap stain).

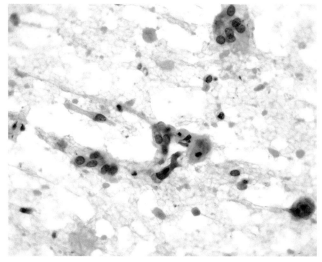

Figure 3.53. Keratinizing squamous cell carcinoma. Note the markedly abnormal keratinizing cell with a pyknotic nucleus and irregular cytoplasmic processes (Pap stain).

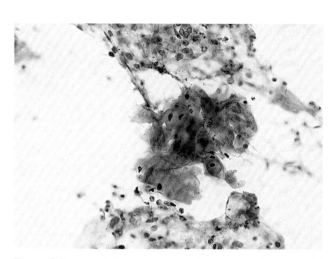

Figure 3.54. Keratinizing squamous cell carcinoma. Separate field (Pap stain).

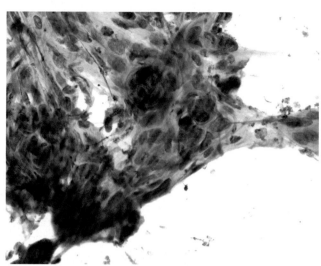

Figure 3.55. Keratin pearls in squamous cell carcinoma of the lung (Pap stain).

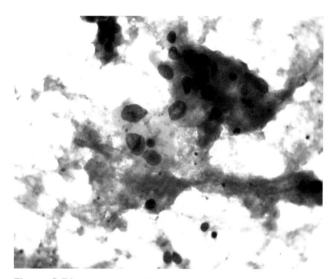

Figure 3.56. Squamous cell carcinoma of the lung. The cells are flat with coarse chromatin and abundant cytoplasm, which has a characteristic greenish-blue "Robin egg blue" color (Diff-Quik stain).

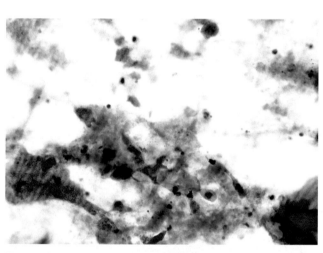

Figure 3.57. Keratinizing squamous cell carcinoma in a background of necrosis. Note the relative paucity of intact, malignant cells in this field (Pap stain).

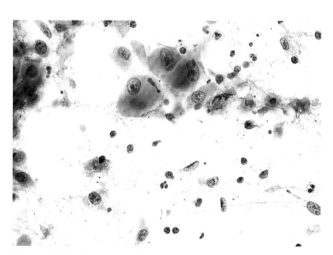

Figure 3.58. Squamous cell carcinoma without obvious keratinization. The cytoplasm is dense and opaque, which is characteristic of squamous differentiation (Pap stain).

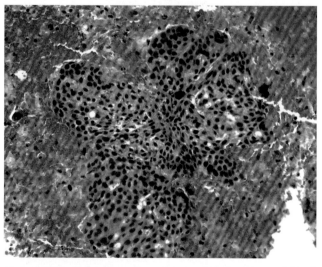

Figure 3.59. Squamous cell carcinoma of the lung in a cell block preparation (H&E).

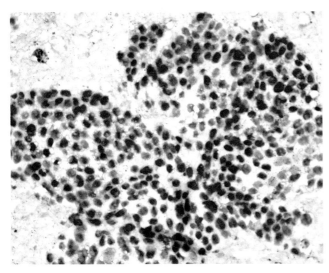

Figure 3.60. Squamous cell carcinoma showing diffuse nuclear p40 expression (red), corresponding to previous cell block (TTF-1/napsin A/p40 triple immunostain).

TABLE 3.2: Morphologic Features of Adenocarcinoma vs. Squamous Cell Carcinoma

Feature	Well to Moderately Differentiated Adenocarcinoma	Squamous Cell Carcinoma
Cohesiveness	Tissue fragments > single cells	Single cells > tissue fragments; often necrotic
Differentiation	Major patterns: • Lepidic: monolayer sheets • Acinar: gland formation • Papillary: papillary fragments • Micropapillary: micropapillae • Solid: 3D clusters Can have mucin production	Keratinization Squamous pearls Intercellular bridges
Nuclei	Round to oval shape Finely granular chromatin Large, central nucleolus Thin nuclear membrane	Irregular, flattened shape Coarsely granular chromatin Small, eccentric nucleolus Thicker nuclear membrane
Cytoplasm	Foamy, vacuolated cytoplasm Indistinct borders	Opaque, "hard" cytoplasm Well-defined borders Irregular and dense cytoplasmic extensions
Immunohistochemistry[22-27]	TTF-1 (nuclear)[a] Napsin A (cytoplasmic)[b] Mucin stains (intracytoplasmic mucin)[b]	p63/p40 (nuclear)[a] CK5/6 (cytoplasmic)[b]

[a]WHO recommended initial panel.
[b]Additional helpful markers.

ADENOSQUAMOUS CARCINOMA

Adenosquamous carcinomas are tumors with separate, well-defined adenocarcinoma and SqCC components (≥10% of each component per the WHO definition[30]). In a cytology preparation, separate populations of glandular and squamous neoplastic cells (features described above) can be seen, depending on the sampling (Figures 3.61 and 3.62). One component may predominate in FNA specimens owing to limited sampling. The presence of a cell block or clot preparation can be helpful, as it can allow for TTF-1 and p40 staining to identify areas of both squamous (p40 positive) and glandular (TTF-1 positive) differentiation. A diagnosis of "adenosquamous carcinoma" is not recommended on cytology samples because the overall proportion of each component cannot be assessed owing to limited sampling. Such cases can be called "non–small cell carcinoma with glandular and squamous features," and molecular testing should be performed.

SAMPLE NOTE: NON-SMALL CELL (POSSIBLE ADENOSQUAMOUS) CARCINOMA

Non–small cell carcinoma with glandular and squamous cell features. See note.

Note: Immunohistochemical studies show that a subset of the neoplastic cells is positive for TTF-1 and napsin A and negative for p40. p40 highlights a separate population of neoplastic cells that are negative for TTF-1 and napsin A. The findings are consistent with a lung primary. A molecular panel, as well as PD-L1 analysis, have been ordered and will be reported as an addendum.

NON–SMALL CELL CARCINOMA

A diagnosis of "non–small cell carcinoma" should be made in cases where the cytomorphology is indeterminate for a squamous or glandular malignancy (and small cell lung carcinoma can be excluded). Most often, these malignancies are very poorly differentiated adenocarcinomas or SqCCs. On an immunostain workup, tumors that are positive for TTF1 (regardless of p63/p40 status) are diagnosed as "non–small cell carcinoma, favor adenocarcinoma." If the tumor is negative for TTF1 and positive for p63/p40, the diagnosis is "non–small cell carcinoma, favor SqCC." Other variations, such as tumors positive for TTF1 and p63/p40 in separate cell populations, should be diagnosed as "non–small cell carcinoma with glandular

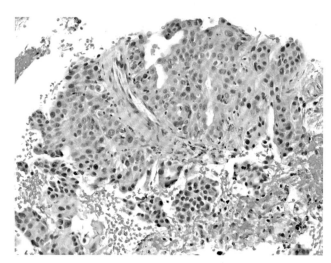

Figure 3.61. Non–small cell carcinoma with glandular and squamous features on a cell block preparation. The clusters of neoplastic cells show features of glandular differentiation, such as vacuolated cytoplasm. However, some areas have dense cytoplasm with well-defined borders suggestive of intercellular bridges, raising the possibility of squamous differentiation. Immunostains are warranted to confirm the morphologic impression (H&E).

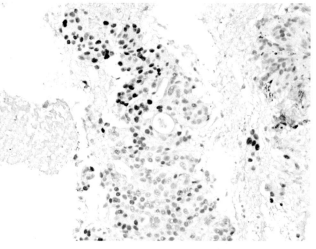

Figure 3.62. Non–small cell carcinoma with glandular and squamous features. There are adjacent glandular (brown nuclear positivity for TTF-1) and squamous (red nuclear positivity for p40) components (TTF-1/napsin A/p40 triple immunostain).

and squamous features," while tumors negative for all markers should be diagnosed as "non–small cell carcinoma, not otherwise specified." A note or comment can be added to provide further details or suggestions. Napsin A and mucin stains can also be helpful adjunct markers for distinguishing adenocarcinomas (Table 3.2).[30-33] Molecular testing should be performed for all of the above diagnoses (Table 3.1) to ensure any patient with a potential diagnosis of adenocarcinoma can be screened for the use of targeted therapy.

SAMPLE NOTE: NON-SMALL CELL CARCINOMA, NOT FURTHER CLASSIFIABLE

Non–small cell carcinoma. See note.

Note: The specimen is scant, and the neoplastic cells show dense cytoplasm and prominent nucleoli in a background of abundant necrosis. There is insufficient material on the cell block preparation for immunohistochemical or molecular studies, precluding further characterization.

MALIGNANT MESOTHELIOMA

Malignant mesotheliomas in the thoracic cavity are malignant neoplasms of the pleura and are typically associated with pleural thickening and unilateral pleural effusions. Cytology specimens can come from pleural effusion fluid or percutaneous FNA of the pleura. However, the sensitivity of pleural fluid cytology for the diagnosis of mesothelioma is only 32% owing to the fact that architectural features (i.e., tissue invasion, full-thickness pleural involvement without zonation, and expansile nodular growth), rather than cytomorphologic features, are most reliable for distinguishing malignant from benign mesothelial proliferations.[34,35] There are three main histologic subtypes of mesothelioma: epithelioid (most common), sarcomatoid, and biphasic (each component comprises >10% of the tumor)[30]; only the epithelioid cells in the epithelioid or biphasic types tend to shed malignant cells into the pleural fluid (see the "Mesothelioma" section under the Serous Effusion Cytopathology chapter).

Cytologically, reactive mesothelial cells may show varying degrees of atypia. Conversely, malignant mesothelial cells can be deceptively bland. Classic features of mesothelial cells, such as intercellular "windows," scalloped edges with a pale, peripheral "lacy skirt" appearance, and round smooth nuclei with abundant cytoplasm may be seen in both benign and malignant mesothelial proliferations. Most often, malignant mesothelial cells appear as epithelioid cells in clusters, sheets, or discohesive single cells; however, in the absence of overt cytologic atypia such as frequent atypical mitoses, this diagnosis is incredibly difficult to make without the support of ancillary studies (Figures 3.63-3.69).

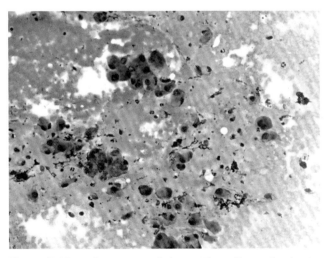

Figure 3.63. Malignant mesothelioma. The cells are discohesive and epithelioid with abundant cytoplasm. There are some binucleate forms, and many cells are plasmacytoid. Immunohistochemistry to confirm mesothelial origin is warranted in these cases (Diff-Quik stain).

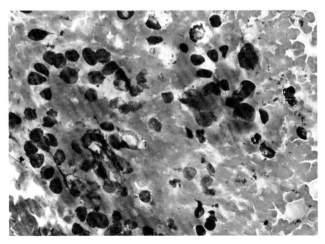

Figure 3.64. Malignant mesothelioma. Note the large binucleated cell seen along with many mononuclear epithelioid cells with pale, fluffy cytoplasm (Diff-Quik stain).

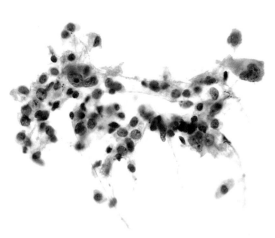

Figure 3.65. Malignant mesothelioma. The cells range from large and atypical with prominent nucleoli to smaller, blander cells (Pap stain).

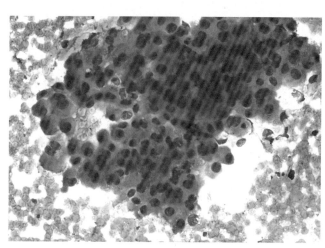

Figure 3.66. Malignant mesothelioma. These neoplastic cells form a large cluster, which raises concern for an adenocarcinoma. However, the nuclei are monotonous, and each cell has abundant cytoplasm (many are plasmacytoid). Careful examination of the periphery of the cluster shows a scalloped border with frilly/lacy edges, which are characteristic of mesothelial cells (Diff-Quik stain).

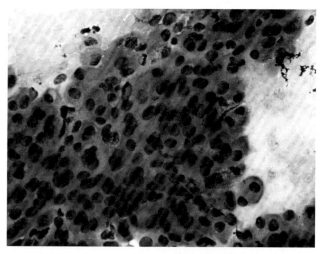

Figure 3.67. Malignant mesothelioma. Note that there is a characteristic dense, fuzzy border at the periphery of the cell cluster, which is characteristic of mesothelial origin (Diff-Quik stain).

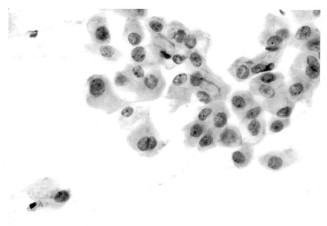

Figure 3.68. Malignant mesothelioma. The cells are loosely cohesive and have low nuclear to cytoplasmic ratios. They can be very difficult to differentiate from adenocarcinomas (Pap stain).

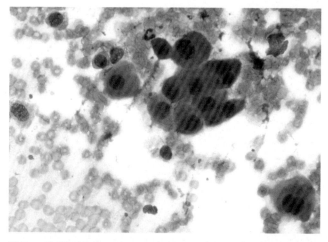

Figure 3.69. Malignant mesothelioma. These cells are bland and may be difficult to distinguish from reactive mesothelial cells but are markedly enlarged compared with adjacent lymphocytes and neutrophils (Diff-Quik stain).

Immunoreactivity for mesothelial markers (e.g., WT1, calretinin, D2-40, CK5/6) can help distinguish mesotheliomas from other types of carcinomas but not from reactive mesothelial cells. In cytology specimens, an immunostain panel of EMA, desmin, BAP1, GLUT-1, and p53 with the following pattern have been shown to be useful ancillary markers to distinguish reactive mesothelial cells from malignant mesothelioma cells: EMA cytoplasmic/membranous positivity (malignant), desmin cytoplasmic/membranous positivity (reactive), BAP1 nuclear loss (malignant), GLUT-1 strong membranous positivity (malignant), and increased p53 expression.[36,37] Furthermore, 40-70% of malignant mesotheliomas show loss of 9p (including *CDKN2A* gene) or 22q (including *NF2* gene), and cytogenetic studies can be used to detect these characteristic deletions; somatic mutations in *CDKN2A*, *BAP1*, *NF2*, and *SETD2* have also been frequently identified in pleural mesotheliomas.[13,38,39] A diagnosis of "atypical mesothelial proliferation" can be rendered in equivocal cases of reactive mesothelial cells versus malignant mesothelioma.

KEY FEATURES of Malignant Mesothelioma

- The specimen is typically hypercellular.
- Morular architecture (large clusters with smooth, scalloped edges), discohesive pattern, or tissue fragments which form bulbous papillary projections
- Intercellular "windows" are created by long microvilli on the surface of mesothelial cells and are a features of both benign and malignant mesothelial cells.
- "Two-toned" cytoplasm (dense central cytoplasm with pale peripheral rim) is a feature seen with both benign and malignant mesothelial cells.
- The cells have moderate to abundant amounts of cytoplasm and may demonstrate cytoplasmic vacuolization.
- The cells are large with round nuclei and regular nuclear contours.
- Binucleation and/or multinucleation may be seen.
- Prominent macronucleoli are suggestive of malignancy.

METASTATIC CARCINOMA

The lungs are a common site of metastasis, and metastatic tumors, such as carcinomas most commonly from the breast, colon, and kidney, are actually more frequently seen than primary lung tumors.[40] It is important to distinguish metastatic carcinoma from primary lung carcinoma, which often involves a combination of recognizing characteristic cytological features (Figures 3.70-3.75), immunohistochemistry, and morphologic comparison with any previous samples from the primary tumor (See Table 5.3 in the Serous Effusion Cytopathology chapter).

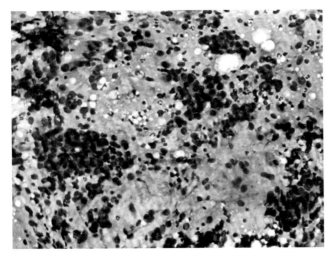

Figure 3.70. Metastatic breast carcinoma to the lung. There are dense clusters of tumor cells and a background of abundant mucin. (Diff-Quik stain).

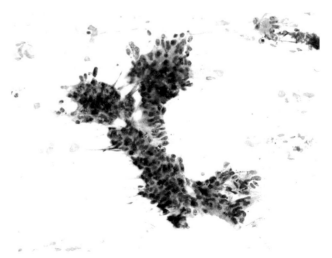

Figure 3.71. Metastatic colon adenocarcinoma to the lung. The glandular cells are columnar and crowded with prominent nucleoli. Note the background dirty necrosis, which is a common but nonspecific finding seen from colonic metastases (Pap stain).

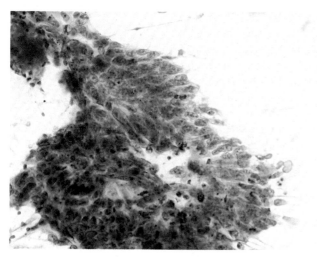

Figure 3.72. High-power view of metastatic colon adenocarcinoma. Note the significantly disorganized architecture and the irregular, elongated, and overlapping nuclei with coarse chromatin (Pap stain).

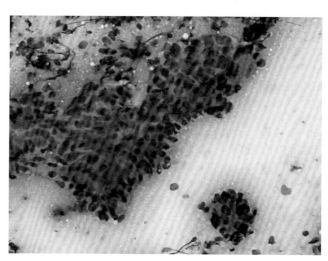

Figure 3.73. Metastatic colon adenocarcinoma to the lung (Diff-Quik stain).

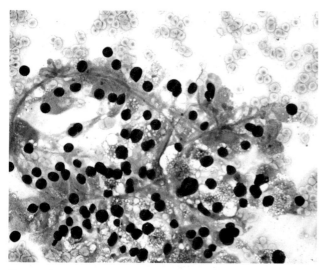

Figure 3.74. Metastatic renal cell carcinoma to the lung. The tumor cells have vacuolated cytoplasm and are loosely attached to fine vascular structures (Diff-Quik stain).

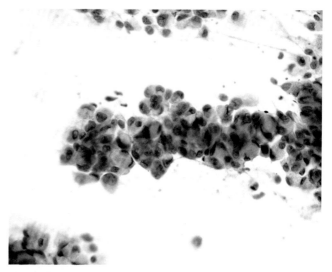

Figure 3.75. Metastatic signet ring cell adenocarcinoma from the stomach. The tumor cells are filled with a large mucin vacuole and an eccentric nucleus pushed to the side (Pap stain).

For example, ductal breast carcinomas often show neoplastic cells in small clusters and present singly with large nucleoli, some with mucin-filled intracellular lumens (Figure 3.70).[41] Breast markers such as GATA-3, mammaglobin, GCDFP-15, ER, and PR can help confirm the diagnosis.[42] Colon adenocarcinomas have palisading tall, columnar cells with hyperchromatic nuclei and a background of "dirty" necrosis (Figures 3.71-3.73).[43] In addition, colon cancers from the hindgut are CK7− and CK20+ (also CDX2+), while lung cancers show the opposite immunoprofile (CK7+, CK20−, also TTF-1+); however, colon cancers arising from the midgut are frequently CK7 positive. Metastatic renal cell carcinomas produce single neoplastic cells and cells in flat tissue fragments. The cytomorphological features vary depending on the subtype, but clear cell renal cell carcinoma represents the overwhelming majority of these cases and characteristically features clear or granular cytoplasm (Figure 3.74).[44]

SQUAMOUS PATTERN

The squamous pattern includes entities that display some degree of squamous differentiation. SqCC and adenosquamous carcinoma, as well as cytologic features of squamous differentiation, are covered in the "Epithelial Pattern" section above.

CHECKLIST: Etiologic Considerations for the Squamous Pattern

☐ Reactive Squamous Atypia/Squamous Metaplasia

☐ Squamous Cell Carcinoma

☐ Adenosquamous Carcinoma

☐ Mucoepidermoid Carcinoma

REACTIVE SQUAMOUS ATYPIA/SQUAMOUS METAPLASIA

Reactive squamous atypia can be seen with any form of lung injury, infectious process, or in the setting of tracheostomy. These squamous cells can demonstrate atypical parakeratosis and appear pleomorphic with enlarged nuclei and prominent nucleoli but still have benign cytologic features: cohesive orderly sheets with minimal nuclear crowding and fine, pale chromatin (Figures 3.76-3.78). Some cases may contain markedly atypical cells suspicious for malignancy (Figure 3.79).

Squamous metaplasia of the bronchial epithelium can occur with chronic irritation. The metaplastic cells usually appear benign, with small, round nuclei and even, pale chromatin. However, degenerated nuclei can become pyknotic and mimic well differentiated SqCC.

SQUAMOUS CELL CARCINOMA

SqCC may share significant overlap with reactive squamous atypia and squamous metaplasia, and thus this diagnosis must be made with caution. Both exfoliative and FNA specimens can sample an area of a large airway that has undergone squamous metaplasia with an overlying reactive changes. SqCC should be more cellular than metaplasia in a well-sampled lesion, and the atypia seen should be convincing for a diagnosis of malignancy if being made for the first time. Helpful features, when present, include cells with irregularly shaped cytoplasm containing rigid projections, pyknotic nuclei with marked hyperchromasia, irregular nuclear borders, and necrosis.

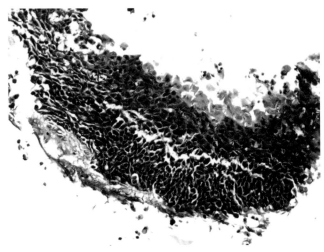

Figure 3.76. Large fragment of metaplastic squamous epithelium with hyperchromatic nuclei. Note that the cells are still arranged in a cohesive, orderly sheet with preserved maturation (Diff-Quik stain).

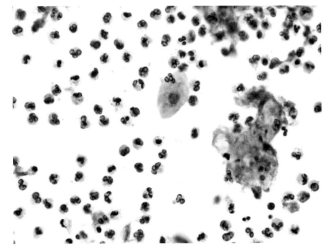

Figure 3.77. Rare reactive atypical squamous cell in a background of abundant acute inflammation (Pap stain).

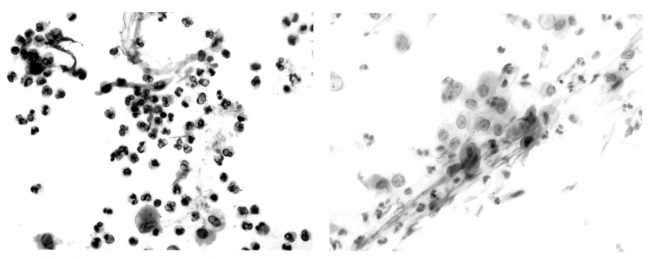

Figure 3.78. Atypical reactive squamous cell with tadpole shape in a background of abundant acute inflammation (Pap stain).

Figure 3.79. Atypical squamous cells suspicious for a squamous cell carcinoma (Pap stain).

SAMPLE NOTE: SUSPICIOUS FOR SQUAMOUS CELL CARCINOMA

Rare markedly atypical squamous cells, suspicious for squamous cell carcinoma. See note.

Note: The specimen contains rare atypical keratinizing cells in a background of abundant bronchial epithelial cells. While the level of atypia seen is concerning for malignancy, the limited number of atypical cells precludes a more definitive diagnosis. A repeat specimen is recommended if clinical concern for a malignancy persists.

ADENOSQUAMOUS CARCINOMA

The squamous component of adenosquamous carcinoma is identical in appearance to pure SqCCs (see the "Squamous Pattern", above). As described above in the "Epithelial Pattern", a separate component of adenocarcinoma must also be identified to suggest this entity, although a definitive diagnosis should not be made on cytology alone.

MUCOEPIDERMOID CARCINOMA

Mucoepidermoid carcinoma is the most common malignant salivary gland tumor but represents only 0.2% of primary lung tumors. In the lung, these tumors arise from the submucosal glands of the trachea and bronchi and tend to cause obstructive symptoms. Mucoepidermoid carcinoma shows clusters of neoplastic squamous cells, mucin-producing glandular cells, and intermediate cells.[45] Importantly, the squamous component of mucoepidermoid carcinomas is non-keratinizing. For suspected cases, molecular analysis can be performed to detect the characteristic *MECT1-MAML2*; t(11;19) translocation.[46,47] See Chapter 2 entitled "Salivary Gland and Cervical Lymph Nodes" for further discussion.

LOOSELY COHESIVE/SINGLE CELL PATTERN

The loosely cohesive/single cell pattern includes a variety of malignant neoplasms, both primary and metastatic to the lungs. These tumors exhibit a discohesive appearance with no appreciable structures and frequent single cells.

CHECKLIST: Etiologic Considerations for the Loosely Cohesive/Single Cell Pattern

☐ Poorly Differentiated Non–Small Cell Carcinoma

☐ Neuroendocrine Tumor

☐ Lymphoma

☐ Metastatic Tumor

POORLY DIFFERENTIATED NON–SMALL CELL CARCINOMA

Adenocarcinomas and SqCCs that do not show overt glandular or squamous differentiation can be classified as poorly differentiated non–small cell carcinoma (Figures 3.80-3.85). In these cases, it is most important to distinguish them from small cell lung carcinoma, which typically has specific cytomorphological features such as nuclear molding, frequent crush artifact, stippled chromatin, scant cytoplasm, and frequent mitoses, apoptotic bodies, and necrotic material (see Neuroendocrine Tumor section below). If cell block material

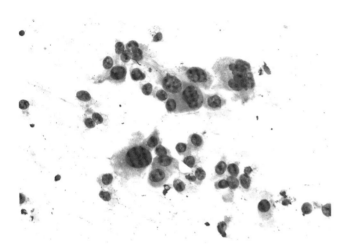

Figure 3.80. Poorly differentiated adenocarcinoma. The markedly atypical malignant cells are loosely cohesive and display significant variations in nuclear size and shape (Diff-Quik stain).

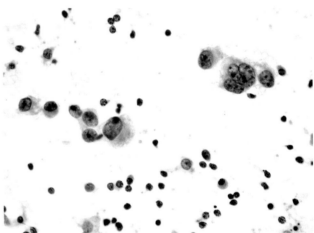

Figure 3.81. Poorly differentiated adenocarcinoma. There are large, single atypical cells with granular cytoplasm and atypical nuclei with coarse, vesicular chromatin (Pap stain).

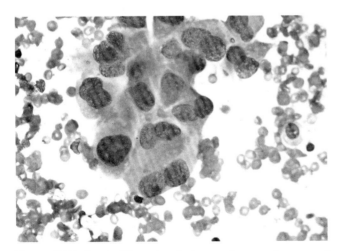

Figure 3.82. Poorly differentiated adenocarcinoma cells arranged in a loosely cohesive cluster (Diff-Quik stain).

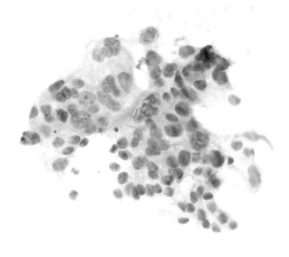

Figure 3.83. Poorly differentiated squamous cell carcinoma demonstrating anisonucleosis and markedly irregular nuclear contours (Pap stain).

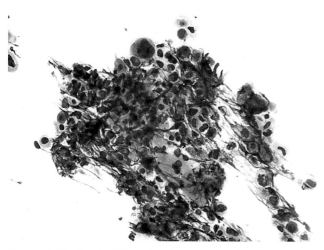
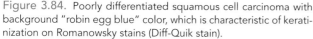

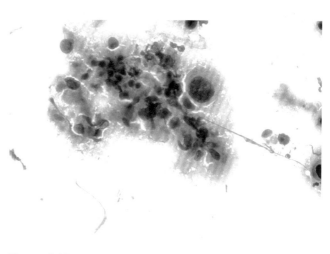

Figure 3.84. Poorly differentiated squamous cell carcinoma with background "robin egg blue" color, which is characteristic of keratinization on Romanowsky stains (Diff-Quik stain).

Figure 3.85. Poorly differentiated squamous cell carcinoma with loosely cohesive, pleomorphic cells with dense cytoplasm (Diff-Quik stain).

is available, immunostains (Table 3.2) may offer additional information, although poorly differentiated carcinomas tend to lose expression of lineage-specific markers. If the tumor subtype cannot be classified, a diagnosis of "non–small cell carcinoma" should be rendered, and molecular testing should be performed.

NEUROENDOCRINE TUMOR

Neuroendocrine tumors of the lung include carcinoid tumors (typical and atypical), small cell lung carcinoma, and large cell neuroendocrine carcinoma (LCNEC).[30] Carcinoid tumors share the neuroendocrine cytomorphology seen in neuroendocrine tumors at other sites: loosely cohesive and single round to oval monotonous, uniform cells with frequently eccentric nuclei and "salt-and-pepper" chromatin (Figures 3.86-3.91). Typical carcinoids have uniformly small, round nuclei, while atypical carcinoids demonstrate greater nuclear pleomorphism, occasional prominent nucleoli, and increased mitoses (2-10 mitoses per 10 high-power fields [HPFs]) and/or focal necrosis.

Small cell lung carcinoma and LCNEC are high-grade neuroendocrine tumors with abundant mitoses and necrosis. Small cell lung carcinoma accounts for up to 25% of primary lung carcinomas and portends a poor prognosis.[48] The tumor cells are relatively small with high N/C ratios, hyperchromatic "smudgy" nuclei, and characteristic nuclear molding (Figures 3.92-3.95). There is often marked crush artifact due to the fragility of the cells,

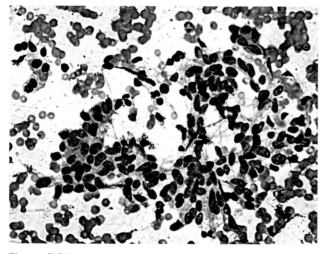

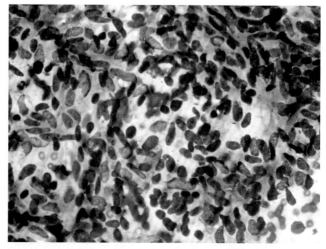

Figure 3.86. Carcinoid tumor. The cells are present in a loosely cohesive cluster and are monomorphic with even, granular chromatin (Diff-Quik stain).

Figure 3.87. Cluster of carcinoid tumor cells with elongated nuclei (Diff-Quik stain).

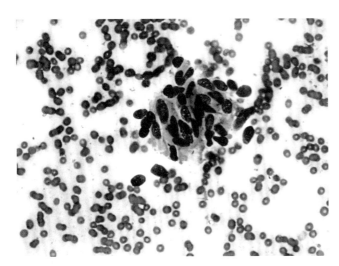

Figure 3.88. Carcinoid tumor present as a loosely cohesive cluster of cells with elongated nuclei (Diff-Quik stain).

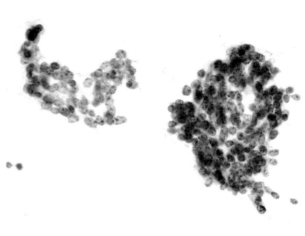

Figure 3.89. Carcinoid tumor. There are loosely cohesive groups of monomorphic, round to oval cells. The chromatin has the characteristic stippled "salt-and-pepper" appearance of neuroendocrine neoplasms (Pap stain).

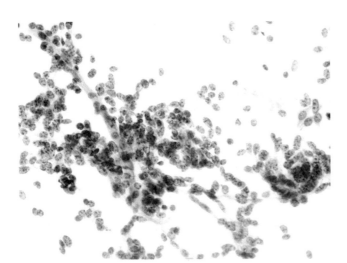

Figure 3.90. Carcinoid tumor. There are many single cells, and the nuclei are monomorphic with coarse, "salt-and-pepper" chromatin. (Pap stain).

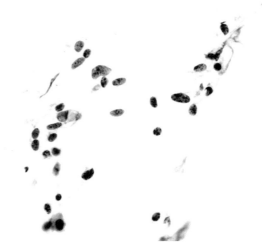

Figure 3.91. Scattered single cells in a carcinoid tumor with naked nuclei (Pap stain).

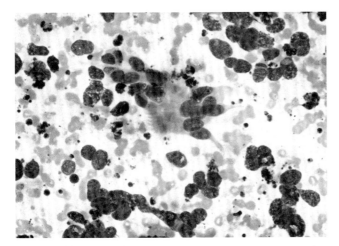

Figure 3.92. Benign ciliated bronchial epithelial cells surrounded by small cell carcinoma. Note the nuclear molding and apoptosis (Diff-Quik stain).

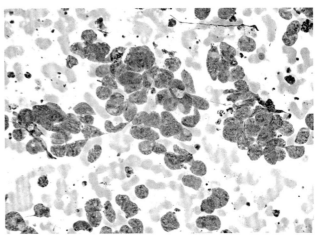

Figure 3.93. Small cell carcinoma. No cytoplasm is appreciable, and the cells mold to one another. There is a background of cellular debris resulting from apoptosis (Diff-Quik stain).

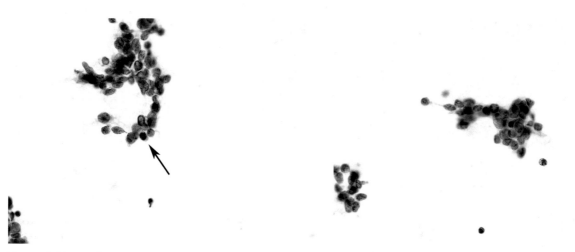

Figure 3.94. Small cell carcinoma. The cells have scant cytoplasm, "salt-and-pepper" chromatin, and mitoses (arrow) (Pap stain).

Figure 3.95. Small cell carcinoma. The cells have "salt-and-pepper" chromatin, high N/C ratios, and show molding (Pap stain).

which appears as linear streaks of chromatin (Figure 3.96). Apoptotic bodies, necrosis, and mitoses are easily seen. Neuroendocrine markers (i.e., chromogranin, synaptophysin, CD56, and INSM-1) are not required to render a diagnosis of small cell lung carcinoma, as many tumors may show minimal positivity. However, they are frequently used to confirm the morphologic impression of small cell lung carcinoma (Figures 3.97-3.99).[49-54] LCNEC classically appears as loose clusters or rosettes of large cells with moderate to abundant cytoplasm, prominent nucleoli, and marked pleomorphism (Figures 3.100-3.103). Large zones of necrosis are often present on histology, and thus, evidence of necrosis may be seen in cytological specimens as well.

KEY FEATURES of Neuroendocrine Tumors
Carcinoid tumor

- The neoplastic cells are present in loosely cohesive clusters and as single cells.
- The neoplastic cells are round to oval with moderate amounts of granular cytoplasm.
- The nuclei have a plasmacytoid appearance (eccentrically placed) with "salt-and-pepper" chromatin.
- Mitoses are absent to rare.
- Necrosis is absent to focal.

Large cell neuroendocrine carcinoma (LCNEC)

- The neoplastic cells are loosely cohesive and larger relative to carcinoid tumors.
- There is marked pleomorphism with irregular nuclear shapes and prominent nucleoli.
- There is moderate to abundant lacy/feathery cytoplasm.
- There are abundant mitoses and necrosis.

Small cell carcinoma (SCLC)

- The neoplastic cells are present in loosely cohesive clusters and/or as dispersed cells.
- The neoplastic cells are relatively small but still 2-3x the size of a lymphocyte.
- The neoplastic cells have high N/C ratio with scant cytoplasm.
- The nuclei are hyperchromatic (often smudgy) with fine, even chromatin and may contain inconspicuous nucleoli.
- Nuclear molding, in which adjacent cells press against one another and compress each other's nuclei, is a classic feature.
- Crush artifact and background debris are often seen.
- There are abundant mitoses, apoptotic bodies, and necrosis.

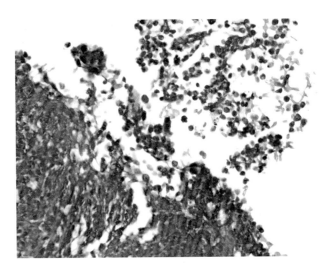

Figure 3.96. Small cell carcinoma with significant crush artifact of the tumor cells (lower left), which is commonly seen with these tumors (H&E).

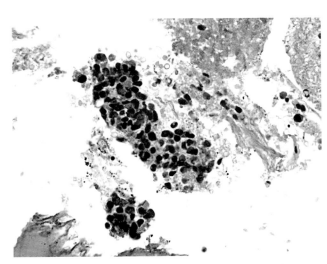

Figure 3.97. Small cell carcinoma on cell block (cell block, H&E).

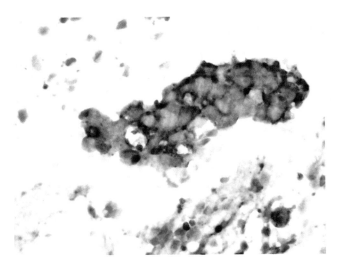

Figure 3.98. Small cell lung carcinoma. Corresponding synaptophysin stain showing diffuse granular cytoplasmic positivity. Neuroendocrine markers may be completely negative, or only focally positive, in many small cell lung carcinomas. (synaptophysin immunostain).

Figure 3.99. Corresponding chromogranin stain showing diffuse granular cytoplasmic positivity. Neuroendocrine markers may be completely negative, or only focally positive, in many small cell lung carcinomas. (chromogranin immunostain).

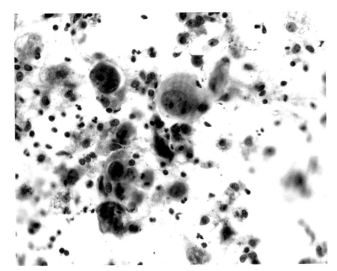

Figure 3.100. Large cell neuroendocrine carcinoma. There are discohesive large malignant cells with moderate amounts of cytoplasm, prominent nucleoli, and marked pleomorphism (Pap stain).

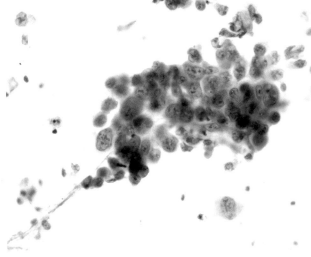

Figure 3.101. Large cell neuroendocrine carcinoma present as a loosely cohesive cluster (Pap stain).

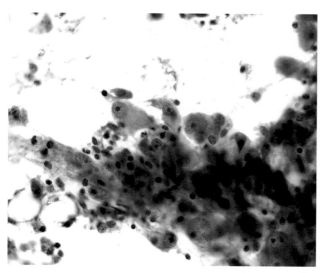

Figure 3.102. Large cell neuroendocrine carcinoma cells with prominent nucleoli and abundant cytoplasm (Pap stain).

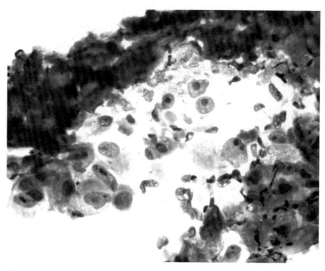

Figure 3.103. Large cell neuroendocrine carcinoma cells with prominent nucleoli present as discohesive single cells (Pap stain).

FAQ: How are neuroendocrine tumors of the lung graded?

Answer: The two criteria formally used to grade neuroendocrine tumors of the lung are (1) mitotic count and (2) amount of necrosis (Table 3.3). However, in small biopsies and limited samples, Ki67 proliferation index is often used as a surrogate grading criteria.[55,56] Grading can be performed on FNA/cell block/ core biopsy material, but there is always the possibility that a higher grade area of the tumor (i.e., with focal mitoses and/or necrosis) was not sampled. A definitive grade does not need to be assigned based on cytology specimens, and a diagnosis of "carcinoid tumor, favor (typical/atypical)" can be rendered.

SAMPLE NOTE : NEUROENDOCRINE TUMOR (CARCINOID TUMOR)

Carcinoid tumor. See note.

Note: The neoplastic cells are plasmacytoid with "salt-and-pepper" chromatin. Mitoses and necrosis are not seen on this limited sample. If this material is representative of the entire lesion, the findings are consistent with a typical carcinoid tumor. However, a higher grade lesion (such as an atypical carcinoid tumor) cannot be entirely excluded.

Reference:
Stoll LM, Johnson MW, Burroughs F, Li QK. Cytologic diagnosis and differential diagnosis of lung carcinoid tumors a retrospective study of 63 cases with histologic correlation. *Cancer Cytopathol.* 2010;118(6):457-467.

TABLE 3.3: Criteria for Grading Neuroendocrine Tumors of the Lung

Grade	Entity	Mitoses per 10 HPF	Necrosis	Ki67 index
Low (G1)	Typical carcinoid	<2	None	<3%
Intermediate (G2)	Atypical carcinoid	2-10	Focal	3-20%
High (G3)	Small cell carcinoma (SCLC) Large cell neuroendocrine carcinoma (LCNEC)	>10	Abundant	>20%

PEARLS & PITFALLS

Distinguishing between high-grade neuroendocrine tumors and NSCLCs (i.e., adenocarcinoma, SqCC) often requires a combination of morphology and immunohistochemistry. Do not rely on immunohistochemistry alone because the results may be difficult to interpret and/or reconcile with morphology in some cases. For example, 65% of LCNECs and >90% of small cell lung carcinomas are TTF-1+; napsin A can be helpful in these TTF-1+ cases because it is only negative in ~2% of adenocarcinomas. In addition, a small percentage of small cell lung carcinomas (<10%) may be negative for one or more neuroendocrine markers. Thus, tumors with definitive morphological features of small cell lung carcinomas can be reported as such.

In addition, 10-20% of NSCLCs show focal positivity with neuroendocrine markers.[57] Again, correlation with morphology is crucial, as tumors with no evidence of neuroendocrine morphology but positive neuroendocrine markers should be classified as "NSCLC with neuroendocrine differentiation." These cases are difficult to classify on cytology alone because architectural neuroendocrine features (e.g., organoid nests, palisading, rosettes, etc.) that can be identified on histology are very helpful for classification.

On the other hand, a diagnosis of LCNEC requires both architectural neuroendocrine morphology and confirmation of synaptophysin and/or chromogranin immunoreactivity.[57] In cases where non–small cell neuroendocrine morphology is present but all neuroendocrine markers are negative, a diagnosis of "NSCLC with neuroendocrine morphology" can be rendered. Consultation with an experienced pulmonary pathologist and/or correlation with histology is highly recommended in equivocal or difficult cases.

LYMPHOMA

Primary lymphomas of the lung are rare. When they occur, the majority are B-cell non-Hodgkin lymphomas, most commonly extranodal marginal zone B-cell lymphoma of mucosa-associated lymphoid tissue (MALT lymphoma), followed by diffuse large B-cell lymphoma (DLBCL).[58,59] However, secondary involvement of the lungs by lymphoma is more common and is seen in up to 50% of patients with both non-Hodgkin and Hodgkin lymphoma.[60] Other hematologic malignancies such as T-cell malignancies, acute leukemia, and myeloma can involve the lungs as well.[61,62]

In general, lymphomas are cytologically discohesive and often exist as a monotonous cell population. Lymphoglandular bodies, which are globular fragments of cytoplasm, can be seen in the background but are nonspecific.[63] MALT lymphoma and other mature B-cell lymphomas are difficult to diagnose by cytology alone because of considerable cytomorphologic overlap between these low-grade lymphomas and a reactive inflammatory process. Thus, flow cytometry to immunophenotype the lymphoid population is crucial to making the diagnosis. Other lymphoid malignancies typically have more distinctive cytological features. DLBCL appears as sheets of large atypical cells with clearly malignant features, such as frequent mitoses, apoptosis, and necrosis (Figures 3.104 and 3.105). Hodgkin lymphoma classically consists of occasional large, atypical binucleate Reed-Sternberg (RS) or RS-like mononuclear cells with large nucleoli in a background of mixed inflammation (Figures 3.106 and 3.107). The inflammatory infiltrate often consists of eosinophils and histiocytes, which may form granulomas.

METASTATIC TUMORS

Some metastatic tumors to the lungs tend to present with a prominent single cell population, including metastatic carcinomas (see the "Metastatic Carcinoma" of the "Epithelial Pattern"), sarcomas, and melanoma (Figures 3.108 and 3.109). In particular, poorly differentiated carcinomas, ductal and lobular breast carcinomas, signet ring cell carcinomas, and others, are characterized by cellular specimens with a loosely cohesive/single cell population of neoplastic cells. Comparison with prior surgical specimens and immunohistochemistry can help further classify a metastatic tumor.

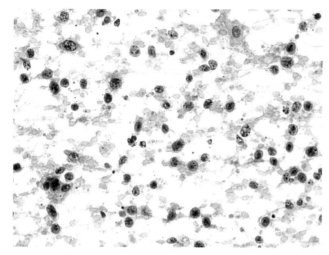

Figure 3.104. Diffuse large B-cell lymphoma in the lung. There is a relatively monomorphic population of discohesive neoplastic cells (Pap stain).

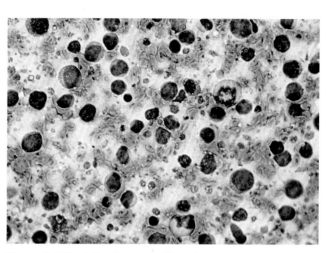

Figure 3.105. Diffuse large B-cell lymphoma in the lung. The scattered neoplastic cells are discohesive and large with atypical mitoses (Diff-Quik stain).

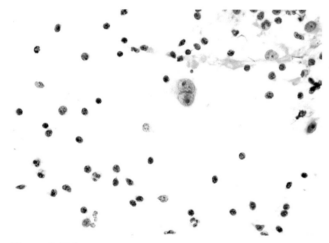

Figure 3.106. Classic binucleated Reed-Sternberg cell in Hodgkin lymphoma of the lung. Note the background mixed inflammatory infiltrate (Pap stain).

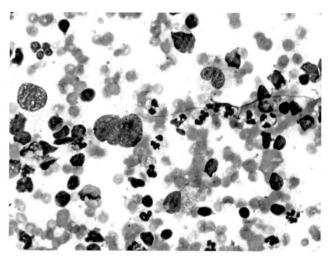

Figure 3.107. Hodgkin lymphoma in the lung. Reed-Sternberg and variant cells are present in a mixed inflammatory background (Diff-Quik stain).

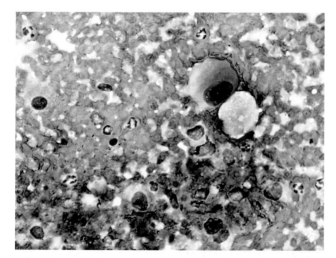

Figure 3.108. Metastatic melanoma to the lung. The malignant cells are discohesive and pleomorphic, often with eccentric nuclei (Diff-Quik stain).

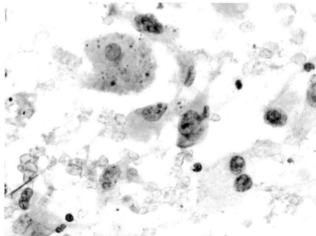

Figure 3.109. Metastatic melanoma to the lung. The large neoplastic single cells contain melanin pigment. The adjacent pulmonary macrophage also contains pigment but has a very small round, bland nucleus (Pap stain).

SPINDLE CELL PATTERN

The spindle cell pattern includes both benign and malignant entities of mesenchymal, neural, and epithelial origin. Some of these lesions may arise within the bronchopulmonary system while others are metastases from distant sites. The differential diagnosis for spindle cell lesions in the pulmonary system is extensive, and small cytologic samples without sufficient cell block material may pose a diagnostic challenge. This section will provide a brief overview of the most relevant spindle cell neoplasms of the lung.

CHECKLIST: Etiologic Considerations for the Spindle Cell Pattern

- ☐ Benign Spindle Cell Tumors
- ☐ Sarcomatoid Carcinoma
- ☐ Malignant Mesothelioma
- ☐ Sarcoma
- ☐ Melanoma
- ☐ Spindle Cell Carcinoid Tumor

BENIGN SPINDLE CELL TUMORS

Inflammatory myofibroblastic tumors (IMT) are spindle cell neoplasms that can arise in many locations and are generally benign but can occasionally be locally aggressive and/or recur after resection.[64] They are genetically defined by anaplastic lymphoma kinase (*ALK*) translocations.[65] IMTs are rarely seen in the lungs and are thought to arise as a result of an excessive inflammatory response; when they occur in the lungs, they typically present as solitary nodules in the periphery of the lung. Cytologically, IMTs consist of bland spindle cells of myofibroblastic origin in an inflammatory background consisting of lymphocytes, plasma cells, eosinophils, and histiocytes (Figures 3.110 and 3.111). Notably, the spindle cells lack overt cytologic atypia and have bland, oval nuclei with small nucleoli; there should be no to rare mitoses. Large "ganglion-like" cells may be present in a small subset of cases.[66] The lack of specific cytomorphologic features and the variable inflammatory and stromal components make diagnosing IMTs extremely challenging on cytology specimens alone. Immunohistochemical stains may be helpful: SMA is usually positive, and ALK1 can be helpful if positive, although 40% of cases are reported to be negative.[67]

Schwannomas are benign peripheral nerve sheath tumors that can occur at many sites, including the lungs. Cytologically, they are composed of cellular, cohesive fragments of spindle cells with "comma-shaped" or "hook-shaped" nuclei (pointed nuclear ends) in a

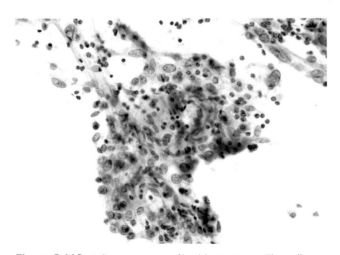

Figure 3.110. Inflammatory myofibroblastic tumor. The cell population consists of bland oval- to spindle-shaped cells mixed with lymphocytes and plasma cells (Pap stain).

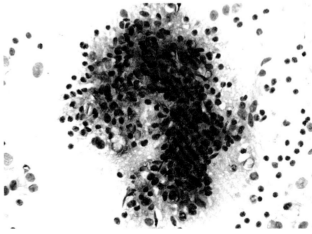

Figure 3.111. Inflammatory myofibroblastic tumor. There is a mixed population of spindle cells and inflammatory cells (Diff-Quik stain).

background of fibrillary stroma. The cells can demonstrate variable anisonucleosis. When all these cytologic features are present, FNA has a high specificity for the diagnosis of schwannoma. The most helpful yet uncommonly encountered diagnostic clue is the presence of Verocay bodies palisading around acellular material. Fortunately, positive immunostaining with S100 protein is sensitive but not specific for distinguishing schwannomas from many other spindle cell neoplasms seen in the lungs.

Solitary fibrous tumors (SFTs) are fibroblastic neoplasms that can occur at various sites, but frequently involve the lungs or pleura.[68] Around 90% of SFTs are benign, slow-growing masses that can be cured by complete excision, although 5-10% behave in malignant/aggressive ways (i.e., local recurrence and/or distant metastasis).[69] Cytologically, they present as variably cellular specimens with a uniform, bland spindle cell population that is frequently present as single cells or naked nuclei. Based on cytology, the differential diagnosis includes monophasic synovial sarcoma, malignant peripheral nerve sheath tumor (MPNST), sarcomatoid mesothelioma, and desmoid fibromatosis, among others. Diffuse, strong nuclear expression with STAT6 immunostaining is a highly sensitive and specific method for establishing the diagnosis, as SFTs are characterized by the *NAB2-STAT6* gene fusion.[70]

SARCOMATOID CARCINOMA

Sarcomatoid carcinomas are poorly differentiated carcinomas that show various forms of sarcomatoid differentiation (Figures 3.112 and 3.113). They are important to distinguish from conventional NSCLCs, sarcomas, and malignant mesotheliomas. Types of sarcomatoid carcinoma that have a spindle cell component include (1) pleomorphic carcinoma, which contains at least 10% malignant spindle cells or giant cells, (2) spindle cell carcinoma, which consists entirely of malignant spindle cells with no specific mesenchymal differentiation, (3) carcinosarcoma, which is a mixture of conventional NSCLC and true sarcoma with mesenchymal differentiation, and (4) pulmonary blastoma, a primitive biphasic tumor composed of glandular and mesenchymal components.[71]

MALIGNANT MESOTHELIOMA

The biphasic and sarcomatoid subtypes of malignant mesothelioma are composed of spindle cells, which can range in cytological appearance from uniform and bland to atypical and pleomorphic. Only the epithelioid cells in the epithelioid or biphasic subtypes tend to shed malignant cells into the pleural fluid; thus, the spindle cell component may only be appreciated in FNA samples of pleural nodules. See the "Malignant Mesothelioma" section under the "Epithelioid Pattern" for further discussion.

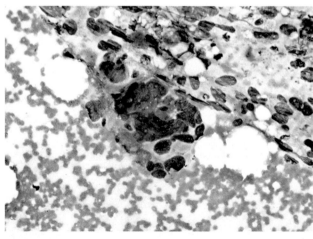

Figure 3.112. Sarcomatoid carcinoma. There are markedly atypical epithelioid and spindle cells that are enlarged and pleomorphic (Diff-Quik stain).

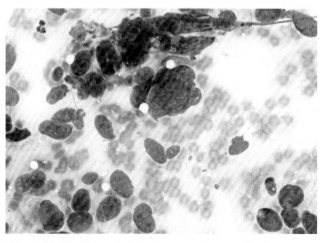

Figure 3.113. Sarcomatoid carcinoma with markedly pleomorphic oval- to spindle-shaped cells (Diff-Quik stain).

SARCOMA

Primary sarcomas of the lung are rare and account for <0.5% of all lung cancers. Most sarcomas in the lung, however, are metastatic in origin; in fact, the lungs are the most common distant site of metastasis for sarcomas.[72,73] The most commonly reported primary pulmonary sarcoma is leiomyosarcoma,[74,75] but well-documented cases also include synovial sarcoma,[76] undifferentiated pleomorphic sarcoma (previously malignant fibrous histiocytoma), chondrosarcoma,[77] epithelioid hemangioendothelioma,[78] Kaposi sarcoma, and rhabdomyosarcoma; very rare entities (<20 reported pulmonary cases each) include liposarcoma, angiosarcoma, MPNST, osteosarcoma, and alveolar soft part sarcoma.[79-81]

Clinical and radiographic correlation to identify or exclude an extrapulmonary primary site is essential to narrow the differential and direct further workup. Cytomorphologically, sarcomas usually consist of cellular fragments of spindle cells and single atypical spindle cells (Figures 3.114-3.119), although the malignant cells may be deceptively bland in certain entities. Furthermore, there is often morphological overlap between multiple entities; thus, as with sarcomas at any site, immunostains and possibly ancillary cytogenetic studies are key to rendering a specific diagnosis.[82]

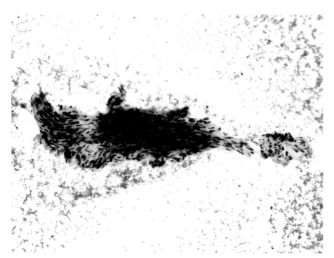

Figure 3.114. Leiomyosarcoma involving the lung. The fragment of malignant spindle cells is cohesive, and the cells stream in parallel within the fragment (Pap stain).

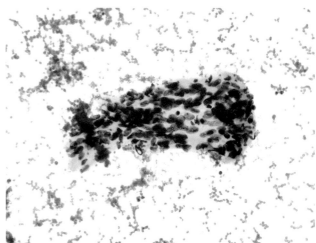

Figure 3.115. Leiomyosarcoma involving the lung. The highly atypical spindle cells are hyperchromatic with coarse chromatin and blunt nuclear ends (Pap stain).

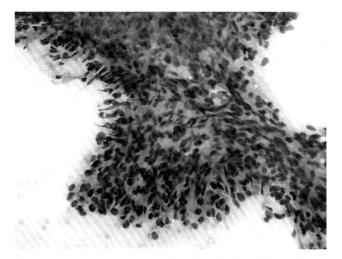

Figure 3.116. Leiomyosarcoma involving the lung. The malignant cells are enlarged and spindle shaped, though they appear more epithelioid at the periphery of fragments (Diff-Quik stain).

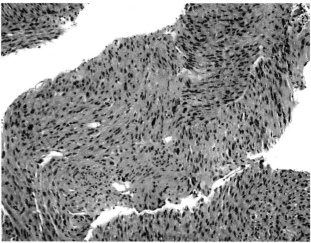

Figure 3.117. Leiomyosarcoma involving the lung. The malignant spindle cells show smooth muscle differentiation and are arranged in perpendicular fascicles (H&E).

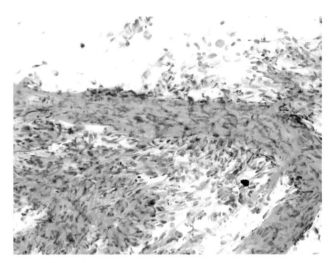

Figure 3.118. Pleomorphic liposarcoma involving the lung. The cells are present in fragments and as single atypical large cells (Pap stain).

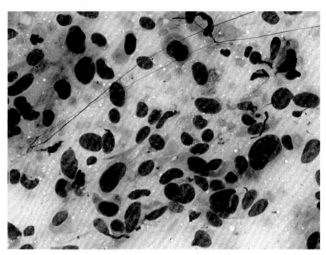

Figure 3.119. High-power view of pleomorphic liposarcoma involving the lung. The spindle cells are markedly pleomorphic and atypical (Diff-Quik stain).

MELANOMA

Melanomas involving the lungs are generally regarded as metastatic lesions even if there is no history/known primary site, as primary cutaneous or mucosal melanomas can spontaneously regress, precluding a definitive diagnosis of primary versus secondary melanoma.[81] Melanoma cells are widely heterogeneous, ranging from epithelioid to spindled in shape, monomorphic to extremely pleomorphic, and may or may not contain pigment (see the "Metastatic Tumors" section under the "Loosely Cohesive/Single Cell Pattern"). Specifically, the spindle cell and desmoplastic melanoma subtypes are characterized by atypical, spindled melanocytes. The diagnosis of malignant melanoma relies on examining a panel of melanocytic markers (i.e., S100 protein, MITF, MelanA, Mart-1, SOX10). A combination of MelanA and trichrome stains has been shown to allow for diagnostic distinction between spindle cell (MelanA positive, trichrome negative) and desmoplastic melanoma (MelanA negative, trichrome positive) when histology is inadequate.[83] Desmoplastic melanomas are usually diffusely and strongly positive for S100 protein and SOX10, but negative (or focal/weak) for the other melanocytic markers.[84,85]

SPINDLE CELL CARCINOID TUMOR

Spindle cell carcinoid tumors are a variant of carcinoid tumor that typically present as well-demarcated tumors in the periphery of the lung, often beneath the pleura. They are usually found incidentally in asymptomatic patients, whom go on to have excellent outcomes. Spindle cell carcinoids are comprised of predominantly spindle cells (≥50% as defined in one study) that are elongated with disorderly growth patterns and have uniform nuclei with fine, granular chromatin.[86] These tumors can present a pitfall in the differential versus bland-appearing mesenchymal tumors such as SFT, synovial sarcoma, and smooth muscle tumors. While these cases can show variable immunoreactivity for broad-spectrum cytokeratin, TTF-1, and vimentin, they should demonstrate positivity for all neuroendocrine markers (i.e., synaptophysin, chromogranin, and CD56).[86,87]

GRANULOMATOUS PATTERN

Granulomatous inflammation consists of nodular aggregates of epithelioid histiocytes mixed with a polymorphous inflammatory infiltrate, with or without coagulative necrosis. In isolation, granulomas are a nonspecific finding. However, in conjunction with clinical history, the presence of granulomas can help narrow the differential diagnosis and direct additional workup. The classic associations with this pattern are tuberculosis and sarcoidosis, but they can also be seen in other fungal infections or in reaction to foreign substances or malignant neoplasms.

☐ Tuberculosis

☐ Sarcoidosis

☐ Fungal Infection

☐ Hodgkin Lymphoma

TUBERCULOSIS

Tuberculosis is classically associated with necrotizing (caseating) granulomas. On cytology, collections of epithelioid histiocytes (i.e., granulomatous inflammation) and Langerhans giant cells are seen, sometimes in a necrotic background with intermixed neutrophils and lymphocytes (Figures 3.120 and 3.121). Mycobacteria cannot be visualized on Papanicolaou or Diff-Quik stains, but the latter can highlight the outlines of the bacilli, imparting the appearance of "ghost bacilli" or "negative images." The diagnosis is confirmed by identifying beaded, red, acid-fast bacilli on a special acid-fast stain and/or by a positive culture for *Mycobacterium tuberculosis*.

SARCOIDOSIS

Sarcoidosis is characterized by nonnecrotizing (noncaseating) granulomas that most often involve the lung and hilar lymph nodes (Figures 3.122-3.127).[88] Although their presence alone is not specific for sarcoidosis, pathologic identification of nonnecrotizing granulomas in the appropriate clinical and radiologic setting can be virtually diagnostic. Other features that are supportive but nonspecific for sarcoidosis are Schaumann bodies (concentrically laminated calcifications) and asteroid bodies (stellate, crystalline inclusions), both of which are found within giant cells. The most important initial step upon encountering nonnecrotizing granulomas is to rule out an infectious etiology by performing special stains for fungus and acid-fast bacilli and correlating with microbiology cultures.

SAMPLE NOTE : GRANULOMATOUS PATTERN, POSSIBLE SARCOIDOSIS

Nonnecrotizing granulomatous inflammation. See note.

Note: In the appropriate clinical and radiologic setting, the findings are compatible with sarcoidosis.

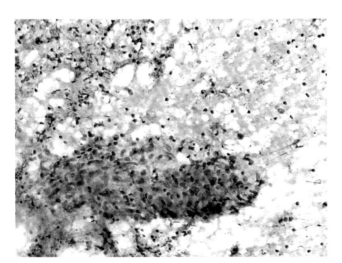

Figure 3.120. Necrotizing granuloma. There is a cluster of epithelioid histiocytes in a dirty necrotic background (Diff-Quik stain).

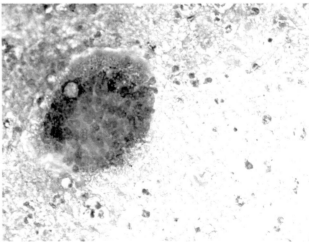

Figure 3.121. Necrotizing granuloma. Abundant necrotic debris in the background of a multinucleated giant cell (Diff-Quik stain).

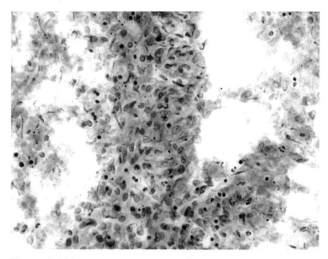

Figure 3.122. High-power view of a necrotizing granuloma. There is a large fragment of epithelioid histiocytes and lymphocytes with granular debris in the background. (Pap stain).

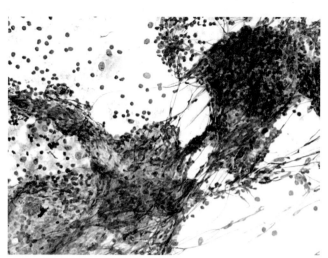

Figure 3.123. Nonnecrotizing granuloma. There are admixed epithelioid histiocytes and lymphocytes, which create a streaking artifact when crushed (Diff-Quik stain).

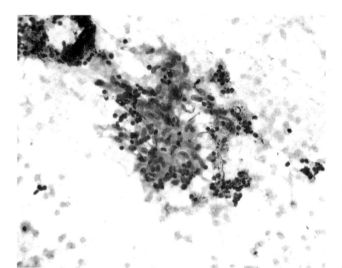

Figure 3.124. Epithelioid and spindle-shaped histiocytes in a nonnecrotizing granuloma (Pap stain).

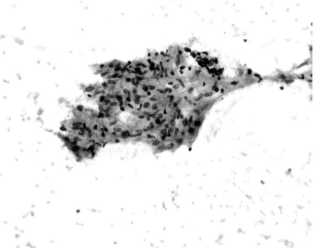

Figure 3.125. Nonnecrotizing granuloma. There is a syncytial appearance to the cluster of histiocytes, with no well-defined cell borders (Pap stain).

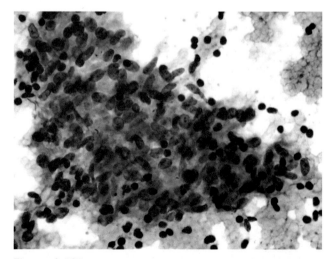

Figure 3.126. High-power view of nonnecrotizing granuloma. There is a tight cluster of histiocytes and scattered lymphocytes at the periphery. Note that the histiocytes have uniform, pale, bland chromatin (Diff-Quik stain).

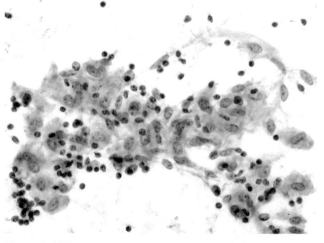

Figure 3.127. High-power view of nonnecrotizing granuloma consisting of admixed histiocytes and lymphocytes (Pap stain).

FUNGAL INFECTION

Fungal infections should always be on the differential when there is granulomatous inflammation (Table 3.4).[93] Microscopic identification of a specific fungal organism confirms the diagnosis (Figures 3.128-3.139), and corroboration with fungal cultures will facilitate speciation in the majority of cases. Some of the most important fungal diseases to be aware of are those caused by dimorphic fungi, which exist as yeasts at 37°C (human body temperature) and molds at colder temperatures; these include histoplasmosis, blastomycosis, coccidioidomycosis, and paracoccidioidomycosis. Invasive aspergillosis, zygomycosis, and candidiasis tend to invade pulmonary tissue and blood vessels, especially in immunocompromised patients.

HODGKIN LYMPHOMA

It is important to distinguish inflammatory processes from Hodgkin lymphoma when a granulomatous background is seen. Hodgkin lymphoma can be associated with a granulomatous reaction; therefore, a careful search for large, atypical Reed-Sternberg (RS) or RS-like cells must be made in cases with granulomatous inflammation (see the "Lymphoma" section under the "Loosely Cohesive/Single Cell Pattern"). Of note, reactive histiocytes may mimic RS/RS-like cells. However, true neoplastic RS/RS-like cells have very large irregular nuclei with prominent, inclusion-like macronucleoli. If cell block material is available, immunopositivity for PAX5 (weak), CD30, and/or CD15 can help distinguish RS/RS-like cells from histiocytes (CD68-positive).

MATRIX-CONTAINING LESIONS

Matrix-containing lesions include those that produce extracellular matrix material, most notably pulmonary hamartoma (benign) and adenoid cystic carcinoma (malignant). Other entities can be matrix containing, such as IMTs or schwannomas; however, the matrix component in these tumors is minimal and does not represent a major cytomorphologic feature required for the diagnosis. This section will focus on matrix-containing tumors found in the lungs, where identification of the matrix component facilitates the diagnosis.

CHECKLIST: Etiologic Considerations for Matrix-Containing Lesions

- ☐ Pulmonary Hamartoma
- ☐ Adenoid Cystic Carcinoma

PULMONARY HAMARTOMA

Hamartomas are the most common benign lung neoplasm and are often found incidentally in the peripheral lung as a well-circumscribed solitary single nodule (uncommonly in a central location or as multiple nodules). Histologically, hamartomas show abnormal growth of normal mesenchymal elements, most commonly cartilage, adipose tissue, and smooth muscle with entrapped ciliated, respiratory-type epithelium. In addition to the normal elements, fibromyxoid cells in a fibromyxoid stroma may be present, representing immature cartilaginous tissue (Figures 3.140 and 3.141). FNA has been shown to have high sensitivity and specificity for diagnosing pulmonary hamartomas,[94] but the presence of mesenchymal components in this location may lead to a misdiagnosis of a malignant sarcoma.

ADENOID CYSTIC CARCINOMA

Adenoid cystic carcinoma is one of the most common salivary gland–type tumor found in the lung, most commonly occurring in the trachea, but also in the major bronchi.[95,96] The tumor cells are small, uniform, and bland, and have round to oval hyperchromatic nuclei with small nucleoli. These cells characteristically form three-dimensional clusters surrounding cores of homogenous, hyaline material, creating an appearance analogous to the microcystic spaces typically seen on histology (Figures 3.142-3.145).[97]

TABLE 3.4: Pulmonary Fungal Infections

Disease	Organism	Location	Cytomorphology	Size (μm)	Cytomorphological Mimics[89]
Cryptococcosis	Cryptococcus neoformans	Worldwide	Yeast Narrow-based budding Gelatinous thick mucoid capsule	5-15	Other endemic fungi, Candida (yeast form)
Histoplasmosis	Histoplasma capsulatum	Americas, especially Ohio and Mississippi river valleys	Yeast, usually intracellular within macrophages; may be extracellular due to macrophage rupture[90,91]	2-5	May be mistaken for Candida (yeast form), P. jirovecii, microcalcifications, or platelets
Blastomycosis	Blastomyces dermatitidis	Americas, especially Ohio and Mississippi river valleys	Yeast Broad-based budding Thick double-layered refractile cell wall Granulomatous inflammatory background	8-20	Other endemic fungi, Candida (yeast form)
Coccidioidomycosis	Coccidioides immitis	Americas, especially southwest United States	Large spherules with thick walls containing endospores Hyphae in 5% of cases[92] Necrotizing granulomatous background	5-100, mean 10-40 (spherules) 2-5 (endospores)	Large fungal organisms
Paracoccidioidomycosis	Paracoccidioides brasiliensis	Central and South America	Yeast Multiple budding ("mariner's wheel")	4-40	
Aspergillosis	Aspergillus sp.	Worldwide	Thick, uniform, septate hyphae with 45-degree angle branching Fruiting bodies associated with calcium oxalate crystals Background typically shows abundant neutrophils and necrosis	3-6	Other filamentous fungi
Zygomycosis	Rhizopus sp. Mucor sp.	Worldwide	Variably sized nonseptate hyphae with 90-degree angle branching ("ribbon-like") Background typically shows abundant neutrophils and necrosis	3-25	Aspergillus, Candida
Candidiasis	Candida sp.	Worldwide	Yeast, can elongate into true or broad-based pseudohyphae ("sausage links")	3-4	May be mistaken for Aspergillus spp. or Cryptococcus spp. (yeast form)

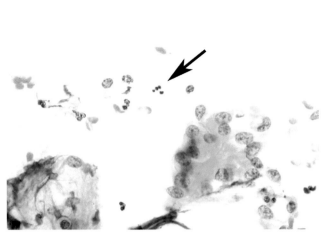

Figure 3.128. *Histoplasma* yeasts within a pulmonary macrophage (arrow). The small, budding yeasts stain dark blue on Pap stain (Pap stain).

Figure 3.129. The presence of *Histoplasma* yeasts is confirmed by silver stain, which show a thin outer capsule (GMS stain).

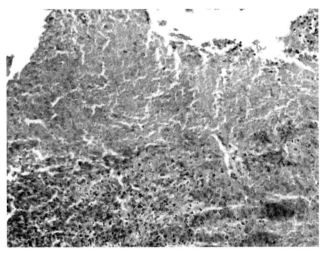

Figure 3.130. Abundant necrotic material in a cell block preparation with many small blue structures, suspicious for infectious organisms (H&E)

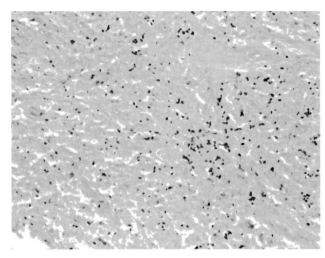

Figure 3.131. Corresponding silver stain of the previous cell block highlights abundant *Histoplasma* yeasts, which have a slightly elongated shape compared with *Cryptococcus* (GMS stain).

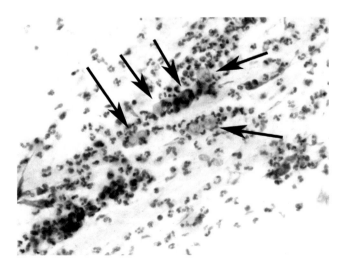

Figure 3.132. Multiple round *Blastomyces* yeast forms (arrows) with a pale, blue-green appearance on Pap stain, in a background of abundant acute inflammation (Pap stain).

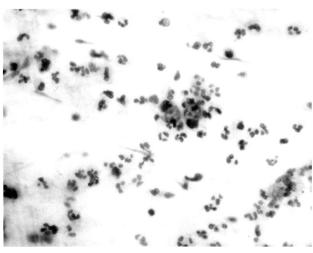

Figure 3.133. *Blastomyces* yeasts with a more purplish color. A double-layered cell wall, which is characteristic of *Blastomyces*, can be appreciated (Pap stain).

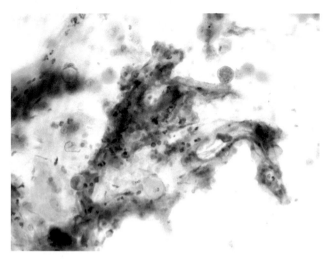

Figure 3.134. Low-power view of multiple *Coccidioides* spherules (pink) in a background of acute and chronic inflammation (Pap stain).

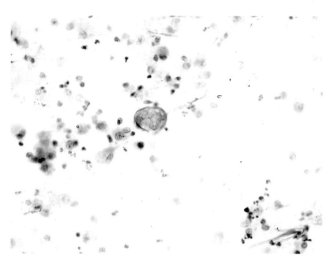

Figure 3.135. *Coccidioides* spherule containing numerous endospores, which appear as translucent balls packed within the thick pink capsule of the spherule (Pap stain).

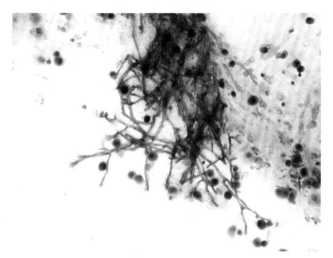

Figure 3.136. *Aspergillus* septate hyphae with uniform width and acute angle branching (Diff-Quik stain).

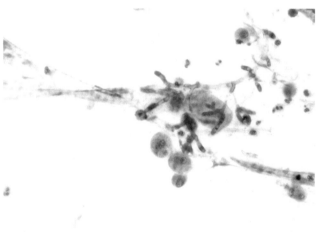

Figure 3.137. *Aspergillus* hyphae admixed with neutrophils and pulmonary macrophages (Pap stain).

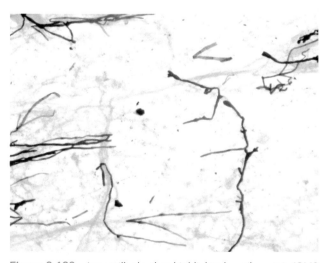

Figure 3.138. *Aspergillus* hyphae highlighted on silver stain (GMS stain).

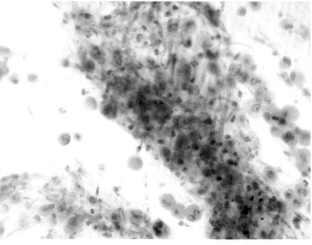

Figure 3.139. Zygomycetes hyphae in a background of inflammation. In contrast to *Aspergillus* hyphae, these are nonseptate with variable widths (Pap stain).

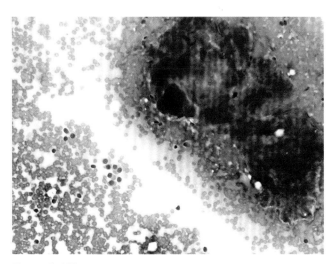

Figure 3.140. Pulmonary hamartoma. Fibromyxoid stroma (upper right) is present in a background of benign epithelial cells (Diff-Quik stain).

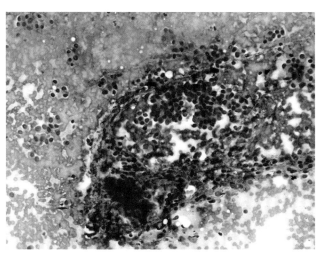

Figure 3.141. Pulmonary hamartoma. There are abundant benign epithelial cells associated with fibromyxoid stroma (Diff-Quik stain).

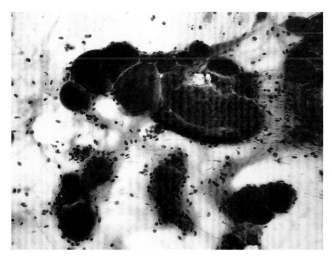

Figure 3.142. Adenoid cystic carcinoma. The cells are basaloid and uniform and form three-dimensional clusters around globules of hyaline material (Diff-Quik stain).

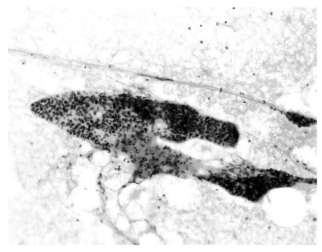

Figure 3.143. Adenoid cystic carcinoma. Basaloid cells form a three-dimensional structure and surround hyaline material. A mixture of matrix material and neoplastic cells should suggest the possibility of a salivary gland neoplasm, though the morphology seen here is not specific for adenoid cystic carcinoma (Pap stain).

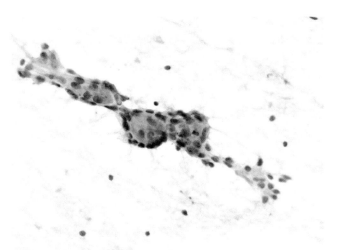

Figure 3.144. Adenoid cystic carcinoma. The small hyperchromatic cells form three-dimensional clusters around a large, homogenous translucent globule (Pap stain).

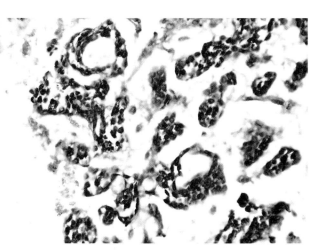

Figure 3.145. Adenoid cystic carcinoma. The microcystic spaces are readily appreciated (cell block, H&E).

EXTRAS

CURSCHMANN SPIRALS

Curschmann spirals are strands of mucus that are characteristically coiled due to their formation as inspissated mucous plugs in the subepithelial mucous gland ducts. Although they are more frequently seen in association with asthma and smoking, they can be seen in other types of specimens and are generally a nonspecific finding. They stain darkly purple on Papanicolaou stain (Figure 3.146).

CHARCOT-LEYDEN CRYSTALS

Charcot-Leyden crystals are orangeophilic rhomboid/needle-shaped crystals formed from the granules within degenerating eosinophils (Figure 3.147 and 3.148). They are seen in patients with allergic conditions such as asthma.

FERRUGINOUS BODIES

Ferruginous bodies are fiber particles encrusted with proteins containing iron salts (i.e. ferroproteins). The fiber is commonly asbestos but can also be other particles/minerals. They are golden brown to black dumbbell-shaped structures on Papanicolaou stain and can be seen within macrophages that have engulfed them (Figures 3.149 and 3.150). The presence of ferruginous bodies should be specifically mentioned in the pathology report to ensure that the patient is screened for mesothelial risk factors, if not already performed.

CORPORA AMYLACEA

Corpora amylacea are spherical, concentrically laminated, noncalcified casts composed of glycoproteins like those seen in benign prostatic glands (Figures 3.151-3.153). They can be seen in conditions associated with pulmonary edema, although they are nonspecific and have no clinical significance.

PSAMMOMA BODIES

Psammoma bodies are concentrically laminated calcifications that are associated with malignant neoplasms (especially those with papillary architecture) as well as benign diseases (e.g., pulmonary alveolar microlithiasis).

AMYLOID

Amyloid can be seen in transbronchial FNAs and appears identical to amyloid deposition in other locations (Figures 3.154 and 3.155).[98] Amyloid is a dense, amorphous, waxy, eosinophilic material with classic "apple green" birefringence under polarized light with Congo red staining.

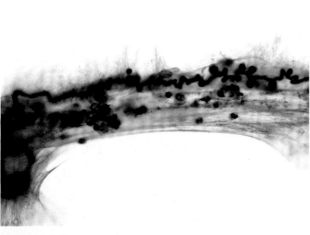

Figure 3.146. Curschmann spiral (dark purple) associated with loose mucus (Pap stain).

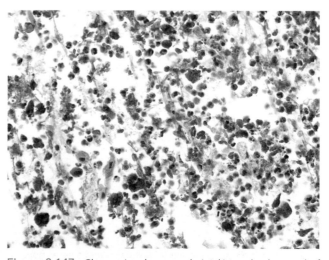

Figure 3.147. Charcot-Leyden crystals (pink) in a background of inflammation, debris, and cellular degeneration (Pap stain).

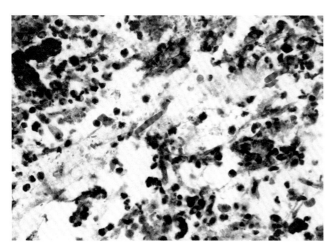

Figure 3.148. Charcot-Leyden crystals (pink) in a background of abundant eosinophils (H&E).

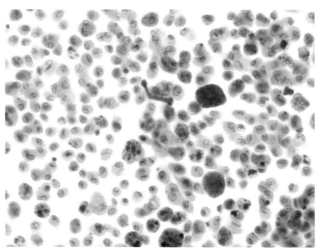

Figure 3.149. Ferruginous bodies (golden brown) in a background of pigmented pulmonary macrophages (Pap stain).

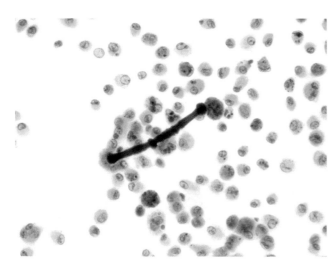

Figure 3.150. Ferrunginous bodies at high magnification (Pap stain).

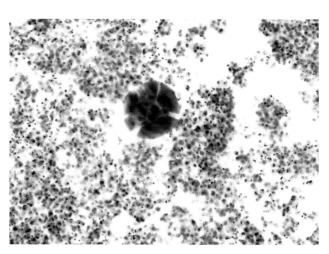

Figure 3.151. Corpora amylacea. The concentric laminations appear as different colors in this case (Pap stain).

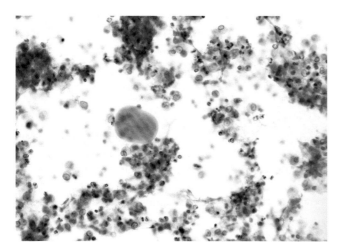

Figure 3.152. Corpora amylacea. This cast appears amorphous and homogenous, with a visible paler rim (Pap stain).

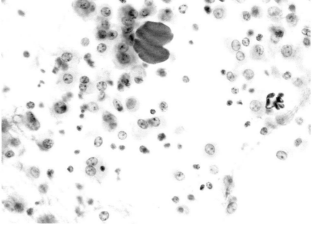

Figure 3.153. Corpora amylacea. This case is orangeophilic without obvious concentric laminations (Pap stain).

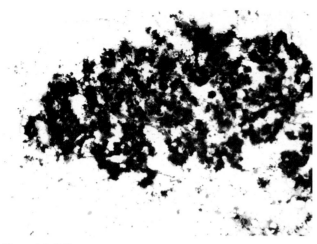

Figure 3.154. Amyloid. The material is dense and amorphous (Diff-Quik stain).

Figure 3.155. Amyloid (Pap stain).

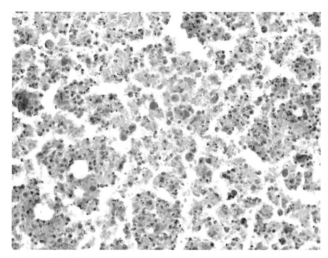

Figure 3.156. Pulmonary alveolar proteinosis. There are scattered, dense, amorphous globules in a dirty, frothy background (Pap stain).

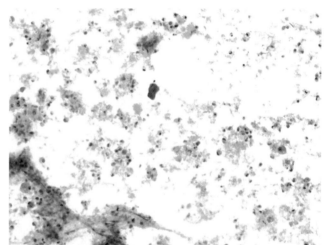

Figure 3.157. Amorphous protein (orangeophilic) in pulmonary alveolar proteinosis (Pap stain).

AMORPHOUS PROTEIN

Amorphous protein, as seen in pulmonary alveolar proteinosis, appears as dense, amorphous, and eosinophilic material in a dirty, hypocellular background (Figures 3.156-3.158). The protein is PAS positive and Oil Red O positive. Amorphous proteins can also be seen in viral infections and *Pneumocystis* pneumonia.[99]

PNEUMOCYSTIS JIROVECII

Pneumonia caused by *Pneumocystis jirovecii* typically presents in immunocompromised individuals and manifests as bilateral pulmonary infiltrates on chest X-ray. The organisms are not visible on Papanicolaou stain, but the associated foamy proteinaceous casts (green) can be seen (Figures 3.159-3.162). Giemsa stains show the cyst outlines and stains the intracystic trophozoites as discrete blue dots. Silver stains highlight the cup-shaped cysts (5-7 μm in diameter).[100]

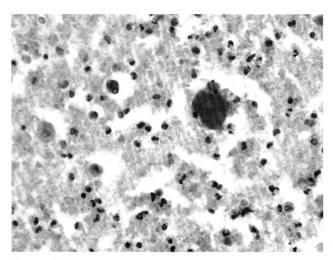

Figure 3.158. Amorphous protein as seen on PAS stain in pulmonary alveolar proteinosis. There is a dirty background of debris, neutrophils, and macrophages (PAS stain).

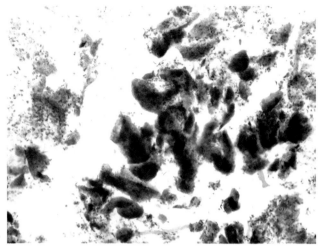

Figure 3.159. Low-power view of specimen from patient with *Pneumocystis* infection. Many frothy, proteinaceous casts can be seen at this power (Pap stain).

Figure 3.160. High-power view of foamy proteinaceous casts associated with *Pneumocystis* infection (Pap stain).

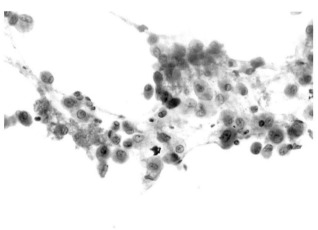

Figure 3.161. *Pneumocystis* infection. Organisms are not visible on Pap stains, but foamy proteinaceous casts are associated with *Pneumocystis* infection and warrant further workup, such as direct immunofluorescence or GMS stain (Pap stain).

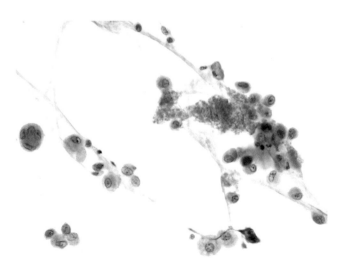

Figure 3.162. *Pneumocystis* infection. Separate field (Pap stain).

NEAR MISSES

INVASIVE ASPERGILLOSIS

Angioinvasive aspergillosis is primarily seen in immunocompromised patients and is difficult to diagnose on pulmonary cytology samples such as BAL. These lesions are characterized by hemorrhagic infarcts, which makes sampling less likely to yield *Aspergillus* hyphae. If no hyphae are visualized, the diagnosis cannot be confirmed. Also, *Aspergillus* can appear translucent ("negative image") on Diff-Quik stains, making the organism even more difficult to identify (Figures 3.163-3.164). Clinical correlation to ascertain the immune status of the patient as well as CT findings can be helpful to make the diagnosis. CT imaging usually shows multiple nodules with halos of ground glass attenuation and areas of segmental consolidation. In these high-risk cases, fungal stains and microbiologic cultures should be performed. Although cytology cannot determine if the aspergillosis is invasive or not, the presence of hyphae in the appropriate clinical and radiologic setting is sufficient to prompt therapy initiation.

PRIMARY SQUAMOUS CELL CARCINOMA VERSUS METASTATIC UROTHELIAL CARCINOMA

The lung is a common site of metastatic disease, and newly diagnosed adenocarcinomas in the lung should be confirmed as having a lung origin when possible, often by proving TTF-1 positivity in the carcinoma cells. The positivity of squamous markers in a newly diagnosed lung carcinoma should not automatically be presumed to indicate a primary SqCC.[101] For instance, in patients with a history of urothelial carcinoma, making a diagnosis of primary SqCC of the lung versus metastatic urothelial carcinoma can be challenging (Figures 3.165-3.170). The cytomorphologic features and immunohistochemical profile of these two tumors can overlap. Urothelial carcinoma is positive for GATA3 and p40/p63 but only positive for uroplakin in approximately half of all metastases. p40/p63 is the confirming immunohistochemical marker for SqCC in the lung, and GATA3 can be positive in 12% of these tumors as well. If GATA3 and uroplakin are both negative, a diagnosis of primary SqCC of the lung can be favored; however, if p40/p63 and GATA3 are both positive and uroplakin is negative, a distinction cannot be made immunohistochemically. Clinicoradiologic correlation to look for multiple lung nodules or other sites of metastatic tumor and/or comparison with the primary tumor (if available) may assist in making the distinction.

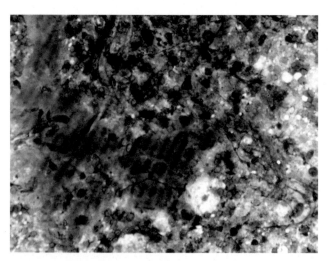

Figure 3.163. *Aspergillus*, seen as a negative image at high magnification (Diff-Quik stain).

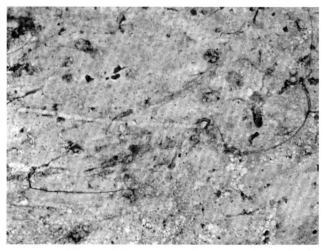

Figure 3.164. *Aspergillus* (separate specimen), seen as a negative image at high magnification (Diff-Quik stain).

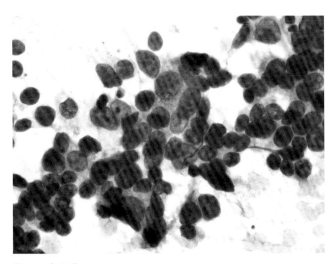

Figure 3.165. Metastatic urothelial carcinoma to the lung. The carcinoma is poorly differentiated, and the cells seen here could also possibly represent a primary lung adenocarcinoma or squamous cell carcinoma (Diff-Quik stain).

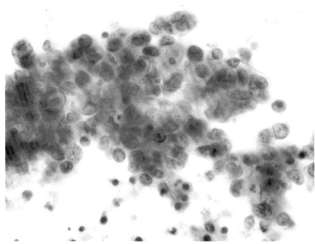

Figure 3.166. Metastatic urothelial carcinoma to the lung. Some cells have dense cytoplasm, and there are spaces between some neighboring cells, suggesting the possibility of squamous differentiation (Pap stain).

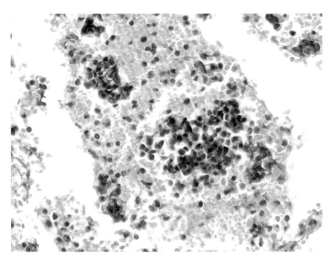

Figure 3.167. Metastatic urothelial carcinoma to the lung. Cell block preparation from the same specimen (H&E).

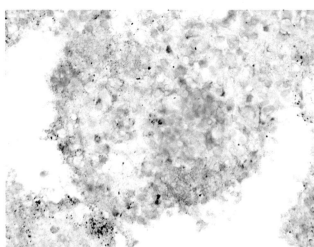

Figure 3.168. Metastatic urothelial carcinoma to the lung. TTF-1 (nuclear marker) is negative in the carcinoma cells. This would be expected in a metastatic adenocarcinoma or primary lung squamous cell carcinoma but does not completely exclude a lung primary adenocarcinoma (TTF-1 immunohistochemical stain).

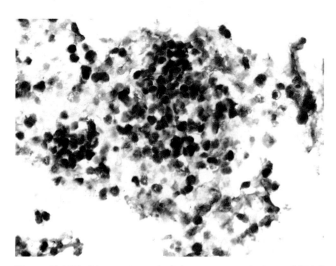

Figure 3.169. Metastatic urothelial carcinoma to the lung. GATA-3 (nuclear stain) is positive in the carcinoma cells. GATA-3 is often positive in breast and bladder adenocarcinomas but can also be positive in some primary lung carcinomas (GATA-3 immunostain).

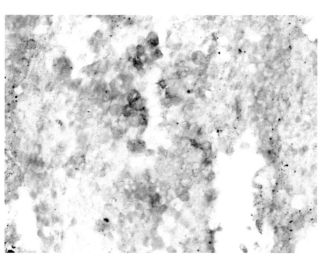

Figure 3.170. Metastatic urothelial carcinoma. The carcinoma cells are focally positive for uroplakin, a specific marker for a urothelial origin. In this case, the patient had a history of invasive urothelial carcinoma. Immunohistochemical results should be interpreted with caution if they conflict with the clinical impression (uroplakin immunostain).

References

1. VandenBussche CJ, Yarmus L, Illei PB. The utility of bronchial brushings in the modern era of flexible bronchoscopy. *J Am Soc Cytopathol.* 2017;6(1):1-7.

2. Russell PA, Wainer Z, Wright GM, Daniels M, Conron M, Williams RA. Does lung adenocarcinoma subtype predict patient survival?: a clinicopathologic study based on the new International Association for the Study of Lung Cancer/American Thoracic Society/European Respiratory Society international multidisciplinary lung adenocarcinoma classification. *J Thorac Oncol.* 2011;6(9):1496-1504.

3. Yanagawa N, Shiono S, Abiko M, Katahira M, Osakabe M, Ogata SY. The clinical impact of solid and micropapillary patterns in resected lung adenocarcinoma. *J Thorac Oncol.* 2016;11(11):1976-1983.

4. Yoshizawa A, Motoi N, Riely GJ, et al. Impact of proposed IASLC/ATS/ERS classification of lung adenocarcinoma: prognostic subgroups and implications for further revision of staging based on analysis of 514 stage I cases. *Mod Pathol.* 2011;24(5):653-664.

5. Rodriguez EF, Dacic S, Pantanowitz L, Khalbuss WE, Monaco SE. Cytopathology of pulmonary adenocarcinoma with a single histological pattern using the proposed International Association for the Study of Lung Cancer/American Thoracic Society/European Respiratory Society (IASLC/ATS/ERS) classification. *Cancer Cytopathol.* 2015;123(5):306-317.

6. Rodriguez EF, Monaco SE, Dacic S. Cytologic subtyping of lung adenocarcinoma by using the proposed International Association for the Study of Lung Cancer/American Thoracic Society/European Respiratory Society (IASLC/ATS/ERS) adenocarcinoma classification. *Cancer Cytopathol.* 2013;121(11):629-637.

7. Bergethon K, Shaw AT, Ou SH, et al. ROS1 rearrangements define a unique molecular class of lung cancers. *J Clin Oncol.* 2012;30(8):863-870.

8. Cancer Genome Atlas Research Network. Comprehensive genomic characterization of squamous cell lung cancers. *Nature.* 2012;489(7417):519-525.

9. Cancer Genome Atlas Research Network. Comprehensive molecular profiling of lung adenocarcinoma. *Nature.* 2014;511(7511):543-550.

10. Drilon A, Wang L, Hasanovic A, et al. Response to cabozantinib in patients with RET fusion-positive lung adenocarcinomas. *Cancer Discov.* 2013;3(6):630-635.

11. Kwak EL, Bang YJ, Camidge DR, et al. Anaplastic lymphoma kinase inhibition in non-small-cell lung cancer. *N Engl J Med.* 2010;363(18):1693-1703.

12. Mok TS, Wu YL, Thongprasert S, et al. Gefitinib or carboplatin-paclitaxel in pulmonary adenocarcinoma. *N Engl J Med.* 2009;361(10):947-957.

13. Monaco S, Mehrad M, Dacic S. Recent advances in the diagnosis of malignant mesothelioma: focus on approach in challenging cases and in limited tissue and cytologic samples. *Adv Anat Pathol*. 2018;25(1):24-30.

14. Peifer M, Fernandez-Cuesta L, Sos ML, et al. Integrative genome analyses identify key somatic driver mutations of small-cell lung cancer. *Nat Genet*. 2012;44(10):1104-1110.

15. Rudin CM, Durinck S, Stawiski EW, et al. Comprehensive genomic analysis identifies SOX2 as a frequently amplified gene in small-cell lung cancer. *Nat Genet*. 2012;44(10):1111-1116.

16. VandenBussche CJ, Illei PB, Lin MT, Ettinger DS, Maleki Z. Molecular alterations in non-small cell lung carcinomas of the young. *Hum Pathol*. 2014;45(12):2379-2387.

17. Rodriguez EF, Monaco SE. Recent advances in the pathology and molecular genetics of lung cancer: a practical review for cytopathologists. *J Am Soc Cytopathol*. 2016;5(5):252-265.

18. Jain D, Roy-Chowdhuri S. Molecular pathology of lung cancer cytology specimens: a concise review. *Arch Pathol Lab Med*. 2018;142(9):1127-1133.

19. Lindeman NI, Cagle PT, Aisner DL, et al. Updated molecular testing guideline for the selection of lung cancer patients for treatment with targeted tyrosine kinase inhibitors: guideline from the College of American Pathologists, the International Association for the Study of Lung Cancer, and the Association for Molecular Pathology. *J Mol Diagn*. 2018;20(2):129-159.

20. Russell-Goldman E, Kravets S, Dahlberg SE, Sholl LM, Vivero M. Cytologic-histologic correlation of programmed death-ligand 1 immunohistochemistry in lung carcinomas. *Cancer Cytopathol*. 2018;126(4):253-263.

21. Skov BG, Skov T. Paired comparison of PD-L1 expression on cytologic and histologic specimens from malignancies in the lung assessed with PD-L1 IHC 28-8pharmDx and PD-L1 IHC 22C3pharmDx. *Appl Immunohistochem Mol Morphol*. 2017;25(7):453-459.

22. Mukhopadhyay S, Katzenstein AL. Subclassification of non-small cell lung carcinomas lacking morphologic differentiation on biopsy specimens: utility of an immunohistochemical panel containing TTF-1, napsin A, p63, and CK5/6. *Am J Surg Pathol*. 2011;35(1):15-25.

23. Terry J, Leung S, Laskin J, Leslie KO, Gown AM, Ionescu DN. Optimal immunohistochemical markers for distinguishing lung adenocarcinomas from squamous cell carcinomas in small tumor samples. *Am J Surg Pathol*. 2010;34(12):1805-1811.

24. Rekhtman N, Ang DC, Sima CS, Travis WD, Moreira AL. Immunohistochemical algorithm for differentiation of lung adenocarcinoma and squamous cell carcinoma based on large series of whole-tissue sections with validation in small specimens. *Mod Pathol*. 2011;24(10): 1348-1359.

25. Rekhtman N, Kazi S. Nonspecific reactivity of polyclonal napsin a antibody in mucinous adenocarcinomas of various sites: a word of caution. *Arch Pathol Lab Med*. 2015;139(4):434-436.

26. Travis WD, Brambilla E, Noguchi M, et al. Diagnosis of lung cancer in small biopsies and cytology: implications of the 2011 International Association for the Study of Lung Cancer/American Thoracic Society/European Respiratory Society classification. *Arch Pathol Lab Med*. 2013;137(5):668-684.

27. Lilo MT, Allison D, Wang Y, et al. Expression of P40 and P63 in lung cancers using fine needle aspiration cases. Understanding clinical pitfalls and limitations. *J Am Soc Cytopathol*. 2016;5(3):123-132.

28. Mukhopadhyay S, Katzenstein AL. Comparison of monoclonal napsin A, polyclonal napsin A, and TTF-1 for determining lung origin in metastatic adenocarcinomas. *Am J Clin Pathol*. 2012;138(5):703-711.

29. Rodriguez EF, VandenBussche CJ, Chowsilpa S, Maleki Z. Molecular genetic alterations in thyroid transcription factor 1-negative lung adenocarcinoma in cytology specimens: a subset with aggressive behavior and a poor prognosis. *Cancer Cytopathol*. 2018;126(10):853-859.

30. International Agency for Research on Cancer, Travis WD, Brambilla E, Burke AP, et al. *WHO Classification of Tumours of the Lung, Pleura, Thymus and Heart*; 2015.

31. Hutchings D, Maleki Z, Rodriguez EF. Pulmonary non-small cell carcinoma with morphologic features of adenocarcinoma or "non-small cell carcinoma favor adenocarcinoma" in cytologic specimens share similar clinical and molecular genetic characteristics. *Am J Clin Pathol*. 2018;149(6):514-521.

32. Ocque R, Tochigi N, Ohori NP, Dacic S. Usefulness of immunohistochemical and histochemical studies in the classification of lung adenocarcinoma and squamous cell carcinoma in cytologic specimens. *Am J Clin Pathol*. 2011;136(1):81-87.

33. Righi L, Graziano P, Fornari A, et al. Immunohistochemical subtyping of nonsmall cell lung cancer not otherwise specified in fine-needle aspiration cytology: a retrospective study of 103 cases with surgical correlation. *Cancer*. 2011;117(15):3416-3423.

34. Renshaw AA, Dean BR, Antman KH, Sugarbaker DJ, Cibas ES. The role of cytologic evaluation of pleural fluid in the diagnosis of malignant mesothelioma. *Chest*. 1997;111(1):106-109.

35. Churg A, Colby TV, Cagle P, et al. The separation of benign and malignant mesothelial proliferations. *Am J Surg Pathol*. 2000;24(9):1183-1200.

36. Cigognetti M, Lonardi S, Fisogni S, et al. BAP1 (BRCA1-associated protein 1) is a highly specific marker for differentiating mesothelioma from reactive mesothelial proliferations. *Mod Pathol*. 2015;28(8):1043-1057.

37. Hasteh F, Lin GY, Weidner N, Michael CW. The use of immunohistochemistry to distinguish reactive mesothelial cells from malignant mesothelioma in cytologic effusions. *Cancer Cytopathol*. 2010;118(2):90-96.

38. Factor RE, Dal Cin P, Fletcher JA, Cibas ES. Cytogenetics and fluorescence in situ hybridization as adjuncts to cytology in the diagnosis of malignant mesothelioma. *Cancer*. 2009;117(4):247-253.

39. Hung YP, Dong F, Watkins JC, et al. Identification of ALK rearrangements in malignant peritoneal mesothelioma. *JAMA Oncol*. 2018;4(2):235-238.

40. Zaman MB, Hajdu SI, Melamed MR, Watson RC. Transthoracic aspiration cytology of pulmonary lesions. *Semin Diagn Pathol*. 1986;3(3):176-187.

41. Ashton PR, Hollingsworth AS Jr, Johnston WW. The cytopathology of metastatic breast cancer. *Acta Cytol*. 1975;19(1):1-6.

42. Ni YB, Tsang JYS, Shao MM, et al. GATA-3 is superior to GCDFP-15 and mammaglobin to identify primary and metastatic breast cancer. *Breast Cancer Res Treat*. 2018;169(1):25-32.

43. Flint A, Lloyd RV. Colon carcinoma metastatic to the lung. Cytologic manifestations and distinction from primary pulmonary adenocarcinoma. *Acta Cytol*. 1992;36(2):230-235.

44. Saleh H, Masood S, Wynn G, Assaf N. Unsuspected metastatic renal cell carcinoma diagnosed by fine needle aspiration biopsy. A report of four cases with immunocytochemical contributions. *Acta Cytol*. 1994;38(4):554-561.

45. Tao LC, Robertson DI. Cytologic diagnosis of bronchial mucoepidermoid carcinoma by fine needle aspiration biopsy. *Acta Cytol*. 1978;22(4):221-224.

46. Tonon G, Modi S, Wu L, et al. t(11;19)(q21;p13) translocation in mucoepidermoid carcinoma creates a novel fusion product that disrupts a Notch signaling pathway. *Nat Genet*. 2003;33(2):208-213.

47. Chiosea SI, Dacic S, Nikiforova MN, Seethala RR. Prospective testing of mucoepidermoid carcinoma for the MAML2 translocation: clinical implications. *Laryngoscope*. 2012;122(8):1690-1694.

48. Travis WD, Rush W, Flieder DB, et al. Survival analysis of 200 pulmonary neuroendocrine tumors with clarification of criteria for atypical carcinoid and its separation from typical carcinoid. *Am J Surg Pathol*. 1998;22(8):934-944.

49. Klimstra DS, Modlin IR, Coppola D, Lloyd RV, Suster S. The pathologic classification of neuroendocrine tumors: a review of nomenclature, grading, and staging systems. *Pancreas*. 2010;39(6):707-712.

50. Maleki Z. Diagnostic issues with cytopathologic interpretation of lung neoplasms displaying high-grade basaloid or neuroendocrine morphology. *Diagn Cytopathol*. 2011;39(3):159-167.

51. Rodriguez EF, Chowsilpa S, Maleki Z. Insulinoma-associated protein 1 immunostain: a diagnostic tool for pulmonary small cell carcinoma in cytology. *Acta Cytol*. 2018:1-6.

52. Rooper LM, Sharma R, Li QK, Illei PB, Westra WH. INSM1 demonstrates superior performance to the individual and combined use of synaptophysin, chromogranin and CD56 for diagnosing neuroendocrine tumors of the thoracic cavity. *Am J Surg Pathol*. 2017;41(11):1561-1569.

53. Thunnissen E, Borczuk AC, Flieder DB, et al. The use of immunohistochemistry improves the diagnosis of small cell lung cancer and its differential diagnosis. An international reproducibility study in a demanding set of cases. *J Thorac Oncol*. 2017;12(2):334-346.

54. Zheng G, Ettinger DS, Maleki Z. Utility of the quantitative Ki-67 proliferation index and CD56 together in the cytologic diagnosis of small cell lung carcinoma and other lung neuroendocrine tumors. *Acta Cytol*. 2013;57(3):281-290.

55. Klimstra DS. Pathology reporting of neuroendocrine tumors: essential elements for accurate diagnosis, classification, and staging. *Semin Oncol*. 2013;40(1):23-36.

56. Pelosi G, Rindi G, Travis WD, Papotti M. Ki-67 antigen in lung neuroendocrine tumors: unraveling a role in clinical practice. *J Thorac Oncol.* 2014;9(3):273-284.

57. Pelosi G, Pasini F, Sonzogni A, et al. Prognostic implications of neuroendocrine differentiation and hormone production in patients with Stage I nonsmall cell lung carcinoma. *Cancer.* 2003;97(10):2487-2497.

58. Habermann TM, Ryu JH, Inwards DJ, Kurtin PJ. Primary pulmonary lymphoma. *Semin Oncol.* 1999;26(3):307-315.

59. Nason KS, Kirchner A, Schuchert MJ, et al. Endobronchial ultrasound-transbronchial needle aspiration for lymphoma in patients with low suspicion for lung cancer and mediastinal lymphadenopathy. *Ann Thorac Surg.* 2016;101(5):1856-1863.

60. Flieder DB, Yousem SA. Pulmonary lymphomas and lymphoid hyperplasias. In: Knowles DM, ed. *Neoplastic hematopathology.* Philadelphia: Lippincott Williams & Wilkins; 2001.

61. Riazmontazer N, Bedayat G. Cytology of plasma cell myeloma in bronchial washing. *Acta Cytol.* 1989;33(4):519-522.

62. Rosen SE, Vonderheid EC, Koprowska I. Mycosis fungoides with pulmonary involvement. Cytopathologic findings. *Acta Cytol.* 1984;28(1):51-57.

63. Bavle RM. Lymphoglandular bodies. *J Oral Maxillofac Pathol.* 2014;18(3):334-335.

64. Meis-Kindblom JM, Kjellstrom C, Kindblom LG. Inflammatory fibrosarcoma: update, reappraisal, and perspective on its place in the spectrum of inflammatory myofibroblastic tumors. *Semin Diagn Pathol.* 1998;15(2):133-143.

65. Lawrence B, Perez-Atayde A, Hibbard MK, et al. TPM3-ALK and TPM4-ALK oncogenes in inflammatory myofibroblastic tumors. *Am J Pathol.* 2000;157(2):377-384.

66. Stoll LM, Li QK. Cytology of fine-needle aspiration of inflammatory myofibroblastic tumor. *Diagn Cytopathol.* 2011;39(9):663-672.

67. Cessna MH, Zhou H, Sanger WG, et al. Expression of ALK1 and p80 in inflammatory myofibroblastic tumor and its mesenchymal mimics: a study of 135 cases. *Mod Pathol.* 2002;15(9):931-938.

68. Vogels RJ, Vlenterie M, Versleijen-Jonkers YM, et al. Solitary fibrous tumor – clinicopathologic, immunohistochemical and molecular analysis of 28 cases. *Diagn Pathol.* 2014;9:224.

69. Lee JC, Fletcher CD. Malignant fat-forming solitary fibrous tumor (so-called "lipomatous hemangiopericytoma"): clinicopathologic analysis of 14 cases. *Am J Surg Pathol.* 2011;35(8):1177-1185.

70. Doyle LA, Vivero M, Fletcher CD, Mertens F, Hornick JL. Nuclear expression of STAT6 distinguishes solitary fibrous tumor from histologic mimics. *Mod Pathol.* 2014;27(3):390-395.

71. Franks TJ, Galvin JR. Sarcomatoid carcinoma of the lung: histologic criteria and common lesions in the differential diagnosis. *Arch Pathol Lab Med.* 2010;134(1):49-54.

72. Crosby JH, Hooeg K, Hager B. Transthoracic fine needle aspiration of primary and metastatic sarcomas. *Diagn Cytopathol.* 1985;1(3):221-227.

73. Travis WD, Travis LB, Devesa SS. Lung cancer. *Cancer.* 1995;75(1 suppl):191-202.

74. Janssen JP, Mulder JJ, Wagenaar SS, Elbers HR, van den Bosch JM. Primary sarcoma of the lung: a clinical study with long-term follow-up. *Ann Thorac Surg.* 1994;58(4):1151-1155.

75. Guccion JG, Rosen SH. Bronchopulmonary leiomyosarcoma and fibrosarcoma. A study of 32 cases and review of the literature. *Cancer.* 1972;30(3):836-847.

76. Yaseen SB, Mustafa F, Rafiq D, Makhdoomi R, Chanda N. Primary pulmonary synovial sarcoma: diagnosis on squash smears. *J Cytol.* 2015;32(1):56-58.

77. Stanfield BL, Powers CN, Desch CE, Brooks JW, Frable WJ. Fine-needle aspiration cytology of an unusual primary lung tumor, chondrosarcoma: case report. *Diagn Cytopathol.* 1991;7(4):423-426.

78. Mhoyan A, Weidner N, Shabaik A. Epithelioid hemangioendothelioma of the lung diagnosed by transesophageal endoscopic ultrasound-guided fine needle aspiration: a case report. *Acta Cytol.* 2004;48(4):555-559.

79. Etienne-Mastroianni B, Falchero L, Chalabreysse L, et al. Primary sarcomas of the lung: a clinicopathologic study of 12 cases. *Lung Cancer.* 2002;38(3):283-289.

80. Keel SB, Bacha E, Mark EJ, Nielsen GP, Rosenberg AE. Primary pulmonary sarcoma: a clinicopathologic study of 26 cases. *Mod Pathol.* 1999;12(12):1124-1131.

81. Leslie KO, Wick MR. *Practical Pulmonary Pathology: A Diagnostic Approach.* Philadelphia, PA: Elsevier/Saunders; 2011.

82. Hummel P, Cangiarella JF, Cohen JM, Yang G, Waisman J, Chhieng DC. Transthoracic fine-needle aspiration biopsy of pulmonary spindle cell and mesenchymal lesions: a study of 61 cases. *Cancer*. 2001;93(3):187-198.

83. Weissinger SE, Keil P, Silvers DN, et al. A diagnostic algorithm to distinguish desmoplastic from spindle cell melanoma. *Mod Pathol*. 2014;27(4):524-534.

84. Chen LL, Jaimes N, Barker CA, Busam KJ, Marghoob AA. Desmoplastic melanoma: a review. *J Am Acad Dermatol*. 2013;68(5):825-833.

85. Ramos-Herberth FI, Karamchandani J, Kim J, Dadras SS. SOX10 immunostaining distinguishes desmoplastic melanoma from excision scar. *J Cutan Pathol*. 2010;37(9):944-952.

86. Tsuta K, Kalhor N, Wistuba II, Moran CA. Clinicopathological and immunohistochemical analysis of spindle-cell carcinoid tumour of the lung. *Histopathology*. 2011;59(3):526-536.

87. Rekhtman N. Neuroendocrine tumors of the lung: an update. *Arch Pathol Lab Med*. 2010;134(11):1628-1638.

88. Spagnolo P, Rossi G, Trisolini R, Sverzellati N, Baughman RP, Wells AU. Pulmonary sarcoidosis. *Lancet Respir Med*. 2018;6(5):389-402.

89. Allison DB, Simner PJ, Ali SZ. Identification of infectious organisms in cytopathology: a review of ancillary diagnostic techniques. *Cancer Cytopathol*. 2018;126(suppl 8):643-653.

90. Blumenfeld W, Gan GL. Diagnosis of histoplasmosis in bronchoalveolar lavage fluid by intracytoplasmic localization of silver-positive yeast. *Acta Cytol*. 1991;35(6):710-712.

91. Gallardo J, Sasal M, Ferreres JC. Diagnosis of histoplasmosis in bronchoalveolar lavage fluid. *Acta Cytol*. 1995;39(3):595-596.

92. Ke Y, Smith CW, Salaru G, Joho KL, Deen MF. Unusual forms of immature sporulating Coccidioides immitis diagnosed by fine-needle aspiration biopsy. *Arch Pathol Lab Med*. 2006;130(1):97-100.

93. Atkins KA, Powers CN. The cytopathology of infectious diseases. *Adv Anat Pathol*. 2002;9(1):52-64.

94. Dunbar F, Leiman G. The aspiration cytology of pulmonary hamartomas. *Diagn Cytopathol*. 1989;5(2):174-180.

95. Houston HE, Payne WS, Harrison EG Jr, Olsen AM. Primary cancers of the trachea. *Arch Surg*. 1969;99(2):132-140.

96. Radhika S, Dey P, Rajwanshi A, Guleria R, Bhusnurmath B. Adenoid cystic carcinoma in a bronchial washing. A case report. *Acta Cytol*. 1993;37(1):97-99.

97. Monaco SE, Khalbuss WE, Ustinova E, Liang A, Cai G. The cytomorphologic spectrum of salivary gland type tumors in the lung and mediastinum: a report of 16 patients. *Diagn Cytopathol*. 2012;40(12):1062-1070.

98. Chen KT. Cytology of tracheobronchial amyloidosis. *Acta Cytol*. 1984;28(2):133-135.

99. Burkhalter A, Silverman JF, Hopkins MB III, Geisinger KR. Bronchoalveolar lavage cytology in pulmonary alveolar proteinosis. *Am J Clin Pathol*. 1996;106(4):504-510.

100. Midgley J, Parsons PA, Shanson DC, Husain OA, Francis N. Monoclonal immunofluorescence compared with silver stain for investigating Pneumocystis carinii pneumonia. *J Clin Pathol*. 1991;44(1):75-76.

101. Nguyen DN, Kawamoto S, Cimino-Mathews A, Illei PB, Rosenthal DL, VandenBussche CJ. Metastatic metaplastic breast carcinoma mimicking pulmonary squamous cell carcinoma on fine-needle aspiration. *Diagn Cytopathol*. 2015;43(10):844-849.

CHAPTER OUTLINE

THE UNREMARKABLE LIVER

The unremarkable liver consists of numerous lobular units composed of a central vein, cords of hepatocytes, and peripheral portal tracts. Portal tracts consist of three separate structures: bile ducts, hepatic artery branches, and a branch of the portal vein (Figures 4.1 and 4.2). The apical surfaces of the hepatocyte cords face the sinusoids, which carries blood from the portal vein and hepatic artery to the central vein. The basal surfaces of the hepatocyte cords form bile canaliculi, which provide a conduit for bile drainage from the hepatocytes to bile ducts that eventually leave the liver.

HEPATOCYTES

Hepatocytes are the predominant liver parenchymal cells. They are large polygonal cells with central, round, variably sized nuclei, prominent nucleoli, and abundant evenly granular cytoplasm (Figures 4.3-4.5). Binucleation/multinucleation and intracytoplasmic lipofuscin pigment are common. Vacuolization of the cytoplasm due to fat or glycogen accumulation is also common and may or may not be pathologic. Benign hepatocytes are present in cytological specimens as single cells or in fragments/trabeculae, typically no more than two cells wide.

BILE DUCT EPITHELIUM

On bile duct brushing samples, normal bile duct epithelium is present as cohesive, flat sheets with evenly spaced nuclei, imparting a honeycomb-like appearance. When sampled by aspiration, the bile duct epithelial cells are usually present in small groups and

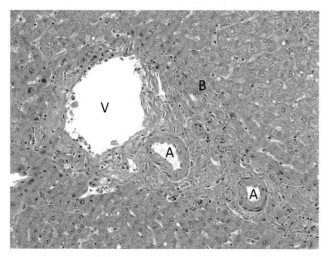

Figure 4.1. Normal portal tract with portal vein (V), multiple hepatic artery branches (A), and a bile duct profile (B) (H&E).

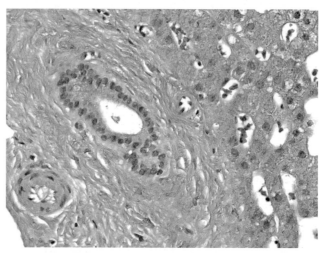

Figure 4.2. High-power view of a benign bile duct within a portal tract and adjacent benign hepatocytes. The bile duct epithelium is composed of cuboidal cells with uniform round nuclei. The hepatocytes are polygonal cells with round nuclei and abundant pink cytoplasm (H&E).

fragments, in contrast to sheets. In both samples, the cells range from low cuboidal to columnar in shape, have round nuclei with smooth nuclear membranes, fine chromatin, and inconspicuous nucleoli, and are smaller than hepatocytes (Figures 4.6-4.9). Bile duct epithelial cells are commonly seen in nonneoplastic liver aspirates but should be absent in hepatic adenomas and hepatocellular carcinomas (HCCs).

KUPFFER CELLS

Kupffer cells are specialized macrophages lining the liver sinusoids. In aspirate smears, Kupffer cells have ovoid or elongated nuclei and scant cytoplasm and are often attached to hepatocytes. They may contain vacuolated cytoplasm and hemosiderin pigment.

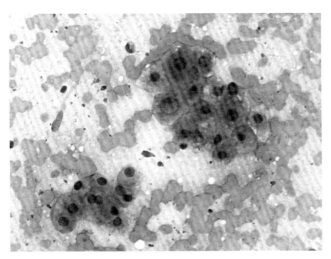

Figure 4.3. Fragments of benign hepatocytes. Some nuclear size variation and occasional binucleation is normal (Diff-Quik stain).

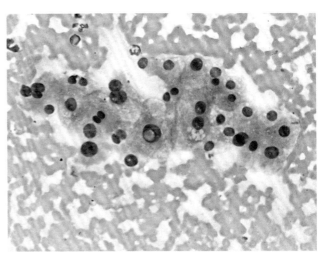

Figure 4.4. Benign hepatocytes, one of which contains an intranuclear inclusion (Diff-Quik stain).

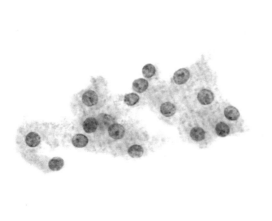

Figure 4.5. Benign hepatocytes. Distinct nucleoli can be seen in normal hepatocytes (Pap stain).

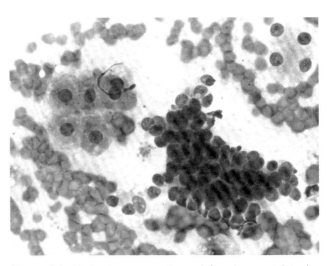

Figure 4.6. Benign hepatocytes (upper left and upper right) adjacent to benign ductal epithelium (lower right). Hepatocytes have abundant cytoplasm and lower nuclear to cytoplasmic ratios, as compared with the ductal epithelium (Diff-Quik stain).

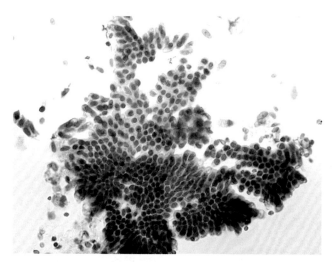

Figure 4.7. Benign ductal cells are arranged in an evenly spaced monolayer with a honeycomb-like appearance (Pap stain).

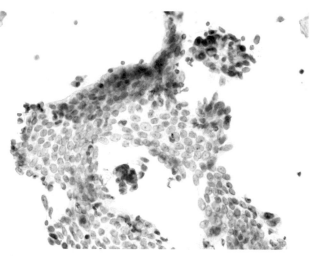

Figure 4.8. Monolayer of benign bile duct epithelium. Note that the cells have pale bland chromatin and are evenly spaced (Pap stain).

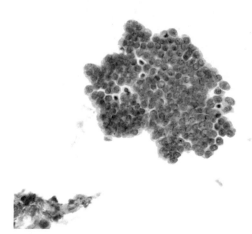

Figure 4.9. Uniform cells in a sheet of benign bile duct epithelium (Pap stain).

HEPATOCELLULAR PATTERN

The hepatocellular pattern includes benign/reactive and neoplastic lesions composed primarily of hepatocytes, which can range from bland-appearing to cytologically atypical. This pattern includes hepatocellular carcinoma (HCC) and its variants, which are malignant neoplasms derived from hepatocytes.

CHECKLIST: Etiologic Considerations for the Hepatocellular Pattern

☐ Focal Nodular Hyperplasia

☐ Regenerative Nodules

☐ Hepatic Adenoma

☐ Hepatocellular Carcinoma (HCC), Well to Moderately Differentiated

☐ Fibrolamellar Hepatocellular Carcinoma (HCC)

☐ Hepatoblastoma

FOCAL NODULAR HYPERPLASIA

Focal nodular hyperplasia (FNH) is a benign tumor-like lesion mainly found in females (80-95%) in the third or fourth decade that is thought to result from a hyperplastic response to vasculopathies.[1-3] These lesions have no malignant potential and usually present asymptomatically as a solitary (sometimes multifocal) mass. Radiologic correlation can be very helpful, as FNH nodules characteristically have a central stellate scar that can be appreciated on magnetic resonance imaging. Cytologically, FNH smears show normal hepatocytes and/or fragments of bile duct epithelium without significant cytomorphologic changes. Fragments of bland spindle cells intermixed with metachromatic stroma and other normal cell types may also be seen (Figures 4.10-4.13).[4,5] FNH can be difficult to distinguish from regenerating nodules in cirrhosis and hepatic adenomas. However, in the absence of a clinical history of cirrhosis, which affects the liver diffusely, along with the lack of substantial cytologic atypia point to a diagnosis of FNH. To differentiate FNH from hepatic adenomas, it is important to identify bile duct epithelium in the sample, as bile ducts are absent in hepatic adenomas. However, bile duct epithelium may not be present in an undersampled FNH nodule.

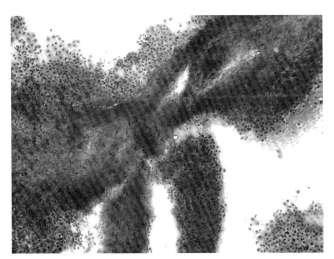

Figure 4.10. Low-power view of focal nodular hyperplasia, which contains a mixture of benign hepatocytes and fibroblasts/fibrosis (Diff-Quik stain).

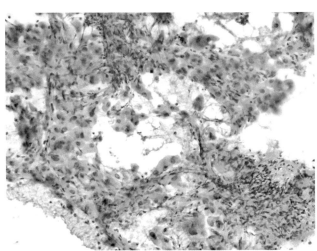

Figure 4.11. Focal nodular hyperplasia. Benign hepatocytes are intermixed with fibroblasts, which traverse across the hepatocytes (Pap stain).

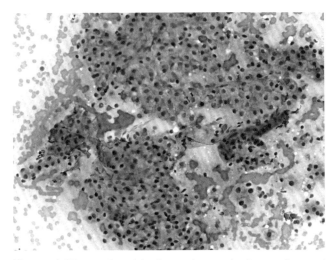

Figure 4.12. Focal nodular hyperplasia with sheets of normal hepatocytes (Diff-Quik stain).

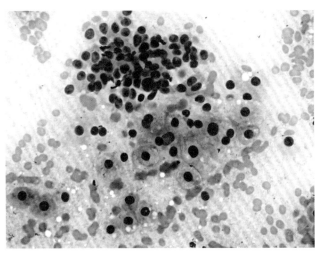

Figure 4.13. Focal nodular hyperplasia with adjacent benign hepatocytes and ductal cells. Note that the benign hepatocytes have no nuclear atypia or pleomorphism, and there is no necrosis or mitoses, which can be seen in cirrhosis (Diff-Quik stain).

REGENERATIVE NODULES

Regenerative nodules in the liver are generally seen in association with cirrhosis, where the normal liver architecture is transformed by bands of bridging fibrosis, resulting in nodules of regenerating hepatocytes. Regenerating hepatocytes range in appearance from normal to atypical, the latter of which includes enlargement, pleomorphism, prominent nucleoli, increased mitoses, and binucleation (Figures 4.14 and 4.15). As patients with cirrhosis are at increased risk for developing HCC, it can be diagnostically challenging to distinguish a regenerative cirrhotic nodule (especially >2 cm) from well differentiated HCC (Table 4.1). The presence of severely atypical cytomorphological features in the sampled hepatocytes supports a diagnosis of HCC.[6-8]

A cytologically similar entity is nodular regenerative hyperplasia, which is a rare form of benign liver hyperplasia associated with portal hypertension in the absence of cirrhosis, in which the liver parenchyma is diffusely transformed into small regenerative nodules.[9]

HEPATIC ADENOMA

Hepatic adenomas are rare benign neoplasms of hepatocytes usually seen in young women with a history of oral contraceptive use longer than 5 years.[10] They are highly vascular and can rupture through the liver capsule and result in life-threatening peritoneal hemorrhage. In addition, malignant transformation to HCC can rarely occur.[11] On histology, hepatic

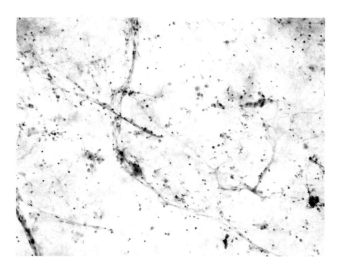

Figure 4.14. Low-power view of regenerative nodule in cirrhosis. Small thin fragments and scattered benign-appearing hepatocytes are seen in a background of fibrotic strands and lymphocytes (Pap stain).

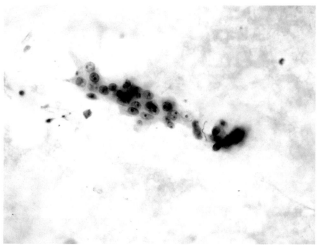

Figure 4.15. High-power view of regenerative nodule in cirrhosis. The regenerating hepatocytes in this fragment have prominent nucleoli and increased nuclear to cytoplasmic ratio but no architectural features to suggest malignancy (i.e. endothelial wrapping, transgressing vessels, etc.) (Pap stain).

TABLE 4.1: Morphologic Features of Benign vs. Malignant Hepatocytes

Benign/Regenerating Hepatocytes	Malignant Hepatocytes
Polymorphous variation	Monomorphic atypia
Normal nuclear to cytoplasmic ratio	Increased nuclear to cytoplasmic ratio (in well to moderately differentiated HCC)
Fragments/clusters of normal hepatocytes with normal trabecular thickness (2 cells thick)	Thickened trabeculae of varying thickness (>2 cells thick)
No to minimal endothelial wrapping of hepatocytes	Endothelial wrapping of hepatocytes
	Atypical naked nuclei

adenomas characteristically lack portal triads and contain naked arterioles without associated bile ducts. Correspondingly, cytology is notable for large, three-dimensional, cohesive groups of normal-appearing hepatocytes with the absence of bile duct epithelium (Figures 4.16-4.19). Hemorrhage and necrosis can be seen. Again, clinical and radiologic correlation is essential to differentiate hepatic adenomas from FNH and well differentiated HCC, as a definitive diagnosis is often difficult on cytology alone.

HEPATOCELLULAR CARCINOMA (HCC), WELL TO MODERATELY DIFFERENTIATED

HCC is by far the most common primary malignancy of the liver and accounts for 90% of primary liver cancers. In the United States, HCC is primarily seen in the setting of cirrhosis, with common risk factors being alcoholic liver disease and viral hepatitis (hepatitis B or C infection). HCC can present as a solitary mass, multiple masses, or diffuse liver enlargement. Furthermore, there are multiple architectural patterns and histologic variants of HCC, some of which cannot be distinguished on cytology. Based on cytomorphology, HCC can be classified as well differentiated, moderately differentiated, and poorly differentiated

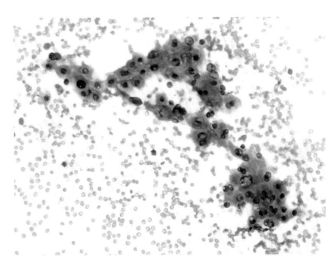

Figure 4.16. Hepatic adenoma. The smear is cellular with cohesive fragments of reactive hepatocytes. No bile ducts are seen in this specimen (Diff-Quik stain).

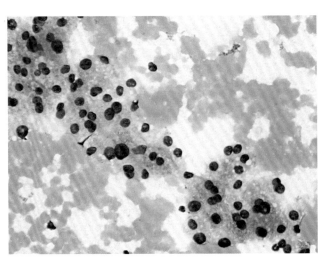

Figure 4.17. Hepatic adenoma. The hepatocytes are benign-appearing with binucleation, moderate anisonucleosis, and abundant granular/vacuolated cytoplasm (Diff-Quik stain).

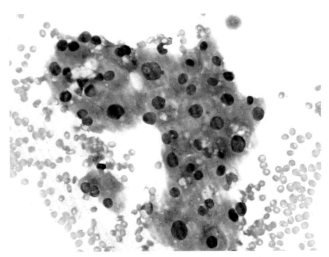

Figure 4.18. Hepatic adenoma. A thick fragment of benign-appearing hepatocytes is seen. Bile accumulation within hepatocytes may be seen, but bile ducts are not present within the lesion (Diff-Quik stain).

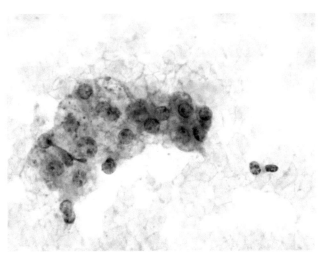

Figure 4.19. Hepatic adenoma. The hepatocytes are benign-appearing with abundant vacuolated cytoplasm (Pap stain).

tumors. In contrast to poorly differentiated HCC (see the "Poorly Differentiated/Epithelioid Pattern"), well to moderately differentiated HCCs have recognizable hepatocytic differentiation but may be more monotonous appearing with mild cytomorphologic atypia such as increased nuclear to cytoplasmic (N/C) ratio, prominent macronucleoli, and disorganized nuclear crowding within sheets (Figures 4.20-4.35).[6,12-14] Multinucleation and mitoses are increased in HCC but can also be seen in benign hepatocytes. Glypican-3 is a marker that is more likely to be positive in HCC than in benign hepatocytes, and may help support a diagnosis of well differentiated HCC when positive.[15]

KEY FEATURES of Well to Moderately Differentiated HCC

- The specimen often has high cellularity.
- The specimen contains isolated cells and naked nuclei.
- Thickened trabeculae (>2 cells thick) may be seen.
- Trabeculae may be surrounded by small vessels ("endothelial cell wrapping").
- Capillaries may traverse through neoplastic tissue fragments ("transgressing vessels").
- The neoplastic cells may form pseudoglandular (acinar) structures.
- The neoplastic cells demonstrate an increased N/C ratio.
- The neoplastic cells contain enlarged nuclei with prominent macronucleoli.

FAQ: Is this population of hepatocytes on FNA benign or malignant?

Answer: A specimen consisting entirely of hepatocytes may also be seen when a lesion of interest was not sampled, resulting in the presence of only benign hepatocytes. In the case of a missed lesion, the specimen should not be very cellular and only contain rare hepatocytes. Normal hepatocytes may be present as single cells and in small fragments. Rare fragments of benign ductal epithelium may also be seen. A highly cellular specimen containing predominantly hepatocytes is suggestive of a proliferative process and the adequate sampling of lesional tissue. Hepatocytes with atypical features (prominent nucleoli, dispersed small cells, thickened hepatocytic fragments with or without endothelial cell wrapping) raise the suspicion for HCC. A well differentiated HCC may be impossible to definitively diagnose on cytologic material alone, although convincing immunoreactivity with glypican-3 favors a malignant process. In cases that are not definitively malignant by cytomorphology, a core biopsy is recommended.

SAMPLE NOTE: HEPATOCELLULAR PATTERN, ATYPICAL CELLS

Atypical hepatocyte proliferation. See note.

Note: The specimen contains predominantly hepatocytes. The cells form small trabecular fragments and are also present as individually dispersed cells in the background. Some fragments are encircled by endothelial cells. While this architecture is suggestive of a hepatocytic neoplasm, a tissue biopsy is required for a definitive diagnosis. The patient's history of chronic hepatitis C is noted. The differential diagnosis includes hepatocellular carcinoma, regenerative nodule, focal nodular hyperplasia, and hepatic adenoma.

Reference:
Bottles K, Cohen MB. An approach to fine-needle aspiration biopsy diagnosis of hepatic masses. *Diagn Cytopathol*. 1991;7(2):204-210.

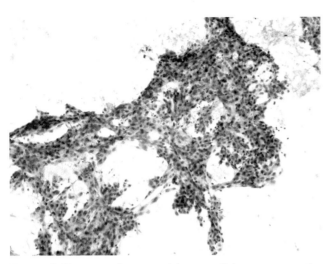

Figure 4.20. Well differentiated hepatocellular carcinoma. The smear is highly cellular and contains sharply outlined trabecular groups (Pap stain).

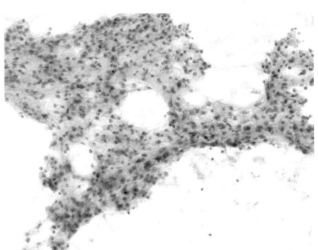

Figure 4.21. Well differentiated hepatocellular carcinoma (Pap stain).

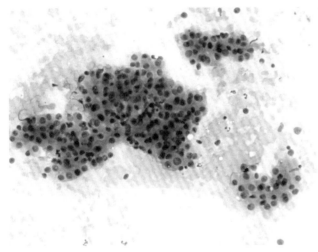

Figure 4.22. Well differentiated hepatocellular carcinoma. There are clusters of tumor cells with clear hepatocellular differentiation, although the nuclear to cytoplasmic ratio is higher. Background solitary tumor cells are naked nuclei stripped of cytoplasm (Diff-Quik stain).

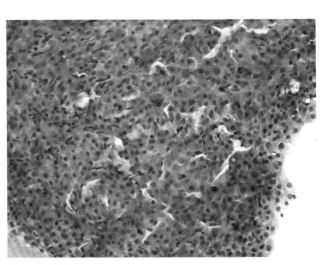

Figure 4.23. Well differentiated hepatocellular carcinoma. Note that the trabeculae are >2 cells thick (Diff-Quik stain).

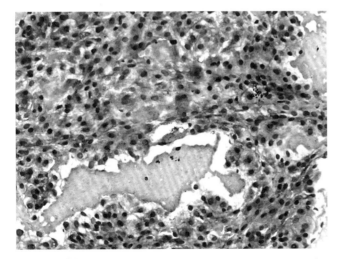

Figure 4.24. Well differentiated hepatocellular carcinoma. The neoplastic cells are monotonous with minimal nuclear atypia, although there is reduced cytoplasm. Note again the thickened trabeculae (Diff-Quik stain).

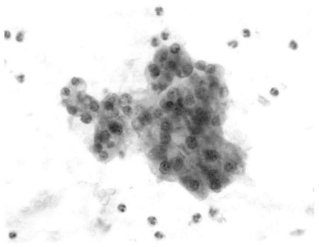

Figure 4.25. Well differentiated hepatocellular carcinoma. The neoplastic cells resemble benign hepatocytes and have regular, uniform nuclei with fine, granular chromatin (Pap stain).

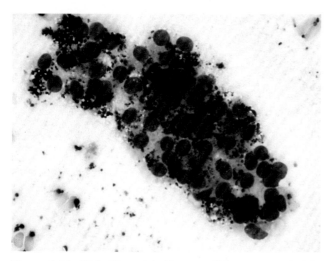

Figure 4.26. Well differentiated hepatocellular carcinoma (HCC). Note the abundant intracellular bile, which may be seen in HCC cells (Diff-Quik stain).

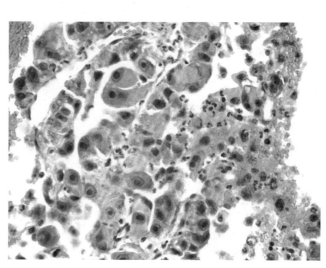

Figure 4.27. Moderately differentiated hepatocellular carcinoma. In this instance, there is increased pleomorphism and nuclear atypia, with eccentric nuclei and very prominent central nucleoli, but the cells maintain some features of hepatocellular differentiation (such as abundant granular cytoplasm) (H&E, cell block).

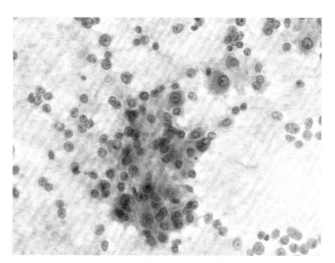

Figure 4.28. Moderately differentiated hepatocellular carcinoma. The smear is very cellular with many naked nuclei, which can be a characteristic of HCC (Pap stain).

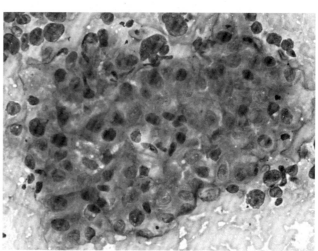

Figure 4.29. Moderately differentiated hepatocellular carcinoma. The neoplastic cells are irregular and pleomorphic with enlarged nuclei and prominent nucleoli (Diff-Quik stain).

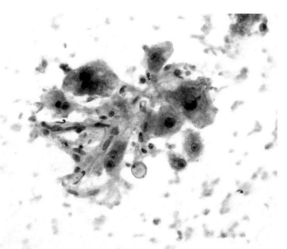

Figure 4.30. Moderately differentiated hepatocellular carcinoma. Note the intranuclear inclusion and intracellular bile (Pap stain).

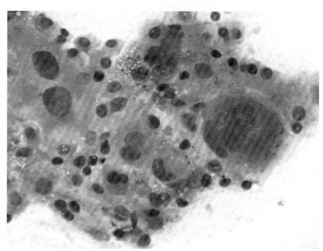

Figure 4.31. Moderately differentiated hepatocellular carcinoma. There is significant pleomorphism with giant multinucleated tumor cells (Diff-Quik stain).

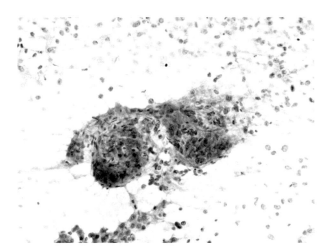

Figure 4.32. Hepatocellular carcinoma. Thickened trabeculae of neoplastic hepatocytes are wrapped by endothelial cells with thin spindle-shaped nuclei (Pap stain).

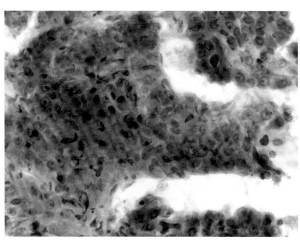

Figure 4.33. Moderately differentiated hepatocellular carcinoma. Note the transgressing vessels through the fragment of neoplastic cells and the endothelial wrapping around the fragments by spindle-shaped nuclei. The neoplastic hepatocytes have increased nuclear to cytoplasmic ratio and prominent nucleoli (Pap stain).

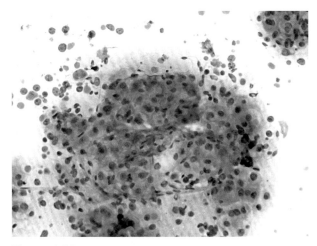

Figure 4.34. Moderately differentiated hepatocellular carcinoma. Note the endothelial wrapping of thickened trabeculae of neoplastic cells (Diff-Quik stain).

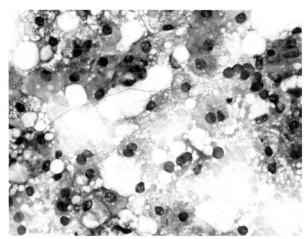

Figure 4.35. Hepatocellular carcinoma. Note that the neoplastic hepatocytes can undergo fatty change, with numerous clear vacuoles within the cytoplasm (Diff-Quik stain).

FIBROLAMELLAR HEPATOCELLULAR CARCINOMA

Fibrolamellar HCC, while conventionally considered a variant of HCC, is now recognized as a distinct entity with a unique clinical presentation and morphology.[17] It occurs in young patients without hepatitis or cirrhosis and has a better prognosis than typical HCC. The neoplastic cells are large, polygonal, and discohesive (singly or in small, loose clusters) with abundant eosinophilic cytoplasm and eccentric nuclei with prominent nucleoli (Figure 4.36). A characteristic feature is lamellar fibrosis, which consists of parallel bands of dense fibrosis around tumor cells (Figure 4.37). The tumor cells are much larger than those of typical HCC, although the N/C ratio is lower (Figures 4.38 and 4.39).[18]

HEPATOBLASTOMA

Hepatoblastoma is the most common pediatric primary liver malignancy, usually seen in children less than 4 years of age but can also occur in older patients.[19] The tumor cells recapitulate the developing embryonal and fetal liver; thus, the cytological pattern is hepatocellular with resemblance to HCC (Figure 4.40). The tumor cells can also show mesenchymal differentiation, and therefore hepatoblastomas are classified into three types: epithelial, mixed epithelial and mesenchymal, and anaplastic (Figures 4.41 and 4.42). The appearance of the immature hepatocytes ranges from anaplastic (small, round, blue cell morphology) to embryonal (hyperchromatic nuclei with coarse chromatin and scant cytoplasm) to fetal (more abundant cytoplasm, most closely resembles hepatocytes) (Figure 4.43). In addition, extramedullary hematopoiesis may be seen.

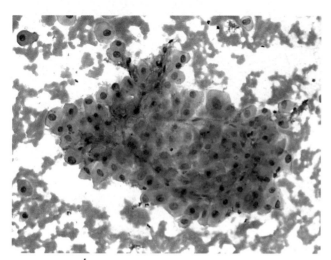

Figure 4.36. Fibrolamellar hepatocellular carcinoma. Note the prominent nucleoli and low nuclear to cytoplasmic ratio (Diff-Quik stain).

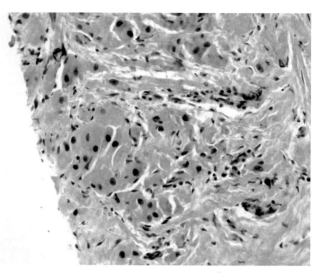

Figure 4.37. Fibrolamellar hepatocellular carcinoma. Note that the neoplastic hepatocellular cells are large with abundant eosinophilic cytoplasm. There is intervening lamellar fibrosis (H&E).

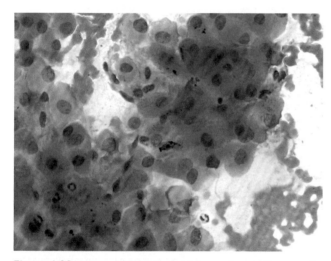

Figure 4.38. Fibrolamellar hepatocellular carcinoma. Compare the large size of the neoplastic cells with the neutrophil (Diff-Quik stain).

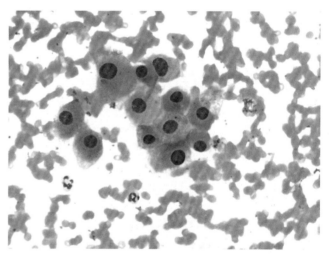

Figure 4.39. Fibrolamellar hepatocellular carcinoma. Compare the large size of the neoplastic cells with the adjacent neutrophils. Note that the cells have low nuclear to cytoplasmic ratio (Diff-Quik stain).

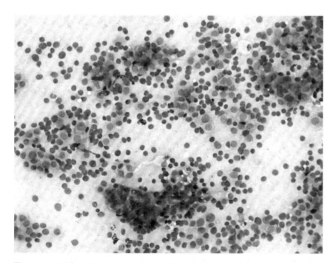

Figure 4.40. Hepatoblastoma. The immature hepatocytes seen here resemble mature hepatocytes, with large round nuclei and abundant cytoplasm (Diff-Quik stain).

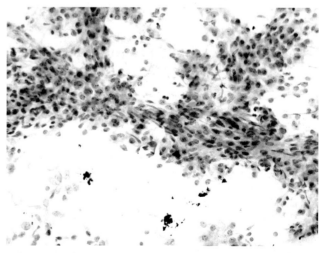

Figure 4.41. Hepatoblastoma, mixed epithelial and mesenchymal type. The epithelioid hepatocellular cells are intermixed with spindled tumor cells that have undergone mesenchymal differentiation (Pap stain).

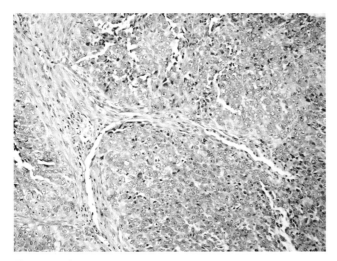

Figure 4.42. Hepatoblastoma, mixed epithelial and mesenchymal type. There are discrete areas of epithelioid immature-appearing hepatocytes and spindled mesenchymal components (H&E).

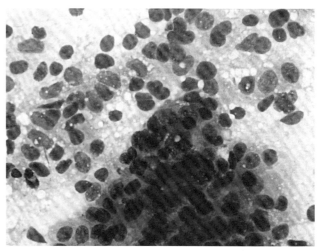

Figure 4.43. High-power view of hepatoblastoma. There is a range of immature hepatocytes, including small, round, blue cells and larger cells that resemble mature hepatocytes (Diff-Quik stain).

GLANDULAR PATTERN

The glandular pattern generally consists of neoplasms of the bile duct. Other glandular-appearing neoplasms in the liver that are not bile duct proliferations raise the consideration of metastatic adenocarcinomas.

CHECKLIST: Etiologic Considerations for the Glandular Pattern

☐ Bile Duct Hamartoma/Adenoma

☐ Cholangiocarcinoma

☐ Metastatic Adenocarcinoma

BILE DUCT HAMARTOMA/ADENOMA

Bile duct hamartomas and adenomas are small (<1 cm), benign intrahepatic nodules composed of well-formed bile ducts within mature fibrous stroma.[20] Bile duct hamartomas (von Meyenburg complex) can be found anywhere scattered throughout the liver, while bile duct adenomas are solitary subcapsular nodules. Cytological specimens are hypocellular due to fibrosis and contain cohesive sheets of benign, orderly, columnar bile duct epithelial cells (Figures 4.44 and 4.45). The ductal cells do not exhibit any atypical features and are therefore cytologically distinct from cholangiocarcinomas and metastatic adenocarcinomas.

CHOLANGIOCARCINOMA, WELL TO MODERATELY DIFFERENTIATED

Cholangiocarcinoma is the second most common primary malignancy of the liver after HCC, accounting for 5-15% of primary liver cancers.[11] They can arise anywhere in the biliary tract from the ampulla of Vater to the small intrahepatic bile ducts. Most commonly, cholangiocarcinomas occur in the extrahepatic bile ducts or near the junction of the right and left hepatic ducts as they bifurcate into the common hepatic duct.[21] Clinically and radiologically, HCC and intrahepatic cholangiocarcinomas can sometimes be difficult to distinguish. However, cytomorphologically, cholangiocarcinomas are gland-forming tumors

Figure 4.44. Low-power view of bile duct hamartoma. The smear is paucicellular and contains small clusters of benign bile duct epithelial cells. No hepatocytes are present in the specimen (Pap stain).

Figure 4.45. High-power view of bile duct hamartoma. The smear consists entirely of benign duct epithelial cells that have an orderly arrangement and no atypical features (Pap stain).

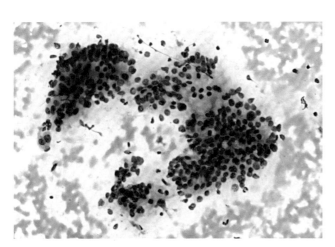

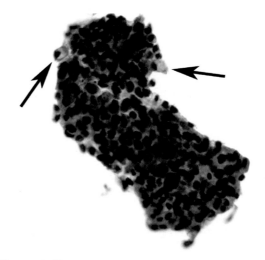

Figure 4.46. Well differentiated cholangiocarcinoma. There are cohesive, crowded clusters of neoplastic cells with glandular differentiation (Diff-Quik stain).

Figure 4.47. Well differentiated cholangiocarcinoma. The neoplastic cells in this cluster are hyperchromatic, and some contain vacuolated cytoplasm (arrows). Note the glandular formation (lower right) (Pap stain).

composed of atypical cuboidal to columnar cells arranged in sheets, not the polygonal hepatocyte-derived cells of HCC in a trabecular pattern (Figures 4.46-4.51). In equivocal cases, staining for cytokeratins on a cell block can help make the distinction: cholangiocarcinomas can be positive for the "odd-numbered" cytokeratins CK7 and CK19, while HCCs tend to be positive for the "even-numbered" CK8 and CK18.[22] Other helpful stains include glypican-3 and arginase, which are relatively sensitive and specific for HCC, and mucicarmine, which may be positive in some cholangiocarcinomas but are negative in HCCs.

KEY FEATURES of Cholangiocarcinoma

- The malignant cells form cohesive cell clusters, crowded sheets, and/or isolated cells.
- The malignant cells demonstrate marked pleomorphism.
- Variation in nuclear size (anisonucleosis) of more than 4:1 between neighboring cells is considered a specific feature for malignancy.
- The malignant cells may have prominent nucleoli.
- The malignant cells have increased N/C ratio with nuclear enlargement.
- Vacuolated and/or mucinous cytoplasm may be present, which can decrease the N/C ratio.

FAQ: Is this bile duct brushing cytology specimen diagnostic of adenocarcinoma?

Answer: Brushing procedures involve physical forces that disrupt epithelium and cause alterations in morphology. Furthermore, exfoliative specimens can sample a large surface area and contain rare lesional cells in a background of abundant benign epithelium. This epithelium may be reactive and simulate a proliferative process. Importantly, patients may have a history of a stent or cholangitis, either of which can result in marked reactive atypia. For these reasons, it is recommended to be cautious and use a higher threshold to make the diagnosis of adenocarcinoma on a brushing specimen as compared with an FNA specimen. Scant fragments of atypical cells in a background of otherwise benign-appearing ductal epithelium should not be considered diagnostic of malignancy. It can be helpful to compare malignant cells with background reactive ductal epithelium. To avoid the possibility of a false-positive diagnosis, one should find singly dispersed markedly atypical cells in the background—a very specific finding of adenocarcinoma in this setting.

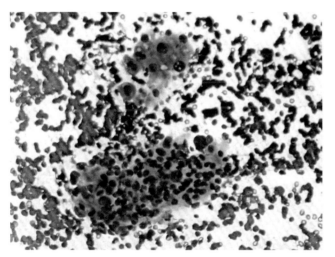

Figure 4.48. Moderately differentiated cholangiocarcinoma. Compare the cholangiocarcinoma cells (bottom), which are pleomorphic and crowded and include many small, ovoid nuclei to the benign hepatocytes (top), which have round nuclei with abundant cytoplasm (Diff-Quik stain).

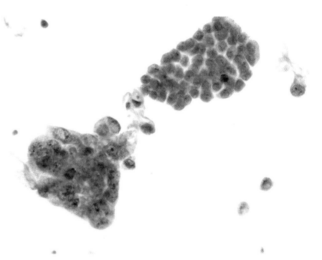

Figure 4.49. Moderately differentiated cholangiocarcinoma (lower left) adjacent to benign ductal epithelium (upper right). The neoplastic cells are enlarged with coarse chromatin, prominent nucleoli, and increased nuclear to cytoplasmic ratio. The organized honeycomb structure is lost, and the nuclei are overlapping (Pap stain).

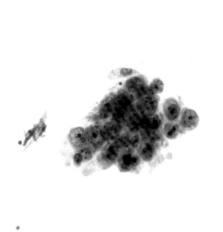

Figure 4.50. Moderately differentiated cholangiocarcinoma. The neoplastic cells are overlapping and have coarse chromatin, prominent nucleoli, and high nuclear to cytoplasmic ratios (Pap stain).

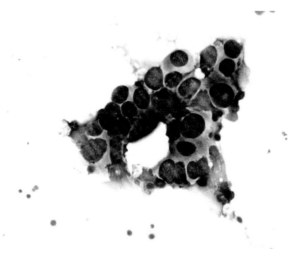

Figure 4.51. Moderately differentiated cholangiocarcinoma. These tumors are often desmoplastic, and thus the specimens may be of low cellularity (Diff-Quik stain).

METASTATIC ADENOCARCINOMA

Metastatic adenocarcinoma often enters into the differential diagnosis of cholangiocarcinoma, as both are malignant gland-forming tumors, and the liver is a common site for metastatic disease owing to its rich blood supply. The most common primary tumor site of origin is the gastrointestinal (GI) tract, with other common sites including the lung, breast, and pancreas (Figures 4.52-4.55). A thorough clinical evaluation for a non-hepatic primary tumor and imaging studies are necessary to exclude a metastasis. If a prior pathology specimen is available from a known primary, morphologic comparison can be very helpful. In the setting of an unknown primary, a combination of cytomorphological features and immunohistochemical profile characteristic to certain tumors may narrow down the list of likely primary sites. Of note, cholangiocarcinomas and pancreatic ductal adenocarcinomas (PDACs) cannot be distinguished cytomorphologically or immunophenotypically, as both are positive for CK7 and occasionally for CK20 and can show overexpression of p53 and loss of SMAD4/DPC4.[23,24]

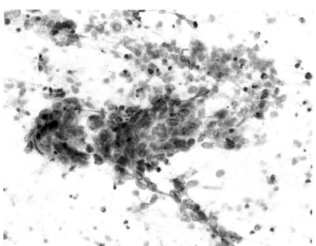

Figure 4.52. Metastatic colon adenocarcinoma to the liver. The neoplastic cells are in a crowded cluster. Note the abundant granular debris comprised of degenerating nuclear material and necrotic cellular contents, commonly referred to as "dirty necrosis" (Pap stain).

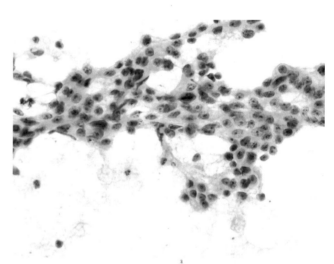

Figure 4.53. Metastatic breast ductal adenocarcinoma to the liver. The neoplastic cells are forming glandular structures with lumens. Note the prominent red central nucleoli (Pap stain).

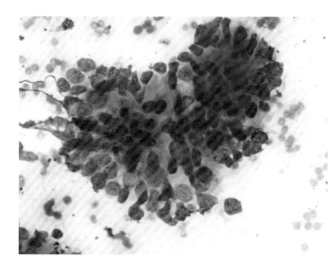

Figure 4.54. Metastatic prostatic adenocarcinoma to the liver. The neoplastic cells are forming glandular (acinar) structures. The site of origin cannot be determined on cytology alone; patient history and/or ancillary immunostains would be needed (Diff-Quik stain).

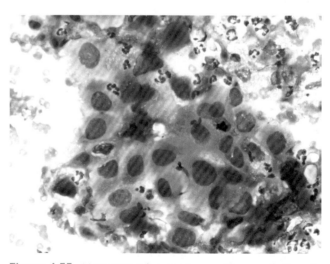

Figure 4.55. Metastatic adenocarcinoma. The neoplastic cells are relatively uniform, and gland formation can be appreciated (Diff-Quik).

POORLY DIFFERENTIATED/EPITHELIOID PATTERN

The poorly differentiated/epithelioid pattern includes poorly differentiated primary hepatic malignancies such as poorly differentiated HCC and cholangiocarcinoma, metastatic poorly differentiated carcinomas, and other epithelioid neoplasms. A common trend among these lesions is their overtly malignant appearance and loss of recognizable features characteristic of their cell of origin, which makes it difficult to distinguish between these poorly differentiated neoplasms. In these cases, immunostains which confirm the cell origin are especially helpful.

CHECKLIST: Etiologic Considerations for the Poorly Differentiated/Epithelioid Pattern

☐ Hepatocellular Carcinoma (HCC), Poorly Differentiated

☐ Cholangiocarcinoma, Poorly Differentiated

☐ Metastatic Carcinoma, Poorly Differentiated

☐ Epithelioid Hemangioendothelioma and Angiosarcoma

HEPATOCELLULAR CARCINOMA (HCC), POORLY DIFFERENTIATED

Poorly differentiated HCC no longer has recognizable features of hepatocyte differentiation, such as polygonal shape, centrally placed nuclei, and trabecular architecture. The neoplastic cells appear increasingly atypical and bizarre, with marked pleomorphism, irregular round to ovoid nuclei, indistinct cell borders, and scant cytoplasm (Figures 4.56-4.59). The cells are dispersed in a more haphazard fashion with many single cells (Figure 4.60). Multinucleation and cytoplasmic bile are rare. Immunohistochemical markers of hepatocyte differentiation—cytoplasmic expression of HepPar-1, glypican-3, arginase-1—can help distinguish HCC from other poorly differentiated carcinomas (Figure 4.61).[15,25] Of note, HepPar-1 tends to be negative in poorly differentiated HCC, while glypican-3 tends to be positive in poorly differentiated HCC.[26]

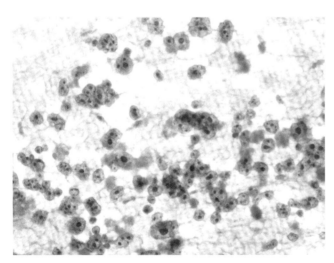

Figure 4.56. Poorly differentiated hepatocellular carcinoma. The neoplastic cells are naked nuclei that have prominent nucleoli and are present singly and in small clusters, without trabeculae formation (Pap stain).

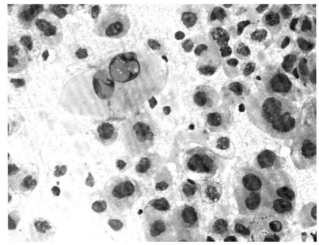

Figure 4.57. Poorly differentiated hepatocellular carcinoma. Binucleated cells are usually rare in poorly differentiated hepatocellular carcinoma but can be seen. The cells are markedly pleomorphic and atypical and are dispersed as single cells (Diff-Quik stain).

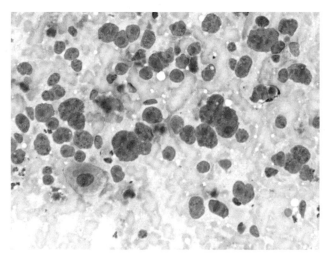

Figure 4.58. Poorly differentiated hepatocellular carcinoma. The nuclei are bizarre with multiple nucleoli, coarse chromatin, and irregular nuclear borders (Diff-Quik stain).

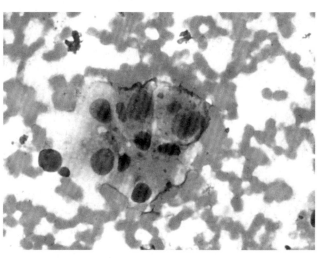

Figure 4.59. Poorly differentiated hepatocellular carcinoma. This small cluster of atypical epithelioid cells does not show clear hepatocytic differentiation. There are eccentric nuclei with nuclear fragmentation and prominent nucleoli (Diff-Quik stain).

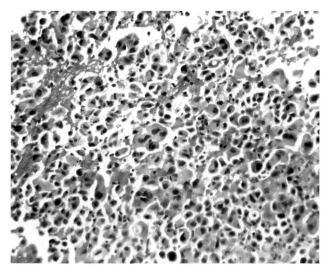

Figure 4.60. Poorly differentiated hepatocellular carcinoma. The cells dispersed singly in a haphazard way and are markedly atypical with bizarre shapes and variably positioned nuclei (cell block, H&E stain).

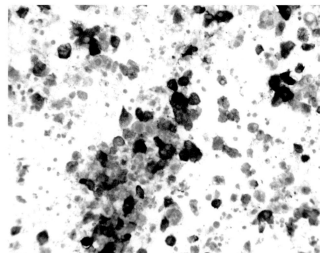

Figure 4.61. Poorly differentiated hepatocellular carcinoma. The tumor cells have strong cytoplasmic expression of arginase, confirming hepatic differentiation (arginase immunostain).

CHOLANGIOCARCINOMA, POORLY DIFFERENTIATED

Poorly differentiated cholangiocarcinoma can lose its glandular differentiation and appear as markedly enlarged, pleomorphic, single cells without organized architecture (Figures 4.62-4.65). Cholangiocarcinoma will not express hepatocytic markers and is typically CK7 positive, with possible expression of the GI tract markers CDX2 and SATB2, as well as possible loss of SMAD4/DPC4 expression. Unfortunately, these staining patterns can be seen with metastases from other upper GI tract and pancreatic adenocarcinomas. However, albumin RNA in situ hybridization is a sensitive and highly specific marker for tumors of hepatic origin, thus distinguishing intrahepatic cholangiocarcinoma from other metastatic adenocarcinomas to the liver (Figures 4.66 and 4.67).[27]

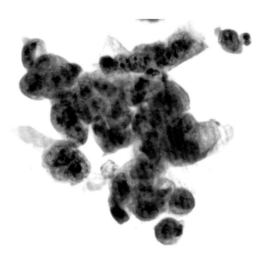

Figure 4.62. Poorly differentiated cholangiocarcinoma. The neoplastic cells are large, epithelioid, and pleomorphic with coarse chromatin. There is some semblance of glandular formation, but no well-formed lumens (Pap stain).

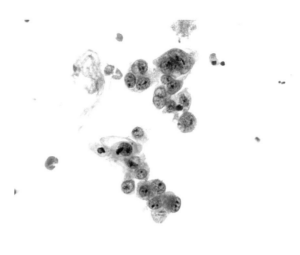

Figure 4.63. Poorly differentiated cholangiocarcinoma. The neoplastic cells are loosely cohesive. Note the cytoplasmic vacuolization (Pap stain).

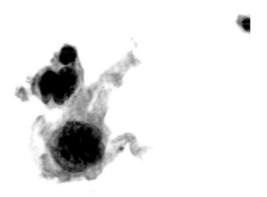

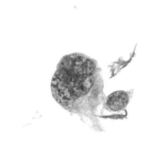

Figure 4.64. Single highly atypical cells in poorly differentiated cholangiocarcinoma. The larger cell is multinucleated with hyperchromasia, coarse chromatin, and prominent nucleoli (Pap stain).

Figure 4.65. Single highly atypical cells in poorly differentiated cholangiocarcinoma. The chromatin is coarse, and the nuclear border is irregular with many folds (Pap stain).

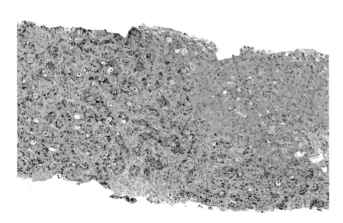

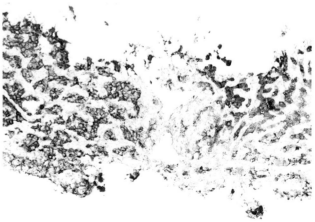

Figure 4.66. Poorly differentiated adenocarcinoma (left) adjacent to normal liver tissue (right). The differential diagnosis is between intrahepatic cholangiocarcinoma versus metastatic adenocarcinoma (H&E).

Figure 4.67. Albumin RNA in situ hybridization (which is highly specific for primary liver tumors) from the same case shows diffuse positivity in both the tumor cells (left) and benign hepatocytes (right). This confirms the diagnosis of intrahepatic cholangiocarcinoma (albumin in situ hybridization).

METASTATIC CARCINOMA, POORLY DIFFERENTIATED

Poorly differentiated metastatic carcinoma is an important consideration when faced with a poorly differentiated malignancy in the liver because metastatic carcinomas are more common than primary HCCs and intrahepatic cholangiocarcinomas (Figures 4.68-4.71). As always, a detailed clinical history and careful clinical and radiologic evaluation are essential for identifying a possible primary tumor. If prior histology of a primary tumor is available, morphologic comparison with the current cytologic specimen can be very helpful. In the case of an unknown primary and nonspecific cytomorphological features, ancillary studies, such as immunostains, may help point to a site of origin.

EPITHELIOID HEMANGIOENDOTHELIOMA AND ANGIOSARCOMA

Epithelioid hemangioendothelioma and epithelioid angiosarcoma are rare malignant tumors of endothelial cells. Epithelioid hemangioendotheliomas have intermediate aggressiveness,[28] while angiosarcomas are more aggressive. Cytomorphologically, the epithelioid variant of angiosarcoma and epithelioid hemangioendotheliomas cannot be distinguished,

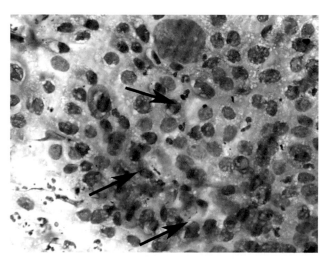

Figure 4.68. Metastatic poorly differentiated carcinoma. The cells are epithelioid and pleomorphic with large atypical cells. There is a hint of glandular formation (arrows), and the site of origin was found to be the colon (Diff-Quik stain).

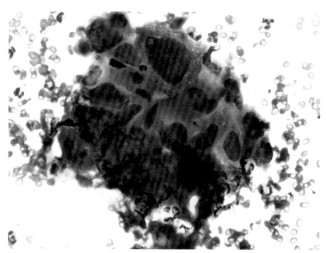

Figure 4.69. Metastatic poorly differentiated carcinoma. The neoplastic cells are large, pleomorphic, and cohesive but with no definite features of differentiation (Diff-Quik stain).

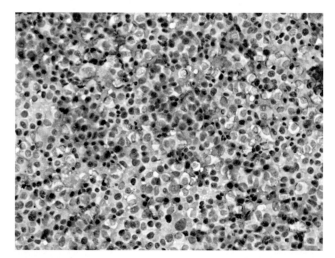

Figure 4.70. Low-power view of metastatic high-grade neuroendocrine tumor. The smear is filled with sheets of epithelioid cells with no discernable architecture. The cells have round to oval nuclei with speckled chromatin and moderate amounts of cytoplasm (Diff-Quik stain).

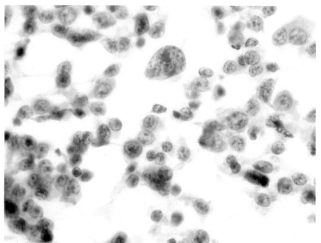

Figure 4.71. High-power view of metastatic high-grade neuroendocrine tumor. The atypical cells are present as scattered cells and are pleomorphic but overall round to oval with prominent nucleoli and coarse speckled chromatin (Pap stain).

although some studies have shown that angiosarcoma cells tend to be larger and more atypical.[29] Features shared between the two entities include epithelioid cells, eccentric nuclei, and intracytoplasmic lumens (Figures 4.72-4.75).[30] These neoplasms may be difficult to distinguish from carcinomas, especially if the cytomorphologic features of vascular differentiation (e.g., intracytoplasmic lumens) are absent or go unnoticed. Immunostains for endothelial markers CD34, CD31, FLI-1, and/or ERG on cell block material can help confirm the diagnosis of a vascular neoplasm.[89] In addition, nuclear expression of CAMTA1 can be seen in the majority of epithelioid hemangioendotheliomas, while it is generally negative in other epithelioid mesenchymal neoplasms.

KEY FEATURES of Epithelioid Hemangioendothelioma and Angiosarcoma

- The specimen may be paucicellular and contain only rare tumor cells.
- Small amounts of metachromatic stroma can be seen associated with tumor cells (Diff-Quik stain).
- The tumor cells exist primarily as dispersed single epithelioid cells with some cohesive cell clusters.[31]
- The tumor cells sometimes contain intracytoplasmic lumina containing red blood cells and/or neutrophils.[31]
- The tumor nuclei usually have membrane irregularities and/or grooves and contain prominent nucleoli.[31]
- The tumor cells are frequently binucleated or multinucleated.

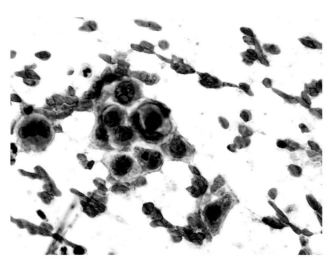

Figure 4.72. Epithelioid angiosarcoma in the liver. The large, epithelioid cells are present as small fragments and single cells and demonstrate intracytoplasmic lumens with a "cell-in-cell" morphology (Pap stain).

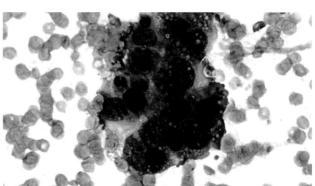

Figure 4.73. Epithelioid angiosarcoma in the liver. The large, epithelioid cells have eccentric nuclei and abundant vacuolated cytoplasm with phagocytosed cells (Diff-Quik stain).

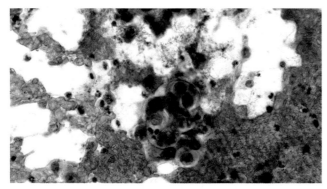

Figure 4.74. Epithelioid angiosarcoma in the liver. Within the cluster of atypical epithelioid cells, there is an intracytoplasmic lumen containing a red blood cell (Pap stain).

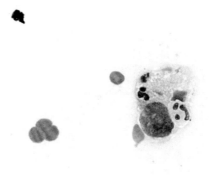

Figure 4.75. Epithelioid angiosarcoma in the liver. The smear is paucicellular with an occasional single large epithelioid cell that has engulfed neutrophils and a red blood cell (Pap stain).

PAUCICELLULAR/CYSTIC PATTERN

Specimens with the paucicellular/cystic pattern may be virtually acellular and/or can be composed predominately of macrophages (with or without cells arising from a cyst lining) and debris. When cyst-lining cells are present, they may be too few to sufficiently characterize, making a definitive diagnosis problematic. The presence of granular debris does not necessarily indicate tumor necrosis, although cellular necrosis is concerning for malignancy. If infection is a concern, material may be sent for microbiologic studies during on-site evaluation. The creation of a cell block from the cyst contents may provide further diagnostic clues and allow for special stains or immunohistochemical studies.

CHECKLIST: Etiologic Considerations for the Paucicellular/Cystic Pattern

☐ Benign Cysts

☐ Hemangioma

BENIGN CYSTS

Benign cysts of the liver can be solitary or multifocal and unilocular or multilocular. They are usually lined by a single layer of benign biliary-type cuboidal or columnar epithelium. The aspirated cyst fluid is hypocellular and may not contain cyst-lining epithelium. The presence of cystic macrophages (macrophages containing cytoplasmic pigment representing hemosiderin breakdown products) confirms the sampling of cystic fluid. When present, the epitheliallining cells are typically scant, bland, and cytomorphologically nonspecific, often resulting in a nondiagnostic specimen. Specific benign cysts include the ciliated foregut cyst, which may produce specimens with ciliated respiratory-type columnar cells and mucoid material, and bile duct cystadenoma, which may produce specimens with bland, cuboidal cells forming papillary structures.[32,33]

HEMANGIOMA

Hemangiomas are the most common benign tumors of the liver and are usually asymptomatic. When detected incidentally and not recognized as hemangiomas radiologically, they may be aspirated to rule out malignancy. In most instances, only blood is seen on the aspirate, resulting in a nondiagnostic specimen (Figure 4.76). Rarely, aspirates of hemangiomas show bland spindle-shaped endothelial cells with poorly defined cytoplasm, present singly or in larger fragments (Figures 4.77-4.79). A cell block showing dilated vascular spaces can be helpful in making the diagnosis. Clinical and radiologic correlation are important, as well as ensuring that the sample is representative of the lesion.

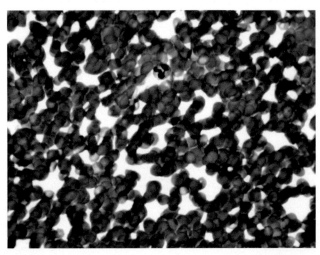

Figure 4.76. Hemangioma. Only blood was sampled in this case, a common finding in the fine-needle aspiration of hemangiomas (Diff-Quik stain).

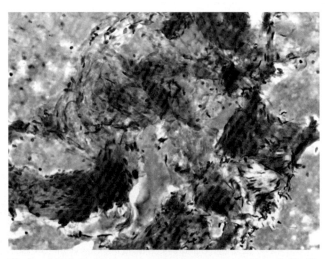

Figure 4.77. Hemangioma. Fragments of bland, spindled cells stream in a syncytial pattern (Diff-Quik stain).

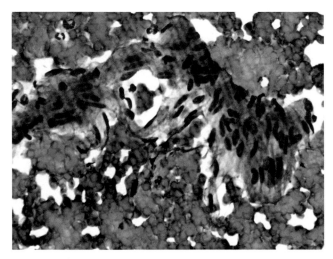

Figure 4.78. Hemangioma. Fragment of bland, spindled endothelial cells in a background of blood (Diff-Quik stain).

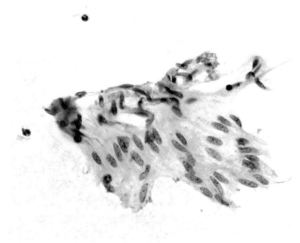

Figure 4.79. Hemangioma. Fragment of bland, spindled endothelial cells with fine, even chromatin and indistinct cell borders (Pap stain).

SINGLE CELL/DISPERSED PATTERN

The single cell/dispersed pattern consists of highly cellular specimens composed predominantly of single discohesive cells. In some instances, tissue fragments or loosely cohesive clusters of cells may be seen in addition to the discohesive cells. These patterns are typically suggestive of a metastatic neoplasm, poorly differentiated adenocarcinoma, or lymphoproliferative disorder.

CHECKLIST: Etiologic Considerations for the Single Cell/Dispersed Pattern

☐ Poorly Differentiated Carcinoma

☐ Metastatic Melanoma

☐ Metastatic Neuroendocrine Neoplasm

☐ Lymphoproliferative Disorders

POORLY DIFFERENTIATED CARCINOMA

Poorly differentiated carcinomas in some instances may appear as a predominantly discohesive population of cells and only contain rare tissue fragments (Figures 4.80-4.82). Poorly differentiated carcinomas include metastases as well as primary carcinomas (such as HCC and cholangiocarcinoma). These entities are discussed in greater detail under the "Poorly Differentiated/Epithelioid Pattern."

METASTATIC MELANOMA

Melanoma consists of individually dispersed cells, although in some instances a specimen may be so cellular that the individual cells appear to form fragments. A melanoma cell typically has abundant cytoplasm, a round eccentrically placed nucleus with regular borders, and a prominent nucleolus (Figures 4.83-4.85). Melanoma can be distinguished from other entities in this pattern using immunostains; S100 protein is usually diffusely positive, and other melanoma-specific markers (i.e. Sox10, HMB-45, Melan-A) may be expressed; these findings are not usually seen in the other entities. Melanoma is usually negative for cytokeratins, hematopoietic markers, and neuroendocrine markers.

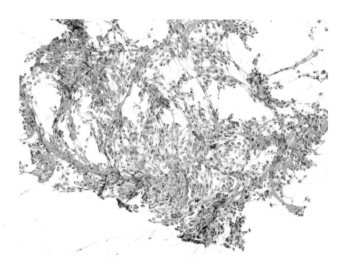

Figure 4.80. Metastatic urothelial carcinoma to the liver. The cells are arranged in a papillary, loosely cohesive fashion with central fibrovascular stalks (Pap stain).

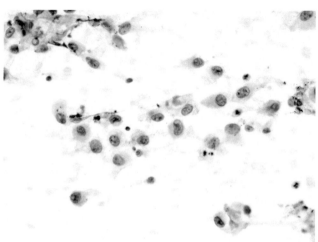

Figure 4.81. Metastatic urothelial carcinoma to the liver. The individual neoplastic cells are dispersed with round to oval nuclei (some with grooves) and moderate amounts of cytoplasm (Pap stain).

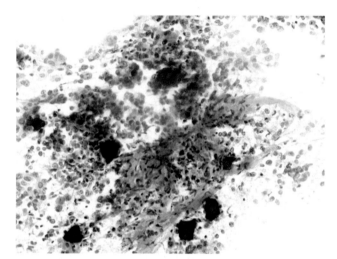

Figure 4.82. Metastatic ovarian high-grade serous carcinoma to the liver. The neoplastic cells are present in loosely cohesive clusters and scattered singly. Note the prominent red nucleoli and psammoma bodies (Pap stain).

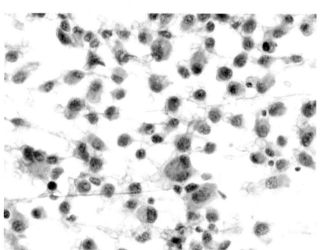

Figure 4.83. Metastatic melanoma to the liver. The neoplastic cells are dispersed and present as single atypical cells with eccentric nuclei. No definitive pigment is seen (Pap stain).

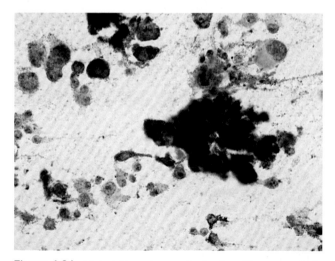

Figure 4.84. Metastatic melanoma to the liver. These neoplastic cells display all the classic features of melanoma: eccentric nuclei (upper right), prominent red nucleoli, and abundant melanin pigment (Pap stain).

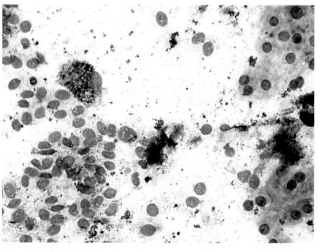

Figure 4.85. Metastatic melanoma to the liver. Compare the neoplastic cells, some of which are large and contain abundant pigment, with benign hepatocytes (right) (Diff-Quik stain).

METASTATIC NEUROENDOCRINE NEOPLASM

Neuroendocrine neoplasms from the GI tract and pancreas may metastasize to the liver, particularly carcinoid tumors from the ileum, cecum, and ascending colon.[34] As with other metastatic lesions, they typically present as multiple lesions scattered throughout the liver. The cytomorphological features are those characteristic of neuroendocrine cells: generally monomorphic with round to oval eccentric nuclei containing finely stippled "salt-and-pepper" chromatin, moderate to abundant cytoplasm, and present singly or in small clusters (Figures 4.86-4.91). Immunoreactivity to neuroendocrine markers such as synaptophysin, chromogranin A, and/or INSM1 help to confirm the diagnosis, but not the origin, of these neoplasms.

FAQ: What is the primary site of this neuroendocrine tumor in the liver?

Answer: Neuroendocrine tumors found in the liver are assumed to be metastatic processes. Considerations primarily include either a pancreatic neuroendocrine tumor (PanNET) or a carcinoid tumor from the GI tract. Radiologic studies are perhaps the most reliable in identifying the primary site, although immunostains may help suggest a primary site. One study has shown that 65% of PanNET metastases to the liver were positive for Pax-8, while metastases from other sites were all negative for Pax-8. CDX-2 may be positive in GI carcinoid tumors or PanNETs but is negative in pulmonary carcinoid tumors.

LYMPHOPROLIFERATIVE DISORDERS

The most common lymphoproliferative disorders that involve the liver are metastatic lymphomas; primary hepatic lymphomas are extremely rare.[35] Cytology shows a dispersed pattern of monomorphic lymphoid cells with variable nuclear features depending on the type of lymphoma (Figures 4.92 and 4.93). For mature B-cell lymphomas (i.e. follicular lymphoma, small lymphocytic lymphoma, mantle cell lymphoma, and marginal zone lymphoma), the lymphoid cells are predominantly small- to medium-sized lymphocytes with variably irregular nuclei; occasional lymphoid aggregates can be seen. Large B-cell lymphomas such as diffuse large B-cell lymphoma (DLBCL) are composed of predominantly large cells (2.5-5 times the size of a small lymphocyte) with distinct or prominent nucleoli (Figure 4.94). Patients with myeloproliferative disorders may have extramedullary hematopoiesis, which is reflected in cytology specimens by the presence of myeloid precursors, erythroid precursors, and/or megakaryocytes (Figure 4.95).[35] If a lymphoproliferative disorder is suspected, fresh cellular material should be sent for flow cytometry to aid in further classification and/or demonstration of a monoclonal population.

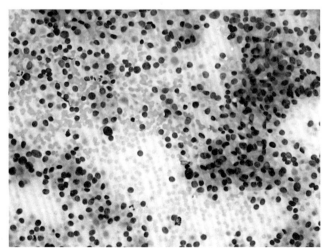

Figure 4.86. Metastatic well differentiated neuroendocrine tumor to the liver. The neoplastic cells are dispersed and monotonous with round nuclei and fine chromatin (Diff-Quik stain).

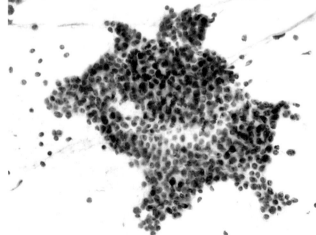

Figure 4.87. Metastatic well differentiated neuroendocrine tumor to the liver. The neoplastic cells are present in a large fragment and as scattered single cells. The speckled chromatin can be appreciated at this power (Pap stain).

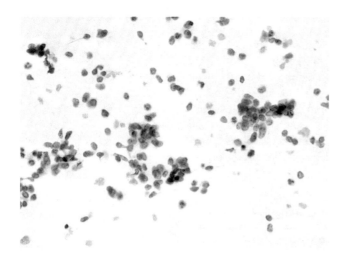

Figure 4.88. Metastatic neuroendocrine carcinoma to the liver. This smear consists predominantly of small clusters and single cells with "salt-and-pepper" chromatin (Pap stain).

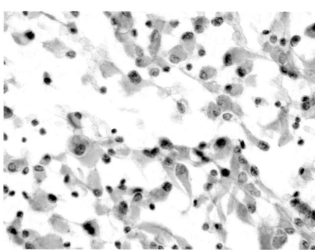

Figure 4.89. High-power view of metastatic well differentiated neuroendocrine tumor to the liver. Note that many of the neoplastic cells have eccentric nuclei and cytoplasmic tails, which are features seen in neuroendocrine neoplasms (Pap stain).

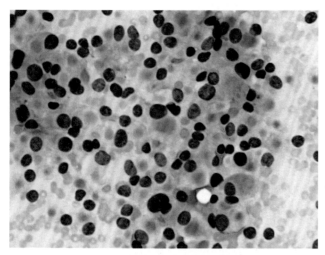

Figure 4.90. High-power view of metastatic well differentiated neuroendocrine tumor to the liver. The neoplastic cells are monotonous with round nuclei and fine, speckled chromatin (Diff-Quik stain).

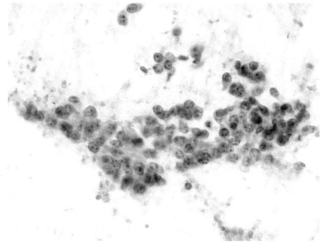

Figure 4.91. Metastatic well differentiated neuroendocrine tumor to the liver. These neoplastic cells are still monotonous with round nuclei but have coarse, condensed chromatin (Pap stain).

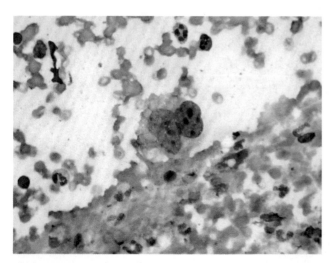

Figure 4.92. Hodgkin lymphoma in the liver. Note the binucleated Reed-Sternberg cell (center) and background of mixed inflammation (Diff-Quik stain).

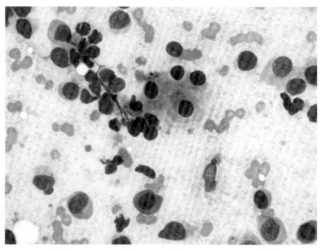

Figure 4.93. Multiple myeloma involving the liver. The neoplastic plasma cells have eccentric nuclei with a perinuclear hof. Compare them with the benign hepatocytes (center) (Diff-Quik stain).

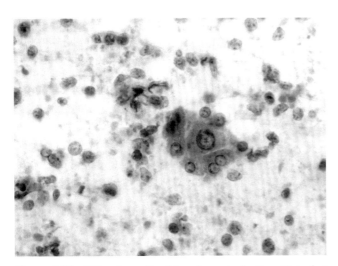

Figure 4.94. Diffuse large B-cell lymphoma in the liver. Note that the largest cells are benign hepatocytes with granular cytoplasm (center), while the neoplastic lymphoid cells are the smaller discohesive cells. Note the necrotic background (Pap stain).

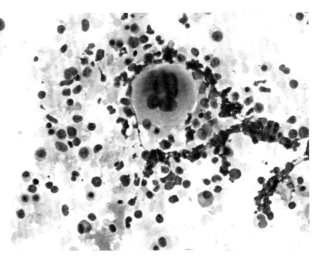

Figure 4.95. Extramedullary hematopoiesis in the liver. These findings are usually seen incidentally or in association with anemia. This smear shows a megakaryocyte and numerous erythroid precursors, which usually reside in the bone marrow (Diff-Quik stain).

SPINDLE CELL PATTERN

The spindle cell pattern includes benign and malignant mesenchymal neoplasms composed of spindle cells that are seen in the liver. Primary hepatic sarcomas are rare, and thus benign spindle cell neoplasms or metastatic disease are high on the differential. Most of these entities, when aspirated, yield paucicellular specimens; this is particularly challenging in situations where immunostains are desired to confirm a particular diagnosis.

CHECKLIST: Etiologic Considerations for the Spindle Cell Pattern

☐ Hemangioma
☐ Angiomyolipoma (AML)
☐ Angiosarcoma
☐ Gastrointestinal Stromal Tumor (GIST)
☐ Leiomyosarcoma
☐ Sarcomatoid Carcinoma

HEMANGIOMA

Hemangiomas are the most common benign tumors of the liver and are composed of spindle cells. Therefore, hemangiomas should be the first diagnostic consideration upon identification of a bland spindle cell lesion in the liver. See the "Paucicellular/Cystic Pattern" for further discussion.

ANGIOMYOLIPOMA (AML)

Angiomyolipomas (AMLs) are benign tumors that most commonly occur in or around the kidney, with the liver being the most common extrarenal site. Hepatic AMLs have similar clinicopathologic features to renal AMLs, presenting at a mean age of 50 years predominantly in females, with most cases discovered incidentally. Most patients have concurrent hepatic and renal AMLs, and a small subset have tuberous sclerosis.[36] These masses are well circumscribed and variable in size. AMLs with high fat content are readily diagnosed radiologically; as a result, only atypical, fat-poor AMLs are subject to biopsy.

On cytology, the presence of all three components—blood vessels, fat cells, and smooth muscle cells—confirms the diagnosis of AML, but often the fat component is absent.[37] The most important and only diagnostic component is the smooth muscle cells, which appear as clusters of spindle cells, combined with variably atypical epithelioid cells with indistinct cell membranes and abundant granular cytoplasm. In addition, around 40% of hepatic AMLs have extramedullary hematopoiesis, which can be a supportive diagnostic feature. The neoplastic smooth muscle cells are positive for smooth muscle actin, HMB-45, and Melan-A, and demonstration of this staining pattern helps to confirm the diagnosis.[36]

ANGIOSARCOMA

Angiosarcoma is the most common primary sarcoma of the liver in adults, but still only accounts for <1% of primary hepatic malignancies.[38] These tumors are associated with cirrhosis, thorium dioxide (Thorotrast) radiographic contrast, industrial exposure to polyvinyl chloride, and arsenic compounds. Angiosarcoma typically presents as multiple hemorrhagic masses with frequent thrombosis and infarction. FNA smears are typically bloody with necrotic debris. The malignant endothelial cells are variably pleomorphic, spindled to epithelioid cells with ill-defined cell borders, elongated hyperchromatic nuclei, and variably abundant, vacuolated cytoplasm. Cohesive clusters and whorls of spindle cells that recapitulate vessels may be seen. Of note, the epithelioid variant of angiosarcoma poses a diagnostic challenge because it is difficult to distinguish this entity from a carcinoma on cytology (see the "Epithelioid Hemangioendothelioma and Angiosarcoma" section of the "Epithelioid/Poorly Differentiated Pattern"). On a cell block, the identification of irregular vascular spaces lined by atypical endothelial cells that are positive for endothelial markers (CD34, CD31, FLI1, and/or ERG) can help confirm the diagnosis of angiosarcoma.

GASTROINTESTINAL STROMAL TUMOR (GIST)

Gastrointestinal stromal tumors (GISTs) are the second most common spindle cell lesion found in the liver, as they often metastasize to the liver from the stomach and small intestine. FNA smears show irregular clusters of spindled to epithelioid cells with bland chromatin and wispy, delicate cytoplasm (Figures 4.96-4.98). Single cells and stripped nuclei can also be seen (Figure 4.99). Immunohistochemical studies are required to confirm the diagnosis, with the neoplastic cells demonstrating immunoreactivity for c-kit (CD117) and/ or DOG1 (Figures 4.100 and 4.101).[39,40]

LEIOMYOSARCOMA

Leiomyosarcomas may metastasize to the liver from the GI tract or retroperitoneum.[41] Cytomorphologically, these tumors consist of dense to loose clusters of spindle cells with centrally located nuclei with blunted ends ("cigar-shaped") and abundant homogeneous, finely granular cytoplasm (Figures 4.102-4.105). Naked nuclei are common, and the amount of atypia (pleomorphism, mitoses, multinucleation) and tumor necrosis increases with tumor grade. Leiomyosarcomas are immunoreactive for desmin, smooth muscle actin, and caldesmon.

SARCOMATOID CARCINOMA

Sarcomatoid carcinoma is a carcinoma that has predominantly spindled morphology and may mimic a malignant spindle cell neoplasm. As carcinomas are more common than sarcomas, sarcomatoid carcinoma should always be kept on the differential diagnosis when encountering a malignant-appearing spindle cell lesion. A pan-keratin panel (such as AE1/AE3 with CAM5.2) helps distinguish sarcomatoid carcinoma from other entities on this list. Sarcomatoid carcinomas should have strong and diffuse expression of keratins, whereas; weak and focal keratin expression can be seen in some sarcomas. Primary HCCs and cholangiocarcinomas may rarely present as sarcomatoid carcinomas and express similar immunomarkers as these entities (see the "Hepatocellular Pattern" and "Cholangiocarcinoma" in this chapter).[42,43] Metastatic sarcomatoid carcinomas may express markers indicating their site of origin.

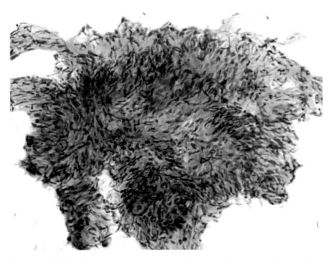

Figure 4.96. Gastrointestinal stromal tumor showing a large cluster of atypical but bland spindled cells (Pap stain).

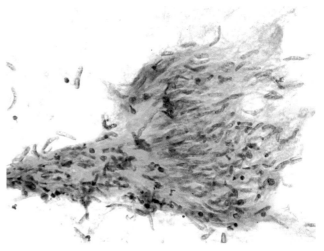

Figure 4.97. Gastrointestinal stromal tumor. Note the bland chromatin and delicate, wispy cytoplasm (Pap stain).

Figure 4.98. Gastrointestinal stromal tumor. The atypical spindled cells in this cluster have delicate, wispy cytoplasm (Diff-Quik stain).

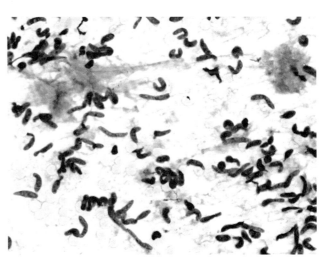

Figure 4.99. Gastrointestinal stromal tumor. Spindled nuclei stripped of cytoplasm are present as single cells in this field (Diff-Quik stain).

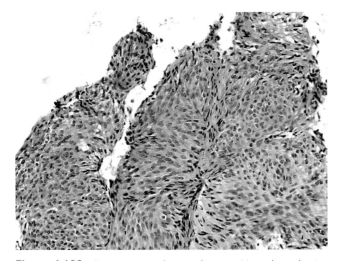

Figure 4.100. Gastrointestinal stromal tumor. Note the cohesive fragments of uniform spindled and epithelioid cells (H&E stain).

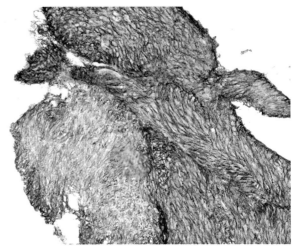

Figure 4.101. Gastrointestinal stromal tumor. The same tumor cells are diffusely positive for DOG-1 (DOG-1 immunostain).

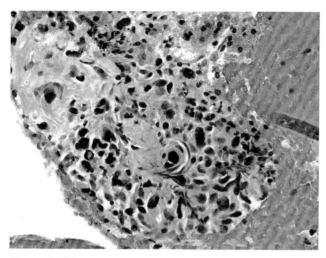

Figure 4.102. Metastatic high-grade leiomyosarcoma to the liver. The neoplastic cells are markedly atypical, with some large, hyperchromatic spindled cells. Apoptotic bodies can be seen (H&E stain).

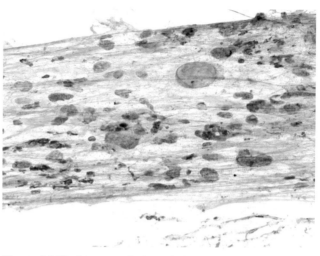

Figure 4.103. Metastatic high-grade leiomyosarcoma to the liver. The neoplastic cells in this loose tissue fragment are spindled and pleomorphic (Pap stain).

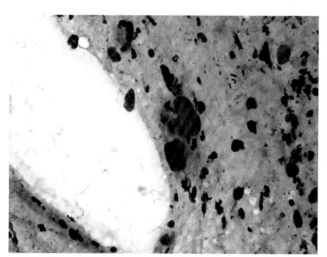

Figure 4.104. Metastatic high-grade leiomyosarcoma to the liver. The neoplastic spindled cells are pleomorphic with large, hyperchromatic nuclei with blunted ends. Naked nuclei are common (Diff-Quik stain).

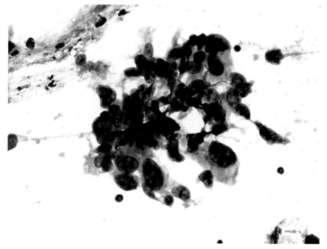

Figure 4.105. Metastatic high-grade leiomyosarcoma to the liver. The neoplastic cells have large, hyperchromatic nuclei with coarse chromatin and fine, granular cytoplasm (Diff-Quik stain).

METASTATIC NEUROENDOCRINE NEOPLASM

Well differentiated neuroendocrine neoplasms such as carcinoid tumors may appear as a population of spindled cells. The tumor cells are often in small fragments and dispersed as single cells in the background. The neoplastic cells are often positive for keratin as well as most neuroendocrine markers (see the "Metastatic Neuroendocrine Neoplasm" section under the "Dispersed Pattern" in this chapter).

EXTRAS

HEPATIC ABSCESS

Hepatic abscesses can be caused by bacteria (most commonly *Streptococcus*, *Staphylococcus*, *Escherichia coli*, *Klebsiella*), fungi (most commonly *Candida*), or the amoeba *Entamoeba histolytica*. Cytological findings include abundant neutrophils, mixed inflammatory cells,

Figure 4.106. Liver abscess. The smear consists of necrotic debris and mixed inflammatory cells (Pap stain).

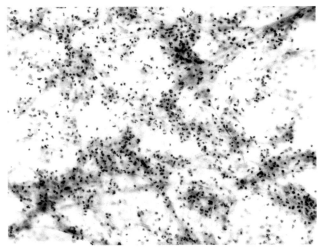

Figure 4.107. Liver abscess. The predominant cells are neutrophils admixed with other inflammatory cells. A careful search for malignant cells should be performed (Pap stain).

necrotic debris, and reactive hepatocytes (Figures 4.106 and 4.107). Special stains for microorganisms (i.e. Gram and silver stains) and correlation with cultures help to identify the offending organism. In amebic abscesses, the cavity is grossly filled with tan-brown "anchovy paste" material. The amoebae are only present in the abscess wall and are not usually seen in aspirated necrotic material. If seen, they resemble histiocytes with small round vesicular nuclei and abundant vacuolated cytoplasm containing phagocytosed red blood cells. Because acute inflammation and/or necrotic debris can also be associated with an undersampled necrotic malignancy, it is important to carefully search for malignant cells.

SAMPLE NOTE: ACUTE INFLAMMATION, POSSIBLE ABSCESS

Predominantly acute inflammation and granular debris. An epithelial component is not definitively identified. See note.

Note: If representative of the entire lesion, the findings would be compatible with the clinical impression of an abscess. Please correlate with microbiologic studies. If the lesion persists after drainage, re-biopsy is indicated.

GRANULOMATOUS INFLAMMATION

Liver granulomas can be caused by infections (most commonly tuberculosis), sarcoidosis, drugs, and neoplasms. Cytology shows clusters of epithelioid histiocytes with elongated nuclei, fine chromatin, and eccentric fibrillar cytoplasm (Figures 4.108 and 4.109). Caseous necrosis is seen in tuberculous granulomas but not with sarcoid or drug-related granulomas. Other inflammatory cells such as lymphocytes, giant cells, and eosinophils (with drug use) may be seen but are nonspecific.

HYDATID CYST

Hydatid cysts are caused by ova from the dog tapeworm *Echinococcus granulosus*, which are passed via a fecal-oral route from dog feces to the human duodenum. From there, the embryo enters the bloodstream and is filtered by the liver, where it develops into a hydatid cyst with an outer laminated membrane and internal cystic layers that contain scolices with hooklets. On cytology, fragments of the laminated membrane, scolices, and/or hooklets can be seen in a background of debris (Figure 4.110).

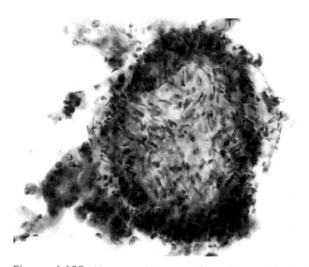

Figure 4.108. Nonnecrotizing granuloma in sarcoidosis. The large, round cluster of histiocytes (granuloma) is adjacent to benign hepatocytes (lower left) (Pap stain).

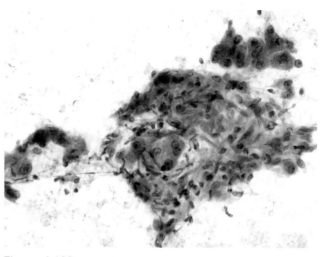

Figure 4.109. Granulomatous inflammation in sarcoidosis. The loose clusters of spindled and epithelioid histiocytes have fine chromatin and fibrillar cytoplasm and are intermixed with lymphocytes and benign hepatocytes (Pap stain).

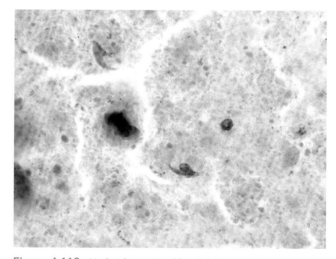

Figure 4.110. Hydatid cyst. Hooklets (pink) are present in a background of debris (Pap stain).

NEAR MISS

THE OVERDIAGNOSIS OF REACTIVE HEPATOCYTES

In general, the aspiration of a neoplastic or proliferative process should yield a cellular specimen. Liver is one organ in which the aspiration of benign tissue can result in numerous reactive hepatocytes present singly and/or in fragments, although the specimen should not be greatly cellular. During on-site evaluation, the presence of many reactive hepatocytes (possibly indicating that the lesion of interest was missed) may result in inadequate sampling being erroneously deemed adequate. Reactive hepatocytes are occasionally mistaken for HCC or adenocarcinoma under intra-procedure time pressure and may emulate the morphology of certain other neoplasms, such as a metastatic melanoma. Hepatocytes typically contain pigment, are polygonal in shape, and have one or two round nuclei. The accurate identification of reactive hepatocytes in a specimen allows for comparison of the hepatocytes to lesional cells.

THE UNREMARKABLE PANCREAS

ACINAR CELLS

Acinar cells are polygonal with abundant coarsely granular cytoplasm and have smooth, round, uniform nuclei with distinct nucleoli (Figures 4.111-4.121). The cytoplasm can commonly develop a vacuolated or clear appearance with degranulation. The cells typically form acinar structures which can mimic the rosette formation seen in some neuroendocrine neoplasms. When sampled by FNA, fragments of varying size maintain the underlying "grape-like" architecture though individual groups of acinar cells and single acinar cells can also be seen (Figure 4.122).[44]

DUCTAL CELLS

Ductal cells range from cuboidal (lining the smaller intralobular ducts) to columnar (lining the larger interlobular ducts) in shape and are typically seen as strips or sheets with uniform, monotonous, honeycomb-like architecture (Figures 4.123-4.127).[45] Benign ductal cells have smooth nuclear membranes, round, uniform nuclei with inconspicuous nucleoli and delicate, pale cytoplasm. Pancreatic and bile duct brushing specimens contain mostly ductal cells because acinar cells are not sampled using these methods.

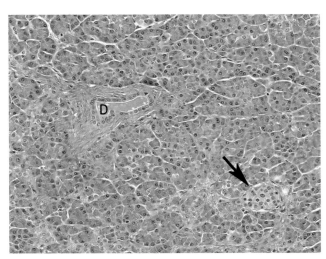

Figure 4.111. Normal pancreatic parenchyma: duct (D) and islet cluster (arrow) in a background of acini (H&E).

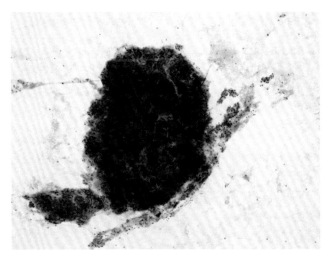

Figure 4.112. A large, benign acinar tissue fragment. Note the uniform, distinct lobules (Pap stain).

Figure 4.113. A large, benign acinar tissue fragment. Note the uniform lobular architecture (Pap stain).

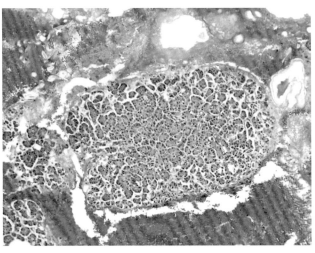

Figure 4.114. Large benign acinar tissue fragment in a background of abundant blood (cell block, H&E).

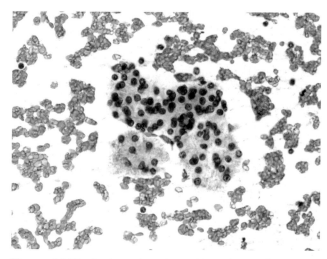

Figure 4.115. Benign acinar tissue. Note their uniform round basally oriented nuclei with delicate, finely vacuolated cytoplasm. Prominent nucleoli can be seen (Pap stain).

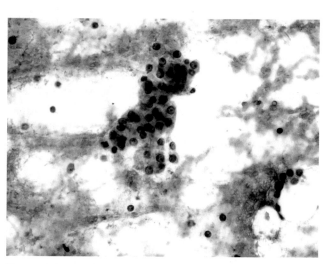

Figure 4.116. Benign acinar tissue. Separate field (Pap stain).

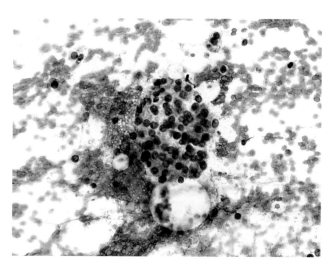

Figure 4.117. Benign acinar tissue. Separate field (Pap stain).

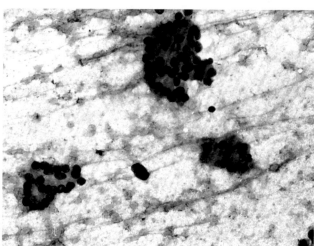

Figure 4.118. Benign acinar tissue. Separate field (Diff-Quik stain).

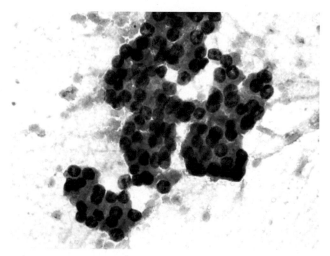

Figure 4.119. Benign acinar tissue. Separate field (Diff-Quik stain).

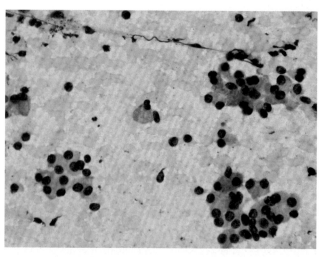

Figure 4.120. Benign acinar tissue. Separate field (Diff-Quik stain).

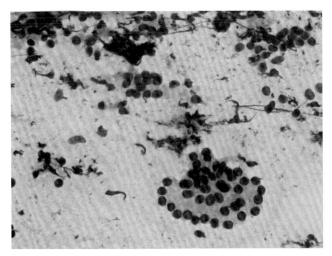

Figure 4.121. Benign acinar tissue. Separate field (Diff-Quik stain).

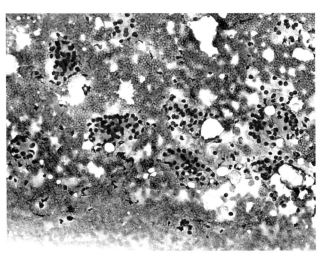

Figure 4.122. Uniform benign acini resembling "clusters of grapes" (Diff-Quik stain).

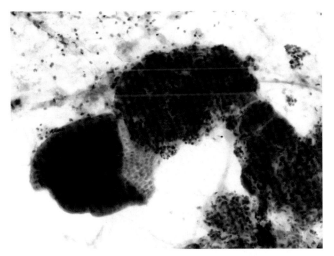

Figure 4.123. Benign acinar tissue fragments adjacent to contaminating benign gastrointestinal (duodenal) epithelium (left) (Pap stain).

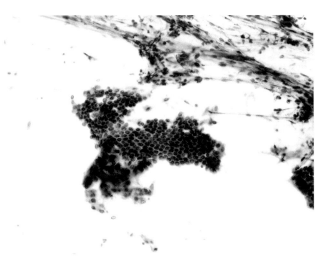

Figure 4.124. Normal pancreatic ductal epithelium. Normal ductal cells are arranged in an evenly spaced monolayer with a "honeycomb" appearance (Pap stain).

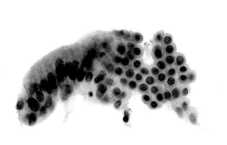

Figure 4.125. Normal pancreatic ductal epithelium. Normal ductal cells can have a "picket fence" arrangement (left half) or "honeycomb-like" appearance (right half), depending on orientation (Pap stain).

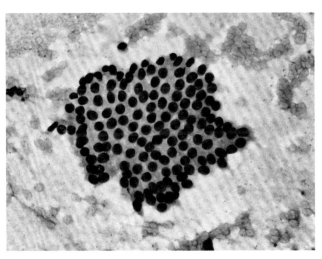

Figure 4.126. Benign ductal epithelium. Note the uniform monolayer of cuboidal cells with round to oval nuclei, smooth nuclear membranes, and well-defined cytoplasmic borders. There is minimal overlapping of nuclei (Diff-Quik stain).

ISLET CELLS

Islet cells are rare and constitute only 1-2% of the pancreatic tissue. They produce hormones that are secreted directly into the bloodstream. Under most circumstances, normal islet cells are rarely sampled by FNA; thus, the presence of a significant population of neuroendocrine cells on FNA is usually indicative of a neoplasm.

GASTROINTESTINAL CONTAMINATION

Depending on the route of the FNA needle during tissue procurement, normal tissue contamination from nearby organs can be seen. Common contaminants include gastric foveolar epithelial cells (during transgastric procedures sampling pancreatic body and tail masses) and duodenal epithelial cells (during transduodenal procedures sampling pancreatic head masses). Duodenal contamination typically contains interspersed goblet cells, which may be absent if the contamination is only present in small fragments (Figures 4.128-4.134). If present in large fragments, gastric "pits" may be seen in the gastric epithelium. GI contamination is often accompanied by mucin containing bacteria and debris. The distinction between normal GI contamination, especially gastric foveolar epithelium, and the lining of a cystic mucinous neoplasm can be difficult. Other infrequently encountered contaminants include mesothelial cells, hepatocytes, adrenal tissue, and renal tubular cells.

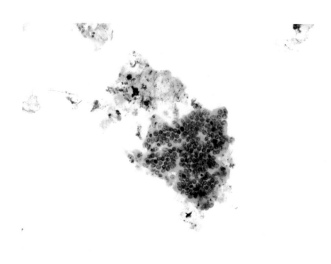

Figure 4.127. Benign bile duct epithelium, which is morphologically similar to pancreatic ductal epithelium. Background bile helps to confirm the biliary origin of this epithelial fragment (Pap stain).

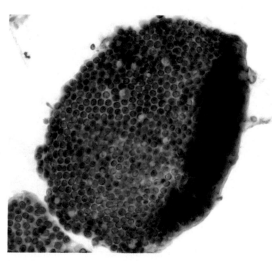

Figure 4.128. Duodenal epithelium contamination, which forms monolayer sheets of columnar cells with interspersed goblet cells. Cells with columnar shapes can be seen at the edge of the fragment (Pap stain).

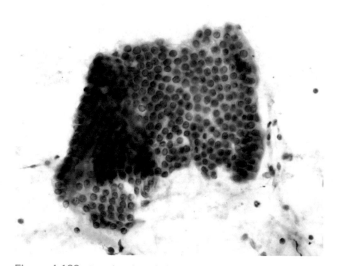

Figure 4.129. Duodenal epithelium contamination. Separate field (Pap stain).

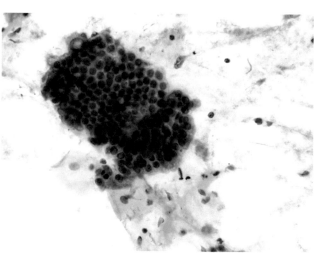

Figure 4.130. Duodenal epithelium contamination. Separate field (Pap stain).

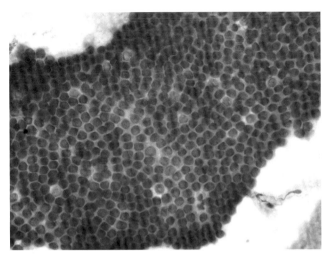

Figure 4.131. Duodenal epithelium contamination. Separate field (Diff-Quik stain).

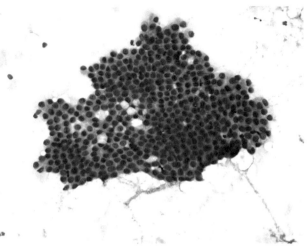

Figure 4.132. Duodenal epithelium contamination. Separate field (Diff-Quik stain).

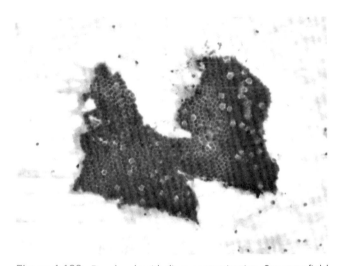

Figure 4.133. Duodenal epithelium contamination. Separate field (Diff-Quik stain).

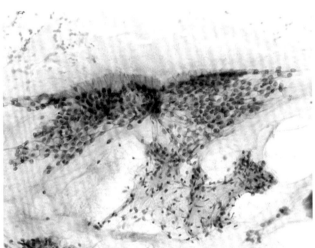

Figure 4.134. Gastric epithelium contamination. Note the "picket fence" arrangement adjacent to "honeycomb" sheets of mucinous foveolar cells, which may be confused with low-grade dysplasia or a mucinous neoplasm of the pancreas (Pap stain).

GLANDULAR/MUCINOUS PATTERN

The glandular/mucinous pattern is seen most often with processes that derive from epithelial linings, primarily that of the pancreatic ductal system. This pattern spans the spectrum from reactive atypia secondary to pancreatitis, to premalignant cystic mucinous neoplasms, to malignancies with glandular components. The cells generally form cohesive tissue fragments or sheets, some of which have a mucinous background or mucinous cytoplasm.

CHECKLIST: Etiologic Considerations for the Glandular/Mucinous Pattern

- ☐ Chronic Pancreatitis/Reactive Ductal Atypia
- ☐ Neoplastic Mucinous Cyst
- ☐ Pancreatic Ductal Adenocarcinoma
- ☐ Adenosquamous Carcinoma
- ☐ Metastatic Adenocarcinoma
- ☐ Gastrointestinal Contamination

CHRONIC PANCREATITIS/REACTIVE DUCTAL ATYPIA

Chronic pancreatitis may be associated with mass-forming fibrosis in its late stage and can thus mimic a neoplastic mass on imaging. Cytologic specimens tend to be hypocellular and often contain fibrotic stromal fragments mixed with bland to atypical ductal epithelium in a background of inflammation (Figures 4.135-4.138). Calcifications are nonspecific but are supportive of chronic pancreatitis in the context of corroborating radiologic findings.[46,47] The reactive ductal atypia can be significant and create difficulty in distinguishing these changes from well differentiated ductal adenocarcinoma. A clinical history of chronic pancreatitis with elevated enzyme levels, gallstones, or an indwelling stent should raise the threshold for malignancy.

FAQ: How should I report a pancreas FNA specimen?

Answer: The Papanicolaou Society of Cytopathology guidelines for standardized terminology in the categorization of pancreatobiliary cytology diagnoses is listed in Table 4.2. While its use is not yet widespread, it is the most commonly used system in North America.[48]

PEARLS & PITFALLS

Autoimmune pancreatitis, specifically lymphoplasmacytic sclerosing pancreatitis (type 1 IgG4-related autoimmune pancreatitis), is a subtype of chronic pancreatitis that is mass-forming and is at risk of being overdiagnosed as malignant. This process is characterized by an infiltrate of lymphocytes and plasma cells with prominent fibrosis (Figures 4.139-4.144). While definitive diagnosis may not be possible on cytology, it is important to raise the possibility of autoimmune pancreatitis and not overinterpret the accompanying cytologic atypia as a malignancy. Autoimmune pancreatitis responds to corticosteroid therapy, and further medical evaluation may preclude unnecessary surgery for the patient.

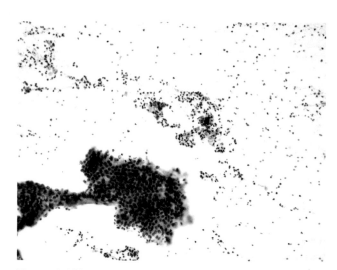

Figure 4.135. Acute on chronic pancreatitis with reactive ductal epithelium. The ductal cells are bland and remain relatively evenly spaced with focal areas of nuclear overlap in a background of acute inflammation (Pap stain).

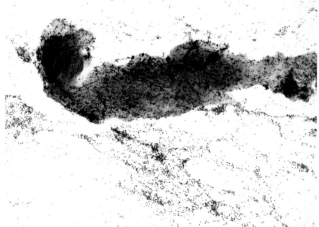

Figure 4.136. Acute on chronic pancreatitis. There is a large fibrotic stromal fragment in a background of acute and chronic inflammation (Pap stain).

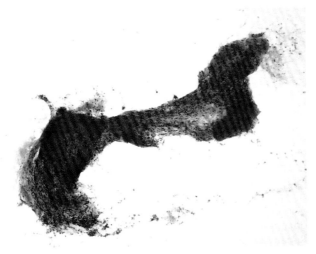

Figure 4.137. Fibrotic stromal fragment in chronic pancreatitis (Diff-Quik stain).

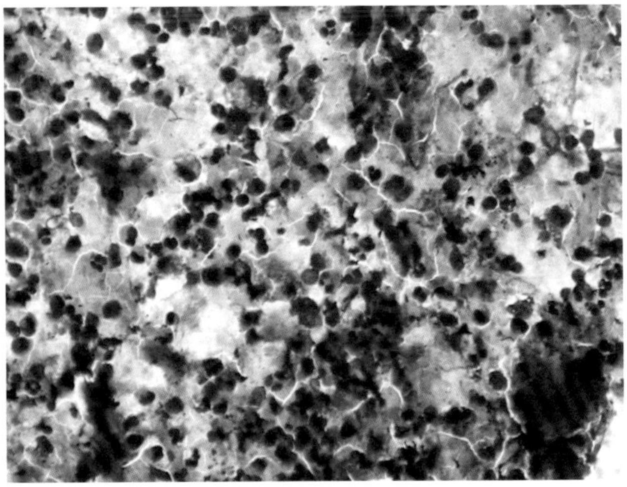

Figure 4.138. Mixed inflammatory infiltrate and calcifications (lower right) in chronic pancreatitis (Diff-Quik stain).

TABLE 4.2: Papanicolaou Society of Cytopathology Guidelines for Standardized Terminology for Pancreatobiliary Cytology

Category	Definition	Risk of Malignancy
I. Nondiagnostic	A nondiagnostic cytology specimen is one that provides no diagnostic or useful information about the solid or cystic lesion sampled (e.g. acellular aspirate of a cyst without evidence of a mucinous etiology, elevated CEA, or *KRAS/GNAS* mutation). **Any cellular atypia precludes a nondiagnostic report.**	
II. Negative (for malignancy)	A negative cytology sample is one that contains adequate cellular and/or extracellular tissue to evaluate or define a lesion that is identified on imaging. Specific diagnoses include benign pancreatobiliary tissue, acute/chronic/autoimmune pancreatitis, pseudocyst, splenule/accessory spleen.	15% false-negative rate for FNA of solid mass Up to 60% false-negative rate for cystic lesions[a]
III. Atypical	There are cells present with cytoplasmic, nuclear, or architectural features that are not consistent with normal or reactive cellular changes of the pancreas or bile ducts and are insufficient to classify them as a neoplasm or suspicious for a high-grade malignancy. The findings are insufficient to establish an abnormality explaining the lesion seen on imaging. Follow-up evaluation is warranted.	44-82%
IVa. Neoplastic: Benign	The cytological specimen is sufficiently cellular and representative, with or without the context of clinical, imaging, and ancillary studies, to be diagnostic of a benign neoplasm (e.g. serous cystadenoma).	
IVb. Neoplastic: Other	The neoplasm is either premalignant, such as intraductal papillary neoplasm of the bile ducts (IPN-B), IPMN, or MCN with low-, intermediate-, or high-grade dysplasia by cytological criteria, or a low-grade malignant neoplasm, such as well differentiated PanNET or SPN.	

(Continued)

TABLE 4.2:   (Continued)

Category	Definition	Risk of Malignancy
V. Suspicious (for malignancy)	The cytologic features raise a strong suspicion for malignancy (mainly PDAC), but the findings are insufficient for a conclusive diagnosis, or tissue is not present for ancillary studies to define a specific neoplasm.	80-96%
VI. Positive/ malignant	A group of neoplasms that unequivocally display malignant cytologic characteristics and include PDAC and its variants, cholangiocarcinoma, acinar cell carcinoma, high-grade neuroendocrine carcinoma (small cell and large cell), pancreatoblastoma, lymphomas, sarcomas and metastases to the pancreas.	>90-95%

[a]However, the absence of high-grade epithelial atypia in pancreatic cyst aspirates has a high negative predictive value for malignancy.

FNA, fine-needle aspiration; IPMN, intraductal papillary mucinous neoplasm; MCN, mucinous cystic neoplasm; PanNET, pancreatic neuroendocrine tumor; PDAC, pancreatic ductal adenocarcinoma; SPN, solid pseudopapillary neoplasm.

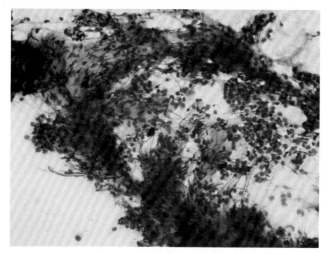

Figure 4.139. Large mixed epithelial and mesenchymal tissue fragments with extensive fibrosis, as seen in autoimmune pancreatitis (Diff-Quik stain).

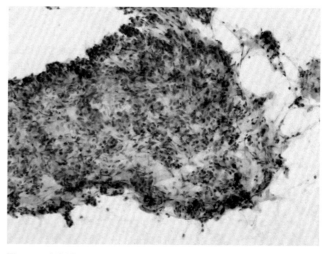

Figure 4.140. Large mixed epithelial and mesenchymal tissue fragments with extensive fibrosis, as seen in autoimmune pancreatitis (Pap stain).

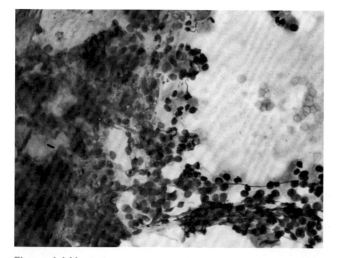

Figure 4.141. Autoimmune pancreatitis. Note the reactive cellular atypia: hyperchromatic, enlarged, overlapping nuclei (Diff-Quik stain).

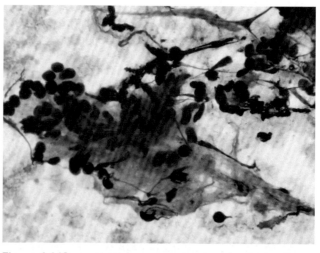

Figure 4.142. Autoimmune pancreatitis. Separate field (Diff-Quik stain).

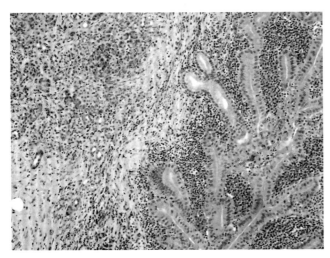

Figure 4.143. Autoimmune pancreatitis, lymphoplasmacytic sclerosing type (type 1). The inflammatory infiltrate is primarily composed of lymphocytes and plasma cells and there is a background of fibrosis (H&E).

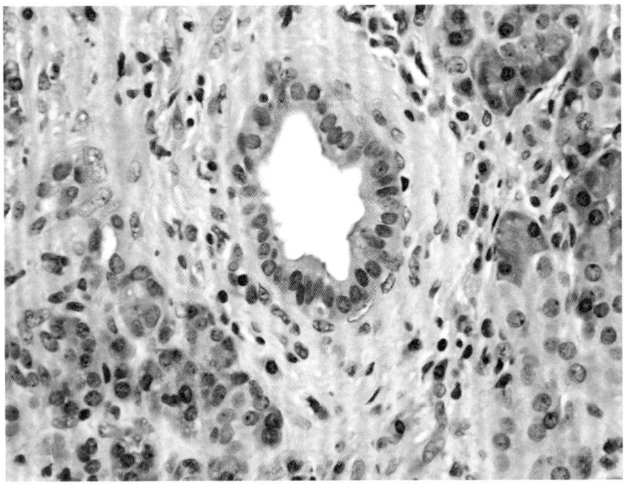

Figure 4.144. Autoimmune pancreatitis, lymphoplasmacytic sclerosing type (type 1). Note the prominent duct-centered fibrosis (H&E).

KEY FEATURES of Chronic Pancreatitis/Reactive Ductal Atypia

- Overall, the specimen is of low to moderate cellularity.
- The specimen contains flat, cohesive sheets of ductal epithelial cells with relatively evenly spaced, uniform, polarized nuclei.
- The atypical cells have even to slightly coarse chromatin and smooth nuclear membranes.
- The atypical cells have low N/C ratios.
- Prominent nucleoli and mitoses may be seen.
- The atypical cells can have enlarged nuclei, but variation in diameter is <4:1.
- The background may contain inflammation, fat necrosis, calcifications, and/or mucoid debris.

FAQ: Is this chronic pancreatitis or adenocarcinoma with desmoplasia?

Answer: False-positive diagnoses of pancreatic lesions on FNA are rare but are often secondary to the presence of chronic pancreatitis. Chronic pancreatitis causes reactive atypia in the ductal epithelium that may overlap with a well differentiated adenocarcinoma. While inflammatory cells and fibrotic tissue fragments may be aspirated, these findings may also be seen in an adenocarcinoma with a desmoplastic reaction. Because chronic pancreatitis is a destructive process, FNA of chronic pancreatitis should yield only rare ductal fragments. The presence of abundant, atypical ductal fragments is more suggestive of an adenocarcinoma than chronic pancreatitis. In the setting of chronic pancreatitis, it is important to not mistake GI contamination for atypical ductal epithelium. Chronic pancreatitis should not cause the markedly atypical changes seen in moderately differentiated or poorly differentiated adenocarcinoma (such as >4:1 nuclear size variation or the presence of singly dispersed markedly atypical cells).

SAMPLE NOTE: GLANDULAR PATTERN, ATYPICAL DUCTAL CELLS

Atypical ductal cells. See note.

Note: There is a population of moderately atypical cells with nuclear enlargement, nuclear crowding, and prominent nucleoli. The overall smooth nuclear membranes and open chromatin suggest atypia secondary to reactive changes. Definitive features of malignancy are not present. While the cellular atypia may raise the suspicion of malignancy, the history of pancreatitis and indwelling stent warrant conservative interpretation.

Reference:
Lin F, Staerkel G. Cytologic criteria for well differentiated adenocarcinoma of the pancreas in fine-needle aspiration biopsy specimens. *Cancer Cytopathol.* 2003;99(1):44-50.

NEOPLASTIC MUCINOUS CYST

Mucinous cysts are diagnosed using the proposed standardized terminology system for pancreaticobiliary specimens from the Papanicolaou Society of Cytopathology based on having one of the following features: 1) thick, colloid-like extracellular mucin, 2) mucinous epithelium, and/or 3) elevated carcinoembryonic antigen (CEA) ≥192 ng/mL (Figures 4.145-4.152).[49-51] In contrast to GI mucin, which contains bacteria, granular debris, and acute inflammatory cells, the mucin aspirated from neoplastic mucinous cysts is "clean," containing few cells except for macrophages. There are two types of neoplastic mucinous cysts that share common cytomorphological features but have distinct clinical and biological characteristics: intraductal papillary mucinous neoplasm (IPMN) and mucinous cystic neoplasm (MCN). Both are stratified into low-/intermediate-grade versus high-grade dysplasia and can be associated with an invasive carcinoma component, which is the most important negative prognostic factor.

Intraductal Papillary Mucinous Neoplasm (IPMN)

IPMN is a grossly visible, mucin-producing epithelial neoplasm that grows within the pancreatic ductal system, often demonstrating a papillary architecture with resultant cystic dilatation. IPMNs are classified into those involving the main pancreatic duct (main duct type), branch ducts (branch duct type), or both (mixed type). They primarily occur in the sixth to seventh decade and comprise 3-5% of pancreatic tumors; 70% arise in the head of the pancreas.[52] High-risk features that may prompt surgical resection include main duct involvement, presence of a mural nodule, and the identification of high-grade dysplasia or invasive carcinoma.[48]

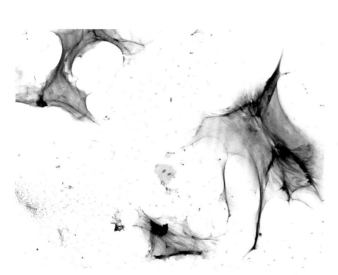

Figure 4.145. Extracellular mucin from a neoplastic pancreatic mucinous cyst (Pap stain).

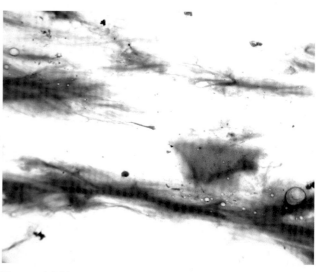

Figure 4.146. Extracellular mucin from a neoplastic pancreatic mucinous cyst (Pap stain).

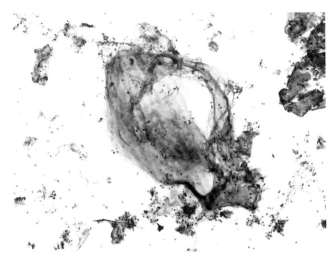

Figure 4.147. Extracellular mucin in a background of acute inflammation and debris from a pancreatic mucinous cyst (Pap stain).

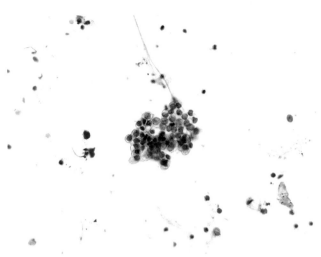

Figure 4.148. Mucinous epithelium with low-grade atypia. Note the clear mucinous cytoplasm and overall intact monolayer organization (Pap stain).

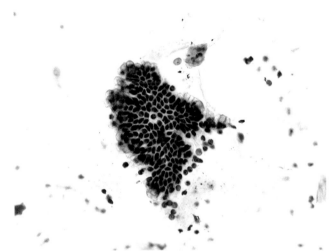

Figure 4.149. Mucinous epithelium with low-grade atypia. The columnar shape and apical mucin can be seen at the edges of the fragment (Pap stain).

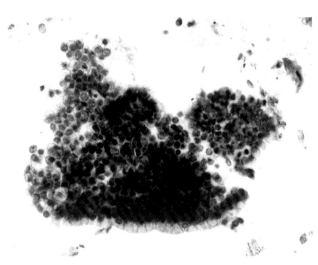

Figure 4.150. Mucinous epithelium with low-grade atypia (Pap stain).

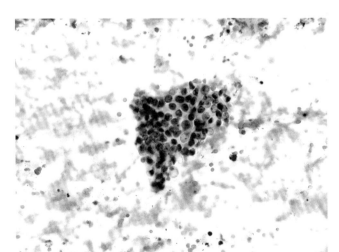

Figure 4.151. Mucinous epithelium with intermediate-grade atypia. Intracellular mucin can still be appreciated in some cells, but there is more cell size variation and nuclear overlapping (Pap stain).

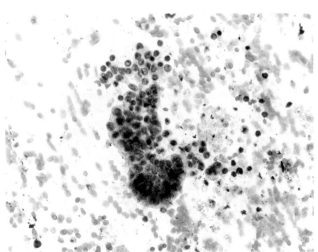

Figure 4.152. Mucinous epithelium with intermediate-grade atypia. It is important to distinguish high-grade atypia from low- to intermediate-grade atypia, but differentiating intermediate- from low-grade atypia is not necessary for clinical prognostication (Pap stain).

Mucinous Cystic Neoplasm (MCN)

MCN is usually a large, solitary, multiloculated, mucin-producing epithelial neoplasm that is defined by the presence of subepithelial ovarian-type stroma. MCNs comprise approximately 6% of pancreatic tumors and occur almost exclusively in women in the fourth to fifth decade; 90% arise in the body or tail of the pancreas. In contrast to IPMNs, surgical resection is recommended for all patients with MCN, as their location in the distal pancreas lends them to less morbid distal pancreatectomy or laparoscopic procedures, and resection removes the need for lifelong surveillance in these relatively young patients.

PEARLS & PITFALLS

The distinction between IPMN and MCN is not possible by cytomorphology alone. When possible, it is important to distinguish MCN from IPMN, as surgical resection is recommended for all patients with MCN irrespective of grade. If a tissue biopsy or forceps specimen is available, look for the presence of subepithelial ovarian-type stroma, which is a defining characteristic of MCN (Figures 4.153-4.155). Immunohistochemistry for estrogen and progesterone receptors, which is positive in the ovarian-type stromal cells, may be considered if morphology is ambiguous.[53-55] If molecular testing is available, the detection of a *GNAS* mutation aids in ruling out MCN.[56]

KEY FEATURES of Neoplastic Mucinous Cysts

- The specimen contains variable amounts of extracellular "clean" mucin (especially thick colloid-like mucin) and/or mucinous epithelium.
- Low-grade atypia: benign-appearing mucinous epithelium in sheets and groups, often indistinguishable from benign gastric epithelium.
- High-grade atypia: small, tight, clusters or isolated atypical epithelial cells, usually smaller than a 12-μm duodenal enterocyte, with increased N/C ratio, irregular nuclear membranes, hyper- or hypochromasia, and variably vacuolated cytoplasm.
- The background may contain cellular debris/necrosis.

FAQ: How is pancreatic cyst fluid analysis used for the diagnosis of pancreatic cysts?

Answer: The current standard of care for the diagnosis of pancreatic cysts involves pancreatic cyst fluid analysis using a combination of cytology and CEA/amylase testing. A CEA ≥192 ng/mL supports the diagnosis of a mucinous cyst. In some institutions, molecular testing is performed on all specimens with sufficient cyst fluid, as the detection of a *KRAS* and/or *GNAS* mutation in mucinous cysts is helpful in cases where cytology and CEA are noncontributory.[57-59] A *GNAS* mutation also supports a specific diagnosis of IPMN.

PEARLS & PITFALLS

As cytology is the best modality for identifying high-risk cysts,[49,50,60] it is important to indicate the presence of low-grade versus high-grade atypia when reporting mucinous cysts, as the latter triages the patient to surgical resection. The three features found to be most accurate for the identification of high-grade atypia were 1) background cellular necrosis, 2) abnormal chromatin pattern (hypo- or hyperchromasia), and 3) increased N/C ratio (Figures 4.156-4.158).[48] New technology, including the Moray micro forceps, can help improve the sampling of the cyst lining and, as a result, improve the detection of high-grade dysplasia and the evaluation of the subepithelial stroma.[61] However, it is important to realize that it is very difficult to distinguish high-grade dysplasia from invasive adenocarcinoma in a cystic pancreatic lesion; thus, one should be extremely cautious in making the diagnosis of adenocarcinoma on FNA of cystic pancreatic lesions.

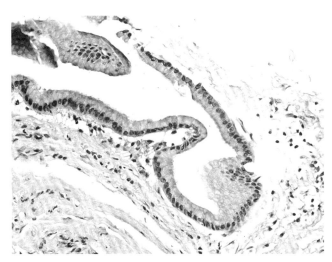

Figure 4.153. Mucinous epithelium with low-grade dysplasia (H&E).

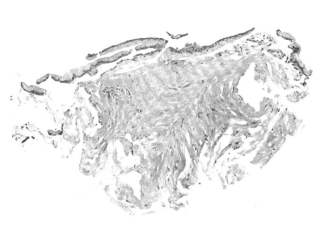

Figure 4.154. Mucinous epithelium with low-grade dysplasia and no underlying ovarian-type stroma, consistent with intraductal papillary mucinous neoplasm (IPMN) (H&E).

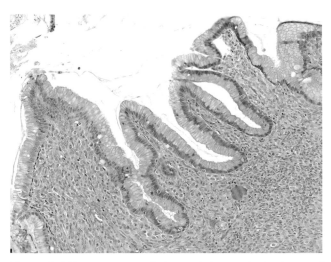

Figure 4.155. Mucinous epithelium with low-grade dysplasia and subepithelial ovarian-type stroma, consistent with mucinous cystic neoplasm (H&E).

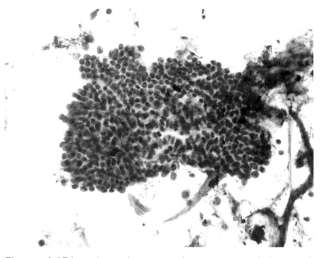

Figure 4.156. A large fragment of mucinous epithelium with high-grade atypia. Note the "drunken honeycomb" architecture, nuclear hyperchromasia, and increased nuclear to cytoplasmic ratio. Intracellular mucin is appreciated in some cells (Pap stain).

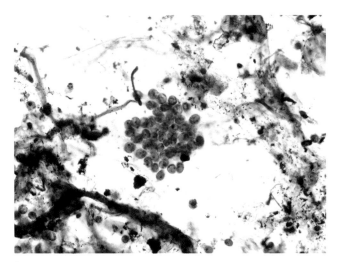

Figure 4.157. Atypical epithelium with high-grade atypia. Note the nuclear overlapping, increased nuclear to cytoplasmic ratio, and prominent nucleoli (Pap stain).

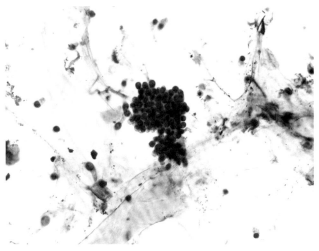

Figure 4.158. Mucinous epithelium with high-grade atypia. Note the nuclear hyperchromasia and increased nuclear to cytoplasmic ratio. Intracellular mucin is appreciated in some cells (Pap stain).

SAMPLE NOTE: MUCINOUS PATTERN, CYSTIC MUCINOUS NEOPLASM

Mucinous epithelium and mucin, consistent with cystic mucinous neoplasm. No high-grade dysplasia is identified. See note.

Note: A mucinous etiology is established by the presence of mucinous epithelial cells and elevated CEA (2485 ng/mL). Molecular analysis is pending and will be reported separately.

PANCREATIC DUCTAL ADENOCARCINOMA

Pancreatic ductal adenocarcinoma (PDAC) is by far the most common tumor of the pancreas and comprises approximately 90% of all pancreatic neoplasms.[62] PDACs most often occur in older individuals aged 60-80 years with a male predominance. The majority of these tumors are located in the pancreatic head and are thus frequently associated with pancreatic and/or bile duct stricture and downstream dilation of the common bile duct and pancreatic duct ("double duct" sign on imaging).[63] Cytologically, the ductal epithelial cells exhibit marked anisonucleosis and are arranged in a more disorganized fashion with variable amounts of mucinous cytoplasm: abundant in well differentiated but scant in more poorly differentiated adenocarcinomas (Figures 4.159-4.174). As mentioned in the Chronic Pancreatitis/Reactive Ductal Atypia section, benign conditions such as chronic pancreatitis (and autoimmune pancreatitis), indwelling stents, inflammatory comorbidities such as primary sclerosing cholangitis and primary biliary cirrhosis, etc. are in the differential diagnosis of PDAC. An accurate diagnosis of adenocarcinoma allows for proper triage of patients to surgical resection, with or without neoadjuvant therapy.

KEY FEATURES of Pancreatic Ductal Adenocarcinoma

- The specimen should be of moderate to high cellularity.
- The malignant cells form irregularly sized and shaped groups with nuclear crowding, overlap, and disrupted organization ("drunken honeycomb" appearance).
- The malignant cells demonstrate nuclear membrane irregularities, hyperchromasia, and coarse chromatin.
- The N/C ratios are increased in the tumor cells.
- In poorly differentiated adenocarcinomas, the background often contains dispersed malignant cells.
- In moderately to poorly differentiated adenocarcinomas, the background often contains necrotic debris.
- Anisonucleosis with >4:1 variation in diameter is a specific feature.

FAQ: How can reactive atypia and ductal adenocarcinoma be distinguished in borderline cases?

Answer: In borderline cases where reactive epithelium appears highly atypical, cytomorphologic features overlap between reactive atypia and ductal adenocarcinoma. Histological examination in the form of a cell block or biopsy can provide architectural or stromal clues, and immunohistochemistry for SMAD4/DPC4 (loss of nuclear expression in approximately half of PDACs) and p53 (overexpression in most PDACs) may be helpful (Figures 4.175 and 4.176). A clinical history of stenting or an inflammatory comorbidity should raise the threshold for malignancy. However, a definitive distinction between reactive atypia and malignancy is not always possible.

ADENOSQUAMOUS CARCINOMA

Adenosquamous carcinoma is the most common variant of PDAC and comprises 3-4% of all pancreatic malignancies.[52] These tumors have variable proportions of glandular and squamous components (Figures 4.177-4.180). The presence of cells with squamous differentiation should raise the possibility of adenosquamous carcinoma (and prompt a careful

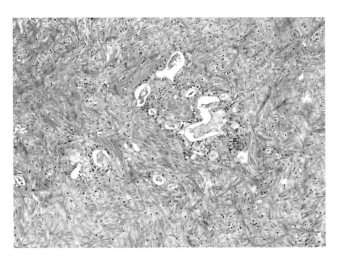

Figure 4.159. Pancreatic ductal adenocarcinoma. Infiltrative neoplastic duct can be seen in a background of markedly desmoplastic stroma (H&E).

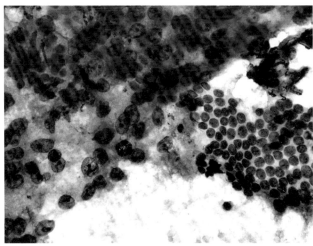

Figure 4.160. Ductal adenocarcinoma cells (left) adjacent to benign ductal epithelium (right). Note that the neoplastic cells are significantly larger with nuclear crowding, overlap, and nuclear membrane irregularities compared with the uniform benign ductal cells (Diff-Quik stain).

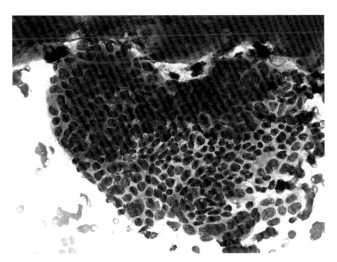

Figure 4.161. Pancreatic ductal adenocarcinoma. A large tissue fragment of atypical epithelium with nuclear enlargement, crowding, hyperchromasia, and pleomorphism (Diff-Quik stain).

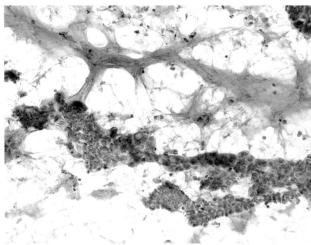

Figure 4.162. Pancreatic ductal adenocarcinoma with abundant background extracellular mucin. Glandular differentiation with central mucin can be seen (Pap stain).

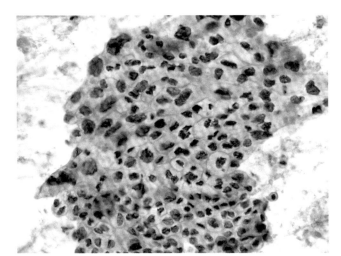

Figure 4.163. Pancreatic ductal adenocarcinoma. Neoplastic epithelial fragment with hyperchromatic nuclei and marked nuclear membrane irregularities (Pap stain).

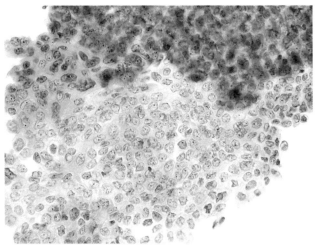

Figure 4.164. Pancreatic ductal adenocarcinoma. Atypical epithelium with nuclear membrane irregularities, distinct nucleoli, and frequent grooves (Pap stain).

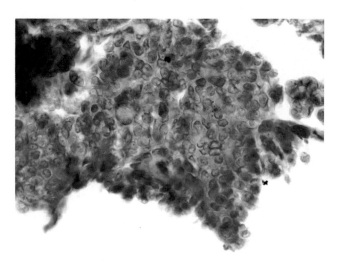

Figure 4.165. Pancreatic ductal adenocarcinoma. The ductal cells are disorderly and abruptly form an intercellular gland containing mucin (Pap stain).

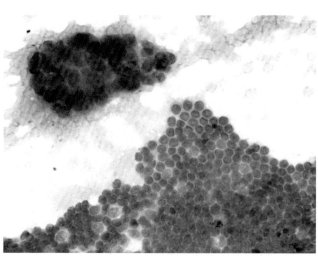

Figure 4.166. A fragment of malignant ductal epithelium (upper left) adjacent to benign duodenal epithelium (lower right) (Diff-Quik stain).

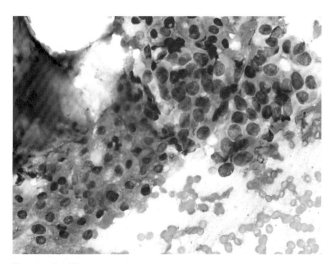

Figure 4.167. A fragment of malignant ductal epithelium (upper right) adjacent to benign hepatocytes (lower left) (Diff-Quik stain).

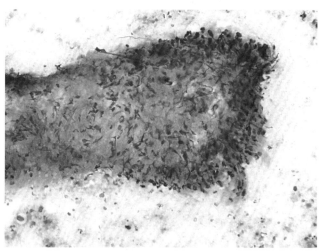

Figure 4.168. A fragment of predominantly fibrous tissue. This represents desmoplasia associated with ductal adenocarcinoma but can be difficult to distinguish from chronic pancreatitis with reactive atypia (Diff-Quik stain).

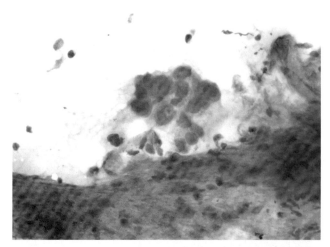

Figure 4.169. Fibrous desmoplastic tissue (bottom) from a ductal adenocarcinoma specimen. A small group of malignant cells is loosely associated with the desmoplastic tissue (Pap stain).

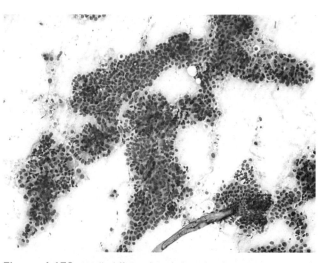

Figure 4.170. Well differentiated ductal adenocarcinoma with mild nuclear and architectural atypia. The nuclei are enlarged with focal crowding and loss of organization (Diff-Quik stain).

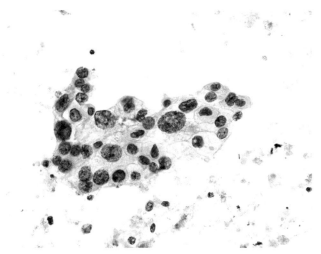

Figure 4.171. Pancreatic ductal adenocarcinoma. This fragment of neoplastic cells demonstrates marked nuclear enlargement, coarse chromatin, and anisonucleosis (>4:1 variation) (Pap stain).

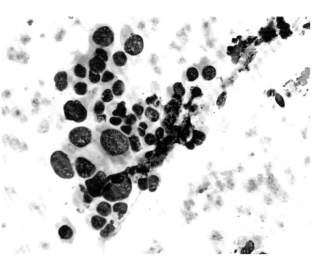

Figure 4.172. Poorly differentiated ductal adenocarcinoma. A group of loosely-cohesive neoplastic cells possesses marked nuclear enlargement and pleomorphism (Pap stain).

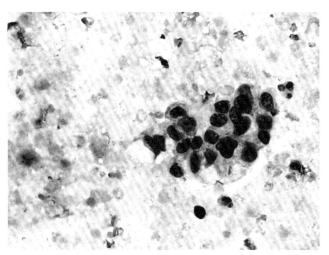

Figure 4.173. Pancreatic ductal adenocarcinoma. A fragment of neoplastic cells can be seen in a background of cellular necrosis (Diff-Quik stain).

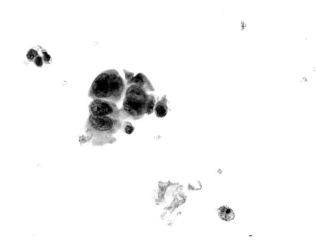

Figure 4.174. Pancreatic ductal adenocarcinoma. These adenocarcinoma cells are enlarged and loosely cohesive. Compare their size with that of the non-neoplastic cells in the upper left (Pap stain).

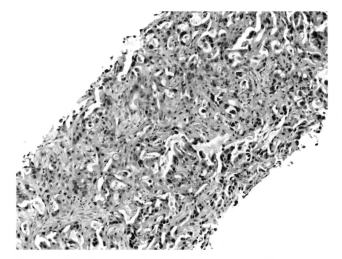

Figure 4.175. Pancreatic ductal adenocarcinoma. A biopsy shows haphazard, infiltrative ducts with minimal intervening stroma (H&E).

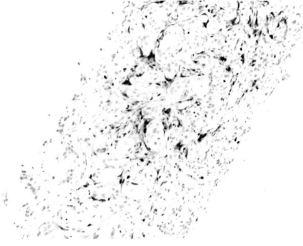

Figure 4.176. A corresponding immunostain for SMAD4 shows complete loss in the neoplastic cells and retention of expression in the nonneoplastic intervening stroma (SMAD4 immunostain).

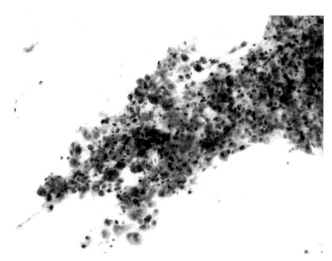

Figure 4.177. Adenosquamous carcinoma. At low magnification, atypical cells can be seen singly and as well as within a necrotic fragment. Many atypical orangeophilic squamous cells are present (Pap stain).

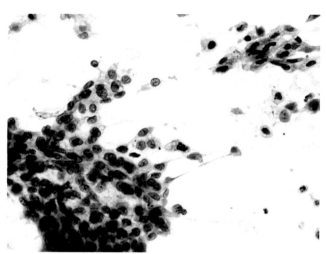

Figure 4.178. Adenosquamous carcinoma. A fragment of atypical ductal-type epithelium (lower left) with glandular formation is adjacent to scattered atypical keratinized cells (upper right) containing hyperchromatic nuclei (Pap stain).

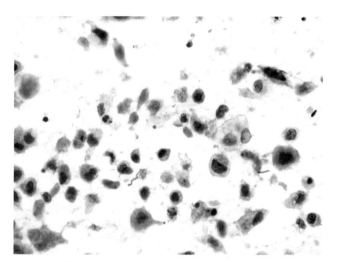

Figure 4.179. Adenosquamous carcinoma. Single atypical keratinized cells with hyperchromatic nuclei and irregular nuclear borders are scattered in a necrotic background (Pap stain).

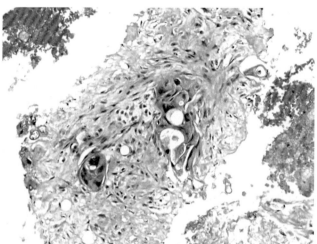

Figure 4.180. Adenosquamous carcinoma. The neoplastic cells show squamous differentiation with hard, glassy eosinophilic cytoplasm. Glandular differentiation was seen in other areas of the neoplasm (H&E).

search for glandular cells), as primary squamous cell carcinoma of the pancreas is extremely rare.[64] However, not all squamous cells detected in a pancreatic specimen are from an adenosquamous or a squamous cell carcinoma. Squamous metaplasia can occur in the extrahepatic bile ducts and should not immediately be overinterpreted as malignant.[65] Additionally, squamous-lined cysts, such as lymphoepithelial cysts, can occur in the pancreas. In both entities, the squamous cells should lack significant atypia. FNA may predominantly sample one component of an adenosquamous carcinoma over another and will therefore not necessarily be concordant with the resection specimen; conventional PDACs can demonstrate areas of focal squamous differentiation. On cytology, the possibility of an adenosquamous carcinoma may be suggested with a diagnosis such as "adenocarcinoma with focal squamous differentiation" or "carcinoma with focal squamous differentiation."

METASTATIC ADENOCARCINOMA

Although PDAC is the most common malignancy of the pancreas, metastatic adenocarcinoma should be considered, especially if any unusual or suggestive features are seen on cytology. The most common primary carcinomas that metastasize to the pancreas are those originating in the lung, breast, and kidney (Figures 4.181 and 4.182).[66]

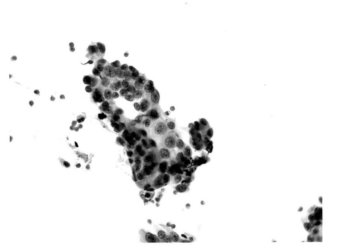

Figure 4.181. Metastatic adenocarcinoma. This fragment contains malignant cells in a glandular formation. Cytomorphologically this could be compatible with a primary pancreatic adenocarcinoma and is generally assumed as such unless ancillary studies or clinicoradiologic impression prove otherwise (Pap stain).

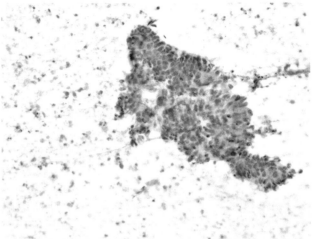

Figure 4.182. Metastatic colon adenocarcinoma to the pancreas. There are fragments of malignant glandular cells in a background of "dirty" necrosis . In this case, some of the elongated nuclei form "picket fence" formations and the cytomorphology strongly suggests a metastatic colorectal adenocarcinoma (Pap stain).

FAQ: Is this a primary pancreatic adenocarcinoma or a metastatic process?

Answer: Most adenocarcinomas found in the pancreas are primary processes and under most circumstances metastasis does not need to be excluded. The most common metastasis to the pancreas is renal cell carcinoma, which does not resemble a pancreatic ductal adenocarcinoma. It is common to find necrosis, focal squamous differentiation, and/or mucin production in pancreatic adenocarcinomas. For patients with a history of metastatic adenocarcinoma, immunostains can be helpful to exclude most breast and lung primaries. It is more difficult to exclude upper GI primaries because they also express CK7 and GI markers (such as CDX2). One potentially helpful marker is SMAD4/DPC4, which demonstrates loss of nuclear expression in up to half of pancreatic adenocarcinomas. The loss of SMAD4/DPC4 expression is strong evidence of a pancreatic primary. If immunostains cannot be performed or are unhelpful, adenocarcinomas are usually assumed to be primary to the pancreas unless there is compelling clinical/radiologic evidence otherwise. As a result, a diagnosis of "adenocarcinoma" may be more appropriate than a diagnosis of "pancreatic adenocarcinoma."

SINGLE CELL/DISPERSED PATTERN

The single cell/dispersed pattern consists of predominantly scattered single cells or small clusters of cells. This patterns consists of some primary pancreatic neoplasms that may morphologically mimic one another, as well as lymphoid proliferations.

CHECKLIST: Etiologic Considerations for the Single Cell/Dispersed Pattern

☐ Pancreatic Neuroendocrine Tumor

☐ Acinar Cell Carcinoma

☐ Pancreatoblastoma

☐ Solid Pseudopapillary Neoplasm

☐ Poorly Differentiated Carcinoma

☐ Lymphoma

☐ Ectopic Spleen (Splenule)

PANCREATIC NEUROENDOCRINE TUMOR (PanNET)

PanNETs represent 1-2% of all pancreatic neoplasms; most PanNETs are nonfunctional.[67] The cells of PanNETs are monomorphic with round to oval eccentric nuclei with finely stippled "salt-and-pepper" chromatin and moderate to abundant cytoplasm, occurring singly and/or in pseudorosettes/small clusters (Figures 4.183-4.186). The most common malignant entity in the differential diagnosis is acinar cell carcinoma because both can have eccentrically placed nuclei, granular cytoplasm, and stripped nuclei. Immunostains can aid the diagnosis by demonstrating neuroendocrine differentiation, with synaptophysin more sensitive than chromogranin A (Figures 4.187 and 4.188).[68] INSM1, a more recently described nuclear marker, has been demonstrated to have greater sensitivity and specificity than synaptophysin and chromogranin.[69] PanNETs can also undergo cystic degeneration and mimic a primary pancreatic cystic neoplasm.

On cytology, an important role is to distinguish well differentiated PanNETs from poorly differentiated pancreatic neuroendocrine carcinomas (PanNECs, discussed below in the "Poorly Differentiated Carcinoma" section). The Ki67 proliferation index is a requirement for grading and can be performed on cell block preparations and core biopsies that are sufficiently cellular,[70] although it must be recognized that a higher grade area may not have been sampled, resulting in discordance with the subsequent resection material.

KEY FEATURES of Well Differentiated PanNETs

- A large proportion of the neoplastic cells are present individually and not strictly seen in fragments.
- The neoplastic cells have a plasmacytoid appearance (eccentrically placed nucleus).
- The neoplastic cells are monomorphic and have round nuclei with regular borders.
- A "speckled" or "salt-and-pepper" chromatin appearance (characteristic of neuroendocrine differentiation) can often be appreciated on Pap-stained smears.
- The neoplastic cells have low N/C ratios.
- Stripped nuclei can often be found in the background.

PEARLS & PITFALLS

While the discohesive nature and plasmacytoid morphology of PanNETs often place them high on a differential diagnosis, some PanNETs may contain additional striking features that can complicate the diagnosis. For instance, lipid-rich PanNETs contain vacuolated cytoplasm that may mimic metastatic renal cell carcinoma (Figures 4.189 and 4.190). Cytoplasmic inclusions of cytokeratin may be present in some tumors, causing a rhabdoid appearance.[71] Despite unusual appearances, PanNET should always be strongly considered when a pancreas FNA specimen demonstrates a discohesive population of neoplastic cells.

FAQ: Is it possible to definitively diagnose a PanNET without confirmatory immunostains?

Answer: Yes. The diagnosis of PanNET can be made without immunostains in the presence of a very cellular population of discohesive, monotonous cells with all the cytomorphologic features of PanNET: plasmacytoid morphology, round nuclei with regular borders, and a neuroendocrine chromatin pattern. Furthermore, a PanNET should be suspected based on imaging studies. A predominance of acinar formations or cohesive tissue fragments as opposed to individually dispersed cells should cause reservation. The presence of papillary fragments containing vessels suggests the possibility of a solid pseudopapillary neoplasm. If stripped nuclei are present, these "nuclei" should be closely examined to ensure they are not actually lymphocytes. Benign acinar tissue and ectopic splenules have been mistaken for PanNETs on FNA, resulting in unnecessary surgery.[72]

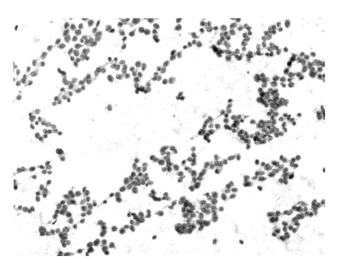

Figure 4.183. Well differentiated pancreatic neuroendocrine tumor. Note the dispersed, discohesive round to oval neuroendocrine cells with "salt-and-pepper" chromatin (Pap stain).

Figure 4.184. Well differentiated pancreatic neuroendocrine tumor with loosely cohesive and dispersed round cells (Pap stain).

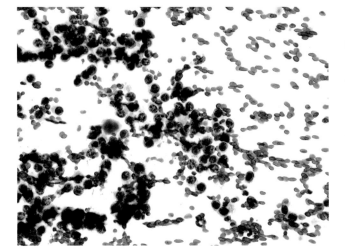

Figure 4.185. Well differentiated pancreatic neuroendocrine tumor (grade 2). The neoplastic cells have stippled chromatin and moderate amounts of cytoplasm, although there are some naked nuclei as well (Pap stain).

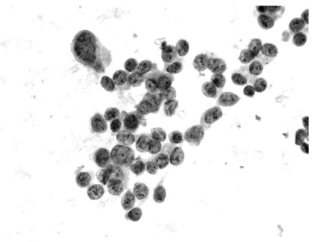

Figure 4.186. Well differentiated pancreatic neuroendocrine tumor (grade 3). The nuclei have the classic stippled chromatin of neuroendocrine cells, but there is marked pleomorphism and increased nuclear to cytoplasmic ratio. Grading can only be performed on adequate tissue (grade 3: >20 mitoses/10 high-power fields, Ki67 >20%) (Pap stain).

ACINAR CELL CARCINOMA

Acinar cell carcinoma is a rare, aggressive tumor and accounts for <2% of all pancreatic neoplasms.[52] The tumor cells are typically seen as isolated cells or small clusters with uniform round to oval nuclei with coarse chromatin and a single prominent nucleolus (Figures 4.191-4.194). The intracytoplasmic zymogen granules impart a delicate granular appearance to the cytoplasm and can also be seen in the background alongside stripped nuclei. Acinar cell carcinomas can be distinguished from benign acinar cells by their discohesive/dispersed nature and loss of the tight, "grape-like" clustering of normal acini. Immunohistochemical detection of specific enzymes produced by acinar cells (i.e. trypsin, chymotrypsin) supports the diagnosis[73] and helps distinguish acinar cell carcinoma from PanNETs and solid pseudopapillary neoplasms. In addition, BCL10 expression has been described as a useful marker for acinar cell differentiation and, in the setting of a pancreatic neoplasm, is specific for acinar cell carcinoma. However, one study demonstrated BCL10 positivity in two of four primary adenosquamous carcinomas, a possible pitfall.[74]

KEY FEATURES of Acinar Cell Carcinoma

- The specimen contains numerous cells present singly and/or in acinar formations.
- The neoplastic cells appear monotonous.

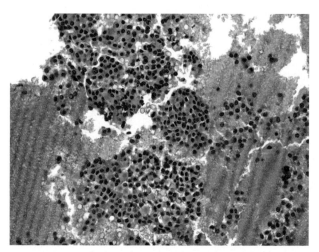

Figure 4.187. Well differentiated pancreatic neuroendocrine tumor (grade 2). The cells are arranged in loosely cohesive clusters and dispersed single cells, and have round, plasmacytoid nuclei (H&E).

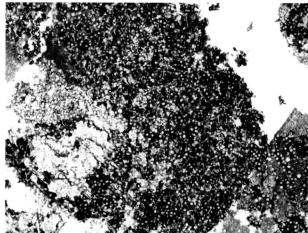

Figure 4.188. A synaptophysin immunostain performed on the same cell block shows diffuse strong positivity, supporting the neuroendocrine differentiation of the tumor (synaptophysin immunostain).

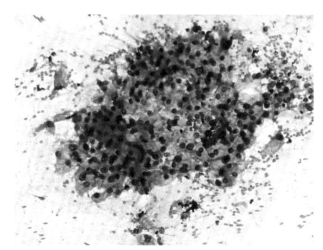

Figure 4.189. Metastatic renal cell carcinoma to the pancreas. There is a loosely cohesive fragment and scattered single neoplastic cells with round nuclei, variably distinct nucleoli, and vacuolated cytoplasm. This appearance can be confused with the lipid-rich variant of pancreatic neuroendocrine tumor (Diff-Quik stain).

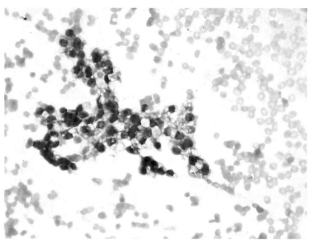

Figure 4.190. Metastatic renal cell carcinoma to the pancreas. The cells are loosely cohesive with clear, finely vacuolated cytoplasm (Pap stain).

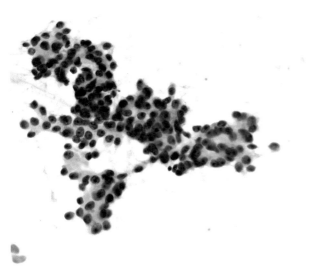

Figure 4.191. Acinar cell carcinoma. Tissue fragment containing loose clusters of neoplastic cells with round to oval nuclei, single prominent nucleoli, and granular cytoplasm (Pap stain).

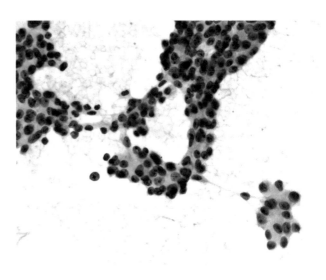

Figure 4.192. Acinar cell carcinoma. Separate field (Pap stain).

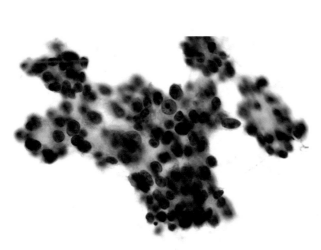

Figure 4.193. Acinar cell carcinoma. Separate field (Pap stain).

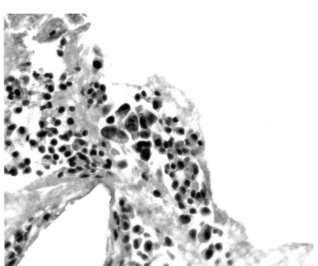

Figure 4.194. Acinar cell carcinoma. Note the discohesive neoplastic cells with oval nuclei with prominent reddish nucleoli and granular cytoplasm (H&E).

- The neoplastic cells usually have prominent nucleoli.
- The neoplastic cells often have a plasmacytoid appearance and abundant, granular cytoplasm, though these features are not specific.
- Diffuse cytoplasmic granular staining with trypsin and/or chymotrypsin (seen in >95% of cases) helps confirm the diagnosis.

PANCREATOBLASTOMA

Pancreatoblastoma is a rare multilineage malignant epithelial tumor that comprises <0.5% of all pancreatic neoplasms and is the most common pancreatic malignancy in children, typically seen in the first decade.[75] Multiple lines of differentiation are seen within the tumor, with a predominant acinar component (that makes it difficult to distinguish from acinar cell carcinoma) and a stromal component with spindle-shaped cells (Figure 4.195). Immunohistochemical stains can be used to highlight the multiple components within the tumor: acinar (trypsin, chymotrypsin), ductal (cytokeratin), and neuroendocrine (synaptophysin, chromogranin). The presence of squamoid morules is pathognomonic and can help distinguish pancreatoblastoma from acinar cell carcinoma.

SOLID PSEUDOPAPILLARY NEOPLASM (SPN)

SPNs are tumors with low malignant potential and account for <2% of all pancreatic neoplasms. The tumor cells are present as single cells and/or in loosely cohesive clusters and classically line myxoid or hyalinized vascular stalks (Figures 4.196-4.198). Cytologically, the cells are uniform with round to oval nuclei that can have nuclear grooves and delicately vacuolated cytoplasm. There is often a background of blood, foam cells, and necrotic debris (Figure 4.199). SPNs harbor activating mutations of the β-catenin gene in >95% of cases,[76,77] resulting in nuclear (and cytoplasmic) accumulation of β-catenin that can be routinely detected by β-catenin immunohistochemistry (Figure 4.200). SPNs may also be positive for neuroendocrine markers such as CD56 and synaptophysin.

KEY FEATURES: Solid Pseudopapillary Neoplasm

- Cells are present both individually as well as in tissue fragments.
- When present, large fragments demonstrate branching vessels with a loosely attached layer of neoplastic cells, resulting in multiple slender papillae which overlap with one another.
- The neoplastic cells are monotonous and can be plasmacytoid in appearance.
- The nuclei are round to oval with regular borders and bland chromatin.

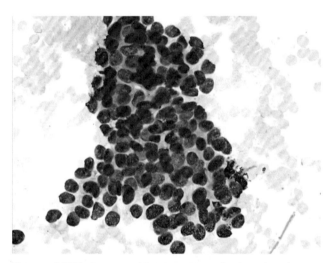

Figure 4.195. Pancreatoblastoma. Note the loosely cohesive, immature-appearing epithelioid cells consistent with acinar differentiation (Diff-Quik stain).

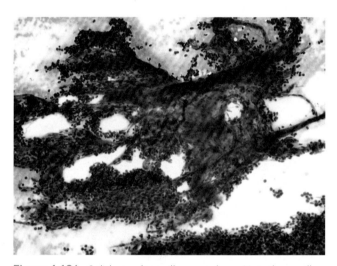

Figure 4.196. Solid pseudopapillary neoplasm. Note the papillary architecture and background of loose clusters and single cells (Diff-Quik stain).

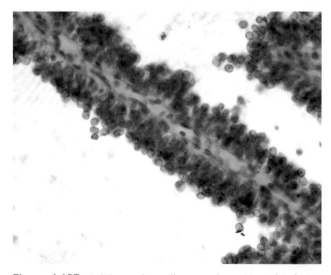

Figure 4.197. Solid pseudopapillary neoplasm. Note the denser layer of monotonous neoplastic cells lining the fibrovascular stalk, with discohesive cells falling off at the edge. The cells have evenly distributed pale chromatin and inconspicuous nucleoli (Pap stain).

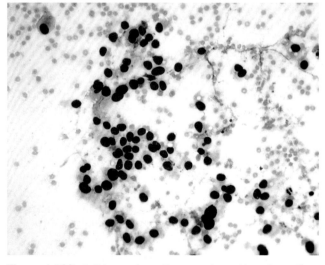

Figure 4.198. Solid pseudopapillary neoplasm. Note the uniform round to oval nuclei with even chromatin and wispy, ill-defined cytoplasm. The cells resemble those seen in a neuroendocrine neoplasm (Diff-Quik stain).

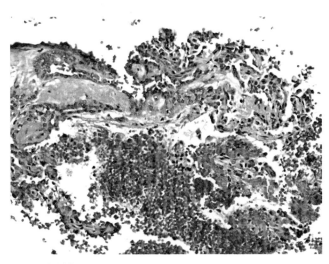

Figure 4.199. Solid pseudopapillary neoplasm. Discohesive neoplastic cells line hyalinized vascular stalks in a background of blood (H&E).

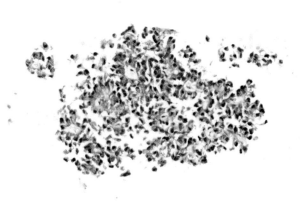

Figure 4.200. Solid pseudopapillary neoplasm with diffuse nuclear and cytoplasmic β-catenin expression (β-catenin immunostain).

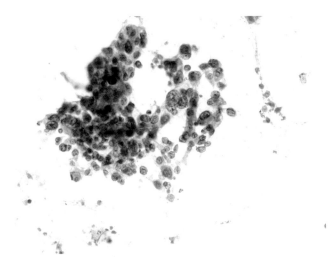

Figure 4.201. Poorly differentiated adenocarcinoma. The loosely cohesive/discohesive cells are markedly atypical and highly pleomorphic without clear glandular differentiation (Pap stain).

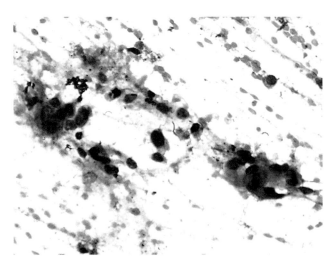

Figure 4.202. Poorly differentiated adenocarcinoma. The markedly atypical cells are present singly and in loose clusters in a background of necrosis (Diff-Quik stain).

POORLY DIFFERENTIATED CARCINOMA

Poorly differentiated carcinomas, such as poorly differentiated ductal adenocarcinomas, anaplastic carcinomas, PanNECs, and poorly differentiated metastatic carcinomas, result in highly cellular cytologic specimens with markedly atypical and discohesive/dispersed cells (Figures 4.201-4.204). The neoplastic cells are often highly pleomorphic with hyperchromatic, large, irregular nuclei and mitoses in a background of necrotic debris. Various cytomorphological features and immunostains may help differentiate the type of carcinoma in some cases.

LYMPHOMA

The most common lymphomas of the pancreas are B-cell non-Hodgkin lymphomas, which may be primary pancreatic lymphomas (rare, <2% of extranodal lymphomas and 0.5% of pancreatic tumors) or secondary lymphomas involving the pancreas (30% of patients with disseminated disease).[78] Cytological features vary depending on the type of lymphoma (Figures 4.205-4.208), and are briefly discussed in the liver "Lymphoproliferative Disorders" section under the "Single Cell/Dispersed Pattern." The primary differential diagnosis is pancreatitis. Thus, if remaining fresh, cellular material is available and a lymphoid neoplasm is suspected, material should be sent for flow cytometry.

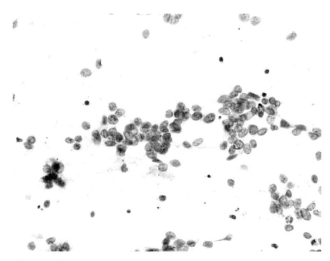

Figure 4.203. Pancreatic neuroendocrine carcinoma. The cells are discohesive with high nuclear to cytoplasmic ratios, variable nuclear shapes, and "salt-and-pepper" chromatin (Pap stain).

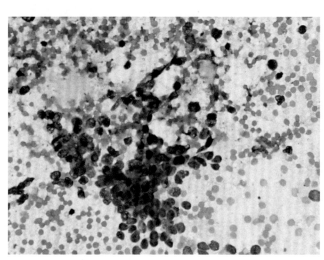

Figure 4.204. Pancreatic neuroendocrine carcinoma. The cells are overall round to oval with stippled chromatin but are large with scant to no visible cytoplasm (Diff-Quik stain).

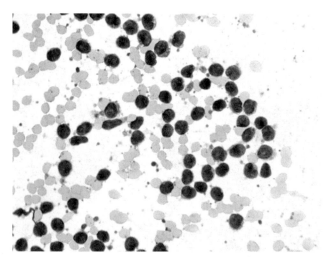

Figure 4.205. Small lymphocytic lymphoma in the pancreas. There is a monomorphic population of small lymphocytes with variably irregular nuclear contours, slightly clumped chromatin, and scant cytoplasm. Lymphoglandular bodies can be seen in the background (Pap stain).

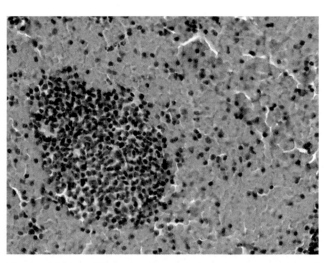

Figure 4.206. Follicular lymphoma in the pancreas. On this cell block, there is an intact follicular lymphoid aggregate with a monotonous population of predominantly small lymphocytes (H&E).

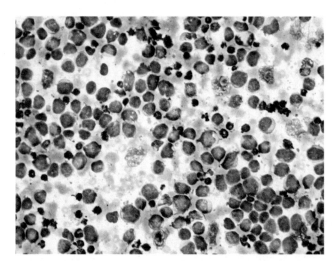

Figure 4.207. Diffuse large B-cell lymphoma in the pancreas. There are sheets of large, malignant lymphocytes with irregular nuclear contours and scant cytoplasm. Note that they are three to five times the size of admixed lymphocytes (Diff-Quik stain).

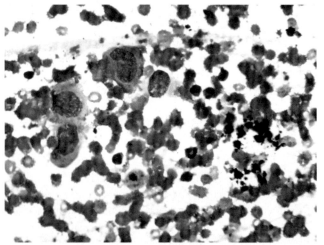

Figure 4.208. Anaplastic large cell lymphoma in the pancreas. Neoplastic horseshoe-shaped "hallmark" cells are present as single cells. Note their enlargement compared with the neutrophils (Diff-Quik stain).

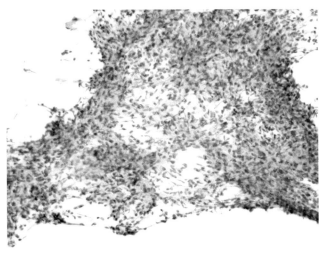

Figure 4.209. Ectopic splenic tissue. Note the stretched lymphocytes (Pap stain).

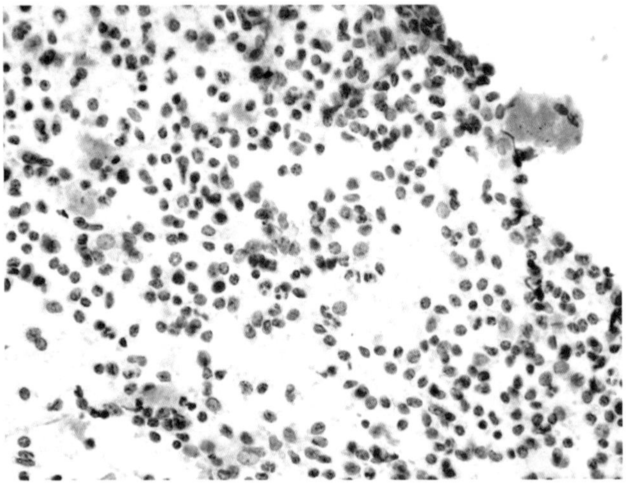

Figure 4.210. Ectopic splenic tissue. Note the benign small round lymphocytes and few interspersed neutrophils (Pap stain).

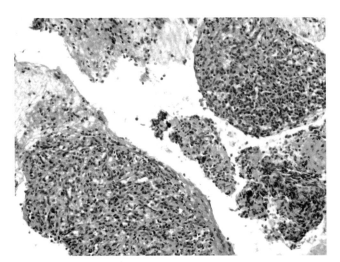

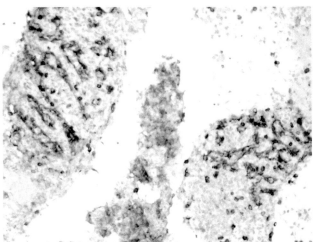

Figure 4.211. Ectopic splenic tissue, which is composed of predominantly lymphocytes (H&E).

Figure 4.212. A CD8 immunostain highlights the thin-walled sinusoids within the nodule of ectopic spleen (CD8 immunostain).

ECTOPIC SPLEEN

Ectopic splenic tissue includes accessory spleen, congenital malformations, and splenosis (focal deposits of autoimplanted splenic tissue secondary to abdominal trauma or splenectomy) and can mimic a PanNET on imaging studies due to high vascularity. Cytology shows abundant small, mature lymphocytes, and immunostains performed on cell blocks may verify the diagnosis by demonstrating CD8+ thin-walled blood vessels (Figures 4.209-4.212).[79,80]

PAUCICELLULAR/CYSTIC PATTERN

The paucicellular/cystic pattern include benign and neoplastic cysts, which generally show sparse cellularity comprised of lining epithelial cells and/or other mixed components such as inflammation or mucin.

CHECKLIST: Etiologic Considerations for the Paucicellular/Cystic Pattern

☐ Squamous-lined Cysts

☐ Pseudocyst

☐ Serous Cystadenoma

☐ Neoplastic Mucinous Cyst

SQUAMOUS-LINED CYSTS

Benign squamous-lined cysts include epidermoid cysts, dermoid cysts, and lymphoepithelial cysts.[81,82] Epidermoid cysts are lined by mature squamous epithelium without atypia and arise in association with intrapancreatic ectopic splenic tissue; dermoid cysts include other germ cell components. Lymphoepithelial cysts are also lined by mature squamous epithelium without atypia; the subepithelial stroma consists of dense, nonneoplastic lymphoid tissue with germinal center formation that may not be well-represented on the FNA material as compared with the squamous epithelial and cystic components. Cytological specimens consist of anucleated and nucleated squamous cells with abundant keratinous debris, with variable cholesterol clefts, lymphocytes, and histiocytes (Figures 4.213-4.216).[83,84]

PSEUDOCYST

Pseudocysts are typically seen in the setting of acute pancreatitis and result from autodigestive damage of pancreatic parenchyma. These cysts lack an epithelial layer and are collections of necrotic material surrounded by a thick, inflammatory fibrous capsule. Pancreatic cyst fluid usually shows a very high amylase level (≥250 U/L).[49] Cytology shows an absence of epithelial cells (aside from possible GI contamination) and can demonstrate mixed polymorphous inflammatory cells, histiocytes, crystalline debris, and yellow hematoidin-like pigment (Figures 4.217 and 4.218).[85] The differential diagnosis includes serous cystadenomas (SCAs) and cystic mucinous neoplasms.

SEROUS CYSTADENOMA (SCA)

SCAs are the most common benign cystic neoplasm of the pancreas and account for 1-2% of pancreatic neoplasms.[86] The goal of preoperative diagnosis is to distinguish these benign cysts from neoplastic mucinous cysts, thus allowing optimal triage of patients to conservative management versus surgical resection. However, the lack of specific cytomorphological features makes diagnosis extremely challenging on cytology alone.[87] SCAs are lined by nonmucinous cuboidal cells with uniform round nuclei (Figures 4.219 and 4.220). Cytoplasmic clearing due to glycogen accumulation can be seen in some cases but should not be mistaken for mucinous epithelial cells, which are columnar with abundant intracellular mucin (Figure 4.221). Most cytologic specimens are hypocellular; epithelial cells are not always present, and the background can be bloody with hemosiderin-laden macrophages (Figure 4.222). A nonspecific or nondiagnostic diagnosis is often rendered. Recently, mutations in the von Hippel-Lindau (*VHL*) gene (3p25) were identified in 67% of sporadic and hereditary SCAs and not found in MCNs.[77] Thus, the detection of a *VHL* mutation in pancreatic cyst fluid supports a diagnosis of SCA.

NEOPLASTIC MUCINOUS CYST

Neoplastic mucinous cysts such as IPMNs and MCNs may appear as paucicellular specimens when the epithelial lining cells are not sampled by the FNA procedure. In the proper clinical/radiologic setting, the presence of "clean mucin" is diagnostic of a neoplastic mucinous cyst, even in the absence of cyst-lining cells (see the "Glandular/Mucinous Pattern").

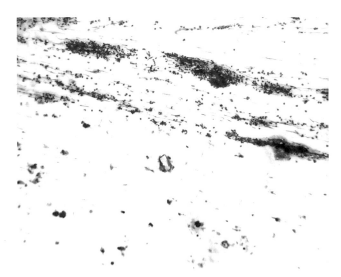

Figure 4.213. Lymphoepithelial cyst. There are abundant crushed lymphocytes and a large cholesterol crystal (center) (Diff-Quik stain).

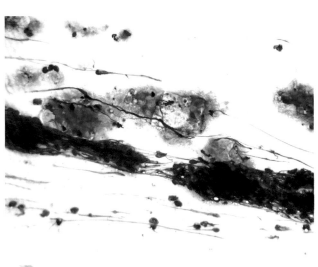

Figure 4.214. Lymphoepithelial cyst. There are abundant crushed lymphocytes, keratinaceous debris, and a large cholesterol crystal (Diff-Quik stain).

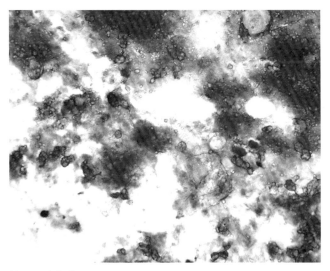

Figure 4.215. Lymphoepithelial cyst with abundant keratinaceous debris and cholesterol crystals. It is important not to confuse this debris with extracellular mucin (Diff-Quik stain).

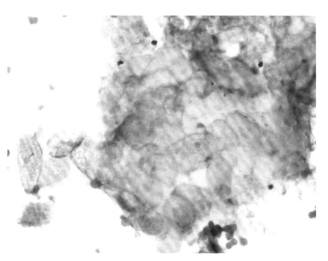

Figure 4.216. Squamous cells from the lining of a lymphoepithelial cyst (Diff-Quik stain).

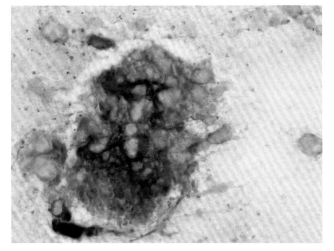

Figure 4.217. Pseudocyst with no epithelial cells, a large cluster of crystals, and mixed inflammation in the background (Pap stain).

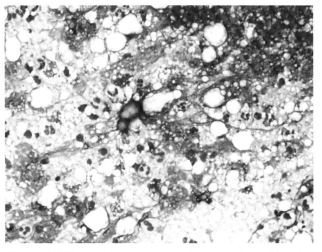

Figure 4.218. Pseudocyst with mixed neutrophilic and lymphocytic inflammation, and crystals (Diff-Quik stain).

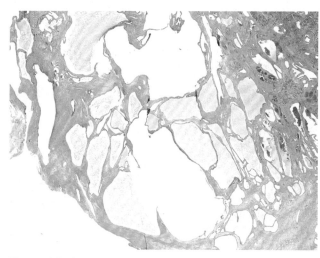

Figure 4.219. Low-power view of serous cystadenoma, which is composed of numerous thin-walled cysts (H&E).

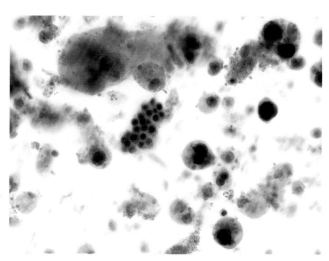

Figure 4.220. Serous cystadenoma. There is a fragment of non-mucinous cuboidal epithelium with uniform round nuclei in a background of abundant hemosiderin-laden macrophages (Pap stain).

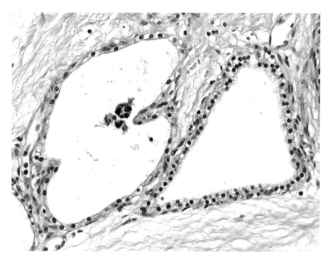

Figure 4.221. High-power view of serous cystadenoma. The cyst is lined by cuboidal cells with uniform round nuclei and cytoplasmic clearing due to glycogen accumulation. Special stains showing that the cytoplasm is PAS+ and PAS/D- help to confirm that the epithelium is serous, not mucinous (H&E).

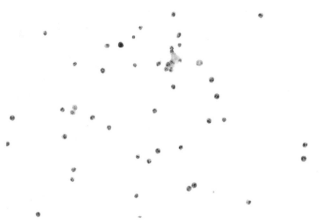

Figure 4.222. Hypocellular specimen from the cyst fluid of a serous cystadenoma. Only scattered neutrophils are seen; no epithelium is present, a typical finding on the fine-needle aspiration (FNA) of serous cystadenoma (SCA) (Pap stain).

SPINDLE CELL PATTERN

Primary mesenchymal tumors of the pancreas are exceedingly rare, although metastatic spindle cell tumors such as GIST, leiomyosarcoma, and others can be seen in the pancreas. Primary sarcomatoid carcinoma of the pancreas is rare but has been described.[88] See the "Spindle Cell Pattern" in the Liver section for further discussion.

EXTRAS

UNDIFFERENTIATED CARCINOMA WITH OSTEOCLAST-LIKE GIANT CELLS

Undifferentiated carcinoma with osteoclast-like giant cells is a variant of ductal adenocarcinoma that is characterized by many large multinucleated cells with abundant cytoplasm and multiple uniform nuclei (benign osteoclast-type giant cells) admixed with smaller pleomorphic mononuclear cells, which are the neoplastic cells (Figures 4.223 and 4.224). The neoplastic cells can occur as single cells or in tissue fragments, with round to irregularly

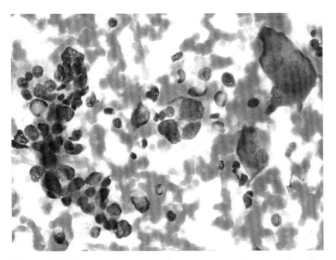

Figure 4.223. Undifferentiated carcinoma with osteoclast-like giant cells. The giant cells have abundant cytoplasm and uniform bland nuclei, while the pleomorphic single cell population in the background is neoplastic (Diff-Quik stain).

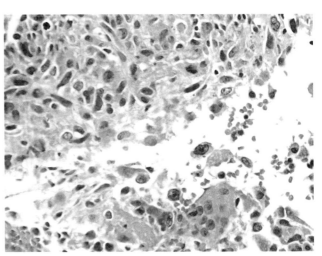

Figure 4.224. Undifferentiated carcinoma with osteoclast-like giant cells. Compare the pleomorphic malignant-appearing cells (top) with the benign multinucleated giant cell (bottom) (H&E).

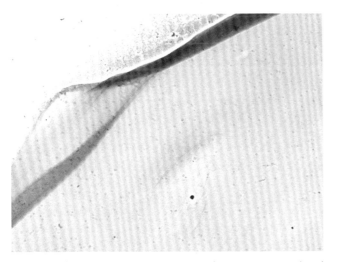

Figure 4.225. Clean mucin. The aspirate of a pancreatic intraductal papillary mucinous neoplasm (IPMN) resulted in abundant clean mucin, from which bacteria, granular debris, and inflammatory cells are absent. Cystic macrophages can sometimes be seen (Diff-Quik stain).

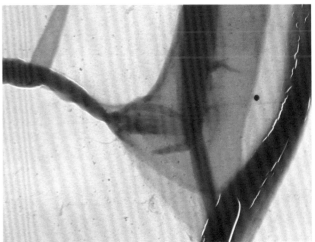

Figure 4.226. Clean mucin. At higher magnification, a cystic macrophage can be seen at the right-hand side of the field (Diff-Quik stain).

shaped nuclei, occasional binucleation, and scant cytoplasm. The presence of these two distinct cell populations is diagnostic of this tumor. The differential diagnosis includes nonneoplastic conditions such as tuberculosis and foreign body–type giant cell reaction, which do not have the population of pleomorphic neoplastic cells.

NEAR MISSES

"CLEAN" VERSUS "DIRTY" MUCIN

Mucin-producing neoplastic cells generally produce sterile mucin ("clean" mucin) which is acellular (Figures 4.225-4.228). After a period of sitting in a cystic space, macrophages may collect in this mucin. The presence of "clean" mucin on FNA can be diagnostic of a mucin-producing neoplasm in the proper clinical/radiologic setting. The mucin present in the GI tract contains inflammatory cells, debris, and bacteria ("dirty" mucin) (Figures 4.229-4.232). An endoscopic procedure may sometimes fail to aspirate a targeted lesion, resulting in abundant GI contamination. In such instances, the presence of abundant "dirty" mucin may give the erroneous impression that a mucinous neoplasm was aspirated. It is therefore worthwhile to closely examine any background mucin in a specimen.

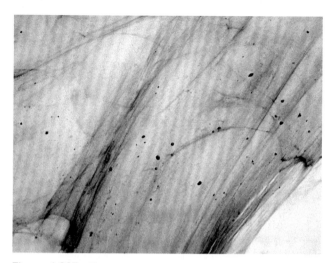

Figure 4.227. Clean mucin. When abundant in an aspirate, clean mucin appears thick on the smear and may be appreciated when smears are created during an on-site evaluation for adequacy. The cells seen here are difficult to identify at low power (Diff-Quik stain).

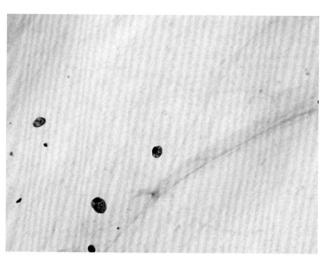

Figure 4.228. Clean mucin. At higher magnification, the cells can be identified as cystic macrophages. They have abundant and foamy cytoplasm (Diff-Quik stain).

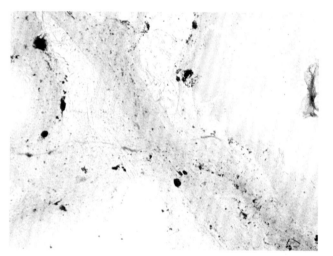

Figure 4.229. "Dirty" mucin. The presence of debris and bacteria in association with mucin suggests the mucin is from the gastrointestinal tract rather than contained in a neoplastic cyst (Diff-Quik stain).

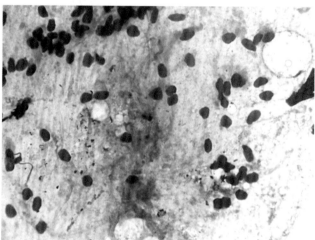

Figure 4.230. "Dirty" mucin. In some cases, it can be difficult to determine whether glandular cells in an aspirate represent the lining of a cystic lesion or gastrointestinal (GI) contamination. In this case, the mucin contains debris and bacteria and is likely a contaminant from the GI tract. Thus, the associated glandular cells are likely GI tract contamination as well (Diff-Quik stain).

GASTROINTESTINAL CONTAMINATION

GI contamination may cause a diagnostic dilemma when GI fragments are erroneously interpreted as representing lesional tissue. During on-site evaluation for adequacy, GI contamination masquerading as mucinous cyst epithelium or even a well differentiated adenocarcinoma may cause inadequate procedures to be inaccurately deemed adequate. The sampling of pseudocysts, which do not contain a true cyst lining, may be complicated by the presence of misinterpreted GI epithelium. GI contamination may contain severe reactive changes which can emulate adenocarcinoma. Small mucinous fragments may contain goblet cells, an important feature that distinguishes GI contamination from pancreatic epithelium in transduodenal procedures (Figures 4.233 and 4.234). The foveolar epithelium contaminating transgastric procedures has similar cytomorphology to neoplastic mucinous epithelium (Figures 4.235 and 4.236). Large fragments may contain the architecture of gastric pits, which is the single most helpful clue.

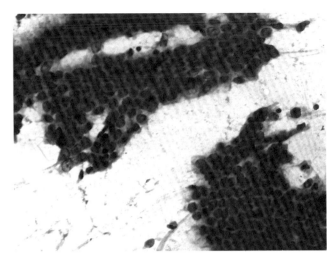

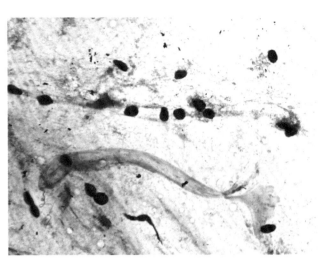

Figure 4.231. "Dirty" mucin. The mucin in the background is thin and contains granular debris and bacteria. The glandular tissue fragments are small and may represent gastrointestinal tract contamination or the mucinous lining of a cystic neoplasm. If doubt exists, the clinical team should be notified that the lesion may not have been adequately sampled (Diff-Quik stain).

Figure 4.232. "Dirty" mucin. Thin mucin with granular debris, bacteria, and stripped glandular cells with degenerative cytoplasm. A Curschmann spiral can be seen in the bottom left-hand side of the field (Diff-Quik stain).

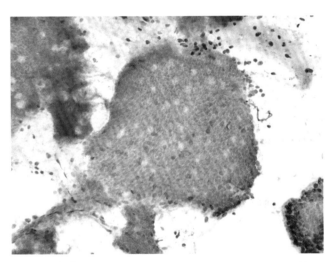

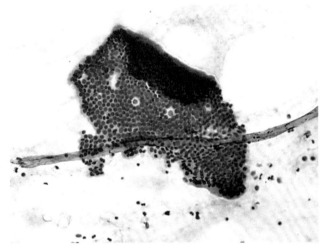

Figure 4.233. Gastrointestinal contamination. Transduodenal fine-needle aspiration (FNA) is often used to sample pancreatic head lesions. Except in small tissue fragments, the presence of goblet cells (seen as the "white holes" in these fragments) should be seen (Diff-Quik stain).

Figure 4.234. Gastrointestinal contamination. An alternate field demonstrating a tissue fragment of benign duodenal epithelium containing goblet cells (Diff-Quik stain).

SAMPLING OF ADRENAL CORTICAL TISSUE

The endoscopic aspiration of a pancreatic tail lesion may miss the lesion and inadvertently sample background elements. In some instances, adrenal cortical tissue may be sampled and result in a cellular specimen which appears neoplastic. When aspirated, adrenal cortical cells appear in fragments and/or as dispersed single cells. The cells typically have round nuclei with regular borders and contain abundant granular or vacuolated cytoplasm (Figures 4.237 and 4.238). Stripped nuclei may also be seen in the background. In some instances, marked variation in nuclear size may be seen, although the nuclei maintain regular borders. If possible, staining with adrenal-specific markers (MART-1, Melan-A, inhibin, SF-1) can help confirm the suspicion of adrenal sampling (Figures 4.239-4.241).

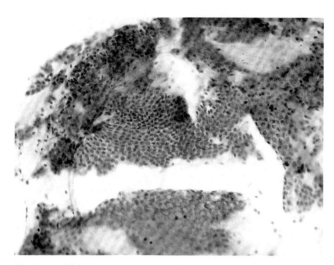

Figure 4.235. Gastrointestinal contamination. Transgastric fine-needle aspiration (FNA) may be used to sample pancreatic body and tail lesions. Gastric foveolar epithelium lacks goblet cells and is cytomorphologically similar to the lining of some cystic mucin-producing neoplasms of the pancreas. Thus, it can be difficult to make a diagnosis that relies on these cells in isolation (Pap stain).

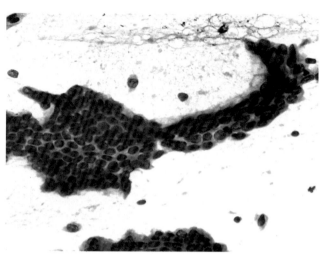

Figure 4.236. Gastrointestinal contamination. An alternate field at higher magnification, demonstrating foveolar gastrointestinal contamination (Diff-Quik stain).

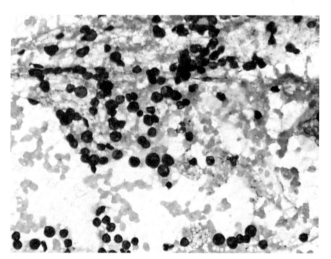

Figure 4.237. Adrenal cortical tissue. Adrenal cortical tissue may be inadvertently sampled during the attempted aspiration of a pancreatic lesion. Sampling of this tissue may yield a very cellular sample and mimic primary pancreatic neoplasms as well as metastatic renal cell carcinoma. The cells often have round, regular nuclei with abundant vacuolated cytoplasm. Anisonucleosis is a common finding, as is the presence of numerous stripped nuclei in the background (Diff-Quik stain).

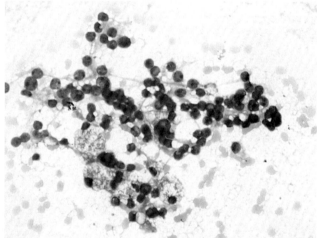

Figure 4.238. Adrenal cortical tissue. Alternate field (Diff-Quik stain).

GASTROINTESTINAL STROMAL TUMOR (GIST)

GIST is often suspected on radiology, especially in organs in which it most commonly arises, such as the stomach. GIST may occasionally arise adjacent to the pancreas and be designated as "pancreas mass" or "peripancreatic mass" on imaging studies. As GIST may not be expected during a pancreatic FNA, the presence of spindled, epithelioid, or a mixture of spindled and epithelioid cells may cause confusion (Figures 4.242-4.245). While GIST is not commonly confused with an adenocarcinoma, less common primary pancreatic neoplasms, as well as other soft tissue neoplasms such as schwannoma, may be considered. Keep GIST in the differential diagnosis when encountering an unusual neoplasm. If possible, dedicated material for immunostaining should be collected.

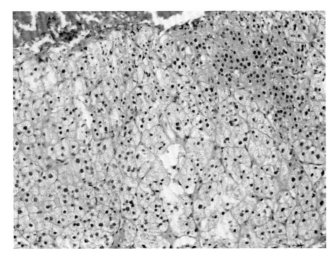

Figure 4.239. Adrenal cortical tissue. The presence of the cells on cell block material is useful, as it often appears similar to adrenal tissue more frequently encountered in tissue sections (H&E).

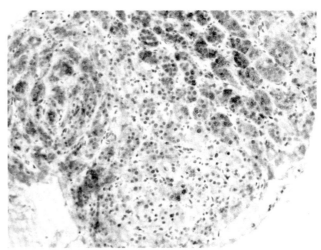

Figure 4.240. Adrenal cortical tissue. Confirmatory immunostains can be performed, as adrenal cortical tissue is positive for HMB-45, Melan-A, SF-1, and inhibin (seen here) (inhibin immunostain).

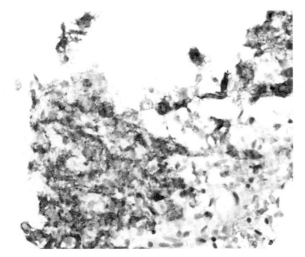

Figure 4.241. Adrenal cortical tissue. (Melan-A immunostain).

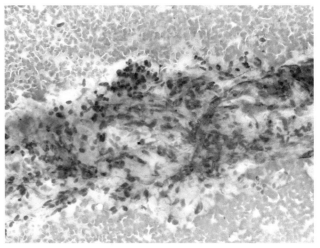

Figure 4.242. Gastrointestinal stromal tumor. GISTs may arise adjacent to the pancreas and mimic a pancreatic neoplasm on imaging studies. GIST should be a consideration when encountering a spindle cell neoplasm of the pancreas. In this field, the cells appear to be a mixture of spindled and epithelioid cells, causing a diagnostic dilemma (Diff-Quik stain).

BENIGN ACINAR CELLS VERSUS PANCREATIC NEUROENDOCRINE TUMOR

Benign acinar cells can be seen in large numbers when a procedure samples benign acinar tissue rather than lesional tissue. A clue to this possibility is the presence of large fragments ("mini-biopsies") of pancreatic parenchyma, in which the grape-like architecture of the acinic tissue is preserved. The background may contain numerous benign acinar cells, present both singly as well as in small acinar structures, which may mimic the rosettes and discohesive nature of a neuroendocrine tumor (Figures 4.246-4.248). In addition to the presence of large fragments of benign pancreatic acinic tissue, fragments of benign ductal epithelium may also be seen, suggesting that a given pass may have missed the lesion and sampled only benign pancreatic parenchyma. Because pancreatic acinar cells do not disperse unless smeared, they are often arranged in a linear fashion. This is in contrast to neuroendocrine neoplasms, in which cells often disperse during aspiration, resulting in a more random dispersion of the cells throughout the background. If there is any doubt that the cells in question may be normal acinar cells, be cautious with the diagnosis.

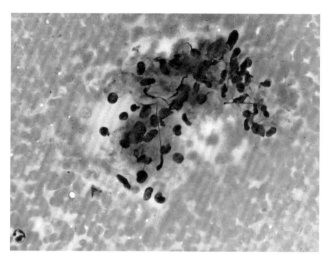

Figure 4.243. Gastrointestinal stromal tumor (GIST). A higher magnification field, demonstrating the spindled and epithelioid nature of this particular GIST (Diff-Quik stain).

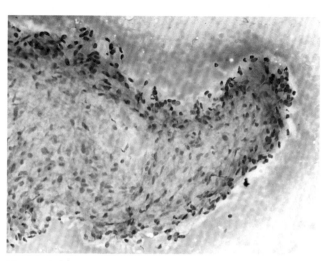

Figure 4.244. Gastrointestinal stromal tumor. Alternate field. The presence of this large tissue fragment suggests lesional tissue was sampled, but the absence of any classic morphologic pattern resulted in a large differential diagnosis, including a nonneoplastic process such as granulomatous inflammation (Diff-Quik stain).

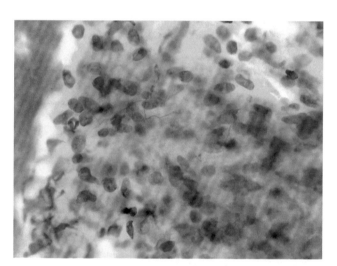

Figure 4.245. Gastrointestinal stromal tumor. Alternate field (Diff-Quik stain).

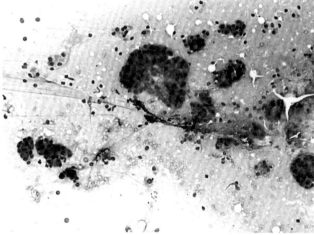

Figure 4.246. Pancreatic acinar tissue. When sampled on fine-needle aspiration (FNA), benign pancreatic acinar tissue can appear as large fragments with grape-like architecture, smaller fragments, and dispersed single cells. The tissue is primarily disrupted during the smearing process, resulting in a linear arrangement of the cells across the slide (Diff-Quik stain).

SPLENULE VERSUS PANCREATIC NEUROENDOCRINE TUMOR

The sampling of ectopic splenic tissue ("splenule") results in a cellular specimen of dispersed lymphocytes, as well as cohesive fragments of lymphocytes trapped in sinusoidal fragments. At low magnification, this picture may be falsely identified as the dispersed pattern seen in a PanNET. The pathologist may be further misguided by the rarity with which splenules are encountered, as well as radiologic studies: both lesions often appear as well-circumscribed lesions in the tail of the pancreas. Close examination should reveal that the cells are lymphocytes, with angulated nuclei and a thin rim of blue cytoplasm (Figures 4.249-4.253). The nuclei of these cells should be smaller than those of neuroendocrine cells, especially on a Diff-Quik preparation. While immunostains can be helpful, cytomorphology alone should be sufficient to exclude a neuroendocrine tumor in this context.

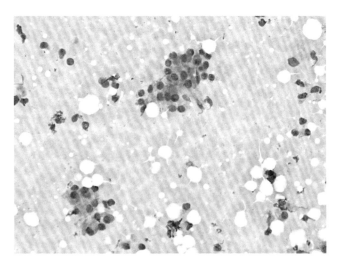

Figure 4.247. Pancreatic acinar tissue. Higher magnification. The acinar cells have abundant, granular cytoplasm and an eccentrically placed nucleus. When a procedure fails to sample lesional tissue, the presence of background benign acinar tissue can be mistaken for a pancreatic neuroendocrine tumor, which can result in unnecessary surgery (Diff-Quik stain).

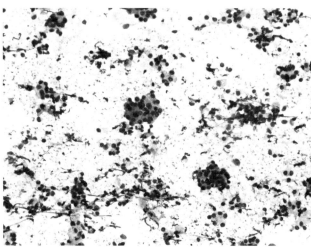

Figure 4.248. Pancreatic acinar tissue. The acinar architecture seen here closely resembles rosette formation in some pancreatic neuroendocrine tumors (PanNETs). The presence of dispersed single cells can also be seen in PanNETs (Diff-Quik stain).

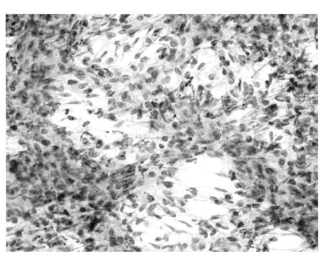

Figure 4.249. Splenule. Fine-needle apiration (FNA) results in both a cohesive and dispersed population of small blue cells (lymphocytes), which can mimic neuroendocrine cells. Bland spindled endothelial cells (seen here intermixed with lymphocytes) which line the sinusoids can also mimic spindle-shaped carcinoid tumors (Diff-Quik stain).

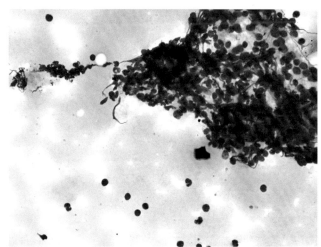

Figure 4.250. Splenule. The lymphocytes dispersed in the background have a thin rim of blue cytoplasm, a feature not seen in most neuroendocrine neoplasms. The lymphocytes form a large fragment in the upper right corner; the chromatin smearing artifact provides a clue that these are lymphocytes and not a well differentiated neuroendocrine neoplasm (Diff-Quik stain).

WELL DIFFERENTIATED ADENOCARCINOMA VERSUS PANCREATIC NEUROENDOCRINE TUMOR

Neuroendocrine neoplasms may form small fragments with an underlying rosette architecture, which may mimic the glandular formation seen in well differentiated adenocarcinomas. Furthermore, when neuroendocrine nuclei are examined at high magnifications on Diff-Quik preparations, the otherwise monotonous-appearing neuroendocrine cells may appear to have irregular nuclear borders and some nuclear size variation (Figures 4.254-4.257). When a specimen contains abundant material, distinguishing between these two processes is not difficult, as well differentiated adenocarcinomas do not have singly dispersed cells whereas neuroendocrine tumors almost always do. While immunostains can help prove a neuroendocrine origin, there are rarely sufficient cells to stain in scant specimens. Exert caution when a lesion does not appear to be adequately sampled.

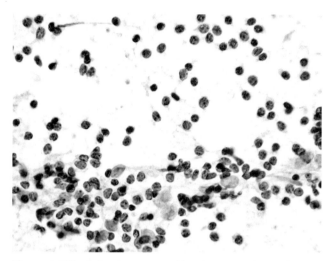

Figure 4.251. Splenule. Dispersed lymphocytes indicates the possibility of either a splenule or an intrapancreatic lymph node. Note the angulation of the nuclei. The chromatin pattern has some similarities to that seen in neuroendocrine neoplasms (Pap stain).

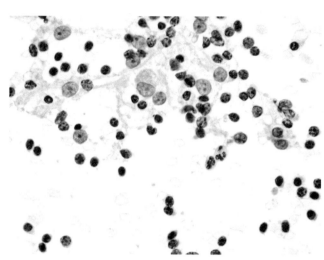

Figure 4.252. Splenule. Alternate field (Pap stain).

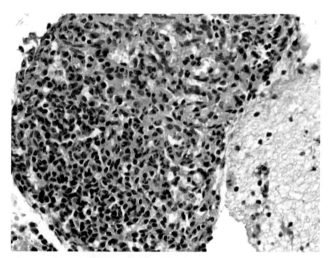

Figure 4.253. Splenule. The creation of cell block material allows better comparison with splenic tissue, which is more commonly seen in surgical specimens. The sinusoids are better appreciated in this tissue fragment than on the conventional smears and are positive by CD8 immunostaining (H&E).

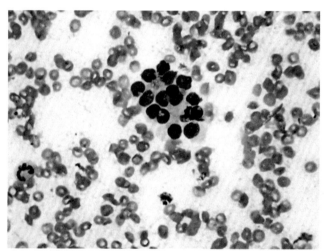

Figure 4.254. Neuroendocrine neoplasm. The cells here form two rosettes which resemble the gland formation seen in some adenocarcinomas (Diff-Quik stain).

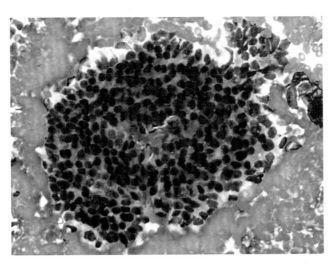

Figure 4.255. Neuroendocrine neoplasm. This large tissue fragment contains many of the features of adenocarcinoma: enlarged nuclei, low nuclear to cytoplasmic ratios, irregular nuclear borders, and anisonucleosis. The specimen was also extremely cellular with few individual cells dispersed in the background (Diff-Quik stain).

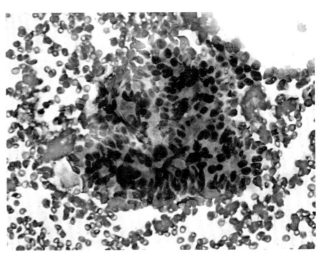

Figure 4.256. Neuroendocrine neoplasm. Alternate field. Note the formation of multiple rosettes, providing the impression of a gland-forming neoplasm (Diff-Quik stain).

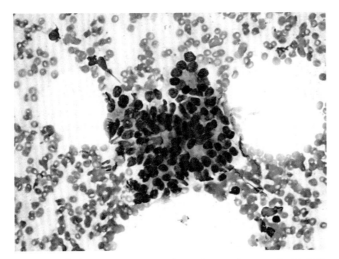

Figure 4.257. Neuroendocrine neoplasm. Alternate field (Diff-Quik stain).

References

1. Nagorney DM. Benign hepatic tumors: focal nodular hyperplasia and hepatocellular adenoma. *World J Surg.* 1995;19(1):13-18.

2. Nguyen BN, Flejou JF, Terris B, Belghiti J, Degott C. Focal nodular hyperplasia of the liver: a comprehensive pathologic study of 305 lesions and recognition of new histologic forms. *Am J Surg Pathol.* 1999;23(12):1441-1454.

3. Wanless IR, Mawdsley C, Adams R. On the pathogenesis of focal nodular hyperplasia of the liver. *Hepatology.* 1985;5(6):1194-1200.

4. Krishnamurthy S, Nerurkar AY. Spindle cell fragments in focal nodular hyperplasia of the liver. A case report. *Acta Cytol.* 2002;46(3):582-584.

5. Ruschenburg I, Droese M. Fine needle aspiration cytology of focal nodular hyperplasia of the liver. *Acta Cytol.* 1989;33(6):857-860.

6. Cohen MB, Haber MM, Holly EA, Ahn DK, Bottles K, Stoloff AC. Cytologic criteria to distinguish hepatocellular carcinoma from nonneoplastic liver. *Am J Clin Pathol.* 1991;95(2):125-130.

7. Lin CC, Lin CJ, Hsu CW, Chen YC, Chen WT, Lin SM. Fine-needle aspiration cytology to distinguish dysplasia from hepatocellular carcinoma with different grades. *J Gastroenterol Hepatol.* 2008;23(7 Pt 2):e146-e152.

8. Yang GC, Yang GY, Tao LC. Distinguishing well-differentiated hepatocellular carcinoma from benign liver by the physical features of fine-needle aspirates. *Mod Pathol.* 2004; 17(7):798-802.

9. Hartleb M, Gutkowski K, Milkiewicz P. Nodular regenerative hyperplasia: evolving concepts on underdiagnosed cause of portal hypertension. *World J Gastroenterol.* 2011;17(11):1400-1409.

10. Gonzalez F, Marks C. Hepatic tumors and oral contraceptives: surgical management. *J Surg Oncol.* 1985;29(3):193-197.

11. Bosman FT, World Health Organization. *WHO Classification of Tumours of the Digestive System.* Lyon, France: IARC Press; 2010.

12. Sole M, Calvet X, Cuberes T, et al. Value and limitations of cytologic criteria for the diagnosis of hepatocellular carcinoma by fine needle aspiration biopsy. *Acta Cytol.* 1993;37(3):309-316.

13. Das DK. Cytodiagnosis of hepatocellular carcinoma in fine-needle aspirates of the liver: its differentiation from reactive hepatocytes and metastatic adenocarcinoma. *Diagn Cytopathol.* 1999;21(6):370-377.

14. Pedio G, Landolt U, Zobeli L, Gut D. Fine needle aspiration of the liver. Significance of hepatocytic naked nuclei in the diagnosis of hepatocellular carcinoma. *Acta Cytol.* 1988;32(4):437-442.

15. Anatelli F, Chuang ST, Yang XJ, Wang HL. Value of glypican 3 immunostaining in the diagnosis of hepatocellular carcinoma on needle biopsy. *Am J Clin Pathol.* 2008;130(2):219-223.

16. Pitman MB, Szyfelbein WM. Significance of endothelium in the fine-needle aspiration biopsy diagnosis of hepatocellular carcinoma. *Diagn Cytopathol.* 1995;12(3): 208-214.

17. Torbenson M. Fibrolamellar carcinoma: 2012 update. *Scientifica (Cairo).* 2012;2012:743790.

18. Perez-Guillermo M, Masgrau NA, Garcia-Solano J, Sola-Perez J, de Agustin y de Agustin P. Cytologic aspect of fibrolamellar hepatocellular carcinoma in fine-needle aspirates. *Diagn Cytopathol.* 1999;21(3):180-187.

19. Bortolasi L, Marchiori L, Dal Dosso I, Colombari R, Nicoli N. Hepatoblastoma in adult age: a report of two cases. *Hepatogastroenterology.* 1996;43(10):1073-1078.

20. Cho C, Rullis I, Rogers LS. Bile duct adenomas as liver nodules. *Arch Surg.* 1978;113(3):272-274.

21. Ishak KG, Goodman ZD, Stocker TJ. *Tumors of the Liver and Intrahepatic Bile Ducts.* Washington, DC: Armed Forces Institute of Pathology; 2001.

22. Stroescu C, Herlea V, Dragnea A, Popescu I. The diagnostic value of cytokeratins and carcinoembryonic antigen immunostaining in differentiating hepatocellular carcinomas from intrahepatic cholangiocarcinomas. *J Gastrointestin Liver Dis.* 2006;15(1):9.

23. Kang YK, Kim WH, Jang JJ. Expression of G1-S modulators (p53, p16, p27, cyclin D1, Rb) and Smad4/Dpc4 in intrahepatic cholangiocarcinoma. *Hum Pathol.* 2002;33(9):877-883.

24. Wang NP, Zee S, Zarbo RJ, Bacchi CE, Gown AM. Coordinate expression of cytokeratins 7 and 20 defines unique subsets of carcinomas. *Appl immunohistochem.* 1995;3(2):99-107.

25. Chu PG, Ishizawa S, Wu E, Weiss LM. Hepatocyte antigen as a marker of hepatocellular carcinoma: an immunohistochemical comparison to carcinoembryonic antigen, CD10, and alpha-fetoprotein. *Am J Surg Pathol.* 2002;26(8):978-988.

26. Wang HL, Anatelli F, Zhai QJ, Adley B, Chuang S-T, Yang XJ. Glypican-3 as a useful diagnostic marker that distinguishes hepatocellular carcinoma from benign hepatocellular mass lesions. *Arch Pathol Lab Med.* 2008;132(11):1723-1728.

27. Ferrone CR, Ting DT, Shahid M, et al. The ability to diagnose intrahepatic cholangiocarcinoma definitively using novel branched DNA-enhanced albumin RNA in situ hybridization technology. *Ann Surg Oncol.* 2016;23(1):290-296.

28. Ishak KG, Sesterhenn IA, Goodman ZD, Rabin L, Stromeyer FW. Epithelioid hemangioendothelioma of the liver: a clinicopathologic and follow-up study of 32 cases. *Hum Pathol.* 1984;15(9):839-852.

29. Cho NH, Lee KG, Jeong MG. Cytologic evaluation of primary malignant vascular tumors of the liver. One case each of angiosarcoma and epithelioid hemangioendothelioma. *Acta Cytol.* 1997;41(5):1468-1476.

30. VandenBussche CJ, Wakely PE Jr, Siddiqui MT, Maleki Z, Ali SZ. Cytopathologic characteristics of epithelioid vascular malignancies. *Acta Cytol.* 2014;58(4):356-366.

31. Murali R, Zarka MA, Ocal IT, Tazelaar HD. Cytologic features of epithelioid hemangioendothelioma. *Am J Clin Pathol.* 2011;136(5):739-746.

32. Kaplan KJ, Escobar M, Alonzo M, Berlin JW. Ciliated hepatic foregut cyst: report of a case on fine-needle aspiration. *Diagn Cytopathol.* 2007;35(4):245-249.

33. Logrono R, Rampy BA, Adegboyega PA. Fine needle aspiration cytology of hepatobiliary cystadenoma with mesenchymal stroma. *Cancer.* 2002;96(1):37-42.

34. Ihse I, Lindell G, Tibblin S. Neuroendocrine tumors metastatic to the liver. In: Holzheimer RG, ed. *Surgical Treatment: Evidence-Based and Problem-Oriented.* Munich: Zuckschwerdt; 2001.

35. Rappaport KM, DiGiuseppe JA, Busseniers AE. Primary hepatic lymphoma: report of two cases diagnosed by fine-needle aspiration. *Diagn Cytopathol.* 1995;13(2):142-145.

36. Tsui WM, Colombari R, Portmann BC, et al. Hepatic angiomyolipoma: a clinicopathologic study of 30 cases and delineation of unusual morphologic variants. *Am J Surg Pathol.* 1999;23(1):34-48.

37. Cha I, Cartwright D, Guis M, Miller TR, Ferrell LD. Angiomyolipoma of the liver in fine-needle aspiration biopsies: its distinction from hepatocellular carcinoma. *Cancer.* 1999;87(1):25-30.

38. Locker GY, Doroshow JH, Zwelling LA, Chabner BA. The clinical features of hepatic angiosarcoma: a report of four cases and a review of the English literature. *Medicine (Baltimore).* 1979;58(1):48-64.

39. Fletcher CD, Berman JJ, Corless C, et al. Diagnosis of gastrointestinal stromal tumors: a consensus approach. *Hum Pathol.* 2002;33(5):459-465.

40. Hwang DG, Qian X, Hornick JL. DOG1 antibody is a highly sensitive and specific marker for gastrointestinal stromal tumors in cytology cell blocks. *Am J Clin Pathol.* 2011;135(3):448-453.

41. Lang H, Nussbaum KT, Kaudel P, Fruhauf N, Flemming P, Raab R. Hepatic metastases from leiomyosarcoma: a single-center experience with 34 liver resections during a 15-year period. *Ann Surg.* 2000;231(4):500-505.

42. Lee DH, Han KH, Ahn SY, et al. Sarcomatoid intrahepatic cholangiocarcinoma: a rare case of primary liver cancer. *J Liver Cancer.* 2016;16(2):139-144.

43. Kakizoe S, Kojiro M, Nakashima T. Hepatocellular carcinoma with sarcomatous change. Clinicopathologic and immunohistochemical studies of 14 autopsy cases. *Cancer.* 1987;59(2):310-316.

44. Klimstra DS, Hruban RH, Pitman MB. Pancreas. In: Mills SE, ed. *Histology for Pathologists.* Philadelphia: Lippincott Williams & Wilkins; 2012:777-816.

45. Collins JA, Ali SZ, VandenBussche CJ. Pancreatic cytopathology. *Surg Pathol Clin.* 2016;9(4):661-676.

46. Kim T, Murakami T, Takahashi S, et al. Ductal adenocarcinoma of the pancreas with intratumoral calcification. *Abdom Imaging.* 1999;24(6):610-613.

47. Samad A, Attam R, Pambuccian SE. Calcifications in an endoscopic ultrasound-guided fine-needle aspirate of chronic pancreatitis. *Diagn Cytopathol.* 2013;41(12):1081-1085.

48. Pitman MB, Centeno BA, Daglilar ES, Brugge WR, Mino-Kenudson M. Cytological criteria of high-grade epithelial atypia in the cyst fluid of pancreatic intraductal papillary mucinous neoplasms. *Cancer Cytopathol.* 2014;122(1):40-47.

49. Brugge WR, Lewandrowski K, Lee-Lewandrowski E, et al. Diagnosis of pancreatic cystic neoplasms: a report of the cooperative pancreatic cyst study. *Gastroenterology.* 2004;126(5):1330-1336.

50. Cizginer S, Turner BG, Bilge AR, Karaca C, Pitman MB, Brugge WR. Cyst fluid carcinoembryonic antigen is an accurate diagnostic marker of pancreatic mucinous cysts. *Pancreas.* 2011;40(7):1024-1028.

51. Pitman MB, Centeno BA, Ali SZ, et al. Standardized terminology and nomenclature for pancreatobiliary cytology: the papanicolaou society of cytopathology guidelines. *Cytojournal.* 2014;11(suppl 1):3.

52. Hruban RH, Pitman MB, Klimstra DS. *Tumors of the Pancreas. Atlas of Tumor Pathology, 4th Series, Fascicle 6.* Washington, DC: American Registry of Pathology; Armed Forces Institutes of Pathology; 2007.

53. Crippa S, Salvia R, Warshaw AL, et al. Mucinous cystic neoplasm of the pancreas is not an aggressive entity: lessons from 163 resected patients. *Ann Surg.* 2008;247(4):571-579.

54. Reddy RP, Smyrk TC, Zapiach M, et al. Pancreatic mucinous cystic neoplasm defined by ovarian stroma: demographics, clinical features, and prevalence of cancer. *Clin Gastroenterol Hepatol.* 2004;2(11):1026-1031.

55. Yamao K, Yanagisawa A, Takahashi K, et al. Clinicopathological features and prognosis of mucinous cystic neoplasm with ovarian-type stroma: a multi-institutional study of the Japan pancreas society. *Pancreas.* 2011;40(1):67-71.

56. Wu J, Matthaei H, Maitra A, et al. Recurrent GNAS mutations define an unexpected pathway for pancreatic cyst development. *Sci Transl Med.* 2011;3(92):92ra66.

57. Chai SM, Herba K, Kumarasinghe MP, et al. Optimizing the multimodal approach to pancreatic cyst fluid diagnosis: developing a volume-based triage protocol. *Cancer Cytopathol*. 2013;121(2):86-100.

58. Pitman MB. Pancreatic cyst fluid triage: a critical component of the preoperative evaluation of pancreatic cysts. *Cancer Cytopathol*. 2013;121(2):57-60.

59. Rosenbaum MW, Jones M, Dudley JC, Le LP, Iafrate AJ, Pitman MB. Next-generation sequencing adds value to the preoperative diagnosis of pancreatic cysts. *Cancer*. 2017;125(1):41-47.

60. Scourtas A, Dudley JC, Brugge WR, Kadayifci A, Mino-Kenudson M, Pitman MB. Preoperative characteristics and cytological features of 136 histologically confirmed pancreatic mucinous cystic neoplasms. *Cancer*. 2017;125(3):169-177.

61. Zhang ML, Arpin RN, Brugge WR, Forcione DG, Basar O, Pitman MB. Moray micro forceps biopsy improves the diagnosis of specific pancreatic cysts. *Cancer Cytopathol*. 2018;126(6):414-420.

62. Hamilton S, Aaltonen L. *Pathology and Genetics of Tumours of the Digestive System*. Lyon, France: IARC; 2000.

63. Gangi S, Fletcher JG, Nathan MA, et al. Time interval between abnormalities seen on CT and the clinical diagnosis of pancreatic cancer: retrospective review of CT scans obtained before diagnosis. *AJR Am J Roentgenol*. 2004;182(4):897-903.

64. Rahemtullah A, Misdraji J, Pitman MB. Adenosquamous carcinoma of the pancreas: cytologic features in 14 cases. *Cancer*. 2003;99(6):372-378.

65. Hoang MP, Murakata LA, Padilla-Rodriguez AL, Albores-Saavedra J. Metaplastic lesions of the extrahepatic bile ducts: a morphologic and immunohistochemical study. *Mod Pathol*. 2001;14(11):1119-1125.

66. Alzahrani MA, Schmulewitz N, Grewal S, et al. Metastases to the pancreas: the experience of a high volume center and a review of the literature. *J Surg Oncol*. 2012;105(2):156-161.

67. Lee DW, Kim MK, Kim HG. Diagnosis of pancreatic neuroendocrine tumors. *Clin Endosc*. 2017;50(6):537-545.

68. Ahmed A, VandenBussche CJ, Ali SZ, Olson MT. The dilemma of "indeterminate" interpretations of pancreatic neuroendocrine tumors on fine needle aspiration. *Diagn Cytopathol*. 2016;44(1):10-13.

69. Tanigawa M, Nakayama M, Taira T, et al. Insulinoma-associated protein 1 (INSM1) is a useful marker for pancreatic neuroendocrine tumor. *Med Mol Morphol*. 2018;51(1):32-40.

70. Klimstra DS. Pathology reporting of neuroendocrine tumors: essential elements for accurate diagnosis, classification, and staging. *Semin Oncol*. 2013;40(1):23-36.

71. Fite JJ, Ali SZ, VandenBussche CJ. Fine-needle aspiration of a pancreatic neuroendocrine tumor with prominent rhabdoid features. *Diagn Cytopathol*. 2018;46(7):600-603.

72. Tatsas AD, Owens CL, Siddiqui MT, Hruban RH, Ali SZ. Fine-needle aspiration of intrapancreatic accessory spleen: cytomorphologic features and differential diagnosis. *Cancer Cytopathol*. 2012;120(4):261-268.

73. Shi C, Klimstra DS. Pancreatic neuroendocrine tumors: pathologic and molecular characteristics. *Semin Diagn Pathol*. 2014;31(6):498-511.

74. Hosoda W, Sasaki E, Murakami Y, Yamao K, Shimizu Y, Yatabe Y. BCL10 as a useful marker for pancreatic acinar cell carcinoma, especially using endoscopic ultrasound cytology specimens. *Pathol Int*. 2013;63(3):176-182.

75. Abraham SC, Wu TT, Hruban RH, et al. Genetic and immunohistochemical analysis of pancreatic acinar cell carcinoma: frequent allelic loss on chromosome 11p and alterations in the APC/beta-catenin pathway. *Am J Pathol*. 2002;160(3):953-962.

76. Reid MD, Lewis MM, Willingham FF, Adsay NV. The evolving role of pathology in new developments, classification, terminology, and diagnosis of pancreatobiliary neoplasms. *Arch Pathol Lab Med*. 2017;141(3):366-380.

77. Springer S, Wang Y, Dal Molin M, et al. A combination of molecular markers and clinical features improve the classification of pancreatic cysts. *Gastroenterology*. 2015;149(6):1501-1510.

78. Low G, Panu A, Millo N, Leen E. Multimodality imaging of neoplastic and nonneoplastic solid lesions of the pancreas. *Radiographics*. 2011;31(4):993-1015.

79. Hutchinson CB, Canlas K, Evans JA, Obando JV, Waugh M. Endoscopic ultrasound-guided fine needle aspiration biopsy of the intrapancreatic accessory spleen: a report of 2 cases. *Acta Cytol*. 2010;54(3):337-340.

80. Schreiner AM, Mansoor A, Faigel DO, Morgan TK. Intrapancreatic accessory spleen: mimic of pancreatic endocrine tumor diagnosed by endoscopic ultrasound-guided fine-needle aspiration biopsy. *Diagn Cytopathol*. 2008;36(4):262-265.

81. Adsay NV, Hasteh F, Cheng JD, et al. Lymphoepithelial cysts of the pancreas: a report of 12 cases and a review of the literature. *Mod Pathol*. 2002;15(5):492-501.

82. Adsay NV, Hasteh F, Cheng JD, Klimstra DS. Squamous-lined cysts of the pancreas: lymphoepithelial cysts, dermoid cysts (teratomas), and accessory-splenic epidermoid cysts. *Semin Diagn Pathol*. 2000;17(1):56-65.

83. VandenBussche CJ, Maleki Z. Fine-needle aspiration of squamous-lined cysts of the pancreas. *Diagn Cytopathol*. 2014;42(7):592-599.

84. Groot VP, Thakker SS, Gemenetzis G, et al. Lessons learned from 29 lymphoepithelial cysts of the pancreas: institutional experience and review of the literature. *HPB*. 2018;20(7):612-620.

85. Gonzalez Obeso E, Murphy E, Brugge W, Deshpande V. Pseudocyst of the pancreas: the role of cytology and special stains for mucin. *Cancer*. 2009;117(2):101-107.

86. Valsangkar NP, Morales-Oyarvide V, Thayer SP, et al. 851 resected cystic tumors of the pancreas: a 33-year experience at the Massachusetts General Hospital. *Surgery*. 2012;152(3 suppl 1):S4-S12.

87. Lilo MT, VandenBussche CJ, Allison DB, et al. Serous cystadenoma of the pancreas: potentials and pitfalls of a preoperative cytopathologic diagnosis. *Acta Cytol*. 2017;61(1):27-33.

88. Alguacil-Garcia A, Weiland LH. The histologic spectrum, prognosis, and histogenesis of the sarcomatoid carcinoma of the pancreas. *Cancer*. 1977;39(3):1181-1189.

89. Doyle LA, Fletcher CD, Hornick JL. Nuclear expression of CAMTA1 distinguishes epithelioid hemangioendothelioma from histologic mimics. *Am J Surg Pathol*. 2016;40(1):94-102.

CHAPTER OUTLINE

THE UNREMARKABLE SEROUS CAVITY SPECIMEN

Serous cavity cytology specimens are exfoliative samples taken from the pericardial space, pleural cavities, and peritoneal cavity. Specimens from the peritoneal cavity may also be further designated as abdominal or pelvic specimens. An effusion is an abnormal amount of fluid present in any serous cavity and contains cells that have naturally exfoliated from the serous lining. A washing specimen is typically taken during surgery, and the physical force of the lavage fluid additionally helps to exfoliate cells.[1] The cellularity of an effusion specimen is variable but usually contains three cellular components: mesothelial cells, lymphocytes, and histiocytes (Figures 5.1-5.20). In an effusion specimen, these three cell populations are usually present as dispersed single cells. In washing specimens, mesothelial cells may also be present as sheets or as collagen balls, which are fragments of collagen lined by a thin layer of mesothelium (Figure 5.21).[2,3]

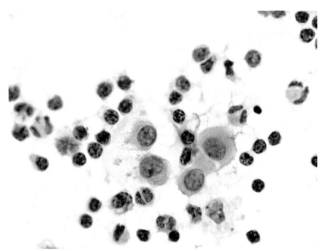

Figure 5.1. Reactive mesothelial cells in a background of lymphocytes. The mesothelial cells have abundant cytoplasm and round nuclei. Here, a small gap (or "window") between the cytoplasm of two adjacent cells helps identify them as mesothelial in origin (Pap stain).

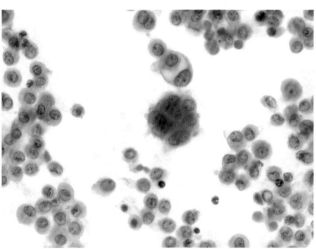

Figure 5.2. A cluster of mesothelial cells among numerous histiocytes. Mesothelial cells tend to have round nuclei with coarse chromatin and/or nucleoli, whereas histiocytes usually have smaller nuclei that may be folded. At the top center, one mesothelial cell appears to "hug" or "wrap" around an adjacent mesothelial cell (Pap stain).

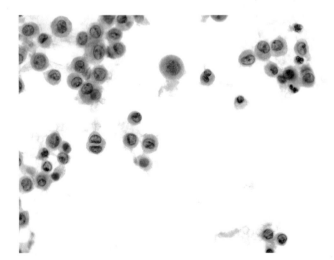

Figure 5.3. Mesothelial cells and histiocytes. A single mesothelial cell (top center) can be seen in a background of numerous histiocytes. The mesothelial cell has dense cytoplasm and a centrally placed nucleus, while the histiocytes have foamy cytoplasm and peripherally placed nuclei (Pap stain).

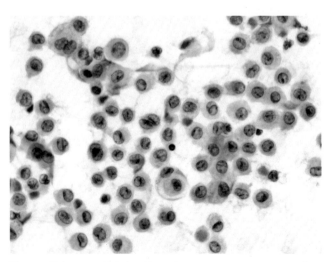

Figure 5.4. Mesothelial cells and histiocytes. Histiocytes often have cytomorphologic overlap with mesothelial cells. Distinguishing features, when present in a given cell, include foamy cytoplasm and an indented or bent nucleus. At least one mesothelial cell is present (top of the field), with a small nucleolus and centrally placed nucleus (Pap stain).

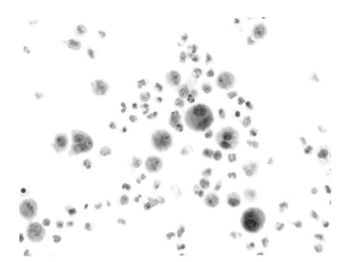

Figure 5.5. Multinucleated mesothelial cells. Many of these mesothelial cells are multinucleated, have prominent nucleoli, and are also larger than the few histiocytes seen at the top left-hand side of the field. Note the two-tone cytoplasm (blue central color and gray peripheral rim), which causes a "lacy skirt" appearance encircling some of the mesothelial cells (Pap stain).

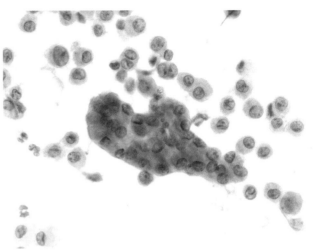

Figure 5.6. Fragment of mesothelial cells. This small fragment contains mesothelial cells, some of which have prominent nucleoli. Histiocytes do not form tissue fragments but may aggregate together into pseudo-fragments (Pap stain).

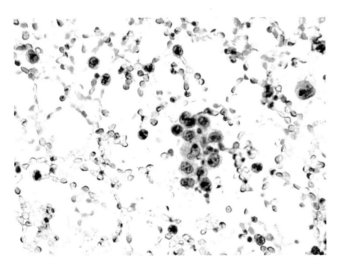

Figure 5.7. Histiocytes. Several histiocytes cluster together in the center of the field. They are easily identified by their curved nuclei (Pap stain).

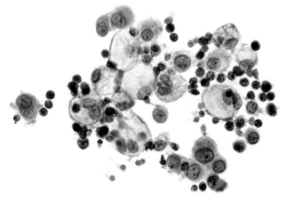

Figure 5.8. Histiocytes and lymphocytes. These histiocytes have vacuolated cytoplasm, and several are binucleated. They are closely associated with lymphocytes, another common resident of serous fluids (Pap stain).

MESOTHELIAL CELLS

Mesothelial cells line all serous cavities and naturally exfoliate into the serous cavity. The underlying cause of an effusion, as well as the increased cavity fluid volume, can contribute to mesothelial proliferation and exfoliation into the fluid.[4] A mesothelial cell is larger than a histiocyte and lymphocyte, has a round to oval nucleus, and has cytoplasm with a two-tone appearance in which the perinuclear area stains more darkly than the periphery (Figures 5.1-5.6). In an effusion specimen, mesothelial cells may form small clusters in which the borders between mesothelial cells are often distinct. In some instances, the border may be open in the center, allowing the background to be seen—this is known as an intercellular "window" that can help identify mesothelial cells.[5] Mesothelial cells are lined by microvilli, which contribute to the

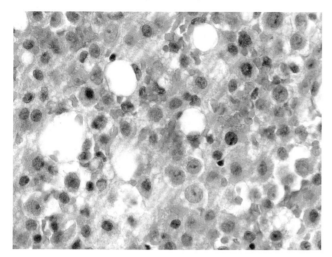

Figure 5.9. Mesothelial cells and histiocytes. This cell block section contains a mixture of histiocytes and mesothelial cells. While it can be challenging to distinguish between them, it is usually not important to identify each individual mesothelial cell and histiocyte in a specimen (Pap stain).

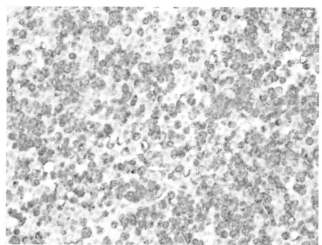

Figure 5.10. CD68 immunostain. A CD68 immunostain was performed on the previous cell block material. This stain identifies histiocytes, which are typically found in greater numbers than mesothelial cells (CD68 immunostain).

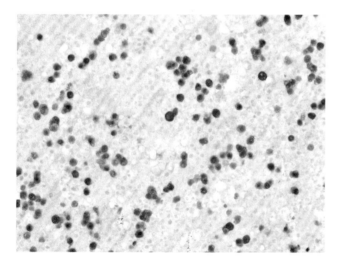

Figure 5.11. Calretinin immunostain. To be interpreted as positive, calretinin should stain both the nucleus and cytoplasm of the cells in question. Calretinin positivity helps establish a mesothelial origin; calretinin is usually negative in most metastatic adenocarcinomas (calretinin immunostain).

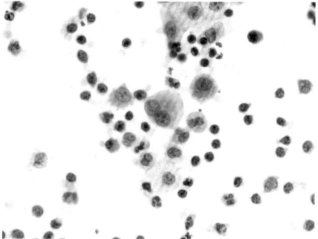

Figure 5.12. Mesothelial cells, histiocytes, and inflammatory cells. The binucleated cell is larger than the adjacent foamy histiocytes and has a "lacy skirt" appearance. These features help identify this cell as a mesothelial cell (Pap stain).

lighter appearance of the cell's outer rim, giving rise to what some call a "lacy skirt" appearance.[6] Reactive mesothelial cells can have greatly varied appearances, which can result in cytomorphologic overlap with malignant processes. Some additional reactive changes include vacuolization, which may cause a signet ring appearance, the engulfment or "hugging" of adjacent mesothelial cells, the development of nucleoli, and the production of mucin.

When present in fragments, mesothelial cells have the same spectrum of cytomorphologic characteristics as single mesothelial cells (Figures 5.17-5.20). Benign fragments have a monolayer architecture in which the fragments appear flat and the cell nuclei are evenly placed within each fragment. The fragments may fold over on themselves but should not form complex three-dimensional structures.

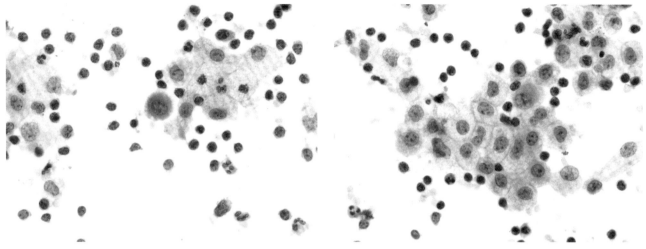

Figure 5.13. Predominantly histiocytes, inflammatory cells, and rare mesothelial cells. The center cell is a mesothelial cell, as identified by its centrally placed nucleus, coarse chromatin, and "lacy skirt" appearance. The histiocytes in the field have foamy cytoplasm, as this specimen was taken from a patient with chylothorax. Mitotic figures (as seen in these two adjacent histiocytes) are frequently seen in serous fluid mesothelial cells and histiocytes (Pap stain).

Figure 5.14. Predominantly histiocytes, inflammatory cells, and rare mesothelial cells. A single mesothelial cell, lacking foamy cytoplasm, stands out in a larger population of histiocytes in this specimen (Pap stain).

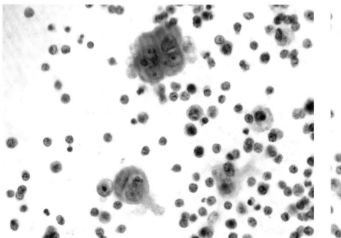

Figure 5.15. Mesothelial cells, histiocytes, and inflammatory cells. Several mesothelial cells form a small cluster. They have prominent nucleoli. In the bottom center field, one mesothelial cell wraps around another (Pap stain).

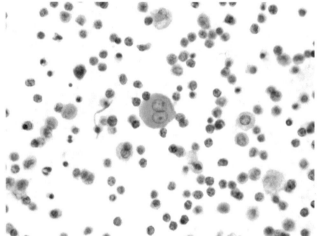

Figure 5.16. Mesothelial cells, histiocytes, and lymphocytes. A single binucleate mesothelial cell (center field) is seen surrounded by smaller histiocytes and numerous lymphocytes (Pap stain).

HISTIOCYTES

Histiocytes are normal residents of the serous cavity (Figures 5.7-5.10). They are larger than lymphocytes and contain more abundant cytoplasm, which may be vacuolated or may contain pigment, most often derived from hemosiderin following the breakdown of red blood cells. Their nuclei can assume many shapes, but the presence of a curved nucleus is the most specific feature of a histiocyte. When the nucleus is round or oval, however, the cells may be difficult to distinguish from mesothelial cells. Specimens can contain varying amounts of histiocytes; in some cases, there is a predominance of histiocytes, which may cause an initial concern for malignancy.[7]

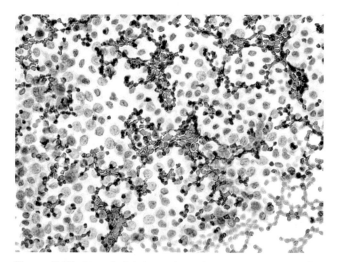

Figure 5.17. Mesothelial sheets. In washing specimens, mesothelial cells may exfoliate as monolayer sheets. This finding should not cause concern for mesothelioma, which is more likely to present as single cells or three-dimensional tissue fragments (Pap stain).

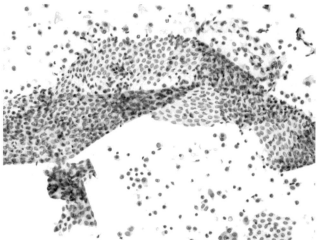

Figure 5.18. Mesothelial sheets. A large exfoliated monolayer sheet has folded over upon itself. The nuclei have slight nuclear border irregularities but generally form a well-organized, honeycomb appearance with little nuclear overlap (Pap stain).

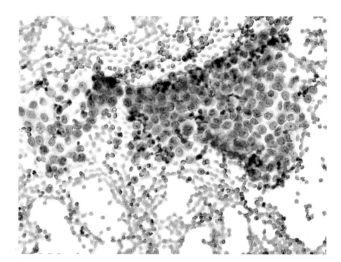

Figure 5.19. Mesothelial sheets. Separate field (Pap stain).

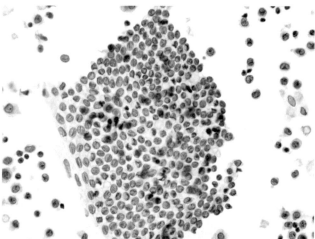

Figure 5.20. Mesothelial sheets. Separate field (Pap stain).

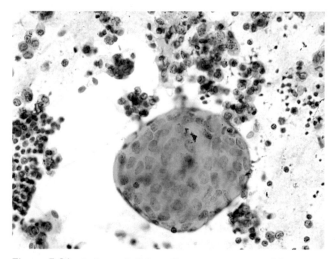

Figure 5.21. Collagen ball. In washing specimens, small fragments of collagen lined by mesothelial cells may be seen. They typically form spheres of varying sizes. While not clinically relevant, they are considered a distractor (Pap stain).

LYMPHOCYTES

Lymphocytes and other mononuclear cells are also normal residents of the serous cavity. Lymphocytes are small cells with round nuclei and a thin rim of cytoplasm. Lymphocytes should be intermixed with mesothelial cells and histiocytes; however, a predominance of lymphocytes (lymphocytosis) is associated with several neoplastic and nonneoplastic pathologic conditions, further detailed later in this chapter.

COLLAGEN BALLS

Collagen balls are fragments of collagen that have been forcibly removed during a serous cavity washing. The collagenous core appears greenish-blue on the Pap stain and has a spherical shape, although elongated and curved shapes can also be seen (Figure 5.21). The balls are lined by a flattened layer of mesothelial cells, seen as small nuclear "bumps" present at regular intervals along the surface. Collagen balls have a distinctive morphology and color and are rarely mistaken for other processes.

SAMPLE NOTE: BENIGN SEROUS FLUID SPECIMEN

Reactive mesothelial cells, histiocytes, and lymphocytes. No malignant neoplasm identified. See note.

Note: The patient's history of breast carcinoma is noted. The reactive mesothelial cells are positive for calretinin. A BerEP4 immunostain is negative. These findings support the above diagnosis.

TISSUE FRAGMENTS PATTERN

The tissue fragments pattern describes the presence of cellular fragments in a background of dispersed mesothelial cells, histiocytes, and lymphocytes. In the case of washing specimens, benign mesothelial sheets should be excluded because they are considered normal background elements. Tissue fragments can have a variety of forms, such as three-dimensional spheres ("cannonballs"), papillary-like structures, and dispersed small cellular fragments.[8] The presence of tissue fragments may represent benign proliferations, neoplastic implants, or a metastatic or invasive malignancy. Proper characterization often requires examination of the cytomorphologic features, ancillary tests such as immunostains, and clinicoradiologic correlation.

CHECKLIST: Etiologic Considerations for the Tissue Fragments Pattern

- ☐ Adenocarcinoma
- ☐ Squamous Cell Carcinoma
- ☐ Noncarcinoma Malignancies
- ☐ Neoplastic Implants
- ☐ Mesothelioma
- ☐ Benign Mesothelial Proliferation
- ☐ Endosalpingiosis
- ☐ Endometriosis

ADENOCARCINOMA

Adenocarcinomas often form three-dimensional, gland-forming structures with mucin production that may be more readily identified on cell block material (Table 5.1).[9] Common features of adenocarcinoma include anisonucleosis, high nuclear to cytoplasmic ratio, prominent nucleoli or coarse chromatin, hyperchromasia, markedly irregular nuclear borders, and large cell size (Figures 5.22-5.90). Under most circumstances, the specimen will be cellular with numerous atypical tissue fragments as well as malignant cells present individually. In contrast to dispersed cells, cells in tissue fragments often retain the architecture and cytomorphology seen at the primary site. Thus, certain cytomorphologic characteristics, when identified, may be useful in elucidating the primary site (Table 5.2).

In patients with a recent history of an aggressive carcinoma, the presence of malignant cells morphologically consistent with the primary site is sufficient for a definitive diagnosis. When the patient has no known history of malignancy, care should be taken to exclude other possibilities before pursuing a workup of an unknown primary. For instance, immunostains should confirm an epithelial origin (membranous staining with BerEP4 or MOC-31) while mesothelial markers (such as calretinin) should be negative.[10-12] The presence of mucin can be confirmed by using special stains for mucin: the most specific special stains for mucin include PAS with diastase or Alcian blue with hyaluronidase because mesotheliomas may produce hyaluronic acid that can cross-react with mucicarmine or stain with

TABLE 5.1: Most Common Malignancy Types in Each Cavity

Site	Most Common Malignancies
Pleural	Lung Breast Lymphoproliferative
Pericardial	Lung Breast Lymphoproliferative
Peritoneal	Ovarian Colorectal Pancreas Uterine Lymphoproliferative Lung Breast

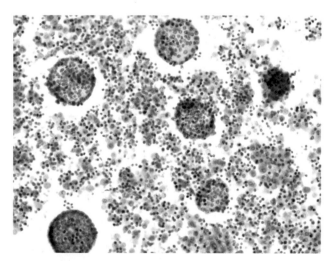

Figure 5.22. Metastatic adenocarcinoma "cannonballs." The presence of "cannonballs" in a fluid specimen can be seen in both metastatic adenocarcinomas as well as some mesotheliomas (Pap stain).

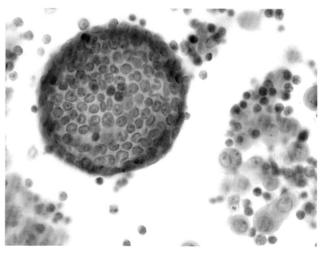

Figure 5.23. Metastatic adenocarcinoma "cannonball." This sphere lacks collagen in the center that would be seen in a collagen ball (Pap stain).

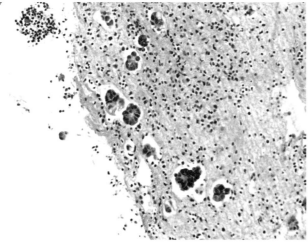

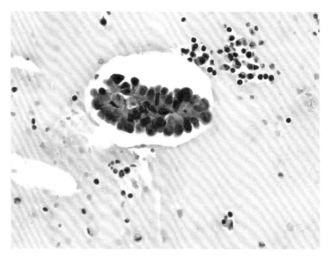

Figure 5.24. Metastatic adenocarcinoma. Cell block preparations often result in a retraction artifact, or "halo," forming around malignant tissue fragments. Here, the cell block material has retracted away from several metastatic gland-forming adenocarcinoma fragments (H&E).

Figure 5.25. Metastatic adenocarcinoma. Separate field at higher magnification (H&E).

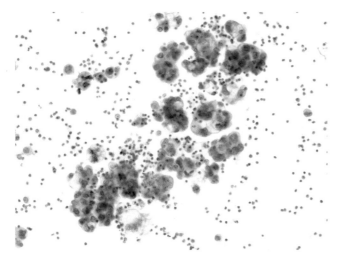

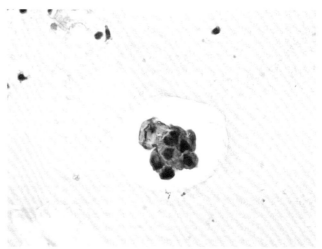

Figure 5.26. Metastatic lung adenocarcinoma. The cells in this field can be identified as adenocarcinoma cells owing to their increased nuclear size, high nuclear to cytoplasmic (N/C) ratios, and anisonucleosis. Some cells have prominent nucleoli and large cytoplasmic vacuoles; the mucin contained in one cell has stained pink on this preparation (Pap stain).

Figure 5.27. Metastatic lung adenocarcinoma. A cell block preparation from the same metastatic lung adenocarcinoma specimen. The morphologic features of adenocarcinoma are not always specific for a site of origin, in which case immunohistochemical studies performed on cell block material can help determine a site of origin (H&E).

Alcian blue in the absence of hyaluronidase.[13] More specific immunohistochemical studies can be performed to confirm a known malignancy or as part of a workup for a cancer of unknown primary (CUP).[14,15] Generally speaking, more sensitive markers should be used before more specific, confirmatory markers (Table 5.3).[16-31]

SAMPLE NOTE: ATYPICAL CELLS ABSENT IN CELL BLOCK MATERIAL

Atypical epithelial cells of uncertain significance. See note.

Note: The patient's history of pancreatic adenocarcinoma is noted. The specimen contains rare atypical cells with enlarged nuclei, irregular nuclear contours, and hyperchromasia. However, the atypical cells are not sufficiently present in the cell block material to allow further characterization.

FAQ: The patient has a history of colorectal cancer, so calretinin and BerEP4 were performed on the cell block material of a pelvic washing specimen to exclude involvement. The majority of the concerning cells and fragments are positive for calretinin, but some fragments have focal staining for BerPE4. How should this be interpreted?

Answer: Reactive mesothelial cells can occasionally demonstrate focal or patchy staining for BerEP4. If the majority of the cells are positive for calretinin and negative for BerEP4, these are likely reactive mesothelial cells. If the BerEP4-positive cells have similar cytomorphology, they are most likely reactive mesothelial cells as well. The presence of focal BerEP4 staining in fragments that are diffusely calretinin positive is a reassuring finding. If any doubt exists, the cells can be diagnosed as atypical, or additional immunostains (in this case, CDX2 or CK20 for a colorectal origin) can be performed to further exclude metastatic colorectal carcinoma.

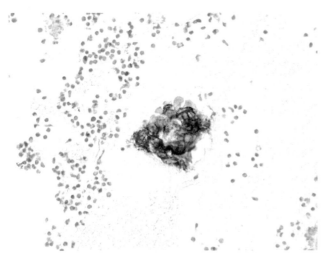

Figure 5.28. BerEP4 does not stain mesothelial cells, histiocytes, or other common benign residents of serous effusions but stains the cytoplasmic membrane of most metastatic adenocarcinomas. This stain was performed on the cell block material of a metastatic lung adenocarcinoma and is positive (BerEP4 immunostain).

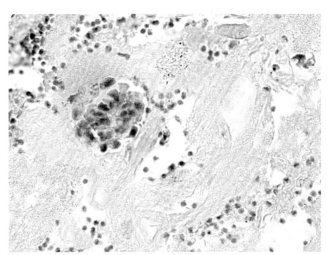

Figure 5.29. Calretinin is negative in most metastatic adenocarcinomas and positive in reactive mesothelial cells that may mimic an adenocarcinoma. The absence of calretinin staining in this atypical tissue fragment, along with positivity for BerEP4, helps confirm a metastatic adenocarcinoma (calretinin immunostain).

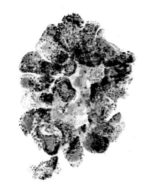

Figure 5.30. The cell block material from this metastatic lung adenocarcinoma is positive for napsin A (granular cytoplasmic staining pattern), a specific finding that helps establish the metastatic adenocarcinoma as having a lung origin (napsin A immunostain).

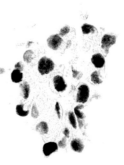

Figure 5.31. TTF-1 is a nuclear stain that is sensitive for lung adenocarcinoma, but it is not as specific for a lung origin as napsin A. The cell block material containing metastatic lung adenocarcinoma shows nuclear positivity for TTF-1 in this field (TTF-1 immunostain).

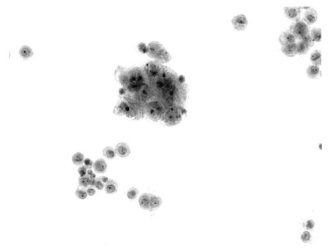

Figure 5.32. Metastatic lung adenocarcinoma. Compared with the background histiocytes and mesothelial cells, the cells in the central cluster have much larger nuclei and coarse chromatin. There is dramatic variation in nuclear size. These features are diagnostic of a metastatic adenocarcinoma but are not specific to the lung (Pap stain).

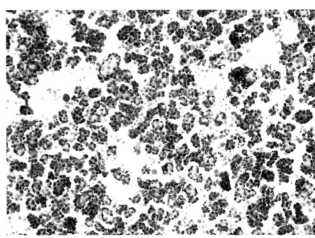

Figure 5.33. Metastatic lung adenocarcinoma. The field is cellular with papillary tissue fragments, and the normal components of a serous fluid are absent. The fragments contain empty spaces, which represent the glandular lumens formed by this adenocarcinoma. This pattern is not specific to a lung origin (Pap stain).

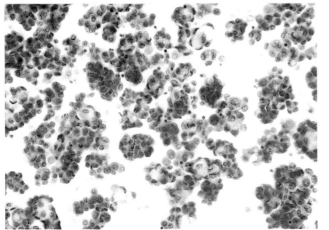

Figure 5.34. Metastatic lung adenocarcinoma. Separate field at higher magnification (Pap stain).

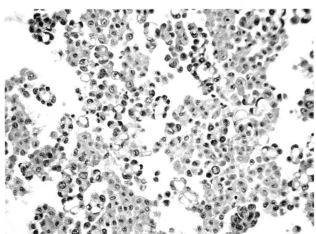

Figure 5.35. Metastatic lung adenocarcinoma. Cell block preparation of the metastatic lung adenocarcinoma seen in Figures 5.33 and 5.34 (H&E).

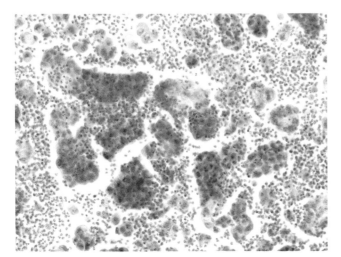

Figure 5.36. Metastatic lung adenocarcinoma. A separate specimen of metastatic lung adenocarcinoma in which the tissue fragments have a papillary appearance. The lung is one of the most common adenocarcinomas to metastasize to the pleural cavity (Pap stain).

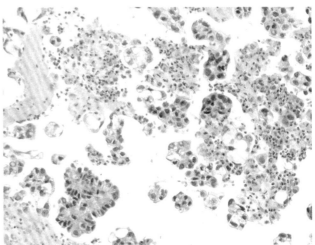

Figure 5.37. Metastatic lung adenocarcinoma. Cell block preparation of the metastatic lung adenocarcinoma seen in Figure 5.36 (H&E).

Figure 5.38. Metastatic lung adenocarcinoma. A separate cell block specimen from a patient with metastatic lung adenocarcinoma. The cells form a central glandular lumen. Note how the cells have dark chromatin, irregular nuclear borders, variation in nuclear size, and vacuolated cytoplasm, all features of adenocarcinoma and not specific for any particular site of origin (H&E).

Figure 5.39. Metastatic breast ductal carcinoma "cannonballs." Breast carcinoma is one of the most common metastases to the pleural fluid, and ductal carcinoma is often associated with "cannonball" formation in fluid specimens (Pap stain).

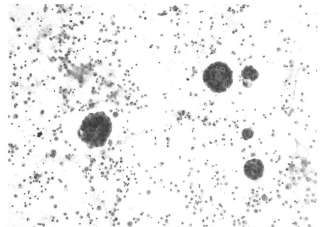

Figure 5.40. Metastatic breast ductal carcinoma "cannonballs." Similar cannonball formation is seen here in a specimen from a different patient with metastatic breast carcinoma (Pap stain).

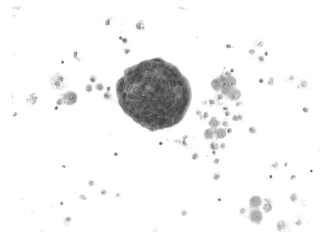

Figure 5.41. Metastatic breast ductal carcinoma "cannonballs." Separate field at higher magnification (Pap stain).

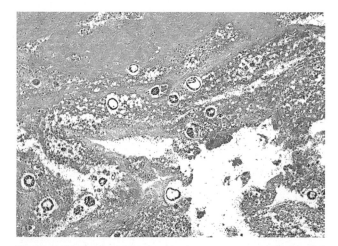

Figure 5.42. Metastatic breast ductal carcinoma "cannonballs." Cell block preparation of the metastatic breast carcinoma seen in Figures 5.40 and 5.41. Note the empty glandular lumens, which would be filled with matrix material in a cannonball-forming mesothelioma (H&E).

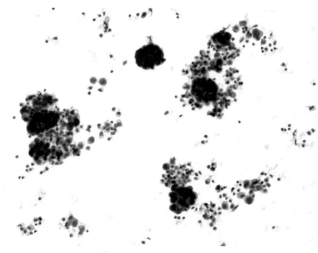

Figure 5.43. Metastatic breast ductal carcinoma. The carcinoma here forms smaller clusters which are less readily identifiable as cannonballs. The cells have little cytoplasm and are quite hyperchromatic, making it difficult to assess their cytomorphologic features (Pap stain).

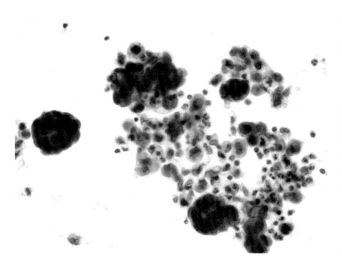

Figure 5.44. Metastatic breast ductal carcinoma. Separate field at higher magnification (Pap stain).

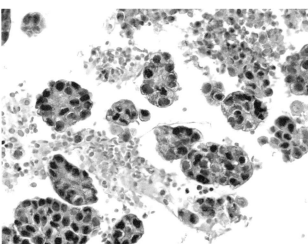

Figure 5.45. Metastatic breast ductal carcinoma. A cell block preparation of the same case (Figure 5.43). Cell blocks are sectioned, allowing better visualization of the malignant cells. The cells have large nuclei with markedly irregular borders and variation in nuclear size, features specific for malignancy but not for a breast origin (H&E).

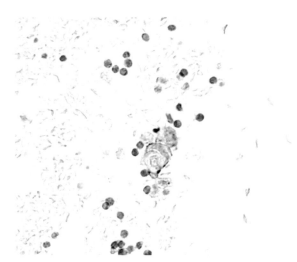

Figure 5.46. A BerEP4 immunostain performed on the same case shows positive membranous staining, helping to confirm the cells as epithelial and nonmesothelial in origin (BerEP4 immunostain).

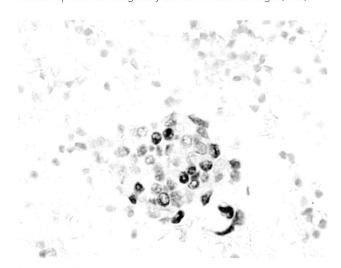

Figure 5.47. An estrogen receptor (ER) immunostain performed on the cell block material is positive (nuclear stain) in the metastatic breast carcinoma cells. Some breast carcinomas may lose ER positivity, and ER may also be positive in other malignancies, including some arising in the gynecologic tract (ER immunostain).

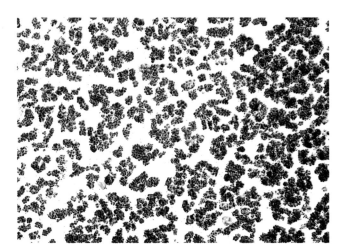

Figure 5.48. Metastatic breast ductal carcinoma. A specimen from a different patient with metastatic breast carcinoma, in which the carcinoma cells form papillary structures (Pap stain).

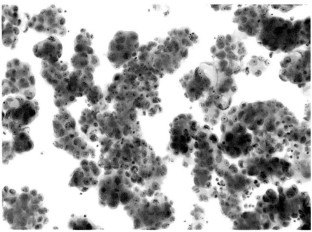

Figure 5.49. Metastatic breast ductal carcinoma. Separate field at higher magnification (Pap stain).

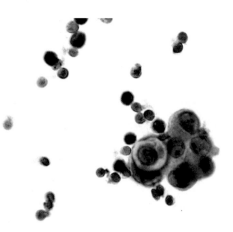

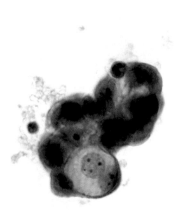

Figure 5.50. Metastatic high-grade serous carcinoma (HGSC). HGSC is a common cause of malignant ascites in women. While not entirely specific, the malignant cells often form fragments with hobnailed edges. The malignant cells are large, have prominent nucleoli, and are often vacuolated (Pap stain).

Figure 5.51. Metastatic high-grade serous carcinoma (HGSC). Separate field, showing one cell containing a large cytoplasmic vacuole (Pap stain).

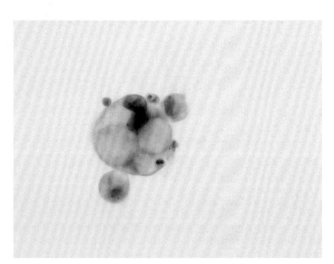

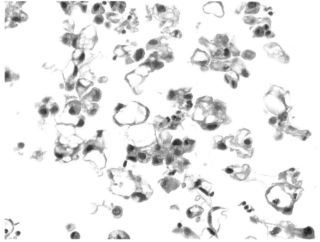

Figure 5.52. Metastatic high-grade serous carcinoma (HGSC). Separate field, showing malignant cells containing multiple large vacuoles that compress the nuclei. The cells are quite large (compared with adjacent neutrophils) and their low nuclear to cytoplasmic (N/C) ratios may be falsely reassuring (Pap stain).

Figure 5.53. Metastatic high-grade serous carcinoma (HGSC). A corresponding cell block preparation of metastatic HGSC. The cytoplasmic vacuolization is a prominent feature on this preparation (H&E).

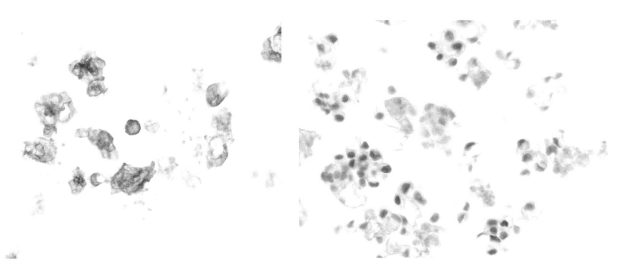

Figure 5.54. Metastatic high-grade serous carcinoma (HGSC). A BerEP4 stain performed on the cell block material confirms that the atypical cells are not histiocytes or mesothelial cells. In abdominopelvic specimens, several nonneoplastic and noncarcinomatous entities can result in BerEP4-positive cells: endosalpingiosis, endometriosis, cystadenofibroma, and implants of low-grade and borderline serous neoplasms, to name a few (BerEP4 immunostain).

Figure 5.55. Metastatic high-grade serous carcinoma (HGSC). Nuclear positivity for Pax-8 in an abdominopelvic specimen strongly suggests a Mullerian origin. However, the differential includes neoplastic and nonneoplastic entities (Pax-8 immunostain).

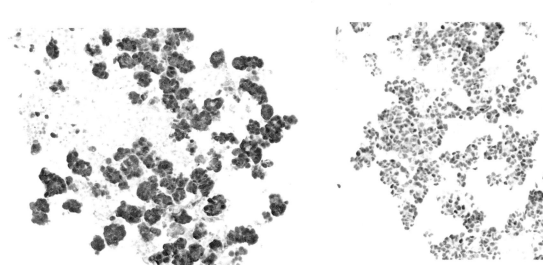

Figure 5.56. Metastatic high-grade serous carcinoma (HGSC). Diffuse cytoplasmic and nuclear immunoreactivity for p16 is a feature of HGSC. While both clear cell carcinoma and HGSC usually demonstrate aberrant p53 expression, clear cell carcinoma should not have diffuse p16 expression (p16 immunostain).

Figure 5.57. Metastatic high-grade serous carcinoma (HGSC). Diffuse nuclear immunoreactivity for p53 is considered to be aberrant and is seen in HGSC as well as clear cell carcinoma, with HGSC being much more common in abdominopelvic specimens. Focal nuclear expression of p53 is not considered aberrant, while complete absence of p53 expression ("null phenotype") is another pattern that is considered to be aberrant (p53 immunostain).

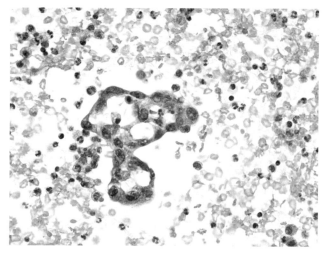

Figure 5.58. Metastatic high-grade serous carcinoma (HGSC). A separate case of metastatic HGSC on a cell block preparation. The tissue fragment contains glandular spaces and could possibly represent a metastasis from the gastrointestinal tract (H&E).

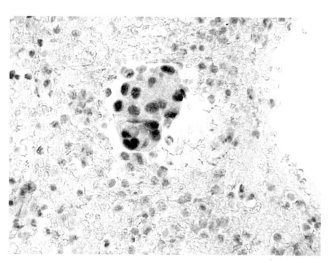

Figure 5.59. Metastatic high-grade serous carcinoma (HGSC). Estrogen receptor (ER) immunostain performed on the same specimen demonstrated diffuse nuclear immunoreactivity. HGSC should demonstrate this pattern, although other neoplasms of the gynecologic tract, as well as breast carcinoma, can show ER positivity (ER immunostain).

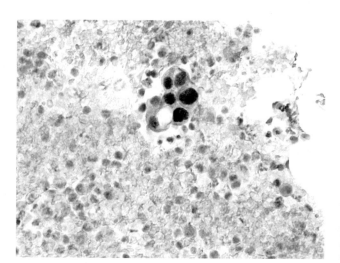

Figure 5.60. Metastatic high-grade serous carcinoma (HGSC). While diffuse nuclear positivity for p53 favors an HGSC (or the rarer clear cell carcinoma), a cell block specimen containing only a few neoplastic cells may limit the interpretation of whether the positive stain is truly "diffuse," or just happens to be positive in the rare assessable cells (p53 immunostain).

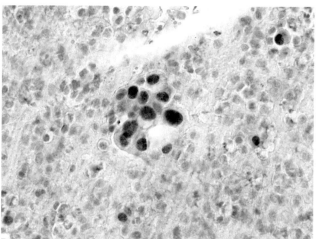

Figure 5.61. Metastatic high-grade serous carcinoma (HGSC). WT1 is another nuclear marker of Mullerian origin but also may be positive in mesothelioma (WT1 immunostain).

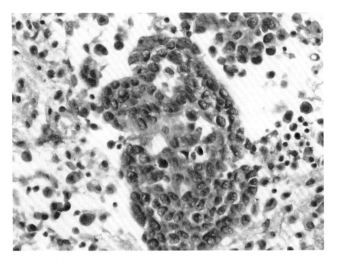

Figure 5.62. Metastatic high-grade serous carcinoma (HGSC). A separate case of HGSC on a cell block preparation. The cells form a large tissue fragment without obvious gland formation or vacuolization. The cells appear atypical and could represent a metastatic adenocarcinoma of unknown origin, or even a mesothelioma (H&E).

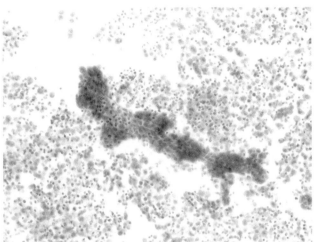

Figure 5.63. Metastatic high-grade serous carcinoma (HGSC). A large tissue fragment of HGSC that has a papillary architecture. The cytomorphology is nonspecific for a site of origin (Pap stain).

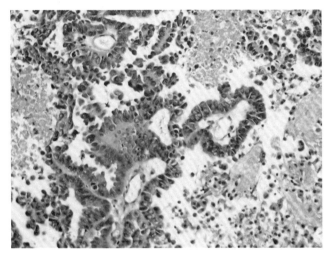

Figure 5.64. Metastatic high-grade serous carcinoma (HGSC). A cell block preparation of the same case, demonstrating prominent papillae with fibrovascular cores (H&E).

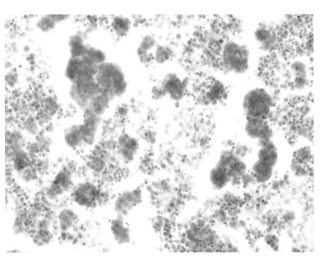

Figure 5.65. Metastatic high-grade serous carcinoma (HGSC). A separate case of HGSC with papillary architecture (Pap stain).

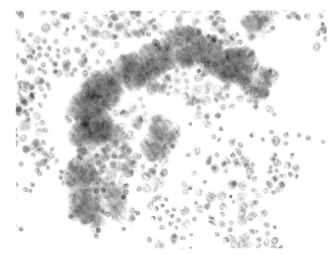

Figure 5.66. Metastatic high-grade serous carcinoma (HGSC). Separate field at higher magnification. Note the cytoplasmic vacuolization and prominent nucleoli that can be identified at this power, features that suggest but do not confirm an HGSC (Pap stain).

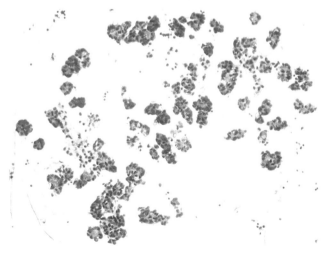

Figure 5.67. Metastatic high-grade serous carcinoma (HGSC). A cell block preparation of the same specimen, demonstrating prominent papillary architecture (H&E).

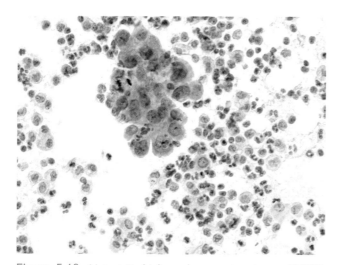

Figure 5.68. Metastatic high-grade serous carcinoma (HGSC). Increased populations of neutrophils are sometimes seen in association with serous carcinoma. However, any neoplasm with necrotic areas may contain numerous neutrophils (H&E).

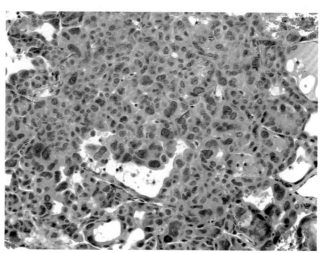

Figure 5.69. Metastatic high-grade serous carcinoma (HGSC). In contrast to low-grade and borderline serous neoplasms, HGSC cells should look overtly malignant. Here, the cells have irregular nuclear borders and great variation in nuclear size. The nuclei are hyperchromatic and large; nuclear to cytoplasmic (N/C) ratios are elevated (H&E).

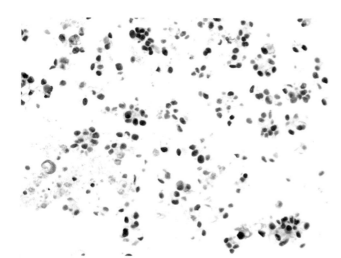

Figure 5.70. Metastatic high-grade serous carcinoma (HGSC). A separate specimen of HGSC with diffuse nuclear immunoreactivity for p53. The negative bystander cells provide an excellent internal control, but also complicate the interpretation of whether some atypical cells may be negative for p53 (p53 immunostain).

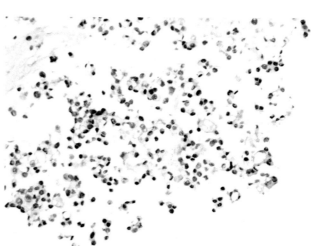

Figure 5.71. Metastatic high-grade serous carcinoma (HGSC). A separate case of HGSC, stained for Pax-8 to demonstrate the number of neoplastic cells. When assessing p53, Pax-8 or BerEP4 can be helpful to assess the proportion of neoplastic to normal cells in a specimen (Pax-8 immunostain).

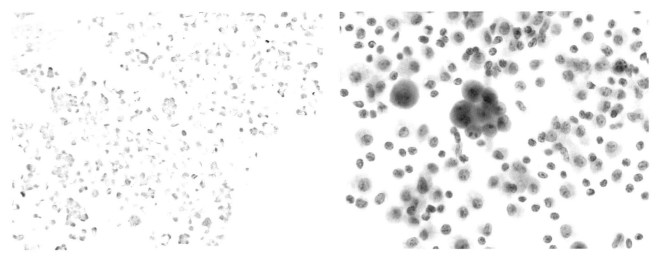

Figure 5.72. Metastatic high-grade serous carcinoma (HGSC). A p53 immunostain was performed on the same case, showing negative p53 expression in a population of Pax-8–positive cells. Absence of p53 expression is compatible with the "null" phenotype and is considered an aberrant form of p53 expression (p53 immunostain).

Figure 5.73. Metastatic high-grade serous carcinoma (HGSC). The specimen contains a small fragment of atypical cells with slight nuclear membrane irregularities and high nuclear to cytoplasmic (N/C) ratios. The cells were positive for Pax-8, and the prominence of nucleoli is more suggestive of a HGSC than a low-grade serous carcinoma or borderline serous tumor. However, tumor grade can be difficult to determine using cytomorphology alone on a limited specimen (Pap stain).

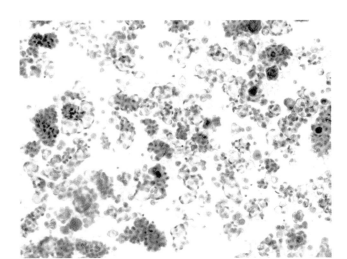

Figure 5.74. Metastatic low-grade serous carcinoma. The specimen is cellular with neoplastic cells within papillary fragments associated with psammoma bodies. Some cells have prominent vacuolization. The nuclei are more monotonous appearing than those seen in high-grade serous carcinoma (Pap stain).

Figure 5.75. Metastatic low-grade serous carcinoma. The neoplastic cells have high nuclear to cytoplasmic (N/C) ratios, but minimal nuclear size variation and only mild nuclear border irregularities (Pap stain).

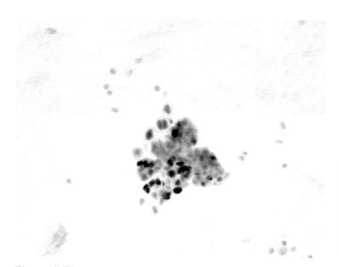

Figure 5.76. Metastatic low-grade serous carcinoma. The tumor cells demonstrate a "wild-type" (patchy) staining pattern for p53, as compared with the aberrant expression pattern expected to be seen in high-grade serous carcinoma (p53 immunostain).

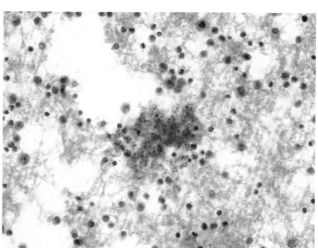

Figure 5.77. Granulosa cell tumor. Granulosa cell tumor often presents with a distinct cytomorphology: cells with elongated nuclei, powdery chromatin, and nuclear grooves. This pattern shares overlap with papillary thyroid carcinoma, which rarely is found metastatic to the peritoneal cavity (Pap stain).

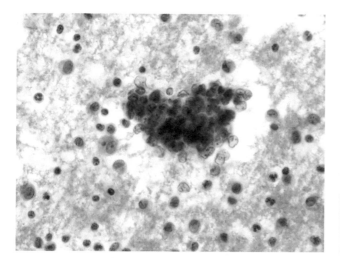

Figure 5.78. Granulosa cell tumor. Separate field. The neoplastic cells have irregular nuclear shapes and little cytoplasm and are haphazardly arranged and loosely cohesive within this fragment. These cells may have exfoliated directly from the tumor, and their presence in a washing specimen does not necessarily indicate the presence of metastatic deposits (Pap stain).

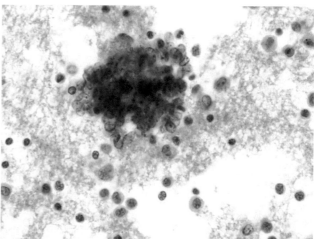

Figure 5.79. Granulosa cell tumor. Separate field (Pap stain).

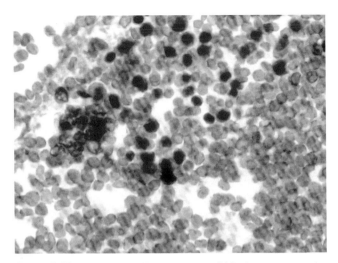

Figure 5.80. Granulosa cell tumor. On a cell block preparation, the granulosa cell tumor cells have similar morphology to what was seen in the Pap stained preparations (H&E).

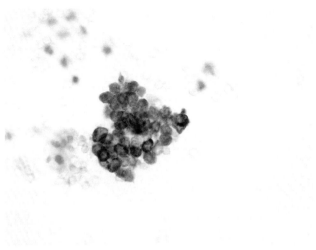

Figure 5.81. Granulosa cell tumor. Positive immunoreactivity for inhibin confirms the diagnosis (inhibin immunostain).

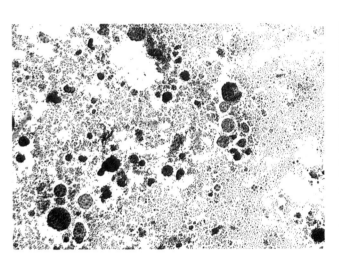

Figure 5.82. Clear cell adenocarcinoma. This patient had clear cell adenocarcinoma, which provided another example of malignant tumor cells forming "cannonballs" in a serous fluid specimen (Pap stain).

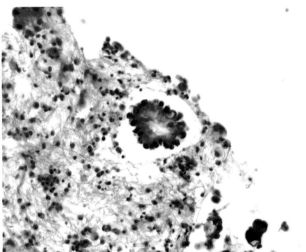

Figure 5.83. Metastatic endocervical adenocarcinoma. This patient had a prior invasive endocervical adenocarcinoma. The adenocarcinoma cells were not seen in the cytospin preparations but could be found on the cell block preparation. Note the presence of the retraction artifact (halo) around the malignant gland-forming cells, which are columnar and morphologically compatible with the patient's history (Pap stain).

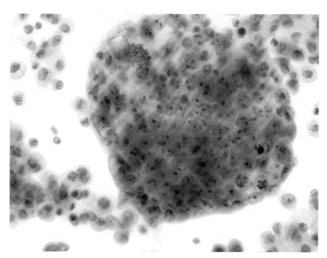

Figure 5.84. Metastatic colorectal adenocarcinoma. The cells in this large fragment have high nuclear to cytolasmic (N/C) ratios, anisonucleosis, irregular nuclear borders, and coarse chromatin. Several mitotic figures can be seen, one of which is highly atypical (Pap stain).

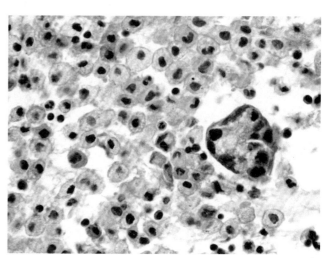

Figure 5.85. Metastatic colorectal adenocarcinoma. A cell block preparation of the same case shows a gland-forming fragment of cells with hyperchromasia, enlarged nuclei, and irregular nuclear borders in a background of predominantly histiocytes (H&E).

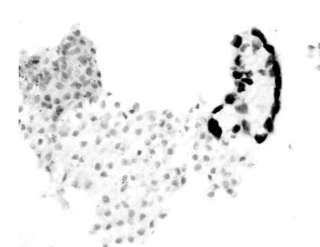

Figure 5.86. Metastatic colorectal adenocarcinoma. The atypical fragment demonstrates nuclear immunoreactivity for CDX2, a marker indicating gastrointestinal differentiation (CDX2 immunostain).

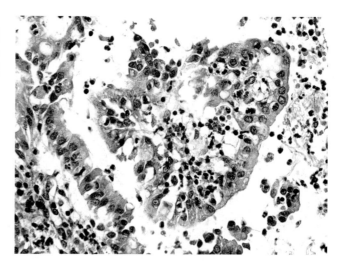

Figure 5.87. Metastatic colorectal adenocarcinoma. A cell block preparation from a different specimen containing a metastatic colorectal adenocarcinoma. The cells are columnar, gland forming, and associated with neutrophils owing to focal necrosis. These cytomorphologic features are suggestive of a colorectal adenocarcinoma (H&E).

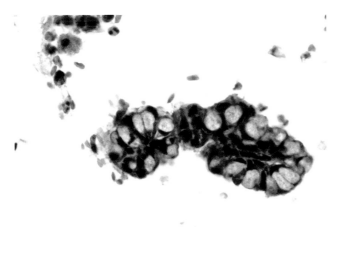

Figure 5.88. Metastatic mucinous adenocarcinoma. A cell block preparation from a separate case of a mucinous adenocarcinoma. The nuclei are hyperchromatic and have markedly irregular contours. When found in a serous effusion specimen, a gastrointestinal or pancreatobiliary primary site should be strongly considered (H&E).

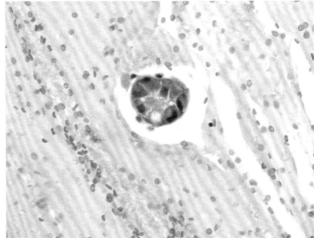

Figure 5.89. Metastatic clear cell renal cell carcinoma. The retraction artifact around this tissue fragment should cause concern for a metastatic carcinoma. The cells have abundant cytoplasm and large nuclei but do not possess specific cytomorphologic features for a site of origin (H&E).

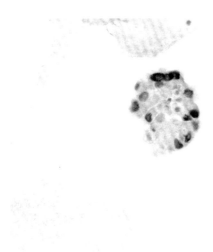

Figure 5.90. Metastatic clear cell renal cell carcinoma. Nuclear immunoreactivity for Pax-8 helped confirm the diagnosis in this patient with a distant history of renal cell carcinoma. In a female patient, Pax-8–positive malignancies may also arise from the gynecologic tract (Pax-8 immunostain).

SQUAMOUS CELL CARCINOMA

Squamous cell carcinoma rarely involves serous effusions but may gain access through direct invasion from an adjacent site (Figures 5.91 and 5.92). One clue aiding the identification of squamous cell carcinoma is the pink-orange color of keratin seen on Pap stained preparations. If keratinization cannot be identified, squamous immunomarkers (such as p40) can be used.[32] It is important to note that squamous differentiation does not indicate a definitive site of origin because squamous cell carcinoma can arise from the lung, cervix, and head and neck; additionally, some adenocarcinomas may undergo squamous differentiation. If the tumor cells are positive for human papillomavirus using ancillary studies (such as in situ hybridization), the site of origin includes the cervix, anus, or head and neck.[33-35]

TABLE 5.2: Neoplasms Associated With Certain Cytomorphologic Features

Cytomorphologic Feature	Suggested Neoplasms
Prominent nucleoli	Renal cell carcinoma Prostate carcinoma Melanoma Hepatocellular carcinoma
Squamous differentiation/keratinization	Squamous cell carcinoma Adenosquamous carcinoma
Gland formation	Adenocarcinoma Adenosquamous carcinoma
Hyperchromatic columnar cells with necrosis	Colorectal adenocarcinoma
Psammomatous calcification	Papillary thyroid carcinoma Neoplasms of Mullerian origin
Pigment	Melanoma Hepatocellular carcinoma
Intranuclear inclusions	Melanoma Papillary thyroid carcinoma
Clear cell features	Renal cell carcinoma Adrenal cortical carcinoma Melanoma
Small round blue cell tumor	Rhabdomyosarcoma Lymphoma Small cell carcinoma Ewing sarcoma Melanoma
Plasmacytoid dispersed cells	Melanoma Plasma cell neoplasm Poorly differentiated adenocarcinoma
Signet ring morphology	Lobular breast carcinoma Gastric adenocarcinoma

Modified From Cowan ML, VandenBussche CJ. Cancer of unknown primary: ancillary testing of cytologic and small biopsy specimens in the era of targeted therapy. *Cancer Cytopathol.* 2018;126:724-737.

NONCARCINOMA MALIGNANCIES

Other malignancies to involve the serous cavity include lymphoma, melanoma, and sarcoma, all of which typically present as a dispersed cell pattern rather than as tissue fragments (see the "'Fourth Cell' Population", below). For other unusual tumors, BerEP4 and MOC-31 expression may be unknown or absent. However, patients usually have a history of malignancy in these cases that can be confirmed if the cells demonstrate a similar immunoprofile and/or cytomorphology. Comparison with previous specimens containing the primary tumor, if available, can be helpful.

NEOPLASTIC IMPLANTS

Neoplasms can form noninvasive implants on the surface of serous cavities and subsequently involve a serous effusion (Figures 5.93 and 5.94). This phenomenon is not infrequent in the peritoneal cavity, where implanted low-grade or borderline serous tumors from the gynecologic tract can form a cellular specimen containing atypical cells. Therefore, caution should be exerted when using the term "metastatic" in peritoneal cavity specimens from female patients, especially when a history of malignancy has not been established or a history of a gynecologic tract neoplasm is known, as gynecologic tract neoplasms are known to form noninvasive

TABLE 5.3: Suggested Markers to Investigate a Cancer OF Unknown Primary

Suggested Priority Marker	Possible Site(s) of Origin	Confirmatory Marker(s)
TTF-1	Lung (87%)	Napsin-A
	Thyroid (63%)	Thyroglobulin (follicular cell origin); PAX-8
GATA-3	Breast (60%)	Mammaglobin; GCDFP-15; ER
	Urothelial (78%)	Uroplakin III; p40 (rule out SqCCa)
PAX-8	Renal (89%)	CD10; RCC
	Thyroid	TTF-1; thyroglobulin (follicular cell origin)
	Gynecologic (Mullerian) (>87%, ovary)	WT-1; ER; diffuse p53 if serous carcinoma
P40 (P63)	Urothelial (61%, p63)	GATA-3; Uroplakin III
	Squamous cell carcinoma	HPV (human papillomavirus) studies if HPV-related
CDX2*	Pancreatobiliary and gastrointestinal tracts (lower > upper)	CK20 (lower tract); SATB2 (lower tract); CK7 (upper tract)
NKX3.1	Prostate (99%)	PSA (99%); PSAP (94%)
DPC4 (SMAD4)	Pancreatic ductal adenocarcinoma and intrahepatic cholangiocarcinoma	Lost in 50%
SALL4	Germ cell tumor (less so in immature teratoma and choriocarcinoma) (100%)	Germ cell panel
HepPar1	Hepatocellular carcinoma	Glypican; arginase
Calretinin	Mesothelioma	WT-1; mesothelioma ancillary studies

Modified from Cowan ML, VandenBussche CJ. Cancer of unknown primary: ancillary testing of cytologic and small biopsy specimens in the era of targeted therapy. *Cancer Cytopathol.* 2018;126:724-737.

implants. For Mullerian tumors, invasion of a serous cavity surface cannot be determined by cytology alone, and serous cavity cytology specimens should be diagnosed as "involved by" a neoplasm rather than using the term "metastatic." Neoplasms of Mullerian origin (e.g., the ovary, fallopian tube, and uterus) are often positive for the Pax-8 immunomarker; if Pax-8 is negative, then further immunostains should be used to exclude other primary sites, such as the gastrointestinal tract.[36] Finally, because endometriosis and endosalpingiosis are also Pax-8 positive, these entities should also be excluded (see below).

MESOTHELIOMA

Historically, the definitive diagnosis of malignant mesothelioma has relied on histological features such as tissue invasion, nodular proliferation, and full-thickness involvement of the pleura as opposed to cytological features. Mesothelioma can take many forms, but cells in effusion specimens tend to appear epithelioid rather than spindled (Figures 5.95-5.105). When present as tissue fragments, mesothelioma may form spherical structures ("cannonballs") containing "ground substance" material consisting of hyaluronic acid (rather than

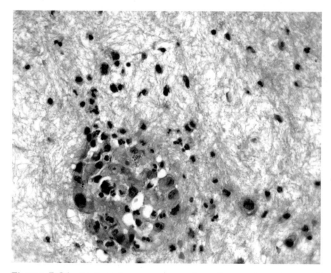

Figure 5.91. Metastatic squamous cell carcinoma. Squamous cell carcinoma rarely involves serous fluid specimens. In this rare case, the patient had a history of primary lung squamous cell carcinoma which involved the pleural fluid (H&E).

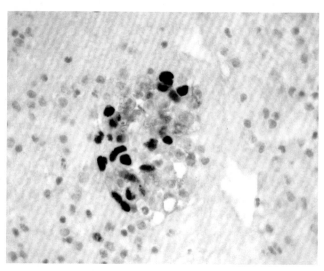

Figure 5.92. Metastatic squamous cell carcinoma. A p63 immunostain was performed on the same specimen, and the carcinoma cells demonstrated nuclear immunoreactivity, confirming squamous differentiation. A pitfall in this interpretation is that adenocarcinomas may sometimes undergo squamous differentiation and become immunoreactive for squamous markers (p63 immunostain).

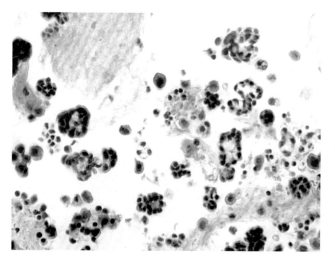

Figure 5.93. Low-grade serous carcinoma. This patient had a primary ovarian low-grade serous carcinoma which was found in the peritoneal washings taken concurrently during surgical removal. The patient was also found to have noninvasive implants within the peritoneal cavity (H&E).

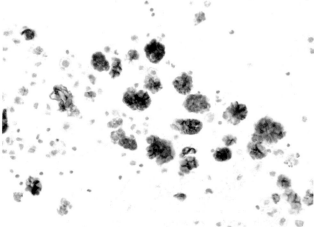

Figure 5.94. Low-grade serous carcinoma. The prior low-grade serous carcinoma was positive for BerEP4. BerEP4 positivity confirms an epithelial origin but does not determine that the positive cells are neoplastic, malignant, or invasive. One must rely on clinical history, cytomorphology, additional ancillary studies, and/or histologic examination to further characterize BerEP4 positive cells (BerEP4 immunostain).

the glands of adenocarcinoma which may contain mucin). Mesothelioma may also form three-dimensional, rigid, branching structures with bulbous ends, which appear distinct from the benign monolayer fragments seen in washing specimens.[37] Mesothelioma may maintain the classic cytomorphologic features of benign mesothelial cells, in which case it must be differentiated from a proliferation of reactive mesothelial cells and mesothelial hyperplasia. This cytomorphologic overlap can be a diagnostic dilemma; as a result, some cytopathologists feel that mesothelioma cannot be definitively diagnosed on a serous cavity effusion specimen alone.

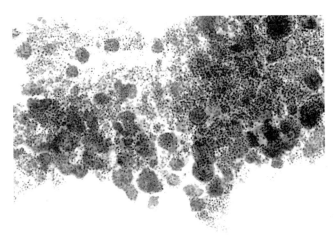

Figure 5.95. Mesothelioma. Mesothelioma may also present as "cannonballs" in a serous fluid specimen, although metastatic breast ductal carcinoma is classically associated with this pattern (Pap stain).

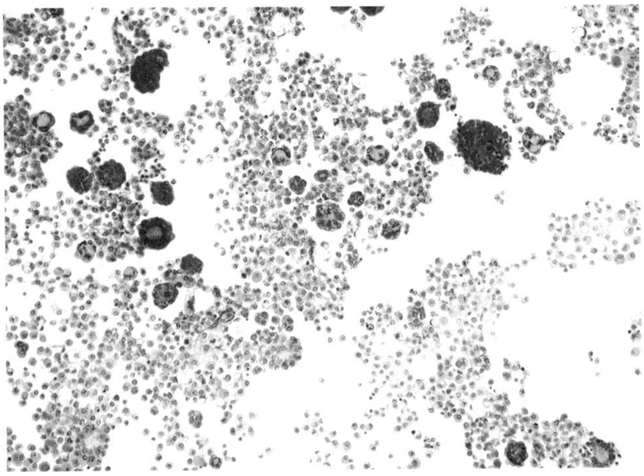

Figure 5.96. Mesothelioma. The mesothelioma cells in this specimen form small spherical structures, some containing central cyan-staining areas which may be mistaken for the gland formation of an adenocarcinoma (Pap stain).

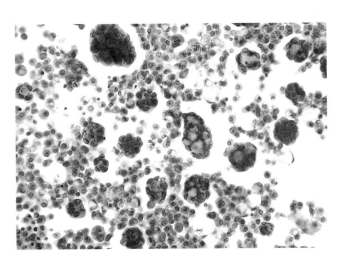

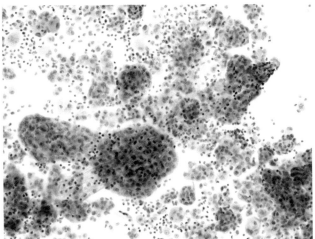

Figure 5.97. Mesothelioma. Separate field at higher magnification (Pap stain).

Figure 5.98. Mesothelioma. This mesothelioma is forming large structures with irregular bulbous projections, another common presentation of mesothelioma in a serous fluid. The cells contain deceiving bland nuclei, which have little size variation, and nuclear to cytoplasmic (N/C) ratios are not concerning. The differential diagnosis includes benign mesothelial hyperplasia (Pap stain).

Currently, the most helpful ancillary tests include the BAP1 immunostain, a specific but insensitive marker whereby loss of nuclear expression is seen in approximately 60% of malignant mesotheliomas, and p16 fluorescence in situ hybridization (FISH), as the homozygous loss of p16 is seen in some mesotheliomas.[38-41] Other common markers used include EMA, desmin, and p53 with the following pattern favoring mesothelioma: EMA diffuse positivity, desmin negative, and increased nuclear p53 expression.[42] In other instances, the cytomorphologic features of mesothelial origin may be lost, in which case mesothelioma must be differentiated from an adenocarcinoma. This distinction is best accomplished by assessing for the positive expression of mesothelial markers (such as calretinin and WT-1) and the absence of epithelial markers (such as BerEP4 or MOC-31).

SAMPLE NOTE: MALIGNANT MESOTHELIOMA

Malignant mesothelioma. See note.

Note: The specimen is highly cellular and contains numerous mesothelial cells in three-dimensional fragments and present singly. The mesothelial cells are enlarged and have prominent nucleoli. Immunohistochemical studies show that the mesothelial cells are positive for calretinin and negative for BerEP4. In addition, BAP-1 staining is lost in the mesothelial cells and retained in background benign cells. These findings are consistent with a malignant mesothelioma.

Reference:
Hwang HC, Sheffield BS, Rodriguez S, et al. Utility of BAP1 immunohistochemistry and p16 (CDKN2A) FISH in the diagnosis of malignant mesothelioma in effusion cytology specimens. *Am J Surg Pathol.* 2016;40(1):120-126.

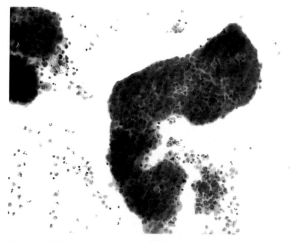

Figure 5.99. Mesothelioma. The mesothelial cells form a cellular papillary fragment; the cells are dark, have irregular nuclear borders, and high nuclear to cytoplasmic (N/C) ratios. A neoplastic process is favored, and adenocarcinoma should be excluded; however, this architecture should cause concern for mesothelioma (Pap stain).

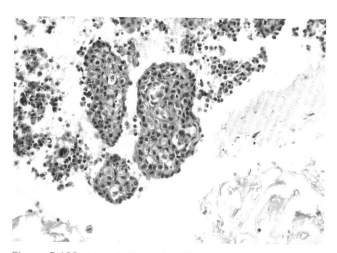

Figure 5.100. Mesothelioma. A cell block preparation of the previous case demonstrates papillary tissue fragments containing cells with irregular nuclei. Without a known history or clinical suspicion for mesothelioma, the odds would incorrectly favor an adenocarcinoma rather than a mesothelioma (H&E).

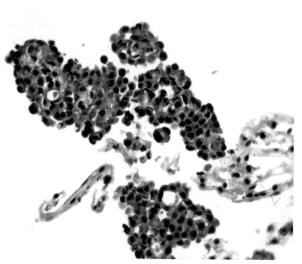

Figure 5.101. Mesothelioma. A separate case of mesothelioma with prominent papillary architecture in the cell block material. Note the hyperchromasia, irregular nuclear borders, and anisonucleosis (H&E).

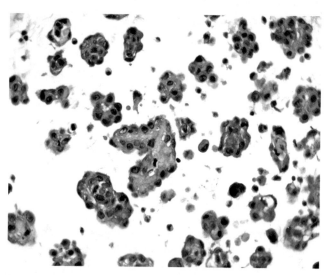

Figure 5.102. Mesothelioma. Separate field (H&E).

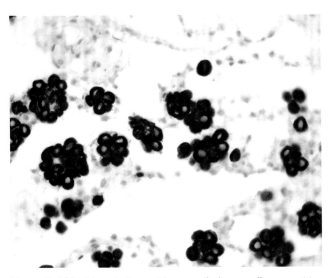

Figure 5.103. Mesothelioma. The mesothelioma cells are positive for CK5/6, a nonspecific finding that favors mesothelioma over an adenocarcinoma (CK5/6 immunostain).

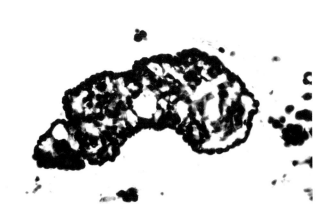

Figure 5.104. Mesothelioma. Strong nuclear and cytoplasmic positivity for calretinin, as seen here, is uncommon in metastatic adenocarcinoma and strongly favors a mesothelioma (calretinin immunostain).

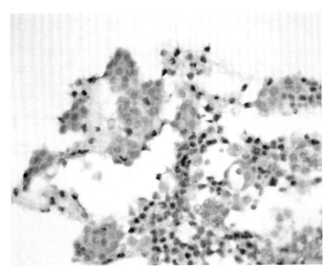

Figure 5.105. Mesothelioma. The nuclear loss of BAP-1 (as seen here in the larger atypical cells) has been shown to be highly specific, but not sensitive, for mesothelioma. The presence of positive nuclear staining in benign bystander cells (seen here) is important to establish as a positive control before providing a definitive diagnosis of mesothelioma (BAP-1 immunostain).

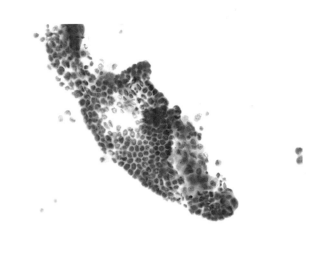

Figure 5.106. Benign mesothelial proliferation. This irregularly shaped fragment of mesothelial cells was found in a serous fluid specimen. While the nuclei are organized within the fragment and no overt features of malignancy can be seen, mesothelioma can often have a deceiving bland appearance and cannot be entirely excluded (Pap stain).

BENIGN MESOTHELIAL PROLIFERATION

Mesothelial cells may proliferate in response to various pathologic processes, and foci of mesothelial hyperplasia may be seen on serous cavity surfaces. These proliferations can result in the presence of numerous mesothelial cells in a serous effusion, sometimes with striking reactive atypia (Figures 5.106-5.111). Once the cells are confirmed as mesothelial in origin with a mesothelial immunomarker, mesothelioma should be excluded through morphologic assessment and/or ancillary studies. If the atypia seen remains concerning and ancillary studies cannot confirm mesothelioma, an indeterminate diagnosis may be the best course of action.

FAQ: Is this mesothelioma or a benign proliferation?

Answer: In the past, the diagnosis of mesothelioma on a fluid specimen was controversial. The availability of two tests with excellent positive predictive values (p16 FISH and BAP1 immunohistochemistry) can increase the confidence of a mesothelioma diagnosis. However, these ancillary tests are not available in most laboratories and rely on an adequate amount of cellularity in a given specimen. Furthermore, even if both tests can be performed, they can both be negative in a fraction of mesothelioma cases. In instances where ancillary tests cannot confirm mesothelioma, a diagnosis of mesothelioma should be made with caution. Other markers have been used to help distinguish reactive mesothelial cells from mesothelioma but lack sensitivity and/or specificity to allow for a definitive diagnosis. For instance, strong nuclear staining for p53, staining with EMA, and/or negative staining for desmin favor mesothelioma.[42] Reactive mesothelial proliferations may yield cellular specimens with markedly atypical mesothelial cells. Specimens containing overtly malignant cells expressing mesothelial markers may be diagnosed as mesothelioma if consistent with the clinicoradiologic impression. Otherwise, a diagnosis of "atypical mesothelial cell proliferation" or "markedly atypical mesothelial cells, suspicious for mesothelioma" should be made.

SAMPLE NOTE: ATYPICAL MESOTHELIAL PROLIFERATION

Atypical mesothelial proliferation. See note.

Note: The specimen contains numerous mesothelial tissue fragments that form irregular, bulbous projections. In addition, atypical cytomorphologic features, such as the presence of prominent nucleoli, can be seen. While these fragments may represent a benign proliferation of mesothelial cells, mesothelioma cannot be entirely excluded. The material is insufficient for further characterization. Please correlate with clinicoradiologic impression; additional sampling may provide material for confirmatory ancillary tests.

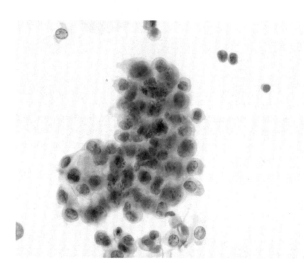

Figure 5.107. Benign mesothelial proliferation. The mesothelial cells have abundant two-tone cytoplasm, common for a mesothelial origin. The nuclei have size variation and some nuclear border irregularities, suggesting the possibility of a mesothelioma, but clinical suspicion was low (Pap stain).

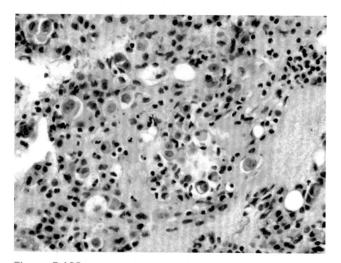

Figure 5.108. Benign mesothelial proliferation. A separate fluid specimen containing numerous enlarged mesothelial cells with prominent nucleoli and binucleation. The abundant, two-tone cytoplasm suggests a mesothelial origin for these cells. Additional workup did not favor a mesothelioma in this patient, and thus these cells were most likely reactive in nature (H&E).

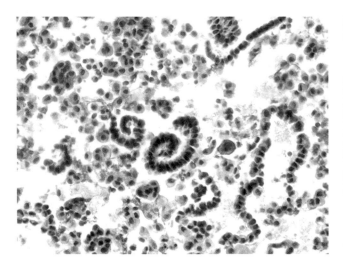

Figure 5.109. Benign mesothelial cells. The specimen contains numerous strips of cells. Given the cellularity of the specimen and lack of any other explanation for the patient's pleural effusion, a workup was conducted (H&E).

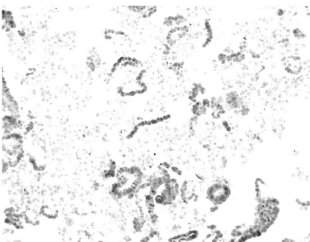

Figure 5.110. Benign mesothelial cells. A calretinin immunostain, positive in both the cytoplasm and nuclei of the atypical cells, helped prove a mesothelial origin and exclude a metastatic adenocarcinoma (calretinin immunostain).

Figure 5.111. Benign mesothelial cells. EMA has been shown to be a sensitive but not specific stain for mesothelioma; most mesotheliomas in fluid specimens are positive for EMA. The negative staining for EMA in this specimen, in addition to the low clinical suspicion for mesothelioma, resulted in a diagnosis of reactive mesothelial cells (EMA immunostain).

ENDOSALPINGIOSIS

Endosalpingiosis is the presence of fallopian tube tissue located outside of the fallopian tubes. This tissue may be present on serous cavity surfaces and shed primarily as small fragments into the fluid. Fallopian tube epithelium may also shed directly into the fluid; however, the distinction with regard to origin cannot be determined in a serous cavity cytologic specimen. The cells are usually columnar with bland nuclear features (Figures 5.112-5.118). When identifiable, a ciliated brush border present on the fragments is highly indicative of their benign nature. When cilia are absent, the cells may be mistaken for a neoplasm of Mullerian origin because they share a similar immunoprofile. In the absence of a known or suspected neoplasm, bland-appearing glandular cells can be noted but should not be overinterpreted as a neoplasm.

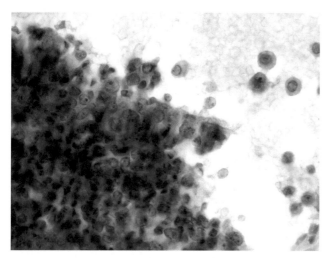

Figure 5.112. Endosalpingiosis. Ciliated epithelial cells may arise from endosalpingiosis or exfoliated from the fallopian tube. While the tissue fragment seen here contains nuclei with markedly irregular borders, the fragment edge is ciliated, and thus the fragment should be dismissed as benign (Pap stain).

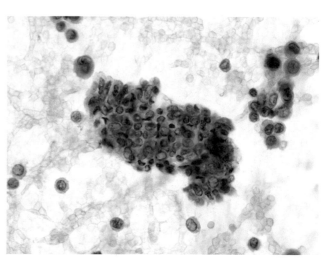

Figure 5.113. Endosalpingiosis. A separate field showing atypical cells associated with columnar cells at the top left edge. While cilia are difficult to identify in this specimen, the columnar cells appear to have a terminal bar and thus the atypia seen should be interpreted with caution. It additionally helps that separate fields (Figure 5.112) contained similar cells with identifiable cilia (Pap stain).

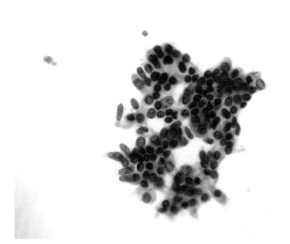

Figure 5.114. Endosalpingiosis. A different specimen containing columnar cells with elongated, bland nuclei and regular nuclear borders. Cilia can be seen attached to some of the cells (Pap stain).

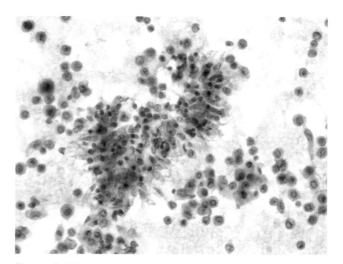

Figure 5.115. Endosalpingiosis. Another fluid specimen containing endosalpingiosis. In this case, the cells are bland and columnar, but cilia are not readily identified. If a workup is undertaken, the cells would be positive for ER, Pax-8, and BerEP4, possibly falsely leading one to a diagnosis of a gynecologic neoplasm (or worse, malignancy!) (Pap stain).

SAMPLE NOTE: BLAND-APPEARING GLANDULAR CELLS

Bland-appearing glandular cells in a background of reactive mesothelial cells, histiocytes, and lymphocytes. Negative for carcinoma. See note.

Note: The patient's high-grade serous carcinoma is noted. Given the bland nature of the glandular cells seen in the peritoneal washing specimen, they are favored to represent a benign process, such as endosalpingiosis.

SAMPLE NOTE: ENDOSALPINGIOSIS

Endosalpingiosis. Background reactive mesothelial cells, histiocytes, and lymphocytes. No malignant neoplasm identified. See note.

Note: Several small fragments of benign-appearing ciliated glandular cells are seen in the specimen. The findings are consistent with endosalpingiosis.

SAMPLE NOTE: ATYPICAL CELLS OF MULLERIAN ORIGIN

Atypical glandular cells of Mullerian origin. See note.

Note: Rare atypical glandular cells are identified. Immunohistochemical studies identify the cells to be positive for BerEP4 and Pax-8 and negative for calretinin. The cells are wild-type for p53. This immunoprofile supports a Mullerian origin. While the atypical cells are favored to represent a benign process, such as endosalpingiosis, involvement by a gynecologic neoplasm cannot be completely excluded.

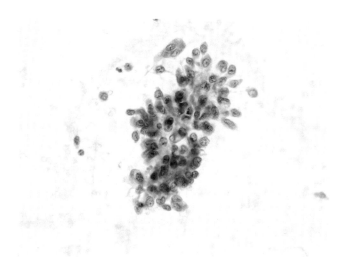

Figure 5.116. Endosalpingiosis. Separate field (Pap stain).

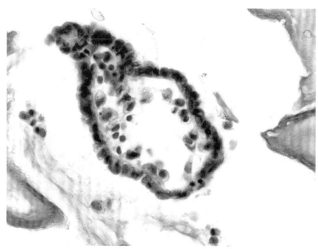

Figure 5.117. Endosalpingiosis. A cell block preparation of the same specimen shows a fragment of columnar cells; several cells are ciliated (H&E).

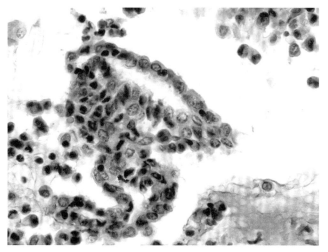

Figure 5.118. Endosalpingiosis. A separate field at higher magnification allows for better identification of terminal bars and cilia (H&E).

ENDOMETRIOSIS

Endometriosis is the presence of endometrial tissue outside of the endometrium. When present on serous cavity surfaces, endometrial cells may shed into the fluid and have a similar appearance to endometrial cells on a liquid-based Pap test (Figures 5.119-5.121). They typically present as small three-dimensional spheres of tightly packed hyperchromatic cells with little cytoplasm. The spheres have a scalloped or hobnailed border. The appearance of the endometrial cells may change depending on the patient's hormonal state. Endometrial cells are often accompanied by blood, which is most often seen as degenerated red blood cells and fibrin or as hemosiderin-laden macrophages. In some instances, degenerated blood and fibrin may be prominent, and the endometrial cells may not be seen. Endometriosis shares a similar immunoprofile as endosalpingiosis, given their common Mullerian origin.

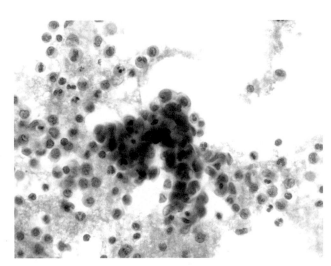

Figure 5.119. Endometriosis. Endometriosis appears similarly to benign endometrial cells on a Pap test. The cells have high nuclear to cytoplasmic (N/C) ratios, appear hyperchromatic, and form clusters with hobnailed edges. These cells may be mistaken for an adenocarcinoma. The background often contains degenerated blood and/or fibrin, a helpful clue (Pap stain).

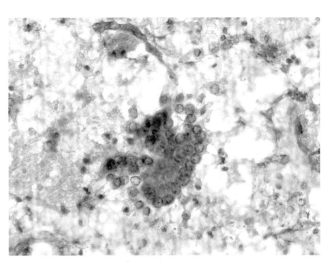

Figure 5.120. Endometriosis. These endometrial cells have high nuclear to cytoplasmic (N/C) ratios, but their chromatin is bland, they have regular nuclear contours, and their nuclei have little size variation. The background is bloody with mostly intact red blood cells, although a traumatic tap could also result in such a background (Pap stain).

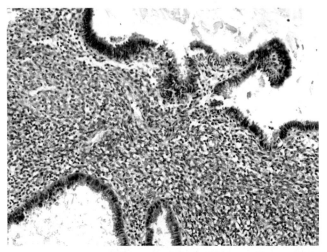

Figure 5.121. Endometriosis. A large fragment of endometriosis was found in cell block material and has similar morphology to secretory endometrium on histology (H&E).

"FOURTH CELL" POPULATION PATTERN

The "fourth cell" population is a population of dispersed cells that differ cytomorphologically from the three cell populations usually seen in a serous cavity specimen (i.e. histiocytes, mesothelial cells, and lymphocytes). The fourth cell population may be overtly malignant and, therefore, diagnostic of metastatic disease when the patient has a known malignancy. If the patient does not have a known malignancy, immunostains may be performed on additionally prepared unstained slides or cell block material to help uncover a site of origin. In some instances, the "fourth cell" population has atypical cytomorphologic features and may represent either a neoplasm or a reactive process. In this case, immunostains specific for mesothelial cells (such as calretinin), histiocytes (such as CD68), and/or epithelial cells (such as MOC-31 or BerEP4) can be performed to better characterize the atypical cells. Finally, a "fourth cell" population may blend in with histiocytes or mesothelial cells and only become apparent once stains are performed.

CHECKLIST: Etiologic Considerations for the "Fourth Cell" Pattern

☐ Metastatic Malignant Neoplasm with Markedly Atypical Cells

☐ "Hidden" Metastatic Malignancy

☐ Neoplastic Implants

☐ Reactive Mesothelial Cells

☐ Mesothelioma

METASTATIC MALIGNANT NEOPLASM WITH MARKEDLY ATYPICAL CELLS

Malignancies may metastasize from various primary sites, with some primary sites being more common in certain serous cavities.[43] For instance, lung adenocarcinoma is the most common metastatic malignancy seen in pleural effusions (Figures 5.122 and 5.123). Carcinomas tend to form fragments rather than dispersed individual cells, but any poorly differentiated carcinoma can present as a single cell dispersed pattern (Figures 5.124-5.133). Other malignancies that may exist predominantly as dispersed cells in serous cavity specimens include melanoma, lobular breast carcinoma, small cell carcinoma and other neoplasms with neuroendocrine differentiation, signet ring

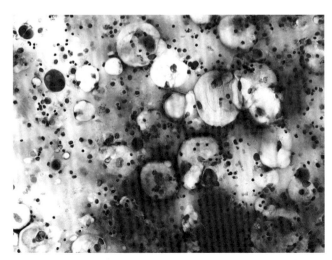

Figure 5.122. Metastatic lung adenocarcinoma. The specimen contains malignant cells which dwarf the surrounding, much smaller mesothelial cells, histiocytes, and lymphocytes. This is an extreme example of overtly malignant cells involving a serous cavity specimen (Diff-Quik stain).

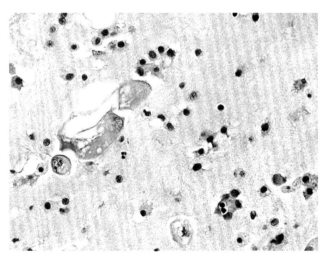

Figure 5.123. Metastatic lung adenocarcinoma. Several enlarged malignant cells have a similar appearance to those seen on the previous preparation (Figure 5.122). It is easy to determine that these cells are malignant, but their cytomorphology provides little clue as to their site of origin (H&E).

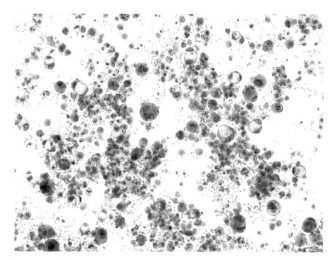

Figure 5.124. Metastatic adenocarcinoma. A separate case of a metastatic adenocarcinoma (primary site undetermined) to a pleural fluid specimen. The cells are present predominantly as single cells and also as cell-in-cell structures. Their cytoplasmic vacuolization is further evidence of their glandular nature (Pap stain).

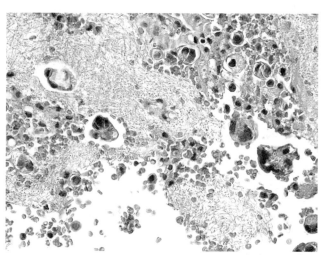

Figure 5.125. Metastatic adenocarcinoma. A cell block preparation of the same case shows single cells and small cellular clusters, some with the retraction artifact that helps identify malignant cells in such preparations. The cells are large and have large, dark nuclei with irregular borders and are therefore easily identifiable as malignant (H&E).

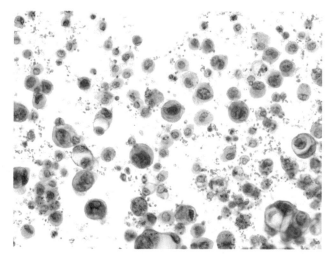

Figure 5.126. Metastatic signet ring adenocarcinoma. This adenocarcinoma has involved the fluid specimen predominantly as single cells rather than forming tissue fragments. Some cells have large mucinous vacuoles which have compressed the nucleus, forming a "signet ring" morphology. In some instances, signet ring cells may blend in with mesothelial cells and histiocytes, but in this case, the cells are too large and their nuclei are too atypical to be benign (Pap stain).

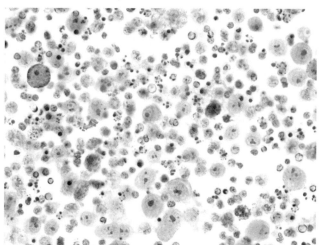

Figure 5.127. Metastatic melanoma. Melanoma often presents as a dispersed population of cells with abundant cytoplasm, eccentrically placed nuclei, and prominent nucleoli. While this cytomorphology is not specific for melanoma, in this case several cells contain green and brown-staining melanin pigment, and the diagnosis can be made even without a history (Pap stain).

cell carcinomas (usually arising from the gastrointestinal tract), lymphomas, and sarcomas.[44-49] While neoplasms tend to retain their original morphology at the serous cavity surface, exfoliated cells floating in serous fluid may appear different. For instance, spindled cells may become more epithelioid once detached from the serous cavity surface.

If the cells are overtly malignant and morphologically consistent with a history of a given malignancy, the specimen can be considered diagnostic. In other cases, immunostains can be performed to confirm a known malignancy or as a workup of a CUP (Table 5.3). If the cells are of indeterminate nature, an initial immunostain workup may begin with calretinin and either BerEP4 or MOC-31, which in most cases will

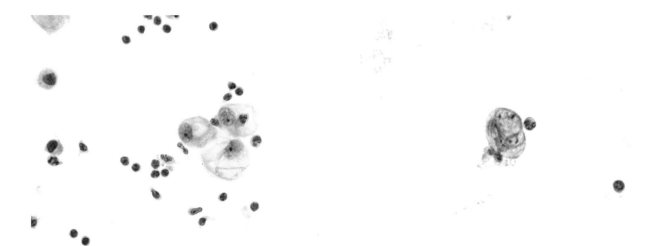

Figure 5.128. Metastatic high-grade serous carcinoma (HGSC). HGSC cells often have abundant, vacuolated cytoplasm. These cells also have enlarged nucleoli and large nuclei, and the cells are much larger than the bystander inflammatory cells in the background (Pap stain).

Figure 5.129. Metastatic high-grade serous carcinoma (HGSC). This highly atypical, multinucleated carcinoma cell was found in a separate case of metastatic HGSC. Compare the cell size with that of the adjacent neutrophil. While this cell has sufficient atypia to be considered malignant, the features are not specific to determine a site of origin (Pap stain).

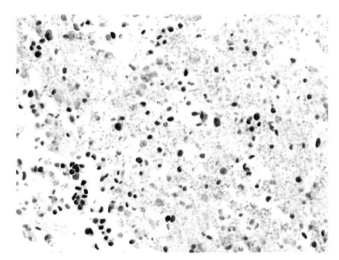
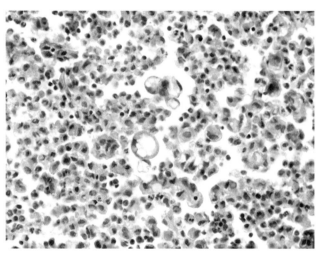

Figure 5.130. Metastatic high-grade serous carcinoma (HGSC). Diffuse nuclear positivity for p53 in ascites and peritoneal washing specimens is most indicative of a HGSC (and, less likely, a clear cell carcinoma). Determining whether p53 is diffuse in a population of singly dispersed carcinoma cells is challenging, as negative staining cells may be missed on the counterstain (p53 immunostain).

Figure 5.131. Metastatic signet ring adenocarcinoma (colorectal origin). Several overtly malignant cells can be seen in this cell block preparation, some with a "signet ring" morphology. This patient had a recent history of invasive colorectal adenocarcinoma (H&E).

identify the cells as mesothelial in origin (calretinin positive) or epithelial in origin (BerEP4 or MOC-31 positive). Cells of mesothelial origin are likely reactive mesothelial cells once mesothelioma is excluded (see "Mesothelioma" under the "Tissue Fragments Pattern"). Cells of epithelial origin may represent benign and subclinical proliferations (such as endosalpingiosis), low-grade neoplasms implanted on a cavity surface (such as a borderline serous tumor), or a metastatic carcinoma (see "Metastatic Adenocarcinoma" under the "Tissue Fragments Pattern"). Unusual tumors, such as sarcomas, may not stain with BerEP4 or MOC-31 and may require additional specific stains for identification. However, in most instances patients will have a known history of disease, which can help aid the workup.

"HIDDEN" METASTATIC MALIGNANCY

Some malignancies are bland-appearing and may appear as a dispersed group of cells that closely resemble reactive mesothelial cells or histiocytes, especially at low magnification (Figures 5.134-5.141). Even at high magnification, the cells may be difficult to identify as a "fourth cell" population. The malignancies that fall into this category usually exist as monotonous dispersed cells with round, regular nuclei, only mild pleomorphism, and ample cytoplasm. Common examples include melanoma, lobular breast carcinoma, and adenocarcinomas with signet ring morphology. Upon immunostaining with specific markers, the "fourth population" becomes obvious. For this reason, it is important to create cell block material and perform immunostains in patients with a history of any of these malignancies.

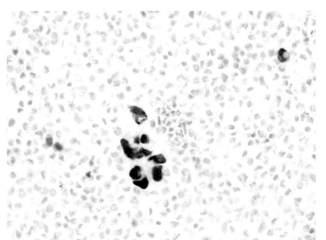

Figure 5.132. Metastatic signet ring adenocarcinoma (colorectal origin). Nuclear positivity for CDX2 helps establish a gastrointestinal (GI) origin. It is more likely to be positive in the lower GI tract but provides sufficient coverage for upper tract and pancreatobiliary primary adenocarcinomas (CDX2 immunostain).

Figure 5.133. Metastatic signet ring adenocarcinoma (colorectal origin). CK20 positivity in a serous fluid most often suggests a lower gastrointestinal tract primary site, especially when CDX2 is also positive (CK20 immunostain).

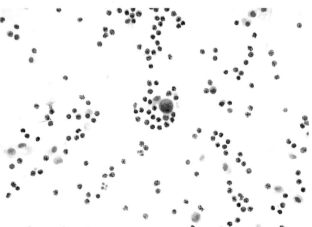
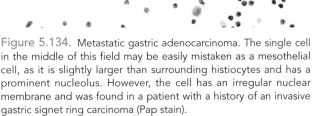

Figure 5.134. Metastatic gastric adenocarcinoma. The single cell in the middle of this field may be easily mistaken as a mesothelial cell, as it is slightly larger than surrounding histiocytes and has a prominent nucleolus. However, the cell has an irregular nuclear membrane and was found in a patient with a history of an invasive gastric signet ring carcinoma (Pap stain).

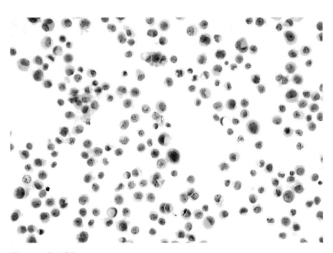

Figure 5.135. Metastatic lobular breast carcinoma. Lobular breast carcinoma can easily be missed in a serous fluid specimen. The cells are singly dispersed and small enough to mimic mesothelial cells. In this case, some histiocytes with curved nuclei can be seen. The majority of the background cells are malignant (Pap stain).

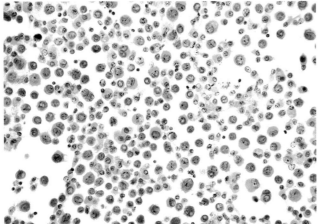

Figure 5.136. Metastatic lobular breast carcinoma. In this separate specimen of metastatic lobular breast carcinoma, the majority of cells present are malignant. The cells have eccentrically placed nuclei and coarse chromatin. Some have irregular nuclear borders and high nuclear to cytoplasmic (N/C) ratios (Pap stain).

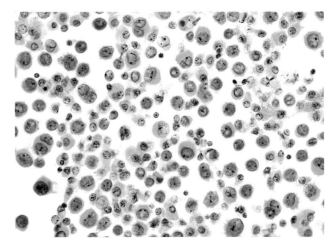

Figure 5.137. Metastatic lobular breast carcinoma. A higher magnification allows better appreciation of the malignant cells' atypical features. Cursory examination at low magnification may not be sufficient in such a specimen (Pap stain).

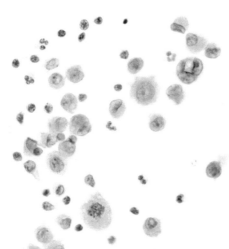

Figure 5.138. Metastatic lobular breast carcinoma. A different specimen containing lobular breast carcinoma. Some of the features present (multinucleation, prominent nucleoli, and mitotic activity) can also be seen in a reactive mesothelial cell population, which is why the creation of cell block material for ancillary studies is important in serous fluid specimens (Pap stain).

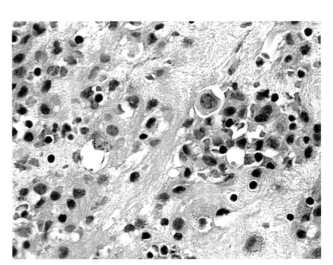

Figure 5.139. Metastatic lobular breast carcinoma. The cell block material created from the same specimen shows several atypical cells, but it is difficult to exclude a population of reactive mesothelial cells without ancillary studies (H&E).

NEOPLASTIC IMPLANTS

Neoplasms can form noninvasive implants on the surface of serous cavities and subsequently involve a serous effusion predominantly as single cells (Figures 5.142 and 5.143). These implants may be invasive or noninvasive and arise from a borderline or malignant neoplasm (discussed further in the "Tissue Fragments Pattern").

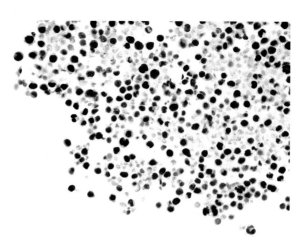

Figure 5.140. Metastatic lobular breast carcinoma. Mammaglobin demonstrates nuclear immunoreactivity in these cells, confirming involvement by the patient's known breast carcinoma. If a history of cancer is unknown, it is best to start with a less specific epithelial marker, such as BerEP4 or MOC-31 (mammaglobin immunostain).

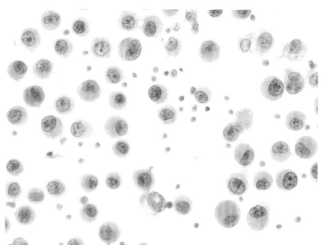

Figure 5.141. Signet ring adenocarcinoma (origin unknown). The specimen appears to contain two populations of cells—lymphocytes and larger cells with abundant cytoplasm. This population may be difficult to identify as foreign when normal histiocytes and mesothelial cells are not found in the background. However, the cells are very large and have nuclear membrane irregularities and coarse chromatin, findings which together are convincing for malignancy (Pap stain).

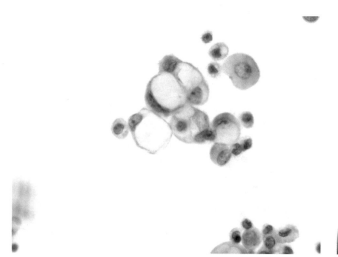

Figure 5.142. Borderline serous tumor. Benign processes as well as processes of uncertain malignant potential can also present as a "fourth" population of single cells in a fluid specimen. In this case, the patient had noninvasive implants from a borderline serous tumor. The tumor cells have vacuolated cytoplasm and small nucleoli, but their nuclear contours are regular. These cells would be positive for BerEP4, Pax-8, and ER and negative for calretinin but do not necessarily represent a malignant process (Pap stain).

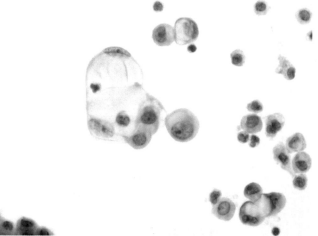

Figure 5.143. Borderline serous tumor. Separate field (Pap stain).

MESOTHELIOMA

Mesothelioma can exist as a dispersed population of markedly atypical cells distinct from the background of reactive mesothelial cells (Figures 5.144-5.155). The cells should be negative for epithelial markers (BerEP4, MOC-31) and positive for mesothelial markers (calretinin). To exclude the possibility of a reactive mesothelial cell proliferation, it is recommended to follow the workup for mesothelioma (discussed in the "Tissue Fragments Pattern").

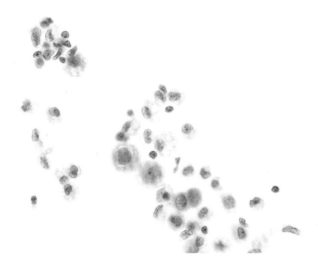

Figure 5.144. Mesothelioma. This patient had an increased number of large mesothelial cells in a pleural fluid specimen, raising suspicion for a mesothelioma, which was later confirmed. However, the mesothelioma cells seen are not overtly malignant and could easily represent a reactive mesothelial population (Pap stain).

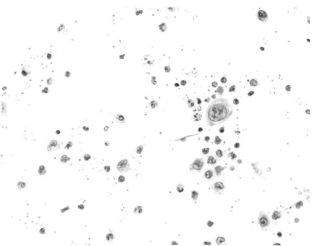

Figure 5.145. Mesothelioma. A separate field shows a single mesothelioma cell that is significantly larger than other cells in the field (Pap stain).

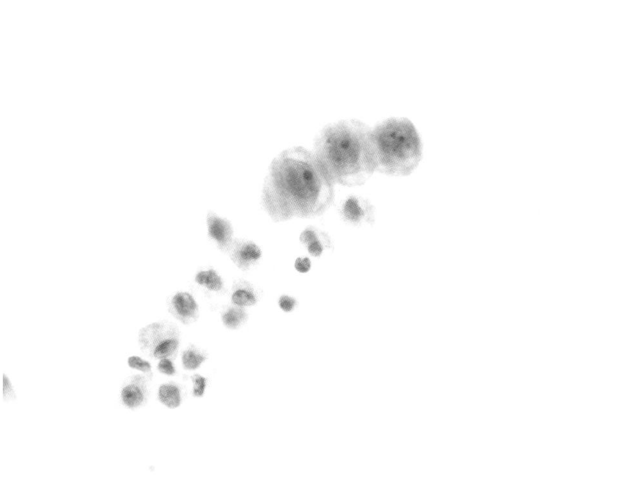

Figure 5.146. Mesothelioma. A separate field with three atypical mesothelial cells with nucleolar prominence (Pap stain).

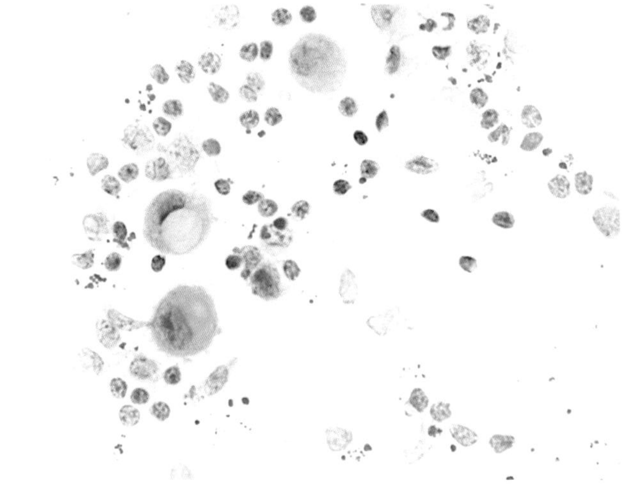

Figure 5.147. Mesothelioma. The mesothelial cells in this specimen "stand out" from the background cells, as they are much larger and have big nuclei. It is difficult to exclude a reactive mesothelial process using cytomorphology alone (Pap stain).

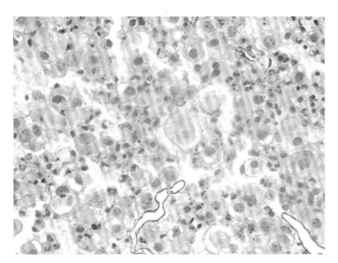

Figure 5.148. Mesothelioma. A cell block preparation of the same case shows a mixture of mesothelioma and background cells. The mesothelioma cells are larger and have prominent nucleoli (H&E).

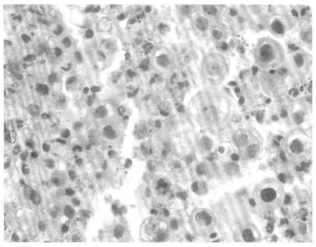

Figure 5.149. Mesothelioma. Separate field (H&E).

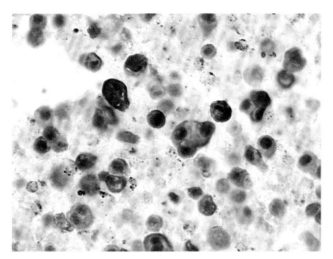

Figure 5.150. Mesothelioma. A calretinin stain highlights the mesothelial cells in the specimen, which are increased in number which suggests at least a reactive population of mesothelial cells and possibly a mesothelioma (calretinin immunostain).

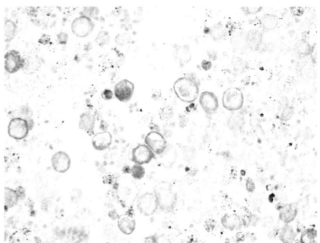

Figure 5.151. Mesothelioma. Positive staining of mesothelial cells by EMA raises concern for, but does not confirm, a mesothelioma. Most mesotheliomas involving fluid specimens are EMA positive, but 10% of reactive mesothelial populations may also be EMA positive (EMA immunostain).

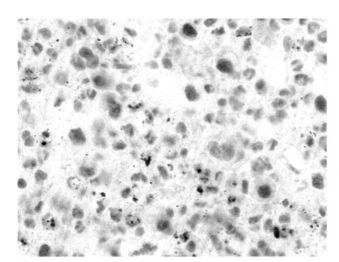

Figure 5.152. Mesothelioma. BAP-1 is retained in background cells as well as some of the atypical mesothelial cells. While its expression is lost in some of the atypical cells, expression in some of these cells precludes a definitive diagnosis of mesothelioma. BAP-1 may be retained in a large minority of epithelioid mesotheliomas (BAP-1 immunostain).

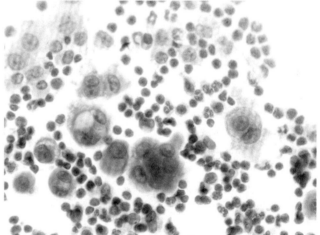

Figure 5.153. Mesothelioma. The specimen contains a large number of mesothelioma cells with increased cell size and prominent nucleoli. Despite being markedly atypical, the cells maintain mesothelial features: abundant cytoplasm, two-tone cytoplasm, and "lacy skirt" morphology (Pap stain).

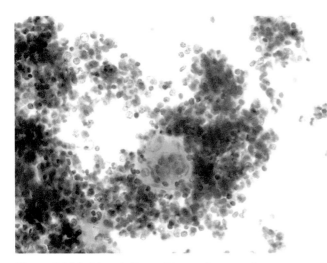

Figure 5.154. Mesothelioma. Giant malignant cells are present in a background of much smaller cells. These large cells could represent a metastatic adenocarcinoma or other malignant process. Staining with a mesothelial marker (such as calretinin) would allow for a definitive diagnosis of mesothelioma (Pap stain).

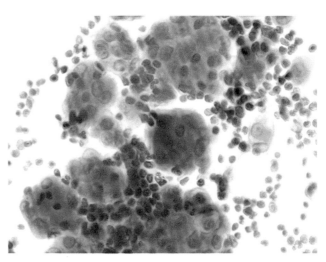

Figure 5.155. Mesothelioma. The specimen contains small clusters and individually dispersed mesothelial cells. The mesothelial cells are present in large numbers and have distinct nucleoli, irregular nuclear borders, and anisonucleosis. The cells are also large in size. If a mesothelial origin can be confirmed on an immunostain, the population is at least suspicious for mesothelioma (Pap stain).

MONOTONOUS DISPERSED CELL PATTERN

The monotonous dispersed cell pattern exists when the normal mixed population of three cell types is not readily seen and one cell type predominates. This occurrence may be due to the expansion of one of the three normal cell populations in response to a disease state or due to a heavy burden of malignant cells from metastatic disease. If the specific cell type seen cannot be definitively identified based on cytomorphology, immunostains can be performed to confirm their origin.

CHECKLIST: Etiologic Considerations for the Monotonous Dispersed Cell Pattern

☐ Metastatic Adenocarcinoma

☐ Histiocyte Proliferation

☐ Reactive Mesothelial Cell Population

☐ Lymphocytosis

☐ Acute Inflammation

☐ Lymphoma

METASTATIC DISEASE

Essentially any metastatic malignancy can form dispersed single cells in serous fluid specimens (Figures 5.156-5.162). As most metastases are adenocarcinomas, positive staining with an epithelial marker (BerEP4 or MOC-31) confirms the diagnosis and allows further workup for a CUP (Table 5.3).

HISTIOCYTE PROLIFERATION

Histiocytes can occasionally predominate in a specimen (Figures 5.163-5.172). While the finding is considered nonspecific, variations in nuclear shape and size may cause initial concern for a metastatic malignancy. Close examination should reveal at least some histiocytes with bent nuclei. The surrounding cells should be of similar size and have a similar chromatin pattern as the more classic-appearing histiocytes. If uncertainty exists, immunostains can be used to identify histiocytes with a specific marker (such as CD68) and exclude metastatic carcinoma (with an epithelial marker).

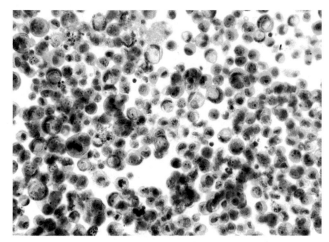

Figure 5.156. Metastatic gastric signet ring carcinoma. This serous cavity specimen has a high burden of disease and essentially every cell seen is overtly malignant. The mucin contained in the cytoplasm is foamy and appears slightly pink on this preparation (Pap stain).

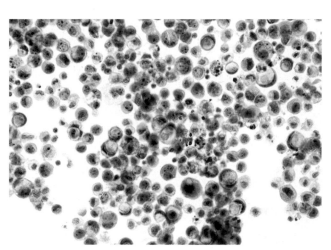

Figure 5.157. Metastatic gastric signet ring carcinoma. Separate field (Pap stain).

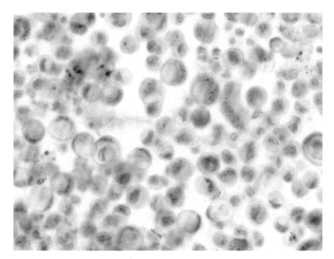

Figure 5.158. Metastatic signet ring carcinoma (origin unknown). A separate specimen is cellular and contains predominantly malignant cells (Pap stain).

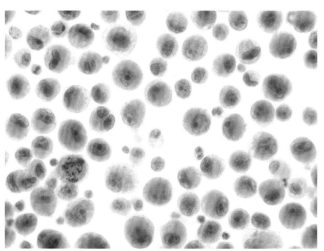

Figure 5.159. Metastatic hepatocellular carcinoma (HCC). This patient had a fibrolamellar variant of HCC which involved the ascites fluid. The specimen consists predominantly of the malignant cells, which have large nuclei with irregular borders and prominent nucleoli (Pap stain).

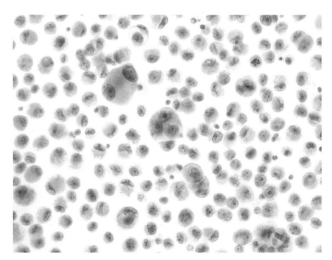

Figure 5.160. Metastatic hepatocellular carcinoma (HCC). Separate field (Pap stain).

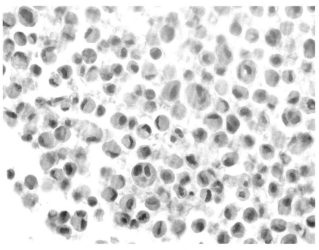

Figure 5.161. Metastatic hepatocellular carcinoma. The cell block preparation of the same case (H&E).

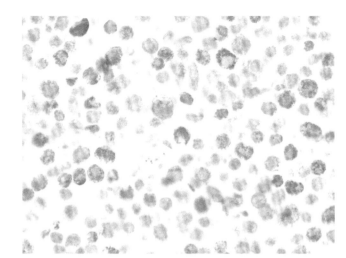

Figure 5.162. Metastatic hepatocellular carcinoma. The majority of the cells in this specimen demonstrated positivity for HepPar1, a marker of hepatocellular origin (HepPar1 immunostain).

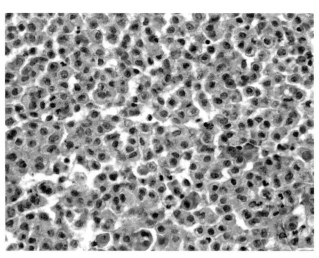

Figure 5.163. Increased histiocyte population. This cell block material demonstrates a monotonous population of cells with abundant, foamy cytoplasm. Some cells have curved nuclei, which help identify them as histiocytes. A histiocytic proliferation in serous fluid specimens is usually reactive and nonspecific but may emulate a neoplastic process (H&E).

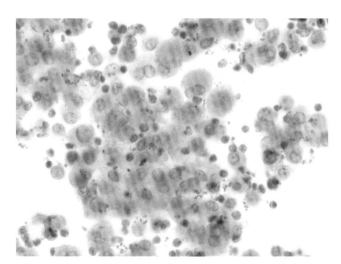

Figure 5.164. Increased histiocyte population. The field contains predominantly histiocytes with abundant cytoplasm. Some cells are binucleated. The nuclei are round or curved and have regular borders and bland chromatin (Pap stain).

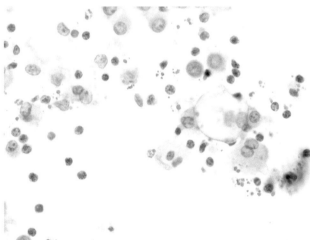

Figure 5.165. Prominent histiocyte population. In this field, the histiocytes are admixed with lymphocytes. One histiocyte has a large vacuole that has made the entire cytoplasm appear clear. This is a visually striking change that can occur in some histiocytes and should be distinguished from vacuoles containing mucin (such as in an adenocarcinoma) or those seen in serous neoplasms (Pap stain).

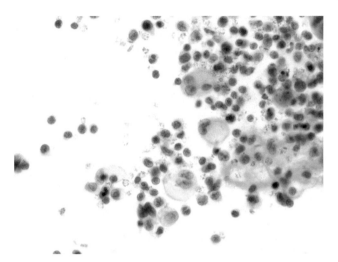

Figure 5.166. Histiocytes and lymphocytes. Separate field demonstrating binucleated histiocytes with bean-shaped nuclei and small nucleoli, some with prominent cytoplasmic vacuolization (Pap stain).

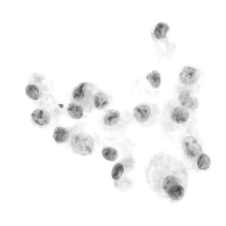

Figure 5.167. Histiocytes. All the cells seen here are histiocytes, some binucleate. Some nuclear border irregularities and nuclear size variation can be seen, which may cause concern for a neoplasm, in which case a CD68 immunostain would confirm these cells as histiocytes. Note the prominent foamy cytoplasm (Pap stain).

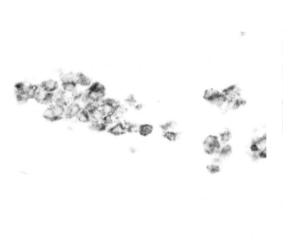

Figure 5.168. Histiocytes. A CD68 immunostain performed on cell block material from the same case demonstrated granular cytoplasmic staining typically seen in histiocytes (CD68 immunostain).

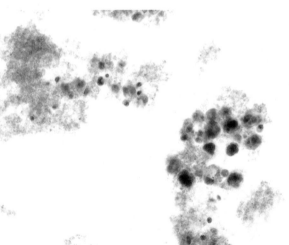

Figure 5.169. Pigment-laden histiocytes. The field contains predominantly histiocytes with a few background lymphocytes. The red granular debris represents degenerated blood that likely had been sitting in the cavity for some time. Several histiocytes have taken up the blood over time, causing their cytoplasm to become pigmented (Pap stain).

REACTIVE MESOTHELIAL CELL POPULATION

Disease processes that irritate the mesothelial lining may cause an increase in the number of mesothelial cells in a serous fluid specimen. Reactive mesothelial cells may exhibit moderate pleomorphism and become enlarged, causing concern for a metastatic carcinoma. The mesothelial origin of the cells can be confirmed with a specific marker (calretinin); the mesothelial cells should be negative for epithelial markers (BerEP4 and MOC-31), although occasionally focal positivity may be seen in reactive mesothelial cells. If any concern for mesothelioma exists, it should be excluded with a proper workup (see the "Tissue Fragments Pattern").

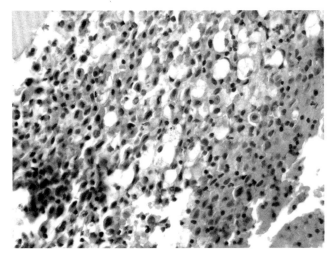

Figure 5.170. Prominent histiocyte population. This cell block contains predominantly histiocytes, some of which can be identified by the large vacuoles that give these cells a "swiss cheese" appearance. The prominence of these vacuoles may cause concern for a mucin-producing adenocarcinoma (H&E).

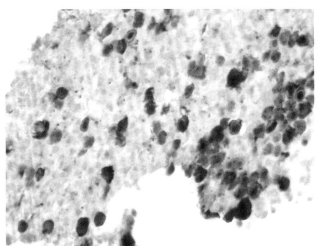

Figure 5.171. Prominent histiocyte population. A calretinin stain was performed on the same material and demonstrates a population of mesothelial cells among the histiocytes, which would be difficult to identify using cytomorphologic features alone (calretinin immunostain).

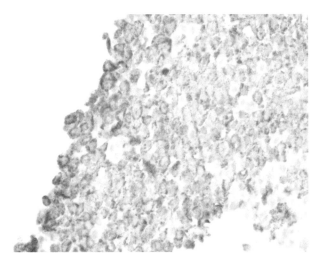

Figure 5.172. Prominent histiocyte population. The CD68 immunostain highlights histiocytes in a granular cytoplasmic fashion. Some cells are negative—presumably the mesothelial cells identified by the calretinin stain in Figure 5.171 (CD68 immunostain).

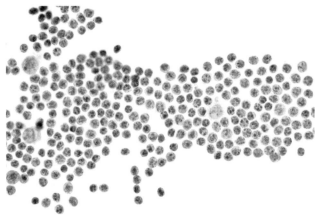

Figure 5.173. Lymphocytosis. Lymphocytosis refers to a predominance of lymphocytes in a given specimen; in some cases, only lymphocytes may be seen. This process usually occurs in pleural fluid specimens and can be associated with tuberculosis, lymphoma, and occult malignancy (Pap stain).

LYMPHOCYTOSIS

Lymphocytosis refers to an increased number of lymphocytes in a specimen (Figures 5.173-5.180). In the case of a serous fluid specimen, lymphocytosis is concerning when the specimen is both cellular and contains a predominance of lymphocytes. The lymphocytes in such situations are small and may either be monotonous or polymorphous. The presence of lymphocytosis may indicate an infectious process or metastatic malignancy that is not otherwise seen in the fluid specimen.[50] In addition, a low-grade lymphoma is difficult to exclude without flow cytometric analysis. For this reason, lymphocytosis should be reported as an atypical finding and requires further workup by the clinical team.

SAMPLE NOTE: LYMPHOCYTOSIS

Lymphocytosis. See note.

Note: The presence of lymphocytosis in a pleural effusion is an atypical finding and is often associated with malignancy, lymphoma, or tuberculosis.

ACUTE INFLAMMATION

The presence of acute inflammation is a nonspecific finding but is often found in patients with an infectious process (Figures 5.181 and 5.182). If a background of granular debris is seen, the cell block material can be stained for infectious agents. However, in most instances, a portion of the specimen should be separately submitted for microbiologic studies. The predominance of acute inflammatory cells should be noted to help the clinical team pursue additional workup.[51]

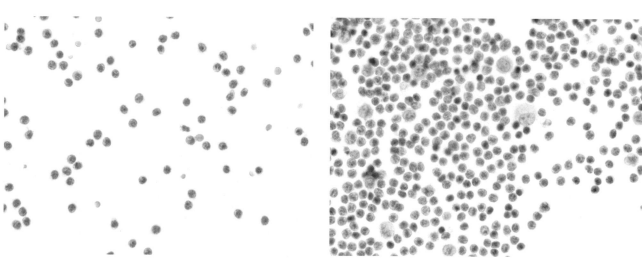

Figure 5.174. Lymphocytosis. This field shows a mixed population of lymphocytes. To exclude lymphoma, a clonal population needs to be demonstrated through immunostains performed on cell block material or, more preferably, flow cytometric analysis (Pap stain).

Figure 5.175. Lymphocytosis. Separate field (Pap stain).

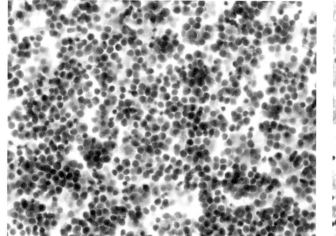

Figure 5.176. Lymphocytosis. Cell block preparation of the same case. Cell block material often demonstrates suboptimal cytomorphology, and in this case, it is difficult to identify the lymphoid nature of this small round blue cell population (H&E).

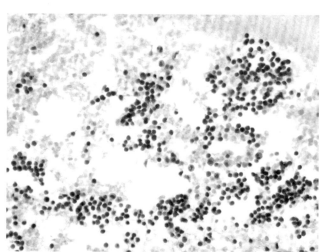

Figure 5.177. Lymphocytosis. A cell block preparation from a different case of lymphocytosis. The lymphocytes are small and most have a thin rim of cytoplasm. While no overt malignancy is identified, a small cell lymphoma cannot be entirely excluded using cytomorphology alone (H&E).

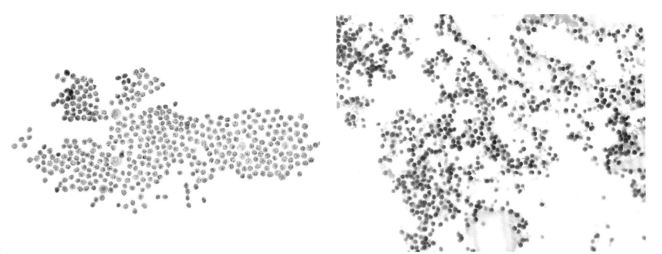

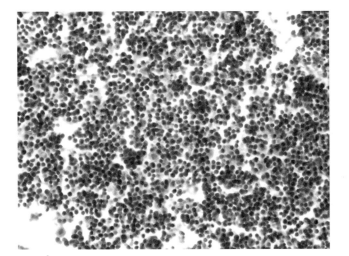

Figure 5.178. Lymphocytosis. The preparation has caused the lymphoid cells to aggregate into a pseudo-fragment. Reactive lymphocytes in fluid specimens often appear more monotonous than lymphocytes taken from a lymph node by fine-needle aspiration (Pap stain).

Figure 5.179. Lymphocytosis. A cell block preparation of the same specimen (H&E).

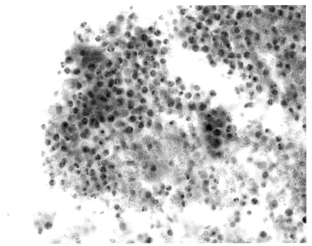

Figure 5.180. Lymphocytosis. Separate field (H&E).

Figure 5.181. Acute inflammation. Acute inflammatory cells are a nonspecific finding in fluid specimens but should be reported if found in significant numbers because they are not normal residents of serous cavities. In this case, the inflammatory cells are mixed with blood but are present in too great a number to simply represent contamination from a bloody tap (Pap stain).

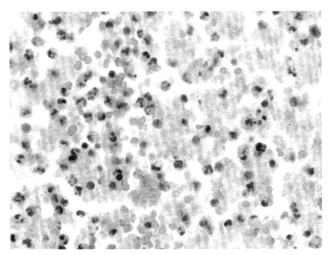

Figure 5.182. Acute inflammation. Acute inflammation is mixed with granular debris and intact red blood cells. The granular debris could represent necrosis or degenerated blood (H&E).

LYMPHOMA

Lymphoma is one of the most common malignancies to involve serous cavity specimens (Figures 5.183-5.196). Lymphomas consisting primarily of small lymphoid cells may intersperse with background benign lymphocytes and may not be identified as a "fourth population" of cells.[52] In all cases where a lymphoproliferative disorder is suspected, a fresh aliquot should be submitted for flow cytometric analysis.[53] Owing to the random distribution of cells in cell block material, it can be difficult to interpret immunostains that would otherwise help establish a clonal lymphoid process; however, large cell lymphomas usually appear atypical and morphologically distinct from the background lymphocytes and can be accurately immunophenotyped. The cells are negative for epithelial (BerEP4, MOC-31) and mesothelial (calretinin) markers and are usually positive for CD45.

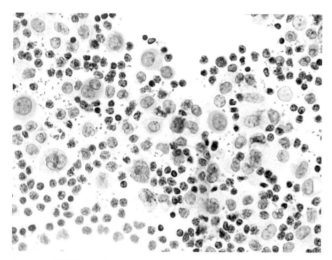

Figure 5.183. Diffuse large B cell lymphoma (DLBCL). Several large atypical cells can be seen with prominent nucleoli and some with multilobated or multinucleated nuclei. The background contains numerous lymphocytes and several mesothelial cells. In this case, the patient had pleural cavity involvement by a DLBCL (Pap stain).

Figure 5.184. Diffuse large B cell lymphoma (DLBCL). In this case, most of the cells in the field represent lymphoma cells. The cells are large, although their size in this field is difficult to determine due to a lack of normal bystander cells. Note the atypical mitosis in the center of the field (Pap stain).

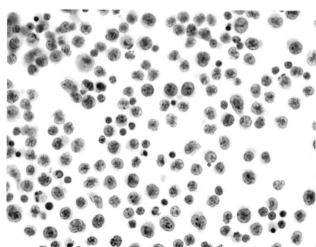
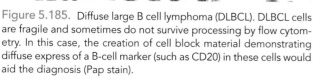

Figure 5.185. Diffuse large B cell lymphoma (DLBCL). DLBCL cells are fragile and sometimes do not survive processing by flow cytometry. In this case, the creation of cell block material demonstrating diffuse express of a B-cell marker (such as CD20) in these cells would aid the diagnosis (Pap stain).

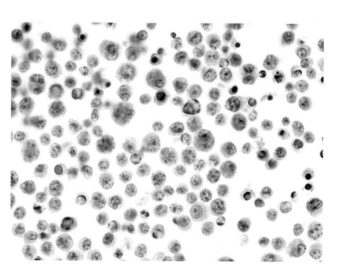

Figure 5.186. Plasma cell neoplasm. This patient had pleural cavity involvement by a plasma cell neoplasm. The cells appear large and vary greatly in size. However, many have an eccentrically placed nucleus as well as prominent nucleoli and/or peripherally clumped chromatin (Pap stain).

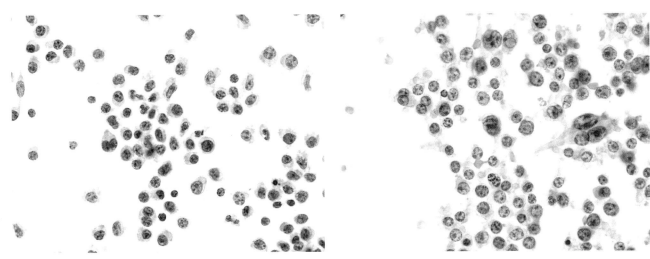

Figure 5.187. Plasma cell neoplasm. A separate specimen containing a neoplastic plasma cell population. Many of the cells have an eccentrically placed nucleus, and some contain prominent nucleoli. Plasma cells can be difficult to identify on the Pap stain, as they are more commonly identified on H&E and/or Wright-stained preparations (Pap stain).

Figure 5.188. Plasma cell neoplasm. Separate field (Pap stain).

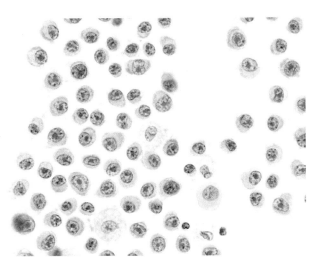

Figure 5.189. Plasma cell neoplasm. A separate specimen containing a plasma cell neoplasm.

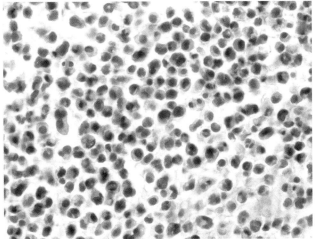

Figure 5.190. Plasma cell neoplasm. A cell block preparation of the same case. A perinuclear hof can be identified in some of the cells, but the section is suboptimal for evaluating chromatin quality (H&E).

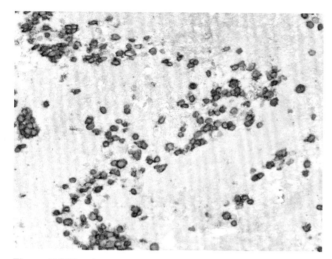

Figure 5.191. Plasma cell neoplasm. A CD138 immunostain shows membranous positivity in the majority of cells confirming the existence of a plasma cell population (CD138 immunostain).

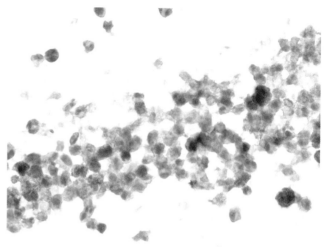

Figure 5.192. Plasma cell neoplasm. A stain for the kappa light chain highlights the majority of the cells in the field, indicating light chain restriction and therefore a clonal process (kappa immunostain).

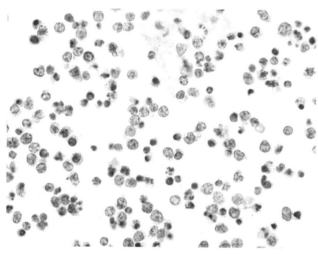

Figure 5.193. Burkitt lymphoma. These lymphoma cells are relatively small but have markedly irregular nuclear contours (Pap stain).

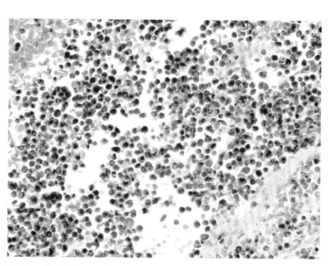

Figure 5.194. Burkitt lymphoma. A cell block preparation of the same specimen (H&E).

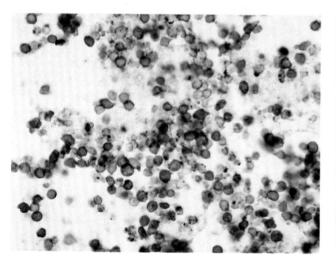

Figure 5.195. Burkitt lymphoma. A CD20 immunostain highlights the majority of the cells in a membranous pattern, indicating a B-cell origin and suggesting against a reactive population of lymphocytes (CD20 immunostain).

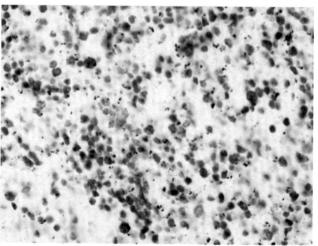

Figure 5.196. Burkitt lymphoma. A large number (>90%) of the lymphoid cells express Ki-67, a proliferation marker. Although not diagnostic of Burkitt lymphoma, a highly proliferative population of small to medium sized B-cells is strongly suggestive of this diagnosis (Ki-67 immunostain).

PSAMMOMATOUS CALCIFICATION PATTERN

Psammomatous calcification appears as blue or purple material that is irregular in shape and size. The calcifications are known as "psammoma bodies" and usually possess concentric lamella. Specimens may contain psammoma bodies associated with cells, naked psammoma bodies, or a mixture of both. Some psammoma bodies may be cracked. When seen in a serous fluid specimen, psammoma bodies suggest the presence of a proliferative process but are not specific for a neoplastic or malignant process, especially in a peritoneal cavity specimen.[54]

CHECKLIST: Etiologic Considerations for the Psammomatous Calcification Pattern

- ☐ Serous Neoplasms
- ☐ Endosalpingiosis
- ☐ Mesothelial Proliferations

SEROUS NEOPLASMS

Serous neoplasms of the gynecologic tract can be associated with psammomatous calcification and typically appear in effusion specimens as small epithelial fragments surrounding psammoma bodies, as well as in small fragments without psammoma bodies (Figures 5.197-5.202). These neoplasms range in behavior from benign (e.g. cystadenoma, cystadenofibroma, adenofibroma, etc.) to borderline to malignant (low-grade and high-grade serous carcinoma). It can be challenging to distinguish these entities on cytologic and cell block material alone because they are all of Mullerian origin and therefore positive for the marker Pax-8. However, the presence of overtly malignant cells favors a carcinoma while bland cytomorphologic features favor a benign neoplasm. If sufficient tumor cells are available for immunostaining, aberrant expression of p53 suggests a high-grade serous carcinoma. Aberrant expression of p53 may either be a null pattern (absence of expression) or diffuse expression.[55] Most importantly, the presence of cells from a serous neoplasm in an effusion specimen should not be definitively considered as a metastatic or invasive process, because the cells may have shed into the fluid from the primary site or a noninvasive implant within the peritoneal cavity.[56] Definitive characterization of such neoplasms requires an excisional specimen, and correlation with such specimens, as well as the patient history, is highly recommended.

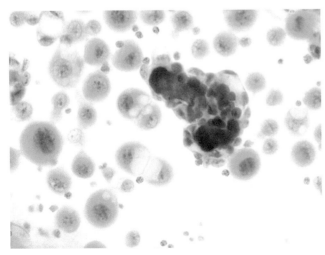

Figure 5.197. Serous borderline tumor. This patient was diagnosed with a noninvasive serous borderline tumor. Most of the large cells seen in the background are tumor cells. Some neoplastic cells are associated with psammomatous calcification (Pap stain).

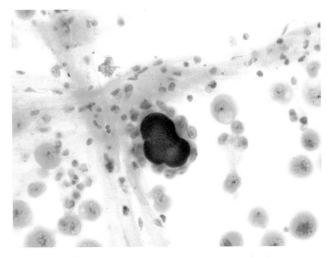

Figure 5.198. Serous borderline tumor. Separate field (Pap stain).

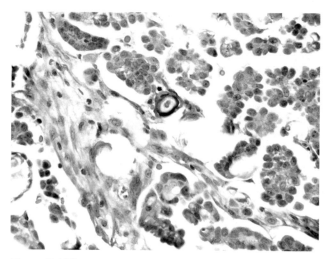

Figure 5.199. Serous borderline tumor. Cell block material of the same case shows bland-appearing neoplastic cells forming papillary structures. Some cells are associated with psammomatous calcification in the center of the field (H&E).

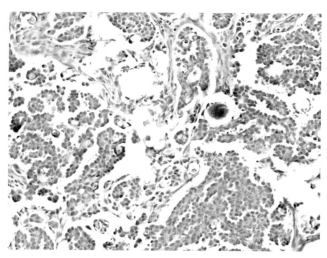

Figure 5.200. Serous borderline tumor. Separate field (H&E).

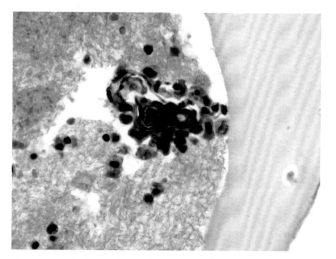

Figure 5.201. Serous borderline tumor. A different case of a serous borderline tumor in a patient with noninvasive implants (H&E).

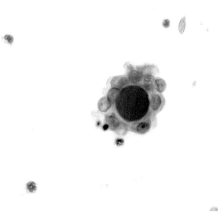

Figure 5.202. Low-grade serous carcinoma. It can be difficult to differentiate between low-grade serous carcinomas and serous borderline tumors on a serous fluid specimen alone. These carcinoma cells are associated with a psammoma body. The tumor was classified as a carcinoma due to invasion found at the primary site; these cells could be from that site or from either invasive or noninvasive implants elsewhere in the peritoneal cavity (Pap stain).

ENDOSALPINGIOSIS

When present on serous cavity surfaces, fragments of bland-appearing ciliated epithelium may be seen in a serous fluid specimen. Endosalpingiosis usually presents as rare fragments, although cases of florid endosalpingiosis resulting in a more cellular specimen have been described.[57] In some instances, the cilia may not be readily identified, and the bland nature of the cells, especially in a patient with no known neoplasm, suggests that endosalpingiosis is likely. Because this process is common and subclinical, the first identification of endosalpingiosis may be made on a fluid specimen. It is generally considered a benign process, but it may initially be concerning for a clinically relevant gynecologic neoplasm given that it will be positive for both Pax-8 and epithelial markers (BerEP4 and MOC-31).

FAQ: What is the significance of psammomatous calcification in a washing specimen?

Answer: The presence of psammomatous calcification in a washing specimen is nonspecific and should be correlated with the patient's history and the cytomorphology of any cells associated with the psammomatous calcification. However, studies have shown that psammoma bodies found in pericardial and pleural fluid specimens were usually associated with malignancy. In peritoneal fluids, psammoma bodies were associated with benign processes 36% of the time.[54] These benign processes included cystadenofibroma, papillary mesothelial hyperplasia, endosalpingiosis, and endometriosis. In patients without suspicion for or a history of malignancy, psammomatous calcification should not be overinterpreted, especially if any associated cells are bland-appearing or lacking (Figures 5.203-5.206).

SAMPLE NOTE: PSAMMOMATOUS CALCIFICATION

Bland-appearing glandular cells and associated psammomatous calcification in a background of reactive mesothelial cells, histiocytes, and lymphocytes. Negative for carcinoma. See note.

Note: The presence of psammomatous calcification in a peritoneal washing specimen is often associated with benign processes, such as endosalpingiosis, cystadenofibroma, papillary mesothelial hyperplasia, or endometriosis.

Reference:
Parwani AV, Chan TY, Ali SZ. Significance of psammoma bodies in serous cavity fluid: a cytopathologic analysis. *Cancer Cytopathol.* 2004;102(2):87-91.

MESOTHELIAL PROLIFERATIONS

Papillary mesothelial hyperplasia and other mesothelial proliferations may be associated with psammoma bodies. The cells are typically bland and may have features suggestive of a mesothelial origin (Figures 5.207 and 5.208). The cells will be positive for mesothelial markers (calretinin) and negative for epithelial markers. If there is any concern for mesothelioma, a mesothelioma workup should be performed (see the "Tissue Fragments Pattern").

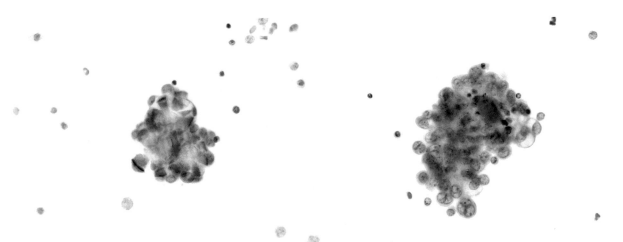

Figure 5.203. Cystadenofibroma. The psammoma bodies seen here have cracked during processing, giving them the appearance of crushed eggshells. The patient had a concurrent resection of an ovarian cystadenofibroma, which can cause this finding. The nuclei are bland, with granular chromatin and regular nuclear borders (Pap stain).

Figure 5.204. Cystadenofibroma. Numerous bland cells are associated with psammomatous calcification. Some of the cells are vacuolated, a feature seen in serous neoplasms regardless of grade as well as cells from cystadenofibroma (Pap stain).

Figure 5.205. Cystadenofibroma. A cracked psammoma body is seen associated with one bland-appearing epithelial cell. The presence of psammoma bodies in ascites fluids or peritoneal washings can be associated with both nonneoplastic and neoplastic processes (Pap stain).

Figure 5.206. Psammomatous calcification. In some instances, the presence of psammomatous calcification cannot be explained. Patients may have subclinical endosalpingiosis which can also form psammomatous calcification. Without a population of atypical cells to assess, a diagnosis cannot be made (H&E).

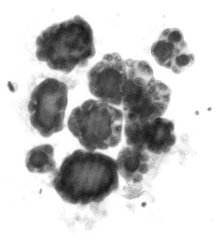

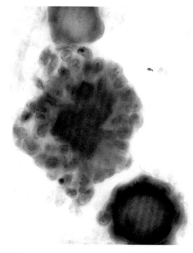

Figure 5.207. Mesothelial cell proliferation. On pleural biopsy, this patient had an atypical proliferation of mesothelial cells associated with psammomatous calcification. The corresponding fluid specimen demonstrated mesothelial cells with prominent nucleoli surrounding psammoma bodies (Pap stain).

Figure 5.208. Mesothelial cell proliferation. Separate field (Pap stain).

BLOODY PATTERN

The bloody pattern is defined by an abundance of red blood cells, either fresh or degenerated, which may obscure other cells in the specimen. If cells are present but cannot be assessed due to obscuring blood, a note should be provided that the specimen is either unsatisfactory or that the diagnosis is limited due to obscuring blood.

CHECKLIST: Etiologic Considerations for the Bloody Pattern

☐ Traumatic Tap

☐ Hemothorax, Hemopericardium, and Hemoperitoneum

☐ Endometriosis

☐ Fibrinous Effusion

TRAUMATIC TAP

In a traumatic tap, the specimen contains numerous intact red blood cells and little else. A traumatic tap indicates that the procedure may not have successfully accessed the serous cavity, especially if a small volume is submitted to the laboratory (Figures 5.209 and 5.210). Degenerated blood or blood clot, however, suggests a pathologic hemorrhage, indicating that the cavity may have been properly accessed.

HEMOTHORAX, HEMOPERICARDIUM, AND HEMOPERITONEUM

Patients with a hemothorax may have a mixture of intact and degenerated red blood cells, as well as a background of fibrin and granular debris. It is unlikely that the specimen will contain only intact red blood cells unless the procedure is performed early in the disease process. It is, therefore, important to note the presence of degenerated blood and/or fibrin and not simply dismiss the specimen as "blood only." "Lines of Zahn" may be seen in older clots that have begun to organize. As cancer can be the cause of hemorrhage, such specimens should be carefully examined for malignant cells.[58]

ENDOMETRIOSIS

Endometriosis refers to the presence of endometrial tissue outside of the endometrium (see "Endometriosis" under the "Tissue Fragments Pattern"). Endometriomas may bleed, resulting in both endometrial cells and degenerated blood in the serous cavity (Figures 5.211-5.221). If the endometrial cells have not shed before specimen procurement, the specimen may contain degenerated blood and lack the diagnostic endometrial cells. Given their hyperchromatic appearance and immunoreactivity for Pax-8 and epithelial markers, endometrial cells may initially cause concern for a clinically relevant gynecologic neoplasm involving the serous cavity. Therefore, cytomorphologic identification together with the bloody background can prevent a suboptimal diagnosis.

FIBRINOUS EFFUSION

A fibrinous effusion may occur as a consequence of any process that allows protein leakage into a serous cavity (exudative effusions), including malignancy, infection, and autoimmune disease. When destructive, these processes result in the presence of red blood cells, necrotic debris, and inflammatory cells. Fibrin enters the cavity where it clots around these exudative elements to form a fibrinous exudate (Figures 5.222-5.224). While much of the necrotic debris may be washed away in liquid-based preparations, specimens demonstrate

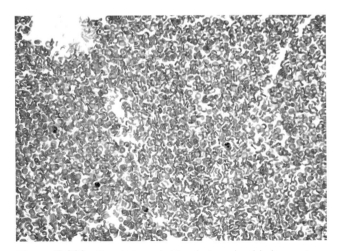

Figure 5.209. Bloody tap. A bloody tap should demonstrate peripheral blood components—predominantly intact red blood cells and rare white blood cells, as seen here. Degenerated blood with fibrin is more suggestive of blood that has been present in a body cavity (Pap stain).

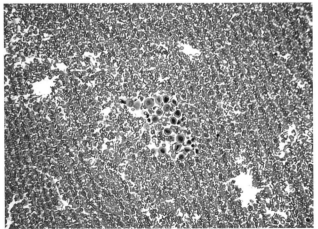

Figure 5.210. Bloody tap. Rare mesothelial cells, histiocytes, and lymphocytes have been diluted by peripheral blood during a bloody tap. While this could also occur with active bleeding into a serous cavity, usually some degenerated blood would be found (Pap stain).

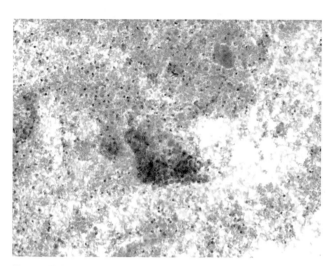

Figure 5.211. Endometriosis. Endometriosis may present as predominantly degenerated blood, a nonspecific finding. The presence of endometrial cells (seen here) allows for a more specific diagnosis, as well as an explanation for the background blood cells (Pap stain).

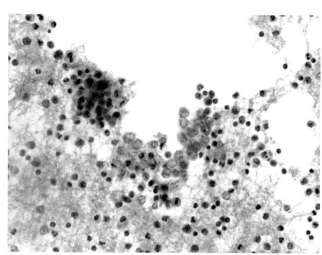

Figure 5.212. Endometriosis. Endometrial cells may have different morphologies depending on the patient's hormonal state. Here, the cells have high nuclear to cytoplasmic (N/C) ratios and irregular nuclear borders, which may cause concern for a malignant process if one does not consider the possibility of endometriosis. The background of degenerated blood provides a clue (Pap stain).

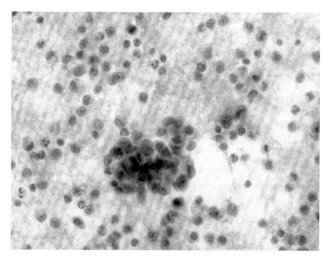

Figure 5.213. Endometriosis. Separate field (Pap stain).

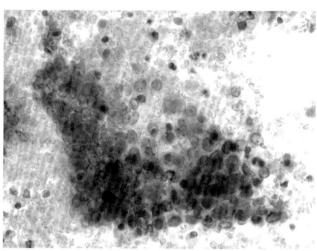

Figure 5.214. Endometriosis. Separate field (Pap stain).

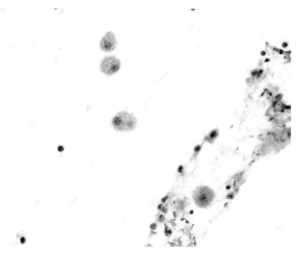

Figure 5.215. Endometriosis. A separate field shows the presence of pigmented macrophages. The green pigment is an indication that hemoglobin has been ingested and broken down. This finding is non-specific and may be found in any condition which causes chronic bleeding into a serous cavity (Pap stain).

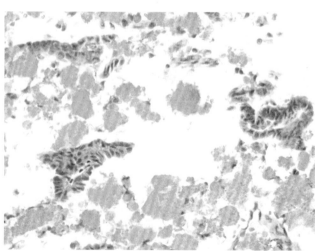

Figure 5.216. Endometriosis. The endometrial glands in this cell block preparation are concerning for a possible metastatic adenocarcinoma. The glands would be positive for BerEP4, Pax-8, and ER and negative for calretinin. The background of degenerated blood should cause one to consider the possibility of endometriosis (H&E).

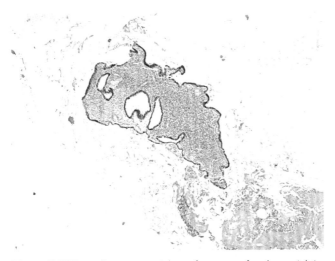

Figure 5.217. Endometriosis. A large fragment of endometrial tissue is seen on a cell block preparation, consistent with a diagnosis of endometriosis (H&E).

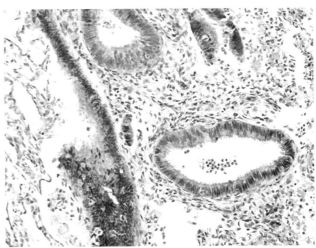

Figure 5.218. Endometriosis. Separate field at higher magnification (H&E).

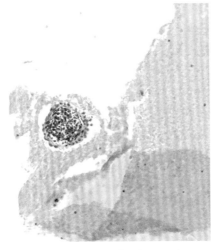

Figure 5.219. Endometriosis. A small cluster of endometrial tissue, with the classic "two-layered" appearance of endometrial glandular cells and underlying stromal tissue (H&E).

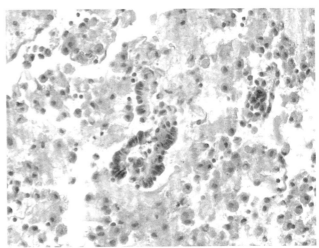

Figure 5.220. Endometriosis. A cell block preparation demonstrating columnar endometrial glandular cells, degenerated blood, and pigmented macrophages (H&E).

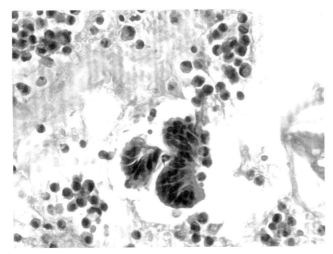

Figure 5.221. Endometriosis. A separate case of endometriosis in which a strip of columnar glandular cells could initially cause concern for a well-differentiated gastrointestinal adenocarcinoma (H&E).

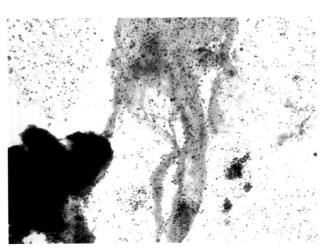

Figure 5.222. Fibrinous effusion. The specimen is cellular, with numerous cells adhered to thick clot material (Pap stain).

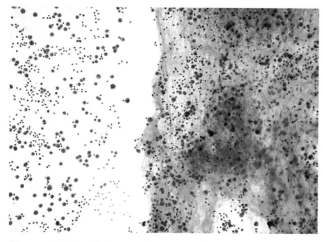

Figure 5.223. Fibrinous effusion. Higher magnification of the same specimen. The background contains predominantly macrophages and acute inflammatory cells. A fibrinous effusion indicates a destructive process, perhaps secondary to infection or autoimmune disease (Pap stain).

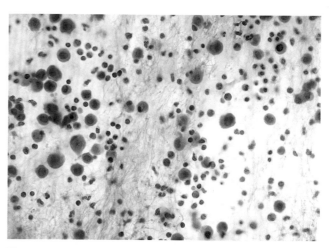

Figure 5.224. Fibrinous effusion. A high-magnification view shows numerous macrophages and inflammatory cells embedded in a fibrinous matrix. This material is thickened and may be difficult to aspirate (Pap stain).

clotted material containing variable proportions of inflammatory cells, degenerated blood, fibrin, and necrotic cells. Necrotic debris may surround the edge of these fragments ("clinging diathesis"). Over time, exudative effusions begin to resolve and harden, becoming difficult to remove. Careful examination of the specimen is required to exclude malignancy, which may be undersampled.[59]

MUCINOUS PATTERN

CHECKLIST: Etiologic Considerations for the Mucinous Pattern

☐ Low-grade Mucinous Neoplasm
☐ High-grade Mucinous Neoplasm

The mucinous pattern simply refers to the presence of mucinous material in the background. Mucin can be difficult to definitively identify on routine cytologic preparations, especially when the mucin is thin and dilute (Figures 5.225-5.228). A specimen may only contain mucin with an absence of any cells or may contain rare background elements such as mesothelial cells. Furthermore, implanted or invasive malignant cells that produce mucin may shed into the fluid and be seen along with the mucinous background.

FAQ: What is *pseudomyxoma peritonei*?

Answer: The presence of mucin in the peritoneal cavity is referred to pseudomyxoma peritonei.[60] The source is typically mucin-producing neoplastic cells implanted in or invading into the peritoneal cavity. Although it is a clinical diagnosis, the presence of mucin in a peritoneal sample can help confirm the clinical impression. Myxoid material seen in the background can be confirmed as mucin using a mucicarmine special stain on cell block or core biopsy material. The World Health Organization classifies pseudomyxoma peritonei into low-grade and high-grade processes which can be classified only on surgical specimens.[61] Because low-grade lesions are associated with low cellularity, they usually present as acellular mucin on cytologic specimens. High-grade lesions are more cellular and have either signet ring morphology or cribiform architecture.

SAMPLE NOTE: ACELLULAR MUCIN

Abundant mucin. See note.

Note: The presence of mucin suggests the presence of a mucinous neoplasm even in a paucicellular specimen. While the differential diagnosis includes the implantation of a low-grade mucinous neoplasm, an invasive mucinous adenocarcinoma cannot be completely excluded. Recommend clinicoradiologic correlation.

Reference:
Yantiss RK, Shia J, Klimstra DS, Hahn HP, Odze RD, Misdraji J. Prognostic significance of localized extra-appendiceal mucin deposition in appendiceal mucinous neoplasms. *Am J Surg Pathol.* 2009;33(2):248-255.

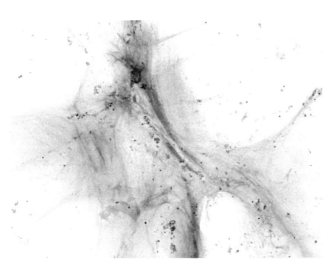

Figure 5.225. Acellular mucin. The presence of mucin in the peritoneal cavity is referred to as *pseudomyxoma peritonei*. This is a clinical diagnosis, but a cytologic correlation may be seen, in which mucin without an obvious cause is aspirated from the pelvic cavity (Pap stain).

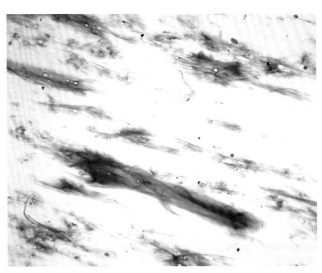

Figure 5.226. Acellular mucin. Mucin containing rare cells. The mucin may be produced by either low- or high-grade neoplasms found in the gastrointestinal tract, especially the appendix. These neoplasms may also implant in the peritoneal cavity and produce mucin. Alternatively, a metastatic mucin-producing adenocarcinoma may cause such a background, but low-grade neoplasms are more likely to produce a specimen of low cellularity (Pap stain).

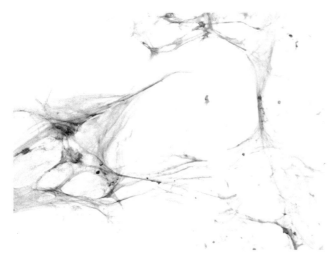

Figure 5.227. Acellular mucin. The cytologic specimen contains a background of mucin and is otherwise acellular; thus, the source of the mucin cannot be determined. This patient was found to have a low-grade mucinous neoplasm arising from the appendix (Pap stain).

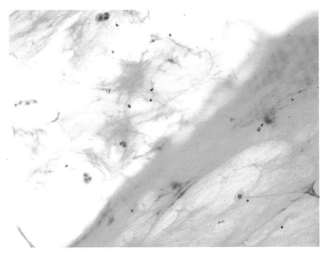

Figure 5.228. Acellular mucin. Separate field. Rare macrophages and inflammatory cells can be seen within the mucinous substance (Pap stain).

LOW-GRADE MUCINOUS NEOPLASM

Low-grade mucinous neoplasms may implant at multiple sites in the peritoneal cavity, which has been called disseminated peritoneal adenomucinosis (DPAM). When this process occurs along with the production of mucin into the peritoneal cavity, the result is peritoneal adenomucinosis (Figures 5.229-5.237). Generally speaking, low-grade mucinous neoplasms are less cellular, although florid lesions have been described. Because these patients have a better prognosis and different treatment option than those with adenocarcinoma, the clinical team should be made aware when a low-grade mucinous neoplasm is in the differential diagnosis.[62,63]

SAMPLE NOTE: DISSEMINATED PERITONEAL ADE-NOMUCINOSIS

Bland glandular cells in a background of mucin. See note.

Note: The differential diagnosis includes a well-differentiated adenocarcinoma as well as the implantation of a low-grade mucinous neoplasm in the peritoneal cavity (disseminated peritoneal adenomucinosis). The presence of invasion cannot be assessed on a cytologic specimen.

Reference:

Ronnett BM, Yan H, Kurman RJ, Shmookler BM, Wu L, Sugarbaker PH. Patients with pseudomyxoma peritonei associated with disseminated peritoneal adenomucinosis have a significantly more favorable prognosis than patients with peritoneal mucinous carcinomatosis. *Cancer.* 2001;92(1):85-91.

Figure 5.229. Low-grade mucinous neoplasm. This patient had a low-grade mucinous neoplasm arising from the appendix. The pelvic cavity sample demonstrated a background of mucin as well as rare, bland-appearing epithelial cells with oval nuclei and regular nuclear borders (Diff-Quik stain).

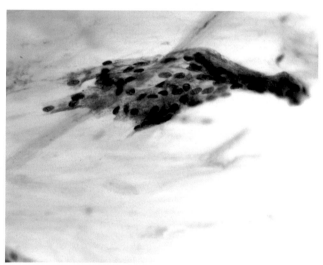

Figure 5.230. Low-grade mucinous neoplasm. A separate patient with disseminated peritoneal adenomucinosis secondary to an appendiceal neoplasm. The cytologic specimen contained only a rare fragment of bland-appearing epithelial cells (Pap stain).

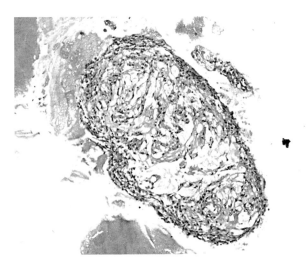

Figure 5.231. Low-grade mucinous neoplasm. A cell block preparation of the same case demonstrates a tissue fragment containing bland-appearing epithelial cells and extruded mucin (H&E).

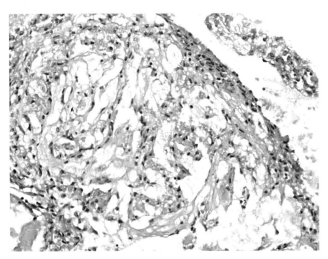

Figure 5.232. Low-grade mucinous neoplasm. Higher magnification of the previous field (H&E).

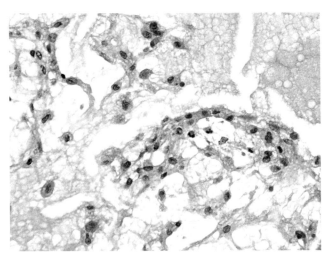

Figure 5.233. Low-grade mucinous neoplasm. Still higher magnification of the previous field. Note the small nuclei with abundant cytoplasm and low cellularity compared with the adjacent mucin (H&E).

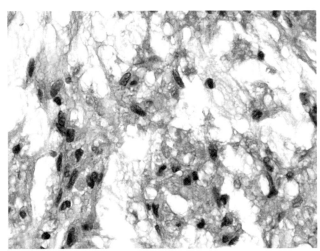

Figure 5.234. Low-grade mucinous neoplasm. Separate field (H&E).

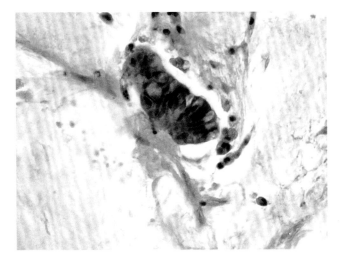

Figure 5.235. Low-grade mucinous neoplasm. A separate case in which the neoplastic cells were only identified in the cell block material. In this case, the cells are more columnar but exist in low numbers and have bland nuclear features: little size variation, regular nuclear contours, and granular chromatin (H&E).

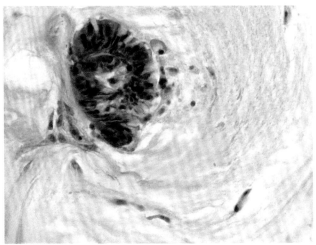

Figure 5.236. Low-grade mucinous neoplasm. Separate field (H&E).

HIGH-GRADE MUCINOUS NEOPLASM

High-grade mucinous neoplasms include mucinous adenocarcinomas and rarely implants from noninfiltrative high-grade neoplasms arising in the appendix or elsewhere in the gastrointestinal tract. A mucinous neoplasm may be considered an adenocarcinoma once it invades into the visceral and peritoneal surfaces, an assessment that can be made only on a surgical specimen (Figures 5.238 and 5.239). However, markedly atypical cytologic features alone may be diagnostic of a high-grade mucinous neoplasm. The tumor cells may form glandular structures, sheets of cells, or be present singly with signet ring or pleomorphic cytomorphology. As opposed to low-grade mucinous neoplasms, which are associated with appendiceal mucinous adenomas, high-grade mucinous neoplasms are more likely to be associated with adenocarcinomas from the appendix or gastrointestinal tract.[64] Generally speaking, high-grade mucinous neoplasms often produce more cellular specimens than low-grade mucinous neoplasms.

SAMPLE NOTE: SUSPICIOUS FOR A MUCINOUS ADENOCARCINOMA

Suspicious for a mucinous adenocarcinoma. See note.

Note: Markedly atypical glandular cells in a background of mucin, suspicious for a mucinous adenocarcinoma. While peritoneal invasion cannot be assessed in a cytologic specimen, the atypical cells possess high-grade features suspicious for a mucinous adenocarcinoma.

Reference:

Ronnett BM, Zahn CM, Kurman RJ, Kass ME, Sugarbaker PH, Shmookler BM. Disseminated peritoneal adenomucinosis and peritoneal mucinous carcinomatosis. A clinicopathologic analysis of 109 cases with emphasis on distinguishing pathologic features, site of origin, prognosis, and relationship to"pseudomyxoma peritonei". *Am J Surg Pathol.* 1995;19(12):1390-1408.

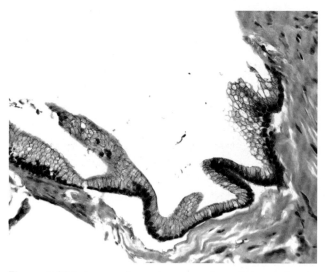

Figure 5.237. Low-grade mucinous neoplasm. This core biopsy demonstrates a noninvasive implant of a low-grade mucinous neoplasm on the peritoneal surface. Noninvasive implants can produce mucin, leading to pseudomyxoma peritonei (H&E).

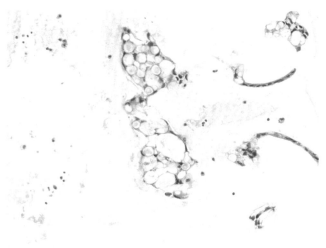

Figure 5.238. High-grade mucinous neoplasm. This colloid carcinoma arose from the colon and is metastatic to the peritoneum. The nuclei cells have higher nuclear to cytoplasmic (N/C) ratios and are hyperchromatic but are still scant compared with the background mucin (H&E).

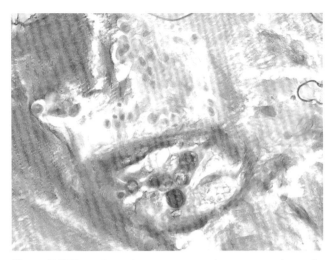

Figure 5.239. High-grade mucinous neoplasm. A special stain for mucin (mucicarmine) stains intracellular and extracellular mucin in a "hot pink" color (mucicarmine special stain).

OTHER

CHYLOTHORAX

If the thoracic duct is obstructed or disrupted, lymph may leak into the pleural cavity. Lymph is a fatty and milky fluid (Figures 5.240-5.243). The lymph is engulfed by macrophages, resulting in the presence of an increased amount of multivacuolated macrophages ("foamy macrophages").[65] Lymph fluid also contains T-lymphocytes, which may appear atypical and cause concern for a lymphoma. When the lymphocytic population predominates, the differential diagnosis overlaps with other causes of lymphocytosis in a pleural fluid (infection, lymphoma, and unsampled malignancy) (see "Lymphocytosis" under the "Single Cell Pattern" for further discussion).

NEAR MISSES

LYMPHOCYTOSIS

Lymphocytosis (a predominance of lymphocytes) in a pleural effusion specimen is considered an abnormal finding (Figures 5.244-5.249). Because lymphocytes are a normal component in benign effusion specimens, lymphocytosis can easily be overlooked. Cell block preparations sometimes yield disparate cell populations compared with other concentration methods; thus, all preparation types created for a given specimen should be examined closely for lymphocytosis. While there is no defined cut-off for a diagnosis of lymphocytosis, the diagnosis should be considered in specimens in which lymphocytes are the predominant cell. The clinical team should more strongly consider the possibility of a lymphoma, carcinoma, or infectious process (such as tuberculosis) when this diagnosis is made.

METASTATIC MELANOMA

Metastatic melanoma can be overlooked in serous fluid specimens because these cells are often singly dispersed and may resemble mesothelial cells (Figures 5.250 and 5.251). In cases in which both mesothelial cells and malignant cells are present, careful examination of

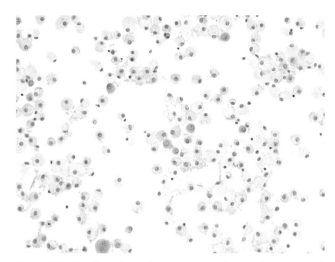

Figure 5.240. Chylothorax. Damage to the thoracic duct can result in the leakage of chyle into the pleural cavity. Numerous foamy histiocytes are seen here, compatible with a clinical impression of chylothorax (Pap stain).

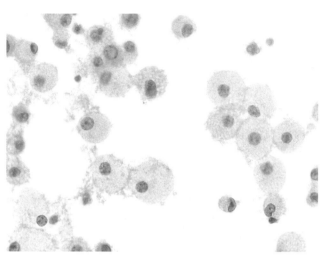

Figure 5.241. Chylothorax. A higher magnification of the same specimen (Pap stain).

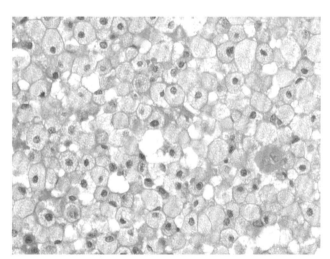

Figure 5.242. Chylothorax. This cell block preparation reveals a predominant population of foamy histiocytes (H&E).

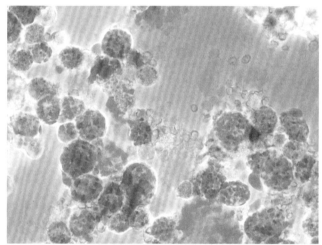

Figure 5.243. Chylothorax. A special stain for lipids (Oil Red O) was performed on an air-dried smear of the same specimen, revealing abundant lipid material (stained red) inside the histiocytes as well as extracellularly (Oil Red O stain).

a specimen at high power often allows differentiation between the two cell populations. In specimens with a higher tumor burden, the majority of cells may be malignant and mimic the "normal" reactive mesothelial cell population. Because melanoma may recur many years after an original diagnosis or initially present as metastatic disease, a panel of immunostains to address this diagnosis may not be ordered initially owing to a low level of suspicion. Furthermore, melanoma is negative for BerEP4 and MOC-31. Therefore, a population of atypical cells negative for both epithelial and mesothelial markers should raise the possibility of metastatic melanoma. Because reactive mesothelial populations can be positive for S100 protein, a panel of multiple melanoma markers (e.g., HMB-45, Melan-A, Sox-10) is usually recommended to make the diagnosis.[66]

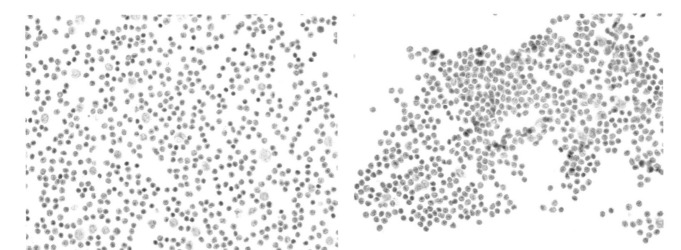

Figure 5.244. Lymphocytosis. Lymphocytosis, a predominance of lymphocytes in the pleural fluid, is considered an atypical finding and should be reported. Patients with lymphocytosis should undergo further workup to exclude lymphoma, tuberculosis, and occult malignancy (Pap stain).

Figure 5.245. Lymphocytosis. Separate field (Pap stain).

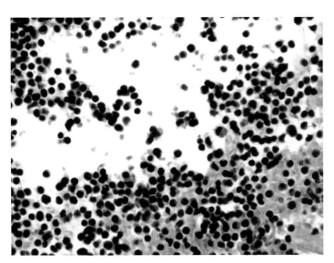

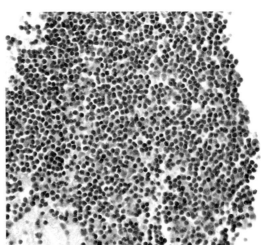

Figure 5.246. Lymphocytosis. A cell block preparation of the same case. Although immunostains can be performed on cell block material to demonstrate a mixture of T and B cells, this does not entirely exclude a subpopulation of clonal B cells (H&E).

Figure 5.247. Lymphocytosis. Separate field (H&E).

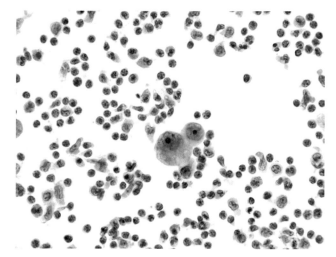

Figure 5.248. Metastatic lung adenocarcinoma in a background of lymphocytosis. This patient had a pleural effusion of unknown etiology. The specimen contained predominantly lymphocytes, but rare malignant cells were identified. Subsequent clinical workup revealed a lung mass (Pap stain).

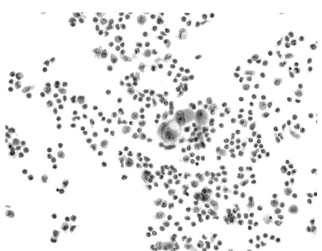

Figure 5.249. Metastatic lung adenocarcinoma in a background of lymphocytosis. Separate field (Pap stain).

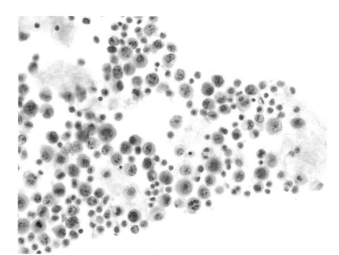

Figure 5.250. Metastatic melanoma. The majority of large cells in this field are melanoma cells, although they are easily mistaken for reactive mesothelial cells. In patients with a history of lobular breast carcinoma, signet ring carcinoma, and melanoma, a cell block should be created and stained with the appropriate markers to exclude metastatic disease, as these cells can be easily missed on routine cytologic preparations (Pap stain).

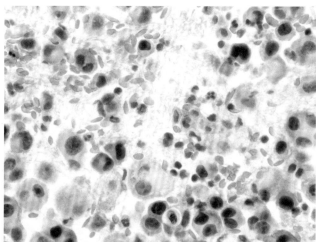

Figure 5.251. Metastatic melanoma. A cell block preparation of the same case provides additional clues that these larger cells may be malignant—they are quite large, some are binucleate, and many have prominent nucleoli. Still, these features could be seen in a reactive mesothelial population (H&E).

References

1. Rodriguez EF, Monaco SE, Khalbuss W, Austin RM, Pantanowitz L. Abdominopelvic washings: a comprehensive review. *Cytojournal.* 2013;10:7.

2. Wojcik EM, Naylor B. "Collagen balls" in peritoneal washings. Prevalence, morphology, origin and significance. *Acta Cytol.* 1992;36(4):466-470.

3. Selvaggi SM. Diagnostic pitfalls of peritoneal washing cytology and the role of cell blocks in their diagnosis. *Diagn Cytopathol.* 2003;28(6):335-341.

4. Hansen RM, Caya JG, Clowry LJ Jr, Anderson T. Benign mesothelial proliferation with effusion. Clinicopathologic entity that may mimic malignancy. *Am J Med.* 1984;77(5):887-892.

5. Murugan P, Siddaraju N, Habeebullah S, Basu D. Significance of intercellular spaces (windows) in effusion fluid cytology: a study of 46 samples. *Diagn Cytopathol.* 2008;36(9):628-632.

6. Yu GH, Sack MJ, Baloch ZW, DeFrias DV, Gupta PK. Occurrence of intercellular spaces (windows) in metastatic adenocarcinoma in serous fluids: a cytomorphologic, histochemical, and ultrastructural study. *Diagn Cytopathol.* 1999;20(3):115-119.

7. Groisman GM, Amar M, Weiner P, Zamir D. Mucicarminophilic histiocytosis (benign signet-ring cells) and hyperplastic mesothelial cells: two mimics of metastatic carcinoma within a single lymph node. *Arch Pathol Lab Med.* 1998;122(3):282.

8. Pereira TC, Saad RS, Liu Y, Silverman JF. The diagnosis of malignancy in effusion cytology: a pattern recognition approach. *Adv Anat Pathol.* 2006;13(4):174-184.

9. Rodriguez EF, Chowsilpa S, Maleki Z. The differential diagnosis in nonlymphoproliferative malignant pleural effusion cytopathology and its correlation with patients' demographics. *Acta Cytol.* 2018;62(5-6):436-442.

10. Bailey ME, Brown RW, Mody DR, Cagle P, Ramzy I. Ber-EP4 for differentiating adenocarcinoma from reactive and neoplastic mesothelial cells in serous effusions. Comparison with carcinoembryonic antigen, B72.3 and Leu-M1. *Acta Cytol.* 1996;40(6):1212-1216.

11. Morgan RL, De Young BR, McGaughy VR, Niemann TH. MOC-31 aids in the differentiation between adenocarcinoma and reactive mesothelial cells. *Cancer.* 1999;87(6):390-394.

12. Nagel H, Hemmerlein B, Ruschenburg I, Huppe K, Droese M. The value of anti-calretinin antibody in the differential diagnosis of normal and reactive mesothelia versus metastatic tumors in effusion cytology. *Pathol Res Pract.* 1998;194(11):759-764.

13. Husain AN, Colby TV, Ordonez NG, et al. Guidelines for pathologic diagnosis of malignant mesothelioma 2017 update of the consensus statement from the international mesothelioma interest group. *Arch Pathol Lab Med.* 2018;142(1):89-108.

14. Cowan ML, VandenBussche CJ. Cancer of unknown primary: ancillary testing of cytologic and small biopsy specimens in the era of targeted therapy. *Cancer Cytopathol.* 2018;126(suppl 8):724-737.

15. Sundling KE, Cibas ES. Ancillary studies in pleural, pericardial, and peritoneal effusion cytology. *Cancer Cytopathol.* 2018;126(suppl 8):590-598.

16. Erickson LA, Papouchado B, Dimashkieh H, Zhang S, Nakamura N, Lloyd RV. Cdx2 as a marker for neuroendocrine tumors of unknown primary sites. *Endocr Pathol.* 2004;15(3):247-252.

17. Ozcan A, Shen SS, Hamilton C, et al. PAX 8 expression in non-neoplastic tissues, primary tumors, and metastatic tumors: a comprehensive immunohistochemical study. *Mod Pathol.* 2011;24(6):751-764.

18. Deftereos G, Sanguino Ramirez AM, Silverman JF, Krishnamurti U. GATA3 immunohistochemistry expression in histologic subtypes of primary breast carcinoma and metastatic breast carcinoma cytology. *Am J Surg Pathol.* 2015;39(9):1282-1289.

19. Gurel B, Ali TZ, Montgomery EA, et al. NKX3.1 as a marker of prostatic origin in metastatic tumors. *Am J Surg Pathol.* 2010;34(8):1097-1105.

20. Brandler TC, Aziz MS, Rosen LM, Bhuiya TA, Yaskiv O. Usefulness of GATA3 and p40 immunostains in the diagnosis of metastatic urothelial carcinoma in cytology specimens. *Cancer Cytopathol.* 2014;122(6):468-473.

21. Bejarano PA, Nikiforov YE, Swenson ES, Biddinger PW. Thyroid transcription factor-1, thyroglobulin, cytokeratin 7, and cytokeratin 20 in thyroid neoplasms. *Appl Immunohistochem Mol Morphol.* 2000;8(3):189-194.

22. Nonaka D, Chiriboga L, Soslow RA. Expression of pax8 as a useful marker in distinguishing ovarian carcinomas from mammary carcinomas. *Am J Surg Pathol.* 2008;32(10):1566-1571.

23. Cimino-Mathews A, Subhawong AP, Illei PB, et al. GATA3 expression in breast carcinoma: utility in triple-negative, sarcomatoid, and metastatic carcinomas. *Hum Pathol.* 2013;44(7):1341-1349.

24. Ozcan A, de la Roza G, Ro JY, Shen SS, Truong LD. PAX2 and PAX8 expression in primary and metastatic renal tumors: a comprehensive comparison. *Arch Pathol Lab Med.* 2012;136(12):1541-1551.

25. Shen SS, Truong LD, Scarpelli M, Lopez-Beltran A. Role of immunohistochemistry in diagnosing renal neoplasms: when is it really useful?. *Arch Pathol Lab Med.* 2012;136(4):410-417.

26. Dragomir A, de Wit M, Johansson C, Uhlen M, Ponten F. The role of SATB2 as a diagnostic marker for tumors of colorectal origin: results of a pathology-based clinical prospective study. *Am J Clin Pathol.* 2014;141(5):630-638.

27. Bhargava R, Beriwal S, Dabbs DJ. Mammaglobin vs GCDFP-15: an immunohistologic validation survey for sensitivity and specificity. *Am J Clin Pathol.* 2007;127(1):103-113.

28. Cao D, Humphrey PA, Allan RW. SALL4 is a novel sensitive and specific marker for metastatic germ cell tumors, with particular utility in detection of metastatic yolk sac tumors. *Cancer*. 2009;115(12):2640-2651.

29. Stoll LM, Johnson MW, Gabrielson E, Askin F, Clark DP, Li QK. The utility of napsin-A in the identification of primary and metastatic lung adenocarcinoma among cytologically poorly differentiated carcinomas. *Cancer Cytopathol*. 2010;118(6):441-449.

30. Kaufmann O, Volmerig J, Dietel M. Uroplakin III is a highly specific and moderately sensitive immunohistochemical marker for primary and metastatic urothelial carcinomas. *Am J Clin Pathol*. 2000;113(5):683-687.

31. Dorfman DM, Shahsafaei A, Chan JK. Thymic carcinomas, but not thymomas and carcinomas of other sites, show CD5 immunoreactivity. *Am J Surg Pathol*. 1997;21(8):936-940.

32. 32 Bishop JA, Teruya-Feldstein J, Westra WH, Pelosi G, Travis WD, Rekhtman N. p40 (DeltaNp63) is superior to p63 for the diagnosis of pulmonary squamous cell carcinoma. *Mod Pathol*. 2012;25(3):405-415.

33. Sotlar K, Köveker G, Aepinus C, Selinka HC, Kandolf R, Bültmann B. Human papillomavirus type 16–associated primary squamous cell carcinoma of the rectum. *Gastroenterology*. 2001;120(4):988-994.

34. Begum S, Gillison ML, Nicol TL, Westra WH. Detection of human papillomavirus-16 in fine-needle aspirates to determine tumor origin in patients with metastatic squamous cell carcinoma of the head and neck. *Clin Cancer Res*. 2007;13(4):1186-1191.

35. Zhang MQ, El-Mofty SK, Dávila RM. Detection of human papillomavirus-related squamous cell carcinoma cytologically and by in situ hybridization in fine-needle aspiration biopsies of cervical metastasis. *Cancer Cytopathol*. 2008;114(2):118-123.

36. Tong GX, Devaraj K, Hamele-Bena D, et al. Pax8: a marker for carcinoma of Mullerian origin in serous effusions. *Diagn Cytopathol*. 2011;39(8):567-574.

37. Whitaker D. Invited review the cytology of malignant mesothelioma. *Cytopathology*. 2000;11(3):139-151.

38. Monaco S, Mehrad M, Dacic S. Recent advances in the diagnosis of malignant mesothelioma: focus on approach in challenging cases and in limited tissue and cytologic samples. *Adv Anat Pathol*. 2018;25(1):24-30.

39. Chiosea S, Krasinskas A, Cagle PT, Mitchell KA, Zander DS, Dacic S. Diagnostic importance of 9p21 homozygous deletion in malignant mesotheliomas. *Mod Pathol*. 2008;21(6):742.

40. Hwang HC, Sheffield BS, Rodriguez S, et al. Utility of BAP1 immunohistochemistry and p16 (CDKN2A) FISH in the diagnosis of malignant mesothelioma in effusion cytology specimens. *Am J Surg Pathol*. 2016;40(1):120-126.

41. Monaco SE, Shuai Y, Bansal M, Krasinskas AM, Dacic S. The diagnostic utility of p16 FISH and GLUT-1 immunohistochemical analysis in mesothelial proliferations. *Am J Clin Pathol*. 2011;135(4):619-627.

42. Hasteh F, Lin GY, Weidner N, Michael CW. The use of immunohistochemistry to distinguish reactive mesothelial cells from malignant mesothelioma in cytologic effusions. *Cancer Cytopathol*. 2010;118(2):90-96.

43. Johnston WW. The malignant pleural effusion. A review of cytopathologic diagnoses of 584 specimens from 472 consecutive patients. *Cancer*. 1985;56(4):905-909.

44. Monaco SE, Dabbs DJ, Kanbour-Shakir A. Pleomorphic lobular carcinoma in pleural fluid: diagnostic pitfall for atypical mesothelial cells. *Diagn Cytopathol*. 2008;36(9):657-661.

45. Beaty MW, Fetsch P, Wilder AM, Marincola F, Abati A. Effusion cytology of malignant melanoma. A morphologic and immunocytochemical analysis including application of the MART-1 antibody. *Cancer*. 1997;81(1):57-63.

46. Abadi MA, Zakowski MF. Cytologic features of sarcomas in fluids. *Cancer*. 1998;84(2):71-76.

47. Chhieng DC, Ko EC, Yee HT, Shultz JJ, Dorvault CC, Eltoum IA. Malignant pleural effusions due to small-cell lung carcinoma: a cytologic and immunocytochemical study. *Diagn Cytopathol*. 2001;25(6):356-360.

48. Niemann TH, Thomas PA. Melanoma with signet-ring cells in a peritoneal effusion. *Diagn Cytopathol*. 1995;12(3):241-244.

49. Sayah M, VandenBussche C, Maleki Z. Epithelioid hemangioendothelioma in pleural effusion. *Diagn Cytopathol*. 2015;43(9):751-755.

50. Yam LT. Diagnostic significance of lymphocytes in pleural effusions. *Ann Intern Med.* 1967;66(5):972-982.

51. Light RW, Erozan YS, Ball WC. Cells in pleural fluid: their value in differential diagnosis. *Arch Intern Med.* 1973;132(6):854-860.

52. Das DK. Serous effusions in malignant lymphomas: a review. *Diagn Cytopathol.* 2006;34(5):335-347.

53. Unger KM, Raber M, Bedrossian CW, Stein DA, Barlogie B. Analysis of pleural effusions using automated flow cytometry. *Cancer.* 1983;52(5):873-877.

54. Parwani AV, Chan TY, Ali SZ. Significance of psammoma bodies in serous cavity fluid: a cytopathologic analysis. *Cancer.* 2004;102(2):87-91.

55. McCluggage WG, Soslow RA, Gilks CB. Patterns of p53 immunoreactivity in endometrial carcinomas: 'all or nothing' staining is of importance. *Histopathology.* 2011;59(4):786-788.

56. Seidman JD, Kurman RJ. Ovarian serous borderline tumors: a critical review of the literature with emphasis on prognostic indicators. *Hum Pathol.* 2000;31(5):539-557.

57. Carlson G, Samuelson J, Dehner L. Cytologic diagnosis of florid peritoneal endosalpingiosis. A case report. *Acta Cytologica.* 1986;30(5):494-496.

58. Ausín P, Gómez-Caro A, Rojo RP, Moradiellos F, Díaz-Hellín V, de Nicolás JM. Spontaneous hemothorax caused by lung cancer. *Arch Bronconeumol.* 2005;41(7):400.

59. Assi Z, Caruso JL, Herndon J, Patz EF Jr. Cytologically proved malignant pleural effusions: distribution of transudates and exudates. *Chest.* 1998;113(5):1302-1304.

60. Shin HJ, Sneige N. Epithelial cells and other cytologic features of pseudomyxoma peritonei in patients with ovarian and/or appendiceal mucinous neoplasms: a study of 12 patients including 5 men. *Cancer.* 2000;90(1):17-23.

61. Panarelli NC, Yantiss RK. Mucinous neoplasms of the appendix and peritoneum. *Arch Pathol Lab Med.* 2011;135(10):1261-1268.

62. Ronnett BM, Yan H, Kurman RJ, Shmookler BM, Wu L, Sugarbaker PH. Patients with pseudomyxoma peritonei associated with disseminated peritoneal adenomucinosis have a significantly more favorable prognosis than patients with peritoneal mucinous carcinomatosis. *Cancer.* 2001;92(1):85-91.

63. Yantiss RK, Shia J, Klimstra DS, Hahn HP, Odze RD, Misdraji J. Prognostic significance of localized extra-appendiceal mucin deposition in appendiceal mucinous neoplasms. *Am J Surg Pathol.* 2009;33(2):248-255.

64. Ronnett BM, Zahn CM, Kurman RJ, Kass ME, Sugarbaker PH, Shmookler BM. Disseminated peritoneal adenomucinosis and peritoneal mucinous carcinomatosis. A clinicopathologic analysis of 109 cases with emphasis on distinguishing pathologic features, site of origin, prognosis, and relationship to "pseudomyxoma peritonei". *Am J Surg Pathol.* 1995;19(12):1390-1408.

65. Kren L, Rotterova P, Hermanova M, et al. Chylothorax as a possible diagnostic pitfall: a report of 2 cases with cytologic findings. *Acta Cytol.* 2005;49(4):441-444.

66. Rasmussen OO, Larsen KE. S-100 protein in malignant mesotheliomas. *Acta Pathol Microbiol Immunol Scand A.* 1985;93(4):199-201.

CHAPTER OUTLINE

THE UNREMARKABLE URINARY TRACT SPECIMEN

It is unusual for a urinary tract specimen to be completely acellular, and even in the absence of disease, a urinary tract specimen will contain at least a few urothelial cells. Additional findings which can be considered normal and of no clinical significance include the presence of rare acute inflammatory cells and bacteria. Voided urine specimens often contain extraurinary contamination, such as mature squamous cells and bacteria. Instrumented specimens, such as those obtained through catheterization or urinary tract washings, typically contain numerous urothelial cells, present as both single cells and fragments.[1,2]

PARABASAL-TYPE CELLS

Parabasal-type cells represent the majority of benign urothelial cells seen in a urinary tract specimen. They are similar in morphology to the parabasal squamous cells seen in cervical Pap test specimens: round to oval in shape with ample dense cytoplasm and a round nucleus with minimal nuclear membrane irregularities (Figures 6.1-6.3).

SQUAMOUS CONTAMINATION

Mature squamous cells often contaminate voided urine specimens but should not be seen in catheterized or instrumented specimens. The cells are large and platelike, are identical to the superficial squamous cells seen on the Pap test, and may occasionally be associated with bacteria (Figures 6.1-6.4). Although cells with squamous differentiation can be native to the urinary tract, such populations usually do not appear as mature squamous cells. The cells often arise from (1) the urethra, which contains nonkeratinizing squamous epithelium distally; (2) squamous metaplasia of the urothelial lining; or (3) a high grade urothelial carcinoma with squamous differentiation.

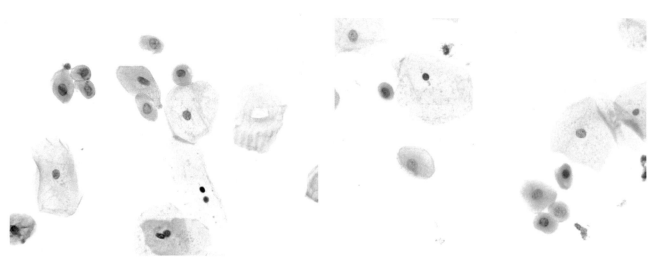

Figure 6.1. Unremarkable urine specimen containing parabasal-type urothelial cells and mature squamous cells. The parabasal cells are small and have dense cytoplasm. The nuclei are round and have regular borders. The chromatin is bland. The nuclear to cytoplasmic (N/C) ratios are low but may approach 0.5 (Pap stain).

Figure 6.2. Unremarkable urine specimen containing parabasal-type urothelial cells and mature squamous cells. Alternate field (Pap stain).

UMBRELLA CELLS

Umbrella cells line the surface of the urothelial tract, display abundant, granular cytoplasm, and contain one to two nuclei, each with a distinct nucleolus. Umbrella cells can sometimes be multinucleated, become greatly enlarged, and/or engulf other cells (Figures 6.5-6.11). Degenerated samples may lead to a loss of umbrella cell cytoplasm, resulting in an increased nuclear to cytoplasmic (N/C) ratio. As a result, these degenerated umbrella cells are sometimes mistaken for atypical urothelial cells (AUC). The presence of granular cytoplasm and round nuclei with nucleoli should help identify these cells as degenerated umbrella cells.

RENAL TUBULAR CELLS

Renal tubular cells (RTCs) occasionally shed into the urine and are sometimes seen in voided urine specimens. Most commonly, RTCs are present in loose clusters and only rarely are found as single, dispersed cells. RTCs have minimal cytoplasm and are smaller than parabasal-type urothelial cells; however, occasionally, RTCs can be large and mimic parabasal-type urothelial cells (Figures 6.12-6.14). It is important to recognize that RTCs have increased N/C ratios due to their minimal cytoplasm and are hyperchromatic at baseline. As a result, RTCs are often overinterpreted as AUC.

CORPORA AMYLACEA

Corpora amylacea are lamellated concretions formed from secretions within the prostate gland. They occasionally can be seen in urinary tract specimens of men and are of no clinical significance (Figure 6.15).

FAQ: How should urinary tract cytology specimens be reported?

Answer: The newly recognized reporting system, *The Paris System for Reporting Urinary Cytology* (TPS), is used worldwide and has standardized the reporting of urinary tract cytology specimens (Table 6.1).[3-6] TPS focuses on assessing a patient's risk for high-grade urothelial carcinoma (HGUC). TPS achieves this goal by noting the presence or absence of HGUC or, in the case of indeterminate findings, assigning either a high-risk or low-risk indeterminate category.

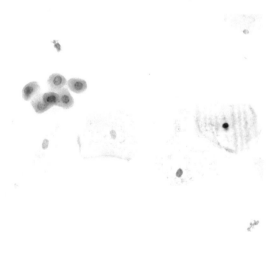

Figure 6.3. Unremarkable urine specimen containing parabasal-type urothelial cells and mature squamous cells. Alternate field (Pap stain).

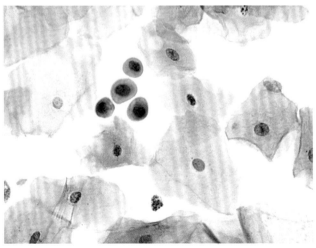

Figure 6.4. Unremarkable urine specimen containing parabasal-type urothelial cells and mature squamous cells. Alternate field (Pap stain).

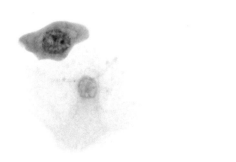

Figure 6.5. Umbrella cell adjacent to a mature squamous cell. Umbrella cells range in size. They have granular cytoplasm, round nuclei with regular borders, and one to two chromocenters (Pap stain).

Figure 6.6. Umbrella cell. Note the granular cytoplasm in this cytoplasm. Umbrella cells may be multinucleated, most commonly with two nuclei. The presence of two nuclei in a cell strongly suggests it is an umbrella cell (Pap stain).

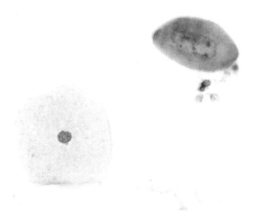

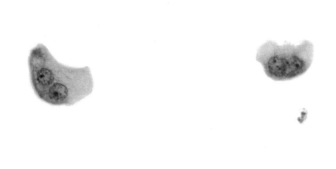

Figure 6.7. Umbrella cell. Alternate field (Pap stain).

Figure 6.8. Two umbrella cells. Note the shared characteristics of the two cells: similar quality of cytoplasm and similar-appearing nuclei (Pap stain).

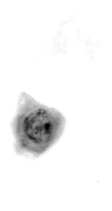

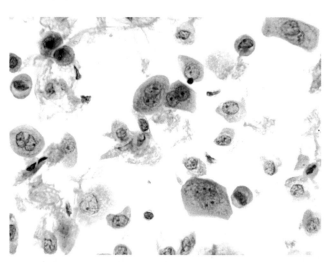

Figure 6.9. Umbrella cell. Alternate field (Pap stain).

Figure 6.10. Numerous umbrella cells. Some specimens may contain numerous umbrella cells, which is a nonspecific finding. Note the variation in cell size. Smaller cells seem to have darker chromatin with higher nuclear to cytoplasmic (N/C) ratios and may be erroneously labeled as atypical urothelial cells (Pap stain).

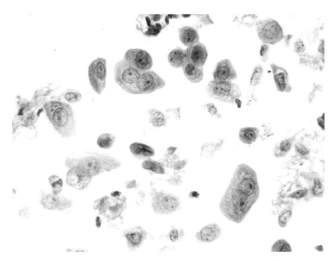

Figure 6.11. Numerous umbrella cells. Alternate field (Pap stain).

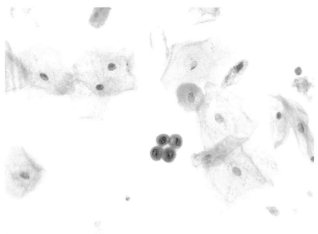

Figure 6.12. Renal tubular cells. Renal tubular cells are small with dense cytoplasm and dark nuclei with nuclear to cytoplasmic (N/C) ratios around 0.5. They form loose clusters containing <10 cells and have a hobnailed appearance to the cluster's edges (Pap stain).

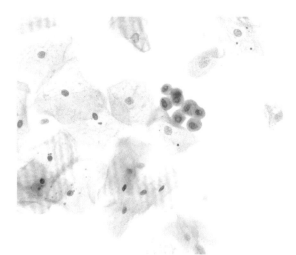

Figure 6.13. Renal tubular cells. Alternate field (Pap stain).

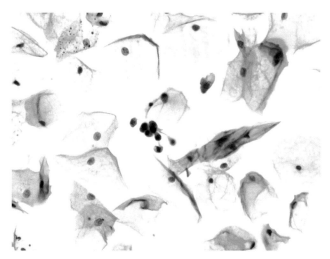

Figure 6.14. Renal tubular cells. These cells are sometimes labeled as atypical urothelial cells or cause concern for small cell carcinoma. However, they are usually only present in small numbers and should not cause great concern for a neoplasm (Pap stain).

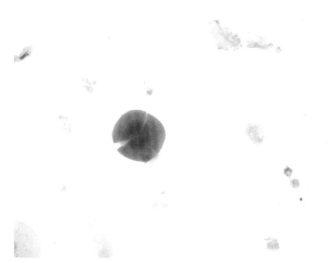

Figure 6.15. Corpora amylacea. A nonspecific finding, corpora are formed in the prostate and appear as acellular material with concentric rings. The cracking artifact seen here is not unusual (Pap stain).

TABLE 6.1: The Paris System for Reporting Urinary Tract Cytology (TPS) Diagnostic Categories

Category	Criteria
Nondiagnostic	No well-defined criteria.
Negative for high-grade urothelial carcinoma (NHGUC)	Features of high-grade urothelial carcinoma are not identified in the specimen.
Atypical urothelial cells (AUC)	Any number of cells in which the nuclear to cytoplasmic (N/C) ratio is >0.5 and one of the below is true: • Mild nuclear border irregularities. • Mild hyperchromasia. • Coarse/clumpy chromatin.
Suspicious for high-grade urothelial carcinoma (SHGUC)	Any number of cells in which the N/C ratio is >0.5, at least moderate to severe hyperchromasia is present, and at least one of the following is true: • Marked nuclear border irregularities. • Coarse/clumpy chromatin. OR Cells meeting the cytomorphologic criteria for the HGUC category in insufficient quantity for a HGUC diagnosis.
High-grade urothelial carcinoma (HGUC)	In an upper tract specimen, at least 10 cells, or in a lower tract specimen, at least 5 cells, in which the following are all true: • N/C ratio ≥0.7. • Marked nuclear border irregularities. • Moderate to severe hyperchromasia. • Coarse/clumpy chromatin.
Low-grade urothelial neoplasm (LGUN)	• The presence of a true urothelial papillary fragment containing a fibrovascular core. • No features that would meet the criteria of an AUC, SHGUC, or HGUC diagnosis.
Other	Important findings that do not fall into the above categories, such as markedly atypical squamous cells and nonurothelial carcinomas.

UROTHELIAL FRAGMENTS PATTERN

Low-grade urothelial neoplasms (LGUNs) and benign urothelial cells usually do not shed as tissue fragments under normal physiologic conditions and, as a result, are typically not present in voided urine specimens. Under the forces of instrumentation, however, urothelial tissue fragments, both benign and neoplastic, may be shed into the urine. High-grade urothelial carcinoma (HGUC) cells tend to be discohesive and more often present as single, dispersed cells rather than in fragments, although fragments of HGUC can be seen in some instrumented specimens.

CHECKLIST: Etiologic Considerations for the Urothelial Fragments Pattern

☐ Benign-Appearing Urothelial Tissue Fragments (BUTFs)

☐ Atypical Urothelial Tissue Fragments (AUTF)

☐ Low-Grade Urothelial Neoplasm (LGUN)

☐ Cohesive High-Grade Urothelial Carcinoma (HGUC)

BENIGN-APPEARING UROTHELIAL TISSUE FRAGMENTS

Benign-appearing urothelial tissue fragments (BUTFs) may be seen in urinary tract specimens of any source. Instrumented specimens inevitably contain BUTFs, as the use of a catheter and/or washing procedure dislodges normal urothelium during specimen procurement. BUTFs contain cells with round nuclei, little size variation, and minimal nuclear border irregularities. The N/C ratios are below 0.5, and the presence of a "cytoplasmic collar"—cytoplasm oriented mostly toward the outer border of the fragment—is considered reassuring (Figures 6.16-6.18). Previously, the conventional wisdom thought the presence of BUTF in voided urine specimens could represent the shedding of urothelium from LGUNs. More recently, however, studies have shown that the presence of BUTFs in voided urine specimens has a low predictive value for LGUN, and in fact, BUTFs are more commonly associated with urolithiasis than neoplasia.[7] In most instances, the cause of BUTFs could not be determined.

FAQ: How should I report numerous urothelial tissue fragments?

Answer: The presence of numerous urothelial tissue fragments is not necessarily associated with the presence of a neoplasm and may be artifactual secondary to instrumentation (even in specimens listed as "voided urine" specimens) or other pathophysiological factors, such as the presence of subclinical urolithiasis. This finding does not have to be reported, and the diagnosis should be based on whether any cytomorphologic atypia present in the tissue fragments is concerning for HGUC.

FAQ: How should I report urothelial tissue fragments in a voided urine specimen?

Answer: While some pathologists previously regarded the presence of urothelial tissue fragments as an abnormal finding that was associated with LGUNs, studies have shown that urothelial tissue fragments in noninstrumented voided urine specimens often have either no identifiable underlying cause or are associated with urolithiasis. The increased risk for LGUN is minimal, and it is not recommended that benign-appearing urothelial tissue fragments be reported. The diagnosis should reflect the presence of any concerning features for HGUC within the fragments.

ATYPICAL UROTHELIAL TISSUE FRAGMENTS

Atypical urothelial tissue fragments (AUTFs) contain mildly atypical features that fall short of a definitive diagnosis of HGUC. Concerning features include cells with hyperchromatic nuclei or irregular nuclear borders (Figures 6.19-6.24). A major cause of AUTFs is urolithiasis, and in such circumstances, this has been labeled "stone atypia."[8] Most patients present with hematuria but may otherwise be asymptomatic. Unless the atypical features are sufficient to merit a diagnosis of *Atypical Urothelial Cells (AUC)* or *Suspicious for High-Grade Urothelial Carcinoma (SHGUC)*, it is best to use a diagnosis of *Negative for High-Grade Urothelial Carcinoma (NHGUC)* and not mention the presence of these fragments (Table 6.1).

FAQ: Are these urothelial tissue fragments atypical or not?

Answer: It can be difficult to assess atypia in urothelial tissue fragments for several reasons. First, intercellular forces alter cell size and shape, making the N/C ratio difficult to determine. In three-dimensional clusters, cellular overlap makes the chromatin appear darker and obscures assessment of the N/C ratio, nuclear borders, and chromatin pattern. HGUC only rarely exists strictly as tissue fragments and single atypical cells should be seen if a specimen contains HGUC. Given the obscuring factors of fragments, it is best to have a higher threshold for making *AUC* or *SHGUC* diagnoses in urothelial tissue fragments with atypia and only diagnose as malignant those fragments displaying overtly high-grade features. In patients with known urolithiasis and no history of urothelial carcinoma, it is wise to altogether disregard mildly atypical fragments.

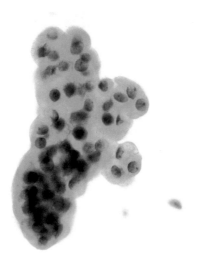

Figure 6.16. Benign urothelial tissue fragment (BUTF). BUTFs may be found in voided or instrumented urine specimens. They have round, regular nuclei with bland chromatin and low nuclear to cytoplasmic (N/C) ratios. Cytoplasm typically lines the edge of the fragment, creating a "cytoplasmic collar" (Pap stain).

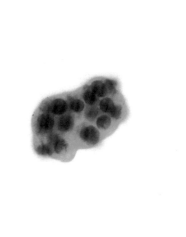

Figure 6.17. Benign urothelial tissue fragment. Alternate field (Pap stain).

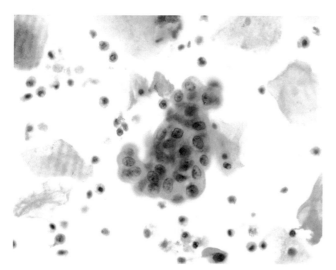

Figure 6.18. Benign urothelial tissue fragment. Alternate field (Pap stain).

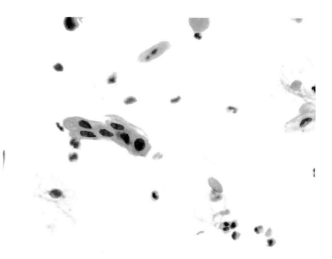

Figure 6.19. Stone atypia. Urolithiasis may cause reactive changes in the urothelium. Affected cells are hyperchromatic and have irregular nuclear borders. The nuclear to cytoplasmic (N/C) ratio typically remains below 0.5 (Pap stain).

LOW-GRADE UROTHELIAL NEOPLASMS

LGUN includes entities such as low-grade urothelial carcinoma (LGUC), papillary urothelial neoplasm of uncertain malignant potential (PUNLMP), and benign urothelial papilloma. Recent studies have determined that urinary tract cytology is neither sensitive nor specific for the detection of LGUN; furthermore, the diagnosis of *LGUN* using urine cytology is not reproducible among pathologists.[9] LGUN exists on a broad cytomorphological spectrum, from lesions that overlap with benign, reactive urothelium to lesions containing areas of focal high-grade cytomorphology.[10] LGUNs are more cohesive than HGUC and rarely spontaneously shed into the urine. As a result, LGUN is most commonly seen in washing or instrumented specimens.

When a LGUN appears in the urine, it may present as a distinct cellular population readily distinguished from benign urothelium. In these cases, the neoplastic cells are often numerous and monotonous.[11] An increased amount of BUTFs may also be seen in a specimen harboring a LGUN, and BUTFs may be difficult to distinguish from neoplastic

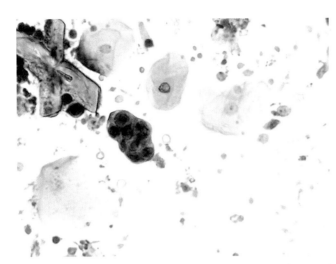

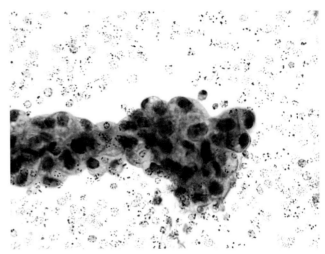

Figure 6.20. Stone atypia. Here, the cells are hyperchromatic and have nuclear to cytoplasmic (N/C) ratios above 0.5. While this meets The Paris System criteria for the *Atypical Urothelial Cells* category, these changes may be dismissed in a patient with known urolithiasis (Pap stain).

Figure 6.21. Stone atypia. Alternate field (Pap stain).

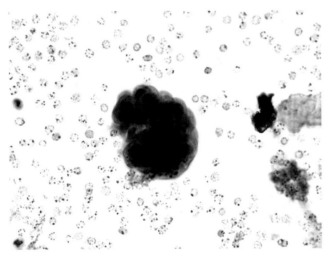

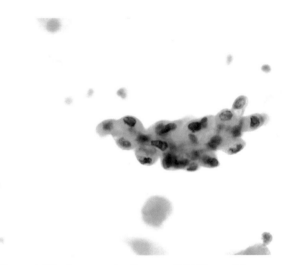

Figure 6.22. Stone atypia. Alternate field (Pap stain).

Figure 6.23. Stone atypia. Alternate field (Pap stain).

urothelial tissue fragments. In specimens with more distinctive morphology, cells may be loosely cohesive, lack the "cytoplasmic collar" seen in BUTFs, have monotonous round to oval eccentrically placed nuclei with regular nuclear borders and small chromocenters, and have N/C ratios that approach 0.5 (Figures 6.25-6.29). Rarely, a tissue fragment containing a fibrovascular stalk can be identified, indicating the presence of a papillary urothelial neoplasm (Figures 6.30 and 6.31). Studies have shown that in some urinary tract specimens from patients with LGUN, rare cells meeting the qualitative requirements for HGUC can be identified in the corresponding or preceding urinary tract specimen. The possible origins of such high-grade cells are not always obvious; these cells may be from focal areas of HGUC within the LGUN, or they may have shed from a synchronous high-grade lesion elsewhere in the urinary tract.[12] If using TPS criteria, it is important to assign a diagnosis based on the presence of high-grade features and not be distracted by low-grade atypia.

While TPS contains the diagnostic category *LGUN*, we recommend caution in its use. Such care is warranted because a LGUN may contain focal areas of HGUC, and these high-grade areas may be underrepresented in a urinary tract specimen. Such lesions may subsequently be diagnosed as HGUC on tissue biopsy if they contain >5% high-grade morphology. The difficulty in separating benign from low-grade malignant cells, paired with the challenge of sampling LGUN and the possibility of focal high-grade carcinoma, makes the diagnosis of *LGUN* very difficult.

KEY FEATURES of Low-Grade Urothelial Neoplasm

- The cytomorphologic features of LGUN are typically only seen in washing/barbotage specimens owing to increased cellular cohesion when compared with high-grade carcinomas, which more readily shed into urine.

- The neoplastic cells are often numerous and monotonous, with an eccentrically placed nucleus 1.5-2.0 times the size of a red blood cell, bland chromatin, and a small chromocenter.

- Cytoplasmic tails may be seen.

- In rare instances, true papillary fragments containing a fibrovascular core lined by the neoplastic cells can be identified.

- LGUN exists on a spectrum, and rare cells with high-grade cytologic features may be seen.

- Specimens should be diagnosed as *AUC* or *SHGUC* only if they have features of HGUC, otherwise, the category *NHGUC* is most appropriate.

FAQ: How should I handle the presence of true papillary urothelial fragments?

Answer: True papillary urothelial fragments are those that contain a fibrovascular core. This finding indicates that some form of urothelial neoplasia, from a benign papilloma to HGUC, was sampled. Accurate grading of such fragments can be difficult on cytology because focal high-grade areas within a lower grade lesion may be absent. The diagnosis should be based on the presence or absence of high-grade features. While TPS allows for a diagnosis of *LGUN*, this diagnosis should be used with caution. Instead, a diagnosis of *NHGUC* is appropriate if no high-grade features are identified.

SAMPLE NOTE: PAPILLARY UROTHELIAL FRAGMENT WITHOUT HIGH-GRADE FEATURES

Negative for High-Grade Urothelial Carcinoma. See note.

Note: A papillary urothelial fragment is identified in the specimen, which indicates the presence of a papillary urothelial neoplasm of undetermined grade. While high-grade features suggestive of a high-grade urothelial carcinoma are not identified, focal areas of a high-grade urothelial carcinoma may not have been sampled in the current specimen.

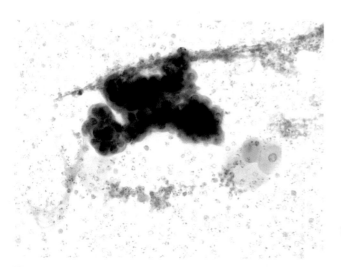

Figure 6.24. Stone atypia. Alternate field (Pap stain).

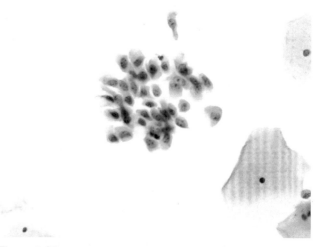

Figure 6.25. Low-grade urothelial neoplasm. The cells are monotonous, with oval-shaped nuclei and regular nuclear borders. The nuclear to cytoplasmic (N/C) ratio is below 0.5. One to two chromocenters are present but not irregular coarse chromatin (Pap stain).

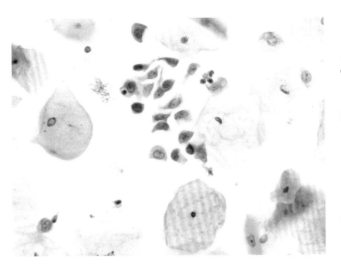

Figure 6.26. Low-grade urothelial neoplasm. Alternate field (Pap stain).

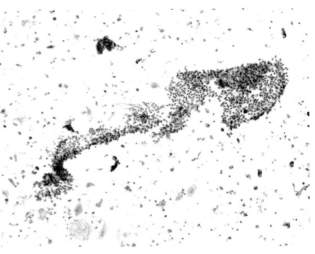

Figure 6.27. Low-grade urothelial neoplasm. The cells form a large papillary fragment without an obvious vascular core. Even at this low magnification, the cells appear neoplastic and monotonous (Pap stain).

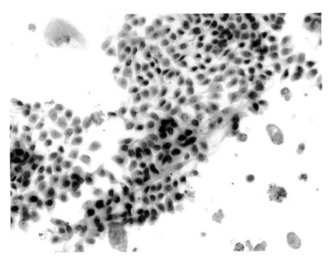

Figure 6.28. Low-grade urothelial neoplasm. Note the eccentrically placed nuclei within these cells. Many have thin, wispy cytoplasmic tails (Pap stain).

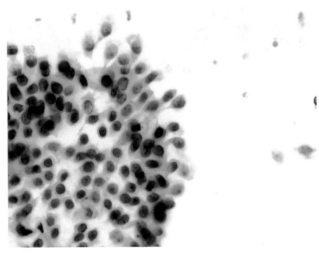

Figure 6.29. Low-grade urothelial neoplasm. Alternate field (Pap stain).

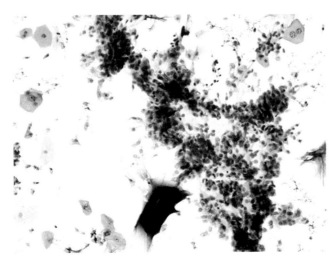

Figure 6.30. Low-grade urothelial neoplasm. The monotonous cells line vascular cores, which are suggested but difficult to see at this magnification. A few cells appear to be "lifting off" from the fragment, and a few are loosely dispersed in the background nearby (Pap stain).

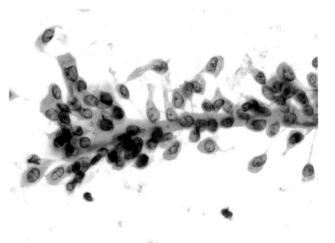

Figure 6.31. Low-grade urothelial neoplasm. The neoplastic cells pull away from the vessel, causing a vase-shaped appearance for some (Pap stain).

COHESIVE HIGH-GRADE UROTHELIAL CARCINOMA

The majority of high-grade urothelial carcinomas (HGUC) will be seen as single, dispersed cells or small clusters in urinary tract specimens regardless of the specimen type. HGUC is significantly less cohesive than LGUN, resulting in both an increased number of neoplastic cells found in voided urine, as well as corresponding areas of denuded epithelium on tissue biopsies. In most instances of HGUC, individual malignant cells are identifiable in the background. It is preferred to assess these individual cells, as the three-dimensional nature of tissue fragments obscures the assessment of the key diagnostic features of HGUC: the N/C ratio, degree of hyperchromasia, chromatin quality, and shape of nuclear borders (see Table 6.1). In instances in which these features can be clearly assessed, the cytomorphologic criteria for classification are the same as those applied to single cells (Figures 6.32-6.41). Interestingly, there is no evidence that fragments of HGUC are more likely to be seen in papillary HGUC lesions compared with carcinoma in situ (CIS) in urinary tract specimens.

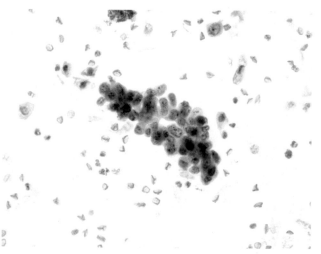

Figure 6.32. Cohesive high-grade urothelial carcinoma (HGUC). The cells have coarse chromatin, high nuclear to cytoplasmic (N/C) ratios, and irregular nuclear borders but are misleadingly small for HGUC. Assessment of these features is best done on single cells rather than cells in fragments. This fragment might best be considered as *Suspicious for High-Grade Urothelial Carcinoma* (Pap stain).

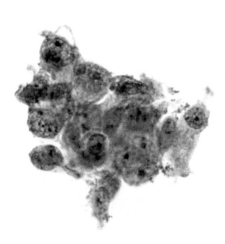

Figure 6.33. Cohesive high-grade urothelial carcinoma (HGUC). HGUC typically forms discohesive cells but may sometimes form small tissue fragments. The cells have high nuclear to cytoplasmic (N/C) ratios, coarse chromatin, and irregular nuclear borders (Pap stain).

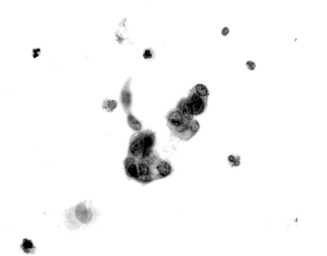

Figure 6.34. Cohesive high-grade urothelial carcinoma. While the chromatin pattern is not so coarse, the chromatin is overall dark and the cells have high nuclear to cytoplasmic (N/C) ratios and irregular nuclear borders (Pap stain).

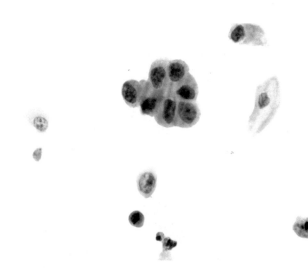

Figure 6.35. Cohesive high-grade urothelial carcinoma. The nuclear to cytoplasmic (N/C) ratio can be difficult to estimate in tissue fragments (Pap stain).

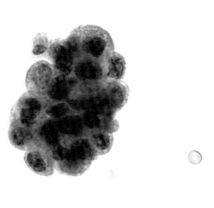

Figure 6.36. Cohesive high-grade urothelial carcinoma. The background is clean in this ThinPrep specimen (Pap stain).

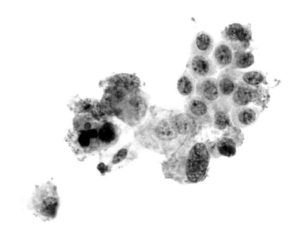

Figure 6.37. Cohesive high-grade urothelial carcinoma. Alternate field (Pap stain).

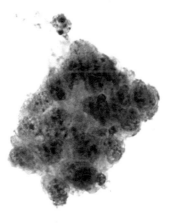

Figure 6.38. Cohesive high-grade urothelial carcinoma. Alternate field (Pap stain).

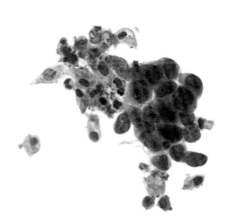

Figure 6.39. Cohesive high-grade urothelial carcinoma. The chromatin is dark, making the coarseness of the chromatin difficult to assess. The nuclear to cytoplasmic (N/C) ratios are high, and very little intervening cytoplasm can be seen in these malignant cells (Pap stain).

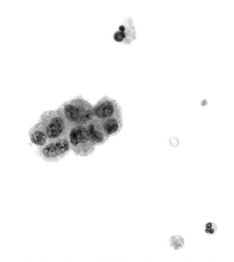

Figure 6.40. Cohesive high-grade urothelial carcinoma. Note the coarseness of the chromatin (Pap stain).

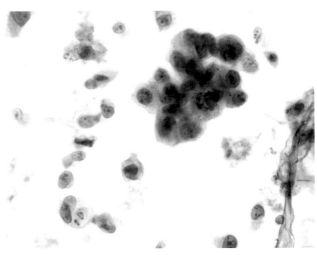

Figure 6.41. Cohesive high-grade urothelial carcinoma (HGUC). A singly dispersed cell (bottom left) has engulfed another cell, which has begun to degenerate. This finding is commonly seen in HGUC but is nonspecific (Pap stain).

DISCOHESIVE PATTERN

A urinary tract specimen containing many dispersed individual cells merits close examination because this is the most common presentation of HGUC. These cells may form a "second population" in a background of normal urothelial cells or may be the predominant population within a specimen. High-power assessment of the cytomorphology of individual cells will reveal whether HGUC can be definitively diagnosed or whether an indeterminate diagnostic category would be more appropriate to risk-stratify a patient for HGUC.

CHECKLIST: Etiologic Considerations for the Discohesive Pattern

☐ Well-Preserved High-Grade Urothelial Carcinoma (HGUC)

☐ *Suspicious for High-Grade Urothelial Carcinoma (SHGUC)*

☐ *Atypical Urothelial Cells (AUC)*

☐ Low-Grade Urothelial Neoplasm (LGUN)

☐ Small Cell Carcinoma

☐ Small Round Blue Cell Tumors

☐ High-Grade Urothelial Carcinoma (HGUC) with a Small Cell Component

---

WELL-PRESERVED HIGH-GRADE UROTHELIAL CARCINOMA

HGUC is typically discohesive, and the malignant cells tend to shed into the urine. Consequently, the examination of voided urine specimens offers excellent diagnostic sensitivity in a noninvasive manner. In an ideal world, the cells would have been recently shed before specimen procurement, with immediate processing and preservation of the specimen. Under these circumstances, well-preserved HGUC cells are readily identified. Well-preserved HGUC cells typically are large, have elevated N/C ratios ($\geq$0.7), and contain coarse, "chunky" chromatin (Figures 6.42-6.47).[13] In rare instances, HGUC may have prominent nucleoli rather than coarse chromatin (see "Prominent Nucleoli Pattern").[14] Despite The Paris System (TPS) requirement that markedly irregular, atypical nuclear borders be present to definitively diagnose HGUC, well-preserved HGUC cells may actually have smooth nuclear borders with only mild nuclear contour irregularities (Figure 6.48). TPS criteria should not be interpreted too literally, because some overtly malignant cells may have low N/C ratios. These cells may still be interpreted as malignant if they contain other features for malignancy and are significantly larger than surrounding cells (Figures 6.49-6.60). For example, HGUC cells may also sometimes have cytoplasmic tails that lower the N/C ratio (Figure 6.61).

KEY FEATURES of Well-Preserved High-Grade Urothelial Carcinoma

- The cells should have N/C ratios of 0.7 or above.
- The chromatin pattern should be coarse ("clumped chromatin").
- The nuclear borders should be markedly irregular.
- Hyperchromasia must be present.
- At least five well-preserved malignant cells should be present in a voided urine specimen, and at least 10 malignant cells should be present in an upper tract (ureter or kidney) washing or brushing specimen.

FAQ: Can I report HGUC when the patient has a concurrent benign tissue biopsy?

Answer: The interpretation of urinary tract cytology specimens should not be overly influenced by biopsy results. The phenomenon of a "false false-negative" result is well known in urinary tract cytopathology. As urinary tract specimens are exfoliative specimens, they may detect lesions that are not recognized until months later. This occurrence is particularly true for carcinoma in situ (CIS) and upper tract lesions, which may not be easily recognized on cystoscopy. In addition, the existence of multifocal and/or multigrade disease may cause discordance. For example, if a low-grade lesion is biopsied, but a separate CIS lesion is not, the urine may contain high-grade cells and be diagnosed as such while the concurrent tissue biopsy is benign. Another common occurrence is the presence of high-grade cells in urine and a completely denuded biopsy with no epithelium present to diagnose malignancy.

FAQ: Can I report HGUC in an upper tract washing specimen?

Answer: A diagnosis of HGUC in an upper tract specimen should be made if the cells present are overtly malignant. However, caution in rendering a malignant diagnosis is imperative because upper tract malignancies may not be as easily biopsied or detected by ureteroscopy and a malignant urinary tract cytology specimen can result in a nephroureterectomy without the step of an intervening tissue biopsy. Partly because of this possible sequence of events, TPS recommends identifying at least 10 well-preserved malignant cells in an upper tract specimen before reporting it as HGUC, as opposed to five cells in bladder specimens.

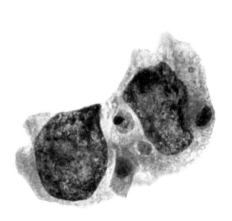

Figure 6.42. High-grade urothelial carcinoma. These two cells are quite large and have engulfed other much smaller cells, some of which have begun to degenerate (Pap stain).

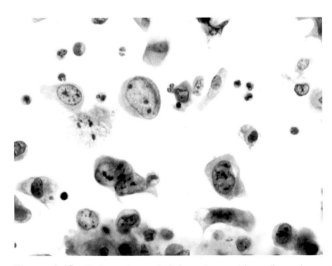

Figure 6.43. High-grade urothelial carcinoma. The cells are large compared with the surrounding cells and have large nuclei. The chromatin is clumped, giving a pale appearance to the remainder of each nucleus (Pap stain).

Figure 6.44. High-grade urothelial carcinoma. The nuclear borders here are regular, but the nuclei are enlarged and demonstrate a coarse chromatin pattern (Pap stain).

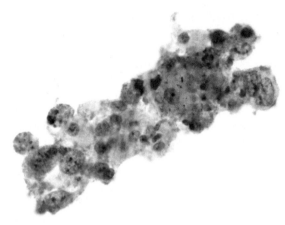

Figure 6.45. High-grade urothelial carcinoma. The malignant cells here are loosely clustered together. Note the variation in nuclear size (Pap stain).

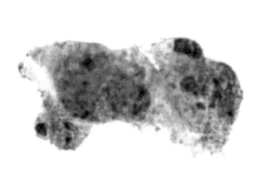

Figure 6.46. High-grade urothelial carcinoma. Several malignant cells form a loose cluster. The nuclear to cytoplasmic (N/C) ratios are difficult to estimate, but the chromatin is coarse and nuclear borders are irregular (Pap stain).

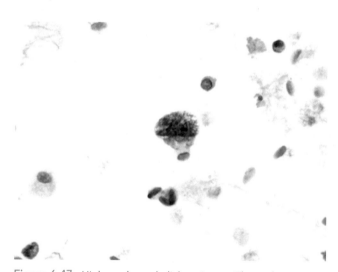

Figure 6.47. High-grade urothelial carcinoma. The nuclear to cytoplasmic (N/C) ratio is elevated, and the nucleus is much larger than the surrounding benign cells (Pap stain).

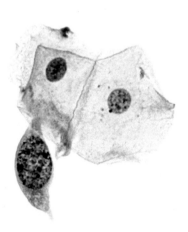

Figure 6.48. High-grade urothelial carcinoma. The nuclear borders are extremely regular in this cell, but all the other features of malignancy are present: high nuclear to cytoplasmic (N/C) ratio, hyperchromasia, and coarse chromatin (Pap stain).

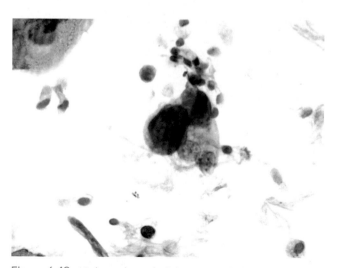

Figure 6.49. High-grade urothelial carcinoma (HGUC). HGUC cells may be multinucleated, but the nuclear atypia distinguishes them from benign umbrella cells, which also may be multinucleated (Pap stain).

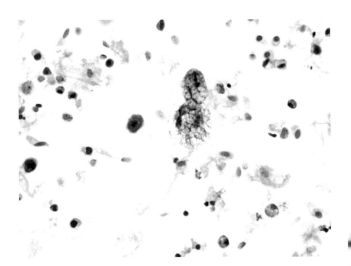

Figure 6.50.   High-grade urothelial carcinoma. This cell has degenerated, and the cytoplasm is no longer intact. The nucleus may be swollen, but the chromatin material is dark and extends over a large area. The finding is highly suspicious for malignancy (Pap stain).

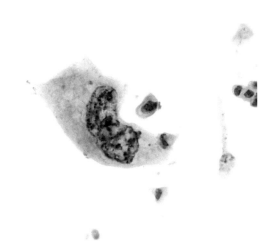

Figure 6.51.   High-grade urothelial carcinoma. The cell emulates an umbrella cell, with granular cytoplasm and binucleation. However, the nuclei are greatly enlarged, have irregular borders, and contain coarse chromatin (Pap stain).

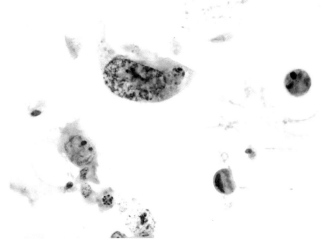

Figure 6.52.   High-grade urothelial carcinoma (HGUC). The nuclear borders are regular, but the coarse chromatin suggests HGUC. A stripped nucleus at the bottom of the field has a similar chromatin pattern and previously belonged to an intact HGUC cell (Pap stain).

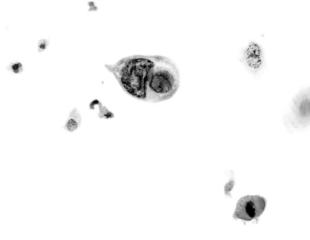

Figure 6.53.   High-grade urothelial carcinoma (HGUC). A "cell-in-cell" pattern may be frequently seen in HGUC. While not entirely specific, the identification of this pattern should cause great concern for HGUC and prompt a careful examination of the entire specimen (Pap stain).

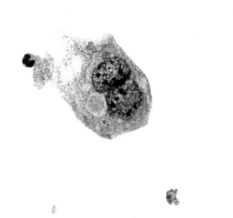

Figure 6.54.   High-grade urothelial carcinoma (HGUC). A binucleate HGUC cell impersonating an umbrella cell. This coarse chromatin pattern should not be seen in umbrella cells (Pap stain).

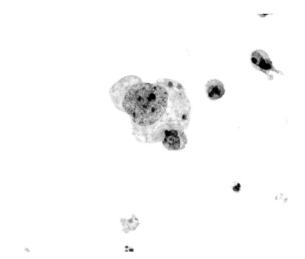

Figure 6.55.   High-grade urothelial carcinoma (HGUC). This cell has a low nuclear to cytoplasmic (N/C) ratio, but the coarse chromatin and large nucleus is concerning for malignancy. Seen alone, this might be best considered *Suspicious for High-Grade Urothelial Carcinoma* (Pap stain).

Figure 6.56. High-grade urothelial carcinoma. The nucleus is more than 10 times the size of a red blood cell, which should cause concern for malignancy. The very low nuclear to cytoplasmic (N/C) ratio is misleading in this instance (Pap stain).

Figure 6.57. High-grade urothelial carcinoma (HGUC). An example of a multinucleated HGUC cell. Note the coarseness of the chromatin (Pap stain).

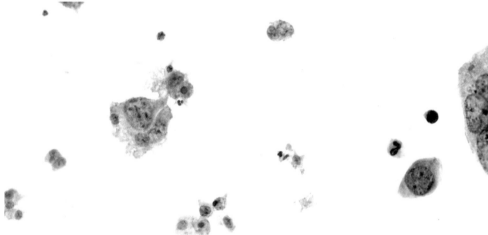

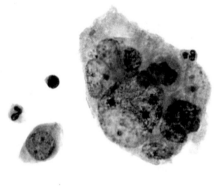

Figure 6.58. High-grade urothelial carcinoma. Alternate field (Pap stain).

Figure 6.59. High-grade urothelial carcinoma. Alternate field (Pap stain).

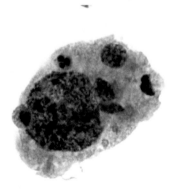

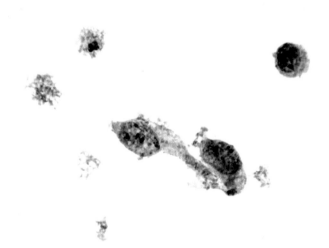

Figure 6.60. High-grade urothelial carcinoma. Alternate field (Pap stain).

Figure 6.61. High-grade urothelial carcinoma (HGUC). While cytoplasmic tails are more frequently associated with low-grade urothelial neoplasms in urinary tract specimens, they can also be seen in HGUC. Their presence causes a lowering of the nuclear to cytoplasmic (N/C) ratio, but all the other characteristics of HGUC are present (Pap stain).

SUSPICIOUS FOR HIGH-GRADE UROTHELIAL CARCINOMA

The *SHGUC* category applies in two situations where atypical cells are insufficient for the diagnosis of malignancy, either in number or in degree of atypia (Figures 6.62-6.75). In the first situation, cells can be identified which meet TPS cytomorphologic criteria for *HGUC* but are insufficient in number. In the second and perhaps more common situation, numerous atypical cells are present, but they do not meet TPS cytomorphologic criteria for *HGUC*. This failure is usually due to degenerative changes, with most cells having N/C ratios between the cutoffs for atypical and malignant cells in TPS (0.5 and 0.7, respectively). The cells usually contain other features of HGUC (irregular nuclear borders, hyperchromasia, and coarse chromatin). The positive predictive values (PPV) of the *SHGUC* and equivalent categories for *SHGUC* varies by institution and follow-up period, but published reports show a range from 37.8-79% within a 6-month follow-up period.[15-18] When the follow-up period is extended, the PPV for this category approaches 95% in some institutions.[18] Early prospective studies have shown that *SHGUC* comprises 2-5% of diagnoses with a rate of malignancy of 55-83% among patients receiving a follow-up cystoscopy and biopsy.[19-21] Patients given a "suspicious" diagnosis are more likely to receive follow-up than those given an "atypical" diagnosis, especially if the ordering physician is not a urologist.[22]

KEY FEATURES of *Suspicious for High-Grade Urothelial Carcinoma*

- The atypical cells should have N/C ratios >0.5, moderately to severely hyperchromatic nuclei, and at least one of the following additional criteria:

  - Coarse, clumped chromatin

  - Markedly irregular nuclear borders

- Rare cells may be overtly malignant and meet all TPS criteria but fail to meet the quantitative threshold of 5 or 10 cells (lower and upper tract specimens, respectively).

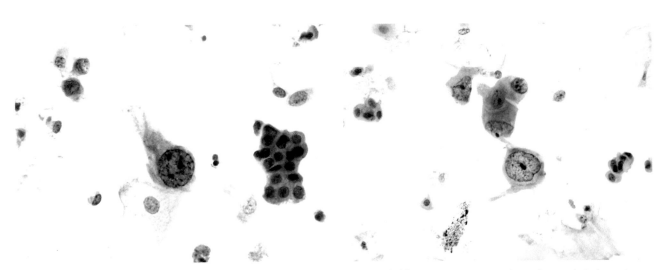

Figure 6.62. Suspicious for high-grade urothelial carcinoma (SHGUC). The cell has a nuclear to cytoplasmic (N/C) ratio of approximately 0.5 but contains other characteristics of malignancy. Experienced pathologists may be comfortable with a diagnosis of HGUC, given the greatly increased nuclear size compared with the surrounding cells (Pap stain).

Figure 6.63. Suspicious for high-grade urothelial carcinoma (SHGUC). The cells have coarse chromatin and irregular borders, but the nuclear to cytoplasmic (N/C) ratios are below 0.7 (Pap stain).

Figure 6.64. Suspicious for high-grade urothelial carcinoma (SHGUC). The specimen is degenerated, and the two suspicious cells at the bottom of the field have disintegrative cytoplasm. However, the nuclei are enlarged and "ink black", a common finding in degenerated HGUC cells (Pap stain).

Figure 6.65. Suspicious for high-grade urothelial carcinoma (SHGUC). The specimen is degenerated, with a single suspicious cell in the center of the field. The cytoplasm is no longer intact, making the nuclear to cytoplasmic (N/C) ratio difficult to assess. However, the coarse chromatin pattern is concerning for HGUC (Pap stain).

ATYPICAL UROTHELIAL CELLS

The goal of the *AUC* category is to identify the subset of patients with an increased risk of HGUC. There is no minimum number of atypical cells required to make a diagnosis of *AUC* in TPS, but the atypical cells should have N/C ratios of at least 0.5.[23-25] In addition, at least one other feature of HGUC should be present: either hyperchromasia, nuclear border irregularities, or coarse chromatin (Figures 6.76-6.80). Care should be taken to exclude benign causes of cellular alterations mimicking neoplasia in normal cells, such as RTCs, BK polyomavirus, and stone atypia.[26] Before TPS, 1.9-30% of urinary tract diagnoses would fall in the "atypical" category, with a variable rate of subsequent malignancy (8.3-37.5%).[6,17,18,23,27-33] While it is uncertain how TPS will ultimately impact the use and performance of the *AUC* category, early prospective data suggest that *AUC* has comprised 15-25% of urinary tract diagnoses, with a 30-50% rate of malignancy among patients receiving a follow-up biopsy.[34,35]

FAQ: Should I report these urothelial cells as atypical?

Answer: To keep *Atypical Urothelial Cells (AUC)* as a diagnosis implying an increased risk of high grade urothelial carcinoma (HGUC), atypical cells should be reported only if they contain features of HGUC. A diagnosis of *AUC* alone has a low associated risk of malignancy, and the diagnosis alone without other findings is not typically a clinically actionable result (but may cause a patient unnecessary trepidation). If the atypical cells have N/C ratios below 0.5 or are degenerated, they should not be reported. In patients with a history of urolithiasis, urinary tract inflammation, and other possible causes of urothelial atypia, mild atypia is best disregarded and the specimen should be reported as *Negative for High-Grade Urothelial Carcinoma (NHGUC)*.

KEY FEATURES of *Atypical Urothelial Cells*
- Atypical cells should be well-preserved without degenerative changes and have a N/C ratio of >0.5, in addition to one of the following:
  - Mild nuclear border irregularities
  - Mild hyperchromasia
  - Coarse/clumpy chromatin

Figure 6.66. Suspicious for high-grade urothelial carcinoma (SHGUC). Alternate field (Pap stain).

Figure 6.67. Suspicious for high-grade urothelial carcinoma (SHGUC). Alternate field (Pap stain).

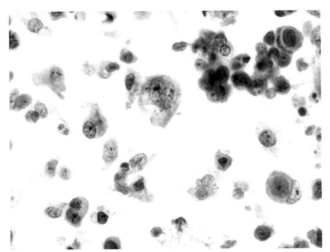

Figure 6.68. Suspicious for high-grade urothelial carcinoma (SHGUC). The field contains many HGUC cells, but the nuclear to cytoplasmic (N/C) ratios are below 0.7. Experienced pathologists may be comfortable diagnosing this specimen as HGUC, given the numerous atypical cells and the coarse chromatin possessed by many of these cells (Pap stain).

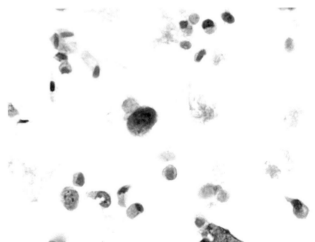

Figure 6.69. Suspicious for high-grade urothelial carcinoma (SHGUC). This cell has only a small amount of cytoplasm left, which forms a square shape. The chromatin is beginning to degenerate, but some chromatin clumps are still identifiable. Several smaller cells in the background are also likely degenerating HGUC cells, although they have fewer features suggestive of HGUC (Pap stain).

LOW-GRADE UROTHELIAL NEOPLASM

Urinary tract washing specimens from LGUN may contain numerous discohesive or loosely cohesive, monotonous, teardrop-shaped cells with small nucleoli and eccentrically placed nuclei in addition to the aforementioned tissue fragments (Figures 6.81-6.86; see the "Urothelial Fragments Pattern").[11,12] Presumably, the unusual morphology of these cells results from their mechanical disruption from the papillary fragment during the procedure. The rare specimens containing a fibrovascular stalk from which the neoplastic cells appear to pull away lend credence to this hypothesis.

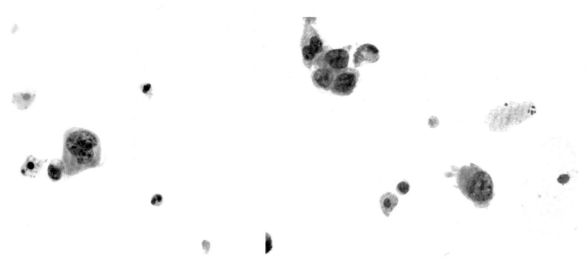

Figure 6.70. Suspicious for high-grade urothelial carcinoma (SHGUC). The cell has a low nuclear to cytoplasmic (N/C) ratio, but the nuclear borders are irregular and the chromatin is coarse. Adjacent smaller degenerating cells have small red inclusions known as Melamed-Wolinska bodies (Pap stain).

Figure 6.71. Suspicious for high-grade urothelial carcinoma (SHGUC). Alternate field (Pap stain).

Figure 6.72. Suspicious for high-grade urothelial carcinoma (SHGUC). Alternate field (Pap stain).

Figure 6.73. Suspicious for high-grade urothelial carcinoma (SHGUC). Alternate field (Pap stain).

SMALL CELL CARCINOMA

Small cell carcinoma is often found in conjunction with metastatic/infiltrative prostate carcinoma or HGUC, but it may also present as a singular malignancy within the bladder.[2,36] The malignant cells are slightly larger than the surrounding inflammatory cells and contain minimal cytoplasm. In liquid-based preparations, cells are typically dispersed with scattered small clusters of loosely cohesive cells (Figures 6.87-6.95). Liquid-based preparations alter the morphological features seen on both cytologic slides and cell block sections with reduced chromatin smearing artifact, minimization of nuclear molding, and geographic necrosis.[37] In specimens with dispersed cells, the tumor cells may blend in with inflammatory background components and be easily overlooked. However, careful high-power examination demonstrates a few distinguishing features of these scattered cells. Small cell carcinoma cells can be compared with the ever-present lymphocytes as an internal control. Such comparison reveals variation in nuclear size beyond that of lymphocytes, the absence of the typical cytoplasmic rim of the lymphocytes, and the key feature of speckled, neuroendocrine-type chromatin. For unknown reasons, necrotic cells of small cell

Figure 6.74. Suspicious for high-grade urothelial carcinoma (SHGUC). A multinucleated HGUC cell. Note the darkness of the chromatin and irregularity to the nuclear borders (Pap stain).

Figure 6.75. Suspicious for high-grade urothelial carcinoma (SHGUC). A large HGUC cell with a nuclear to cytoplasmic (N/C) ratio below 0.7. Although this disqualifies the cell for a diagnosis of HGUC according to The Paris System criteria, the coarse chromatin and large nuclear size (more than 20 times the size of the red blood cells) are diagnostic of HGUC (Pap stain).

Figure 6.76. Atypical urothelial cells. This patient subsequently was found to have high-grade urothelial carcinoma (HGUC). The atypical cells have coarse chromatin, but they have low nuclear to cytoplasmic (N/C) ratios and are only minimally enlarged compared with the adjacent neutrophils (Pap stain).

Figure 6.77. Atypical urothelial cells. Alternate field (Pap stain).

carcinoma often remain intact and create a second population of "ghost cells" scattered across the sample. These ghost cells stain blue on Papanicolaou-stained preparations and, thus, appear as "blue blobs" in the background—in contrast to the eosinophilic color of necrotic cells when stained with H&E.

If necessary, a cell block or additional unstained cytologic slides can be created from any residual specimen and used for confirmatory immunostains (e.g. INSM1, chromogranin, synaptophysin, CD56).[38,39] However, not all small cell carcinomas express these markers. Ki-67 is a useful marker of small cell carcinoma in surgical pathology specimens, as the Ki-67 proliferation rate of small cell carcinoma is typically >90%. In cytologic material, interpretation of Ki-67 becomes problematic owing to admixed benign epithelial cells and inflammatory cells posing as "bystanders" in the background.

As mentioned earlier, small cell carcinoma may arise as a mixed tumor with a second component, and this second component may be underrepresented in a given specimen.[40] TPS recommends that a specimen containing only a small cell component should be classified as *Other:*

Carcinoma with small cell features. If small cell carcinoma is seen along with HGUC or prostate carcinoma, then TPS recommends classification as either *High-grade urothelial carcinoma with a small cell component* or *Other: Prostate carcinoma with a small cell component*, respectively.

KEY FEATURES of Small Cell Carcinoma

- The neoplastic cells are mildly pleomorphic, slightly larger than lymphocytes, and contain minimal to absent cytoplasm.
- The cells are often single but may form small to medium-sized fragments. Other specimens may be comprised exclusively of single cells.
- Cellular necrosis may be seen as dispersed "blue blobs" throughout the background.
- The carcinoma cells contain typical neuroendocrine speckled ("salt-and-pepper") chromatin.
- In liquid-based preparations, the classic features of small cell carcinoma, such as nuclear molding, chromatin streaking artifact, and necrosis, may be reduced.

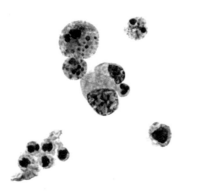

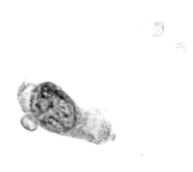

Figure 6.78. Atypical urothelial cells. High magnification of Figure 6.77. Note the red cytoplasmic concretions in the degenerated cells, called Melamed-Wolinska bodies (Pap stain).

Figure 6.79. Atypical urothelial cells. The nuclear to cytoplasmic (N/C) ratio is approximately 0.5, and the cell has coarse chromatin. Because the nucleus is enlarged (10× the size of the adjacent red blood cells), one could argue for a diagnosis of *Suspicious for High-Grade Urothelial Carcinoma*, although nuclear size is not a feature considered by The Paris System (Pap stain).

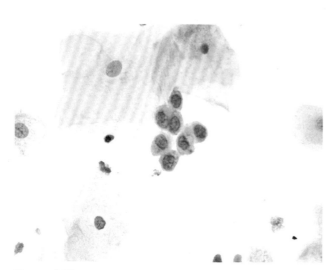

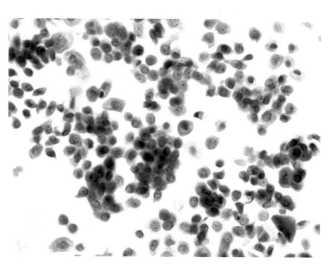

Figure 6.80. Atypical urothelial cells. Small urothelial cells with hyperchromasia and mild nuclear border irregularities. The nuclear to cytoplasmic (N/C) ratios fall between 0.5 and 0.7 (Pap stain).

Figure 6.81. Low-grade urothelial neoplasia (LGUN). The cells are predominantly dispersed and have nuclear to cytoplasmic (N/C) ratios below 0.5. Features of high-grade urothelial carcinoma (HGUC) are lacking: the nuclear membranes are regular, and the chromatin is not coarse (Pap stain).

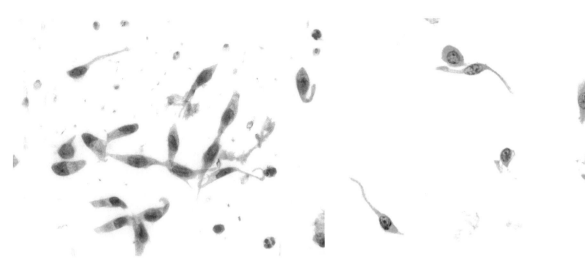

Figure 6.82. Low-grade urothelial neoplasia (LGUN). Alternate field (Pap stain).

Figure 6.83. Low-grade urothelial neoplasia (LGUN). The presence of cytoplasmic tails is often seen with LGUN lesions sampled by washing/barbotage during cystoscopy or ureteroscopy. Note the regular nuclear membranes and bland chromatin (Pap stain).

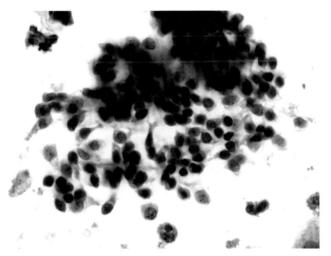

Figure 6.84. Low-grade urothelial neoplasia (LGUN). While LGUN lesions can have focal areas of high-grade morphology, the cells here have nuclei around the same size, bland chromatin, and nuclear to cytoplasmic (N/C) ratios around 0.5 (Pap stain).

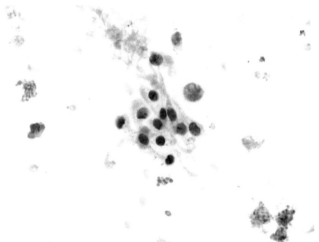

Figure 6.85. Low-grade urothelial neoplasia (LGUN). Alternate field (Pap stain).

SMALL ROUND BLUE CELL TUMORS

Rarely, small round blue cell tumors of renal origin in the pediatric population, such as Wilms tumor (Figures 6.96 and 6.97) or embryonal rhabdomyosarcoma (Figure 6.98), may be seen in urinary tract specimens.[41,42] These patients typically present with a known mass lesion and a distinct clinicoradiologic impression of a renal primary. Tumor sampling, however, is required for a definitive diagnosis. In urinary tract specimens, these neoplastic cells appear similar to those described above for small cell carcinoma in liquid-based preparations.

HIGH-GRADE UROTHELIAL CARCINOMA WITH A SMALL CELL COMPONENT

HGUC sometimes transforms into small cell carcinoma, resulting in a high-grade neoplasm with combined morphology. In most instances, only one component will be seen in the urine specimen. If both components are definitively seen in a urinary tract specimen, then the diagnostic category of *HGUC* is appropriate, with use of the modifier "with a small cell component."

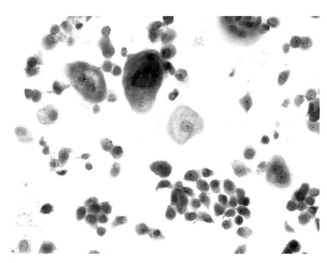

Figure 6.86. Low-grade urothelial neoplasia (LGUN). Alternate field (Pap stain).

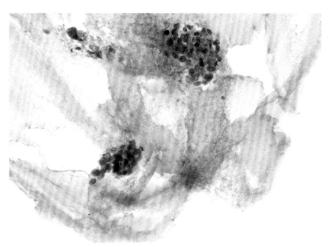

Figure 6.87. Small cell carcinoma. Cell block preparations allow for immunohistochemical studies when the diagnosis is in doubt. However, small cell carcinoma can sometimes be negative for neuro-endocrine markers (chromogranin, synaptophysin, and INSM1). The cells are cytomorphologically compatible with small cell carcinoma, having very little cytoplasm (H&E).

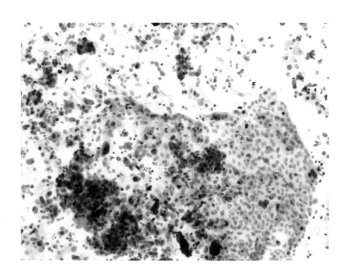

Figure 6.88. Small cell carcinoma. At low magnification, the field is cellular and contains fragments as well as many individually dispersed small cells (Pap stain).

Figure 6.89. Small cell carcinoma. The cells form small discohesive clusters that may mimic renal tubular cells (RTCs) or lymphocytes. However, groups of RTCs are usually smaller and lymphocytes do not form such clusters in urinary tract specimens (Pap stain).

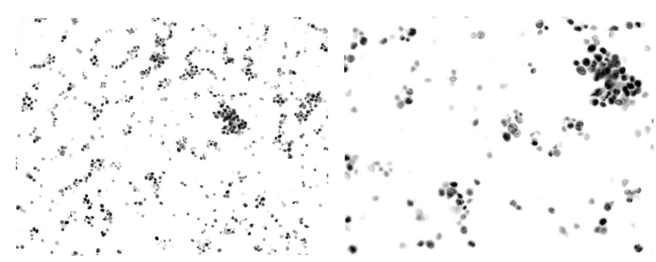

Figure 6.90. Small cell carcinoma. Well-dispersed carcinoma cells emulated a population of lymphocytes at this low magnification. Closer examination will reveal the true nature of these cells (Pap stain).

Figure 6.91. Small cell carcinoma. A higher magnification demonstrates that the cells lack the thin rim of cytoplasm seen in lymphocytes and that the cells are larger than lymphocytes (compare with nearby red blood cells) (Pap stain).

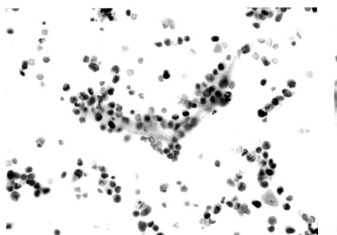

Figure 6.92. Small cell carcinoma. Alternate field (Pap stain).

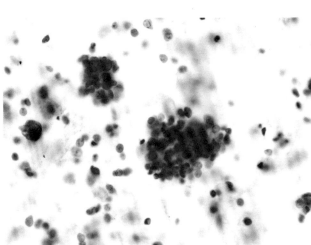

Figure 6.93. Small cell carcinoma. Two loosely cohesive clusters of tumor cells can be seen with numerous dispersed single cells in the background. The chromatin appears pale/speckled in this preparation (Pap stain).

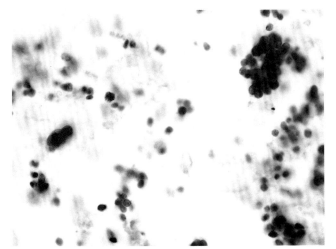

Figure 6.94. Small cell carcinoma. Alternate field (Pap stain).

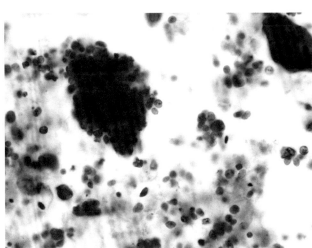

Figure 6.95. Small cell carcinoma. Alternate field (Pap stain).

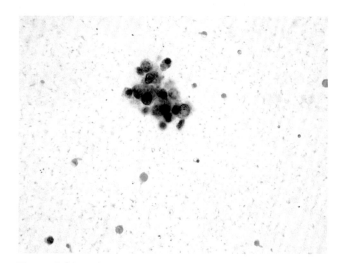

Figure 6.96. Wilms tumor. While uncommon, small round blue cell tumors can sometimes be seen in the urine of affected pediatric patients. Here, the cells are slightly larger than adjacent red blood cells and have very little cytoplasm (Pap stain).

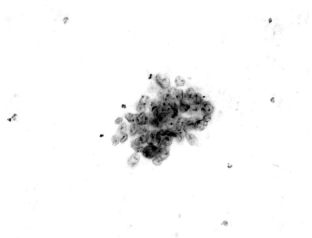

Figure 6.97. Wilms tumor. A cluster of loosely cohesive small round blue cells (Pap stain).

Figure 6.98. Embryonal rhabdomyosarcoma. This is another small round blue cell tumor that can be seen in pediatric patients. Biopsy is typically required for definitive diagnosis (Pap stain).

DEGENERATED PATTERN

Immediate refrigeration or fixation is recommended until further processing of urine samples. Despite this goal, many laboratories receive specimens that have been left at room temperature. Some degree of degeneration is unpreventable. For example, cellular components that have been shed into the urine may have already been exposed to urine at body temperature for several hours before collection. Furthermore, prolonged exposure to room temperature post collection will result in further degeneration of the specimen. Urothelial cells are more susceptible to degeneration than other cells in the urine (e.g., inflammatory cells, squamous cells, etc.). Unfortunately, these changes cause obfuscation, with HGUC cells appearing less malignant and benign cells becoming atypical.

DEGENERATED BENIGN SAMPLE

Urothelial cells are often exposed to urine at body temperature for several hours before collection, resulting in poorly preserved urothelial cell components. Not surprisingly, patients with urinary retention, once catheterized, may provide very cellular specimens containing markedly degenerated cells that mimic degenerated HGUC. While immediate refrigeration or fixation is recommended after collection, many laboratories receive specimens that have been left at room temperature, a practice that results in further degeneration of the specimen. Degeneration in urothelial cells manifests in various morphologies, and some of these could result in an indeterminate diagnosis. Degenerated urothelial cells may have pyknotic nuclei and abundant, vacuolated cytoplasm (Figures 6.99-6.102). In some instances, the cytoplasm may no longer be present and only the stripped, pyknotic nuclei remain. Distinctive intracytoplasmic concretions, known as Melamed-Wolinska bodies, may be seen in benign or malignant cells.[43] These spherical bodies, red or green in color, are believed to arise from swollen lysosomes.

URINARY DIVERSION OR NEOBLADDER SPECIMEN

Following cystectomy, patients often have urinary tract reconstruction using a segment of intestine to form a conduit or neobladder. These patients usually have a history of advanced HGUC and are at high risk of recurrence. Urinary diversion and neobladder specimens are recognizable by the abundance of dispersed, degenerated glandular cells that shed from the mucosa of the intestinal segment. These degenerated benign cells appear hyperchromatic and can obscure the presence of scattered HGUC cells.[44,45] One helpful feature of HGUC in these complex cases is the fact that HGUC cells are typically much larger than the degenerated background cells (Figures 6.102-6.105).

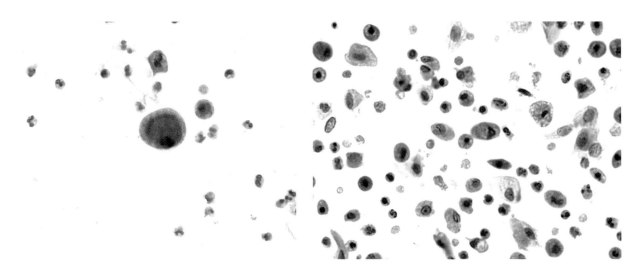

Figure 6.99. Degenerated benign specimen. The two larger cells in this specimen have indistinct boundaries between the nucleus and cytoplasm, one sign that the cells are severely degenerated. Cells such as these should not be assessed for atypia (Pap stain).

Figure 6.100. Degenerated benign specimen. The cells have vacuolated cytoplasm and pyknotic nuclei, but the compressed nuclei do not have the hyperchromasia as would be seen in degenerated high-grade urothelial carcinoma (HGUC) cells. Also, the degenerated cells are smaller than the less degenerated cells in the field (right center) (Pap stain).

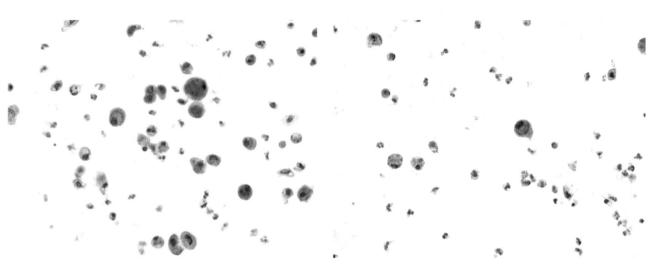

Figure 6.101. Degenerated benign specimen. Alternate field (Pap stain).

Figure 6.102. Degenerated benign specimen. Alternate field (Pap stain).

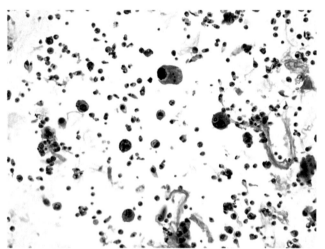

Figure 6.103. Neobladder specimen. The scattered small cells in the background are commonly seen in most patients with neobladders or ileal conduits. The larger cells with large, dark ("ink black"), pyknotic nuclei are degenerated high-grade urothelial carcinoma (HGUC) cells and represent a recurrence in this patient (Pap stain).

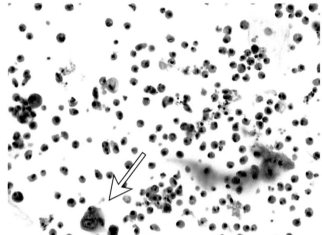

Figure 6.104. Neobladder specimen. Careful examination of the specimen reveals a larger cell with a high nuclear to cytoplasmic (N/C) ratio and irregular borders (arrow). This field is at least suspicious for high-grade urothelial carcinoma (SHGUC) (Pap stain).

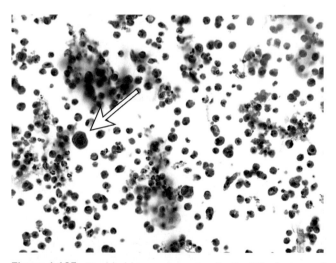

Figure 6.105. Neobladder specimen. A cell with all the features of high-grade urothelial carcinoma (HGUC) (arrow) can be seen among a background of degenerated ileal conduit cells (Pap stain).

DEGENERATED HIGH-GRADE UROTHELIAL CARCINOMA

The prolonged exposure to urine at body temperature that affects benign urothelial cells also alters the appearance of HGUC cells and makes it much more difficult for the pathologist to render a definitive diagnosis. This problem further underscores the need for immediate fixation or refrigeration post collection. Degeneration alters HGUC cells in the same ways as other urothelial cells, with expansion and vacuolization of the cytoplasm and corresponding nuclear pyknosis occurring to varying degrees.[46] The inward condensation of the nucleus causes it to appear coal black (preventing examination of the chromatin pattern) with highly irregular borders. The dark, shrunken nucleus combined with degenerative cytoplasmic expansion results in a lower N/C ratio (Figures 6.106-6.111). For these reasons, most degenerated cells will not meet the criteria for the *HGUC* category put forth in TPS. However, in practice, the presence of numerous individual cells with the above morphology allows for a diagnosis of malignancy. Depending on the comfort level of the pathologist and the clinical situation, it may also be appropriate to make a diagnosis of *SHGUC* in these cases (see *"Suspicious for High-Grade Urothelial Carcinoma*, below).

KEY FEATURES of Degenerated High-Grade Urothelial Carcinoma
- The malignant cells contain degenerated features such as foamy and/or fragmented cytoplasm and pyknotic nuclei, causing lower N/C ratios.
- Despite being compressed, the nucleus contains abundant chromatin and appears "jet black."
- Degenerated malignant cells may be present in great numbers, further supporting the presence of a malignancy.

SUSPICIOUS FOR HIGH-GRADE UROTHELIAL CARCINOMA

Some specimens may contain a high burden of HGUC cells but with significant degeneration. Generally speaking, degenerated HGUC cells contain pyknotic nuclei with sharp nuclear borders and have N/C ratios below 0.7, which precludes a diagnosis of *HGUC* according to TPS (Figures 6.112-6.131).[47]

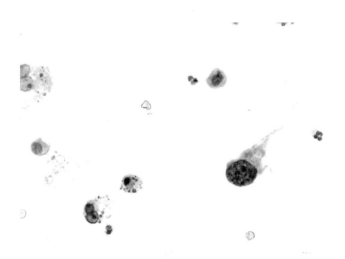

Figure 6.106. Degenerated high-grade urothelial carcinoma (HGUC). The malignant cell's cytoplasm has begun to degenerate, but the nucleus remains intact. Surrounding cells are also degenerated and contain Melamed-Wolinska bodies (Pap stain).

Figure 6.107. Degenerated high-grade urothelial carcinoma (HGUC). This field contains an intact HGUC cell (upper right) and two degenerated HGUC cells in the center of the field. The degenerated HGUC cells have pyknotic "ink black" nuclei with irregular borders (Pap stain).

Figure 6.108. Degenerated high-grade urothelial carcinoma (HGUC). The cytoplasmic borders have become fluffy and somewhat indistinct. The nucleus is extremely dark and has markedly irregular borders (Pap stain).

Figure 6.109. Degenerated high-grade urothelial carcinoma (HGUC). Alternate field (Pap stain).

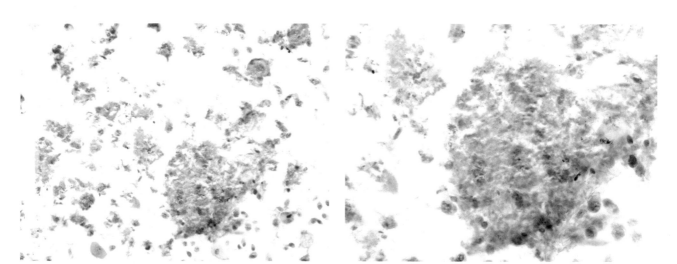

Figure 6.110. Degenerated high-grade urothelial carcinoma (HGUC). This HGUC has become invasive and areas of granular (necrotic) debris can be seen. Numerous malignant nuclei—some degenerated, others somewhat intact—can be seen within the debris (Pap stain).

Figure 6.111. Degenerated high-grade urothelial carcinoma (HGUC). Higher magnification of Figure 6.110 (Pap stain).

BACILLUS CALMETTE-GUÉRIN EFFECT

Intravesical Bacillus Calmette-Guérin (BCG) is used as an effective form of immunotherapy against HGUC. The modified tuberculosis bacterium stimulates an immune response localized within the urinary tract that frequently eliminates noninvasive HGUC and CIS.[48] Specimens from patients with recent BCG therapy are often highly cellular and contain a mixture of inflammatory cells, degenerated benign urothelial cells, debris, and degenerated malignant cells. Multinucleated giant cells and/or granulomatous inflammation may be seen in some instances and are strongly suggestive of recent BCG therapy when a history is not known (Figures 6.132-6.138).[49] Degenerated cells with marked atypia are likely dying HGUC cells and do not necessarily represent active disease. These cells often have abundant, foamy cytoplasm with large, dark nuclei and angulated nuclear borders. It is best not to classify these degenerated atypical cells as *AUC* or *SHGUC* in patients with recent BCG treatment. The same does not apply to viable atypical or malignant cells.

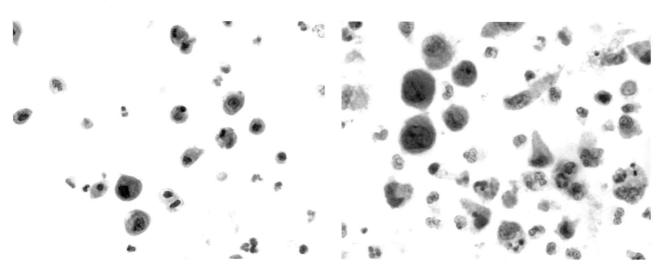

Figure 6.112. Suspicious for high-grade urothelial carcinoma (SHGUC). These HGUC cells have dark pyknotic nuclei with irregular nuclear borders. Despite having nuclear to cytoplasmic (N/C) ratios below 0.5, when numerous cells such as these are seen, it is better to make a diagnosis of at least *SHGUC* (Pap stain).

Figure 6.113. Suspicious for high-grade urothelial carcinoma (SHGUC). The cells in the upper left field have enlarged nuclei, irregular nuclear borders, and dark, coarse chromatin. Most do not have nuclear to cytoplasmic (N/C) ratios of 0.7 and would be classified as *SHGUC* according to The Paris System (Pap stain).

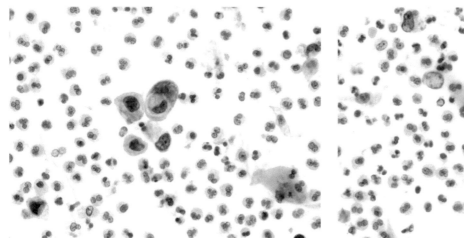

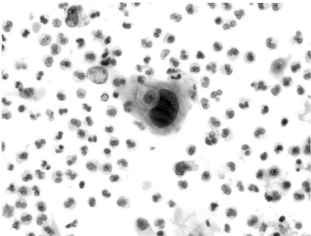

Figure 6.114. Suspicious for high-grade urothelial carcinoma (SHGUC). The four cells in the center of the field are HGUC cells. One cell has engulfed another malignant cell. The cells meet all but one criteria of The Paris System for HGUC: the nuclear to cytoplasmic (N/C) ratios are below 0.7 (Pap stain).

Figure 6.115. Suspicious for high-grade urothelial carcinoma (SHGUC). This cell has a very large, hyperchromatic nucleus. It has engulfed a bystander cell. While the nuclear to cytoplasmic (N/C) ratio is below 0.5, the cell is at the very least suspicious for HGUC (Pap stain).

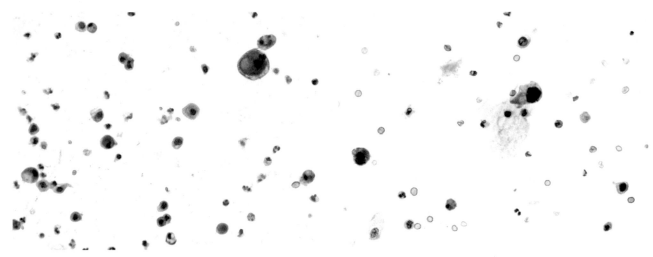

Figure 6.116. Suspicious for high-grade urothelial carcinoma (SHGUC). The cell at the top right is extremely degenerated but has a large nucleus with a high nuclear to cytoplasmic (N/C) ratio. The scattered cells in the background are much smaller, but many are larger than adjacent red blood cells and have hyperchromatic nuclei with irregular borders. The findings are concerning for HGUC (Pap stain).

Figure 6.117. Suspicious for high-grade urothelial carcinoma (SHGUC). The cell in the center has dark chromatin, has irregular nuclear borders, and is quite large compared with adjacent red blood cells. Even though the nuclear to cytoplasmic (N/C) ratio is slightly below 0.5, the cell is at least suspicious for HGUC (Pap stain).

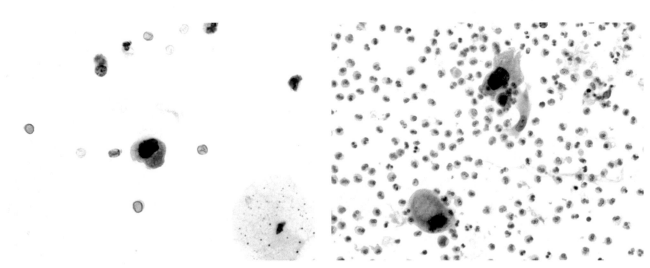

Figure 6.118. Suspicious for high-grade urothelial carcinoma (SHGUC). Alternate field (Pap stain).

Figure 6.119. Suspicious for high-grade urothelial carcinoma (SHGUC). These HGUC cells have abundant cytoplasm which greatly decreases the nuclear to cytoplasmic (N/C) ratio. However, the nuclei are dark, are enlarged, have irregular borders, and should be regarded as at least suspicious for HGUC (Pap stain).

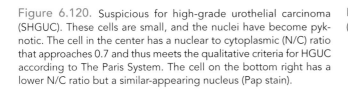

Figure 6.120. Suspicious for high-grade urothelial carcinoma (SHGUC). These cells are small, and the nuclei have become pyknotic. The cell in the center has a nuclear to cytoplasmic (N/C) ratio that approaches 0.7 and thus meets the qualitative criteria for HGUC according to The Paris System. The cell on the bottom right has a lower N/C ratio but a similar-appearing nucleus (Pap stain).

Figure 6.121. Suspicious for high-grade urothelial carcinoma (SHGUC). Alternate field (Pap stain).

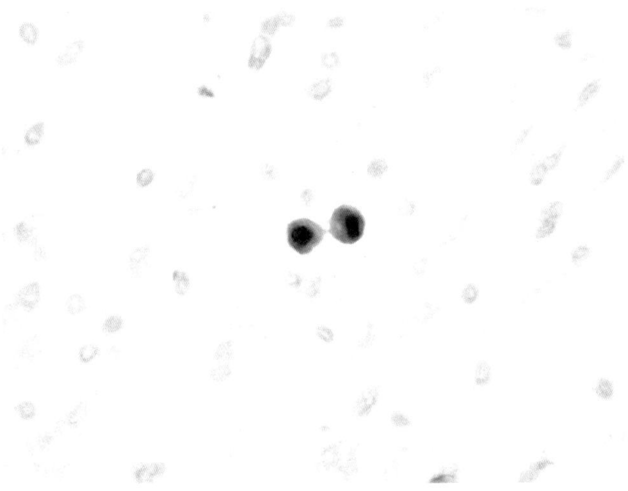

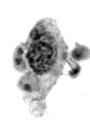

Figure 6.122. Suspicious for high-grade urothelial carcinoma (SHGUC). Alternate field (Pap stain).

Figure 6.123. Suspicious for high-grade urothelial carcinoma (SHGUC). This HGUC cell is degenerating, and the nuclear to cytoplasmic (N/C) ratio is approximately 0.5. It is enlarged and hyperchromatic and has wrinkled nuclear borders and coarse chromatin. Therefore, the diagnosis would be *SHGUC* rather than *AUC* according to The Paris System (Pap stain).

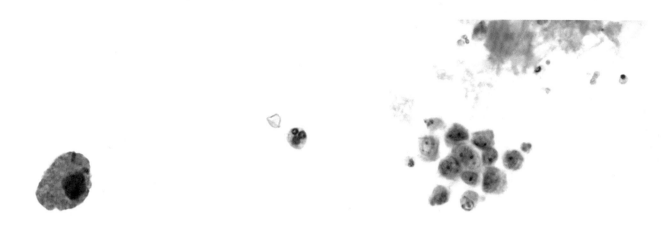

Figure 6.124. Suspicious for high-grade urothelial carcinoma (SHGUC). The cell on the left has degenerative cytoplasm, which has become granular. The nucleus has shrunk and become so dark that the chromatin quality cannot be assessed. Despite the small nuclear to cytoplasmic (N/C) ratio, this cell is best regarded as at least *SHGUC* (Pap stain).

Figure 6.125. Suspicious for high-grade urothelial carcinoma (SHGUC). Numerous cells with fluffy degenerating cytoplasm. The nuclear to cytoplasmic (N/C) ratio is difficult to assess but appears to be less than 0.7 in most of these cells. The nuclear borders are irregular, and the chromatin is clumpy (Pap stain).

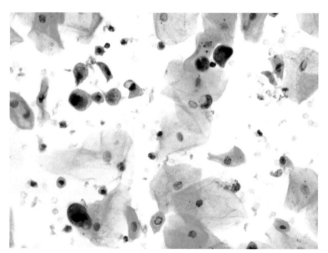

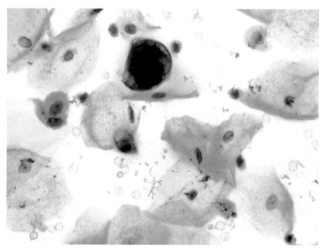

Figure 6.126. Suspicious for high-grade urothelial carcinoma (SHGUC). The hyperchromatic cells in this field demonstrate a spectrum of degenerative changes: in some, the nuclear border can still be seen; in others, the dark chromatin blends into the cytoplasm. The presence of large amounts of dark chromatin raises suspicion for HGUC (Pap stain).

Figure 6.127. Suspicious for high-grade urothelial carcinoma (SHGUC). Alternate field (Pap stain).

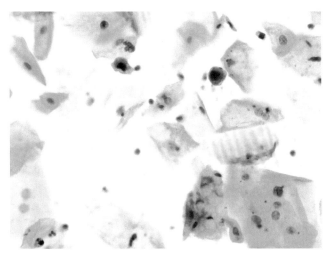

Figure 6.128. Suspicious for high-grade urothelial carcinoma (SHGUC). Alternate field (Pap stain).

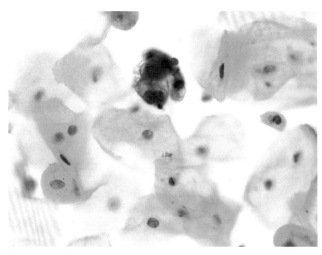

Figure 6.129. Suspicious for high-grade urothelial carcinoma (SHGUC). Alternate field (Pap stain).

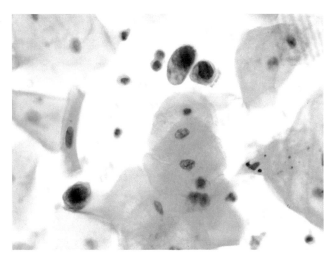

Figure 6.130. Suspicious for high-grade urothelial carcinoma (SHGUC). Alternate field (Pap stain).

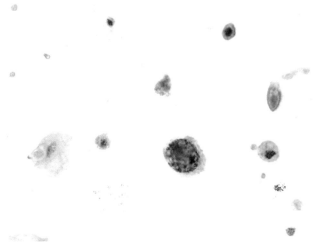

Figure 6.131. Suspicious for high-grade urothelial carcinoma (SHGUC). This degenerating cell has little cytoplasm left, and the chromatin has a ground glass appearance that emulates changes associated with BK polyomavirus. However, the nucleus is much larger (>20×) than nearby red blood cells, raising suspicion for HGUC (Pap stain).

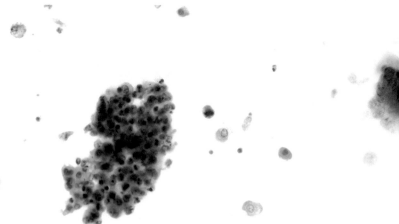

Figure 6.132. Bacillus Calmette-Guérin (BCG) effect. Treatment of high-grade urothelial carcinoma (HGUC) by BCG results in granulomatous inflammation that can sometimes be seen in urinary tract specimens. This fragment represents an aggregate of epithelioid histiocytes. Some cells have curved nuclei, a clue to their nature. When these cells are mistaken for urothelial cells, they may be diagnosed as atypical (Pap stain).

Figure 6.133. Bacillus Calmette-Guérin (BCG) effect. A multinucleated giant cell is ringed by numerous epithelioid histiocytes (Pap stain).

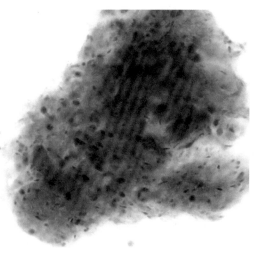

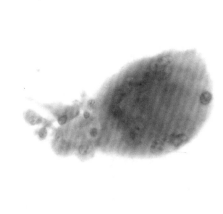

Figure 6.134. Bacillus Calmette-Guérin (BCG) effect. Necrotic debris with associated epithelioid histiocytes and degenerating cells (Pap stain).

Figure 6.135. Bacillus Calmette-Guérin (BCG) effect. A multinucleated giant cell with associated epithelioid histiocytes (Pap stain).

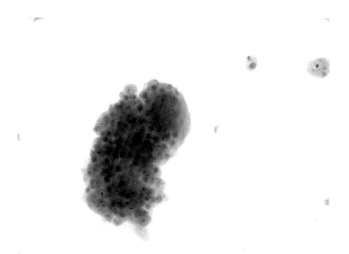

Figure 6.136. Bacillus Calmette-Guérin (BCG) effect. Acellular granular debris, likely representing necrosis (Pap stain).

Figure 6.137. Bacillus Calmette-Guérin (BCG) effect. A multinucleated giant cell with associated epithelioid histiocytes (Pap stain).

BK POLYOMAVIRUS CYTOPATHIC EFFECT

Initial BK polyomavirus infection is usually an asymptomatic disease. Following acute infection, the virus localizes to the kidney and to the urinary tract where it remains latent in most individuals. It is believed that the majority of adults have latent BK infection. If the infection recurs, asymptomatic re-activation of the virus causes a characteristic cytopathic effect seen in urinary tract specimens.[50] In healthy individuals, very few infected cells are seen. In immunosuppressed patients following kidney transplant, the reactivation of BK virus is clinically significant because it can cause kidney damage. As a result, its presence should be considered a critical result and reported as such in transplant patients.[51] Infected cells have dark, round nuclei with chromatin margination combined with small clumps of chromatin and/or stringy peripheral chromatin that give a "spider web" appearance to the nuclei. Infected nuclei also have a central "ground glass" inclusion that can be very helpful in identifying these cells. The cell cytoplasm may be either degenerated or absent (Figures 6.139-6.142). The dark, enlarged nuclei mimic HGUC, and thus, these cells have previously been termed "decoy cells" to caution pathologists not to overdiagnose such cells as malignant.[52,53] As opposed to specimens containing HGUC, benign specimens containing BK virus are less cellular. Additionally, rather than the coarse chromatin seen in HGUC, cells infected with BK virus often have chromatin marginated along the nuclear border and/or a "ground glass" appearance to the chromatin. TPS recommends classifying cells with BK cytopathic effect (CPE) under the *NHGUC* category; however, at least one study has demonstrated that degenerated HGUC cells are difficult to distinguish from benign BK CPE.[54] In addition, some case reports indicate a possible connection between BK polyomavirus and HGUC. Given this uncertainty, the future significance and reporting of BK virus CPE may change.

KEY FEATURES of BK Polyomavirus

- Infected cells are typically present in small numbers in immunocompetent individuals.
- Infected cells contain regular nuclear borders with round or oval-shaped nuclei.
- Infected cells have minimal to absent cytoplasm.
- Infected cells contain homogenously dark chromatin with a "ground glass" appearance and/or peripheral margination of the chromatin resulting in a "spider web" pattern.

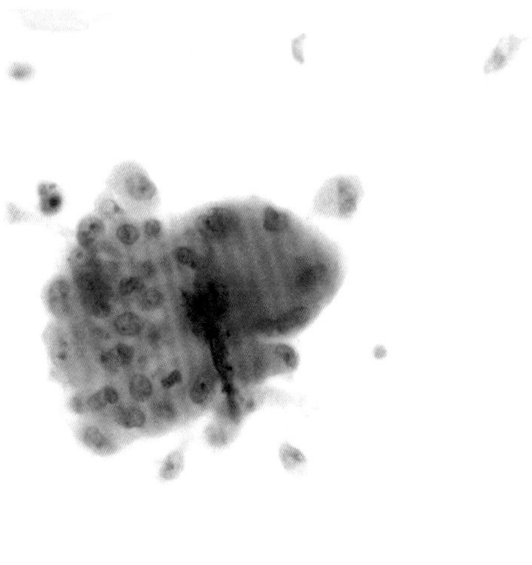

Figure 6.138. Bacillus Calmette-Guérin (BCG) effect. Alternate field (Pap stain).

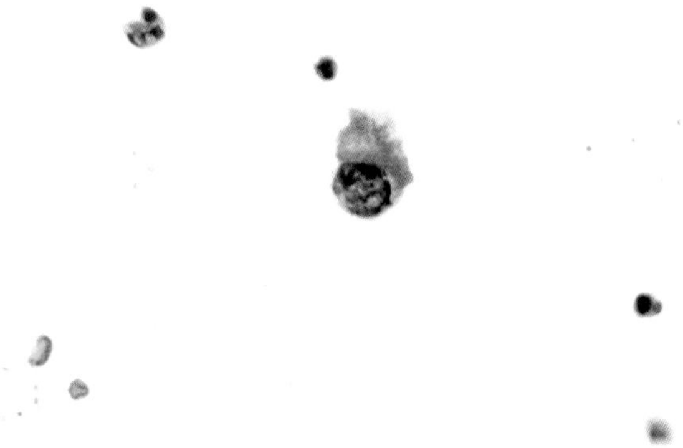

Figure 6.139. BK polyomavirus. BK polyomavirus can induce cellular changes that overlap with high-grade urothelial carcinoma (HGUC). Cells with BK effect usually have very round nuclei with marginated chromatin (Pap stain).

Figure 6.140. BK polyomavirus. Alternate field (Pap stain).

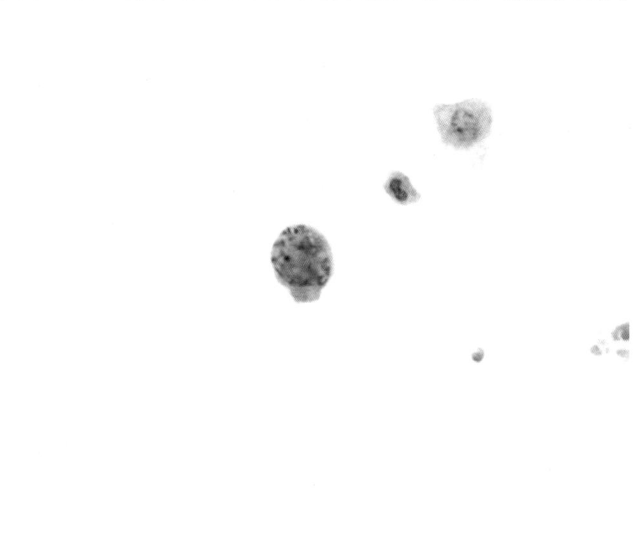

Figure 6.141. BK polyomavirus. BK virus may also cause a "ground glass" appearance to the nucleus, as seen here (Pap stain).

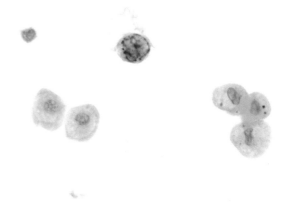

Figure 6.142. BK polyomavirus. Alternate field (Pap stain).

PROMINENT NUCLEOLI PATTERN

Occasionally, a second population of atypical cells with prominent nucleoli may be identified in a urinary tract specimen. Neoplastic urothelial cells may have nucleoli, but in contrast to other cell types (e.g. squamous, glandular), reactive urothelial cells do not tend to have prominent nucleoli. As a result, the presence of prominent nucleoli raises concern for involvement of the urine by a neoplastic process.

CHECKLIST: Etiologic Considerations for the Prominent Nucleoli Pattern

☐ Prostate Carcinoma

☐ Renal Cell Carcinoma (RCC)

☐ High-Grade Urothelial Carcinoma (HGUC) with Prominent Nucleoli

PROSTATE CARCINOMA

Prostate carcinoma is the most common nonurothelial malignancy found in urinary tract specimens. In most instances, the patient will already have a known history of prostate cancer. Tumor cells are present singly or in small fragments. When small fragments are present, the cells are usually arranged in an acinar or cribiform pattern. Prostate carcinoma cells typically have abundant, foamy cytoplasm and an eccentrically located, round nucleus with regular nuclear borders and a single prominent nucleolus (Figures 6.143-6.149). The most common alternative diagnosis to consider is urothelial carcinoma, which occasionally has prominent nucleoli rather than the classic coarse, clumpy chromatin. In such instances, immunostains can help, and a typical panel evaluates GATA-3 and NKX3.1 expression to determine whether the atypical cells are of urothelial and prostatic origin, respectively. An expanded panel, as described below for RCC, may be used if there is suspicion of additional sites of origin.

RENAL CELL CARCINOMA

Renal Cell Carcinoma (RCC) is not usually found in urinary tract specimens, although urine specimens are sometimes submitted during initial workup of a renal mass.[55] When present in urine, RCC cells are typically individual and infrequent. The cells have abundant, granular cytoplasm, round nuclei with regular borders, and prominent nucleoli. RCC cells may share significant cytomorphologic overlap with prostate carcinoma and metastatic melanoma. Confirmation typically requires immunostains, with RCC being positive for PAX-8 (sometimes also positive in upper tract urothelial carcinoma) and negative for GATA-3 (a urothelial marker negative in most forms of RCC), NKX3.1 (a prostate marker), and S100 protein (a nonspecific melanoma marker).[56-58]

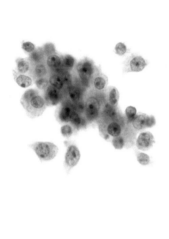

Figure 6.143. Prostate carcinoma. Prostate cancer is the most common extraurinary malignancy to involve urinary tract specimens. The cells usually have abundant foamy cytoplasm, round nuclei with regular borders, and prominent nucleoli (Pap stain).

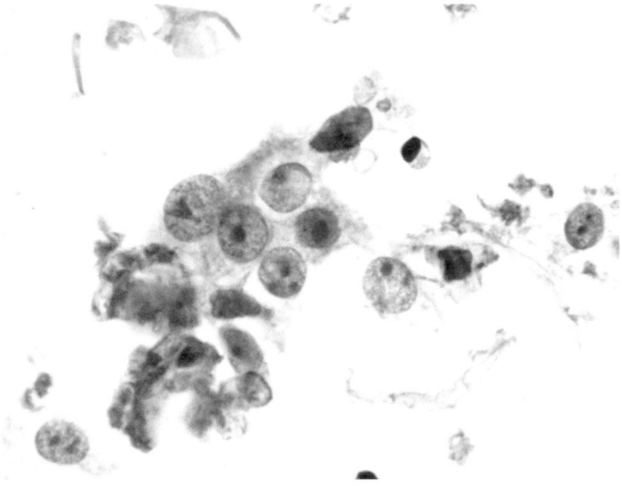

Figure 6.144. Prostate carcinoma. Prostate carcinoma cells in the urine may be present as large fragments, single dispersed cells, or both (Pap stain).

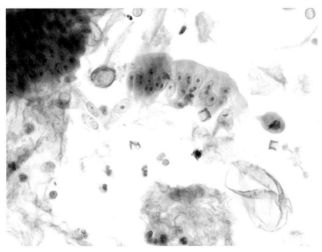

Figure 6.145. Prostate carcinoma. Columnar-shaped cells with prominent nucleoli are an unusual finding in a urinary tract specimen and are consistent with prostate carcinoma (Pap stain).

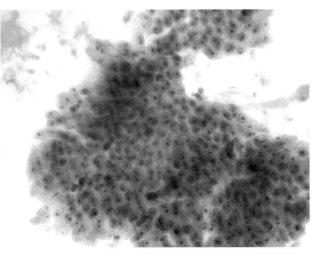

Figure 6.146. Prostate carcinoma. A large fragment of prostate carcinoma cells. The nucleoli are large and a striking feature (Pap stain).

HIGH-GRADE UROTHELIAL CARCINOMA WITH PROMINENT NUCLEOLI

HGUC nuclei are usually either markedly hyperchromatic or contain chromatin that is coarse and clumpy; rarely do a significant number of malignant cells contain prominent nucleoli (Figures 6.150-6.153). If HGUC with classic cytomorphology is present in the background, it is most likely that the patient has dimorphic HGUC with some prominent nucleoli and not two separate cancers presenting at once. If the malignant cells all contain prominent nucleoli, HGUC is still the most likely diagnosis unless the patient has a history of high-grade prostate carcinoma. For a definitive diagnosis, immunostains can be performed, as detailed above for renal cell and prostate carcinomas.

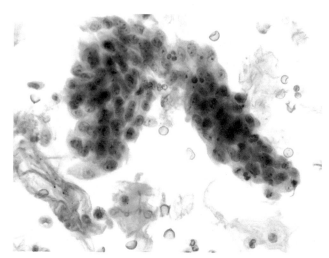

Figure 6.147. Prostate carcinoma. Alternate field (Pap stain).

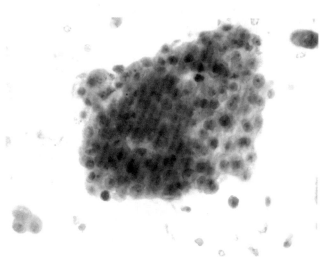

Figure 6.148. Prostate carcinoma. Alternate field (Pap stain).

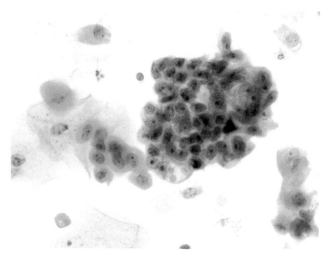

Figure 6.149. Prostate carcinoma. Alternate field (Pap stain).

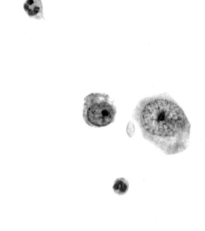

Figure 6.150. High-grade urothelial carcinoma (HGUC) with prominent nucleoli. HGUC may uncommonly demonstrate prominent nucleoli, and thus this feature is not specific for prostate carcinoma. Immunostains are helpful if additional unstained slides or a cell block preparation can be created from the residual material (Pap stain).

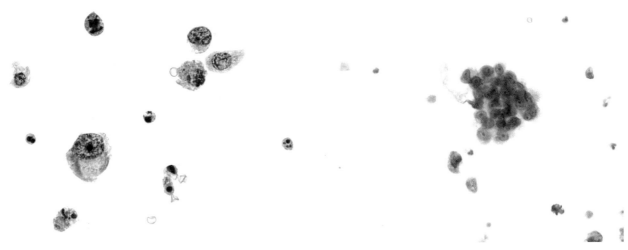

Figure 6.151. High-grade urothelial carcinoma (HGUC) with prominent nucleoli. Alternate field (Pap stain).

Figure 6.152. High-grade urothelial carcinoma (HGUC) with prominent nucleoli. The tumor cells in this fragment have prominent nucleoli, which should raise concern for a prostate carcinoma (Pap stain).

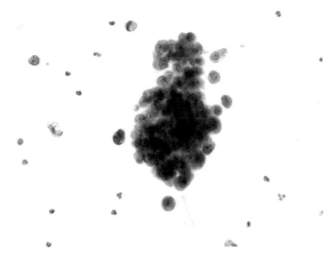

Figure 6.153. High-grade urothelial carcinoma (HGUC) with prominent nucleoli. Alternate field (Pap stain).

SQUAMOUS PATTERN

The squamous pattern here refers to the presence of atypical or malignant cells with squamous differentiation that stand out from other cells in a urinary tract specimen. These cells may arise from areas of squamous differentiation within urothelial lesions or may be an external contaminant of the urine from adjacent sites of origin. Squamous cells within the urine may be few or extensive in number.

CHECKLIST: Etiologic Considerations for the Squamous Pattern

☐ Primary Squamous Cell Carcinoma

☐ HGUC with Squamous Differentiation

☐ Infiltrating Cervical Squamous Cell Carcinoma

☐ Atypical Squamous Cells

PRIMARY SQUAMOUS CELL CARCINOMA

Primary squamous cell carcinoma of the bladder is most common in Egypt and is associated with *Schistosoma haematobium* infection.[59] For unknown reasons, this association is unique to Egypt and is notably absent in other regions endemic for *S. haematobium* infection (such as other parts of the Middle East and Africa). In the United States, primary squamous cell carcinoma of the bladder may be associated with chronic inflammatory states and/or anatomic alterations in the urinary tract.[60] Urothelial carcinoma with squamous differentiation cannot be morphologically distinguished from squamous cell carcinoma arising from other sites that are secondarily involving the urinary tract (such as the cervix). Morphologically, malignant squamous cells in urine display the characteristic morphology of squamous cell carcinoma at other sites: dense cytoplasm with irregular extensions and ink black nuclei with polygonal borders (Figures 6.154-6.165). Keratinizing carcinomas will have pink or orange cytoplasm on Papanicolaou-stained preparations. Necrosis is commonly observed in the background of squamous cell carcinomas. According to TPS, the recommended diagnosis and category is *Other: Carcinoma with squamous differentiation.*

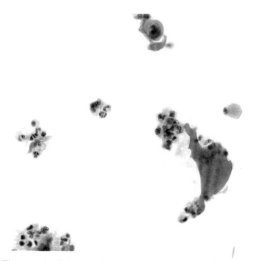

Figure 6.154. Carcinoma with squamous features. There is an irregularly shaped orangeophilic fragment of keratin with dense projections. Fragments such as this should raise concern for squamous cell carcinoma, even if nuclei are absent (Pap stain).

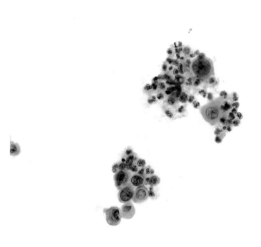

Figure 6.155. Carcinoma with squamous features. Several tumor cells can be seen together with groups of neutrophils. The tumor cells have high nuclear to cytoplasmic (N/C) ratios and coarse chromatin. Some cells have orangeophilic cytoplasm, which indicates squamous differentiation (Pap stain).

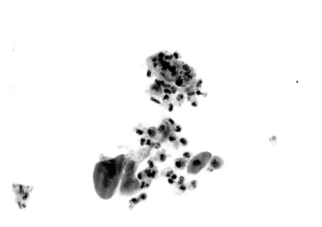

Figure 6.156. Carcinoma with squamous features. Alternate field (Pap stain).

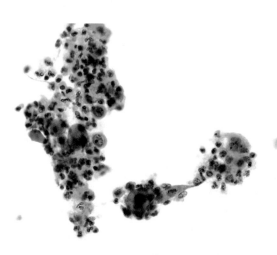

Figure 6.157. Carcinoma with squamous features. Alternate field (Pap stain).

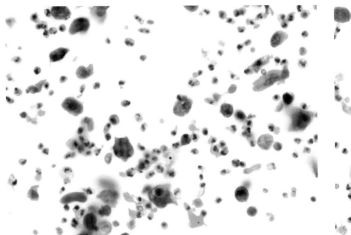

Figure 6.158. Carcinoma with squamous features. Several atypically shaped fragments of keratin can be seen in a background of degenerated urothelial cells. Some of the degenerated cells appear to have dark nuclei, raising the possibility of a high-grade urothelial carcinoma (HGUC) with squamous differentiation (Pap stain).

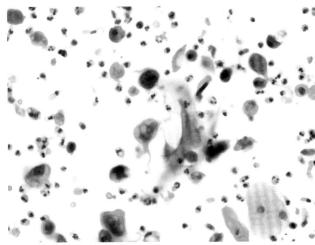

Figure 6.159. Carcinoma with squamous features. Alternate field (Pap stain).

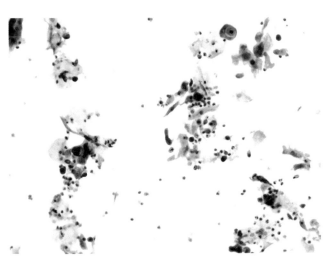

Figure 6.160. Carcinoma with squamous features. Alternate field (Pap stain).

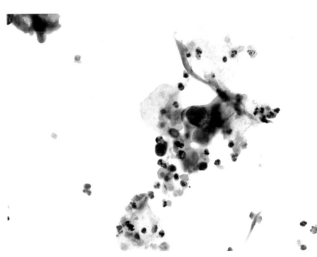

Figure 6.161. Carcinoma with squamous features. Alternate field (Pap stain).

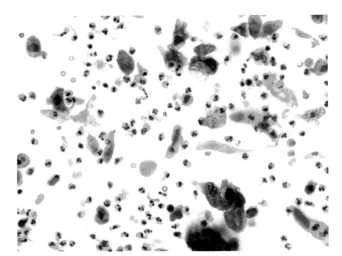

Figure 6.162. Carcinoma with squamous features. Several keratinized cells with large, dark, pyknotic nuclei can be seen. These cells are diagnostic of a carcinoma with squamous features, which may either be a pure squamous cell carcinoma or a high-grade urothelial carcinoma (HGUC) with squamous differentiation (Pap stain).

Figure 6.163. Carcinoma with squamous features. Alternate field (Pap stain).

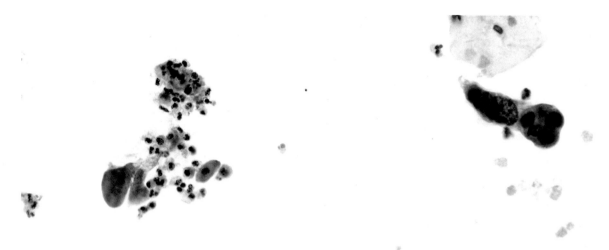

Figure 6.164. Carcinoma with squamous features. The carcinoma cells at the bottom left have very faint–staining nuclei. This finding may be because the keratin is so dense that the nuclear stain does not penetrate well (Pap stain).

Figure 6.165. Carcinoma with squamous features. The keratinized cell has a large nucleus with coarse chromatin and irregular borders. The nuclear to cytoplasmic (N/C) ratio in keratinized cells is sometimes low because the nucleus becomes pyknotic (Pap stain).

HIGH-GRADE UROTHELIAL CARCINOMA WITH SQUAMOUS DIFFERENTIATION

HGUC can develop squamous differentiation, and one or both components may be present in a urinary tract specimen. The presence of malignant cells with squamous differentiation together with HGUC cells implies HGUC with squamous differentiation rather than two separate, simultaneous carcinomas. Typically, only one morphologic component predominates. Regardless of which subtype predominates, TPS recommends a diagnosis of *HGUC with squamous differentiation* in a case where both components are identified.

INFILTRATING CERVICAL SQUAMOUS CELL CARCINOMA

Squamous cell carcinoma may arise at adjacent sites (e.g. anus, cervix, etc.) and subsequently infiltrate the urinary tract. In these instances, the malignant cells appear similar to other squamous cell carcinomas. However, as squamous cell carcinomas from these adjacent sites are usually human papillomavirus (HPV)–related, whereas those arising in the bladder are typically not, immunostains performed on residual specimens can help distinguish the two. HPV-related carcinomas demonstrate diffuse staining for p16 and/or the detection of high-risk HPV by in situ hybridization studies.

It is also possible for adjacent, noninvasive squamous cell carcinomas to contaminate the urinary stream and be present in a voided urinary tract specimen. It is important to include this fact in the diagnosis, so that a clinician does not immediately assume any adjacent carcinoma is invasive. If necessary, procurement of a catheterized specimen will help exclude contamination. In most instances, patients have an established history of squamous cell carcinoma from a nonurothelial site, making a primary squamous cell carcinoma of the bladder unlikely.

ATYPICAL SQUAMOUS CELLS

Like squamous cell carcinoma, atypical squamous cells in a urinary tract specimen may arise either from within the urinary tract or from contamination of the urinary stream (Figure 6.166). Origins include areas of squamous metaplasia within the urinary tract, the urethra, and the genitalia.[61] Depending on the level of atypia, its presence can either be reported in a note following a diagnosis of *NHGUC* or, if appropriate, the *Other* category can be used to report *Atypical squamous cells*. Atypical squamous cells may appear to have koilocytic changes representative of HPV infection associated with genital warts or dysplasia. High-grade squamous intraepithelial lesions (HSILs) may appear as single atypical cells or hyperchromatic crowded groups. It is sometimes difficult to distinguish atypical squamous cells from atypical urothelial cells in these hyperchromatic groups. A follow-up catheterized urine specimen can help isolate the source of the cells by restricting sampling to the urinary tract. Female patients who have not received regular screening for cervical dysplasia should be referred to a gynecologist.[62]

SAMPLE NOTE: ATYPICAL SQUAMOUS CELLS WITH KOILOCYTIC CHANGES

Other: Atypical Squamous Cells. Negative for High Grade Urothelial Carcinoma. See note.

Note: Rare atypical squamous cells with koilocytic changes are identified which may represent contamination from the gynecologic tract. If the patient has not undergone regular screening for cervical dysplasia, a follow-up Pap test is recommended.

Reference:
Owens CL, Ali SZ. Atypical squamous cells in exfoliative urinary cytology: clinicopathologic correlates. *Diagn Cytopathol.* 2005;33(6):394-398.

SAMPLE NOTE: MARKEDLY ATYPICAL SQUAMOUS CELLS

Other: Markedly atypical squamous cells. See note.

Note: Rare markedly atypical squamous cells are identified. These cells may originate from the urinary tract or may represent contamination from outside the urinary tract. The differential diagnosis includes atypical squamous metaplasia and carcinoma with squamous differentiation. A follow-up catheterized specimen may help localize the atypical cells to the urinary tract.

Reference:
Owens CL, Ali SZ. Atypical squamous cells in exfoliative urinary cytology: clinicopathologic correlates. *Diagn Cytopathol.* 2005;33(6):394-398.

PEARLS & PITFALLS

Because the *AUC* category is not strongly predictive of malignancy, many clinicians manage patients as if they had received an *NHGUC* diagnosis. However, repeated "atypical" diagnoses may be concerning to patients and thus should not be made lightly. Before considering a diagnosis of *AUC*, consider the following:

- Does the patient have a history of urolithiasis, or other reasons to cause mild cytomorphologic atypia, that can allow the findings to be dismissed?
- Are the findings truly worrisome for HGUC?
- Could the atypical cells be unusual appearing umbrella cells, renal tubular cells, or other elements sometimes mistaken for atypical urothelial cells?
- If the atypia is mild, is the N/C ratio above 0.5?
- Will a diagnosis of *AUC* change patient management?

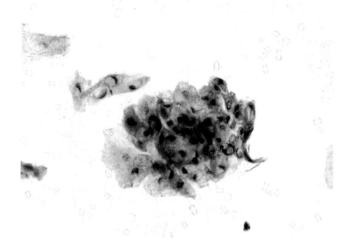

Figure 6.166. Atypical squamous cells. Some cells in this group have pink cytoplasm, indicating squamous differentiation. The nuclei are small, and the nuclear borders are mostly smooth. Atypical squamous cells may originate in the urinary tract where they may represent a benign reactive process or a neoplasm. They may also contaminate the urinary stream during collection from the genital tract and harbor a human papillomavirus (HPV) infection (Pap stain).

GLANDULAR PATTERN

Glandular cells, which may appear as either bland-appearing columnar cells or as three-dimensional clusters of cells, are uncommonly seen in urinary tract specimens. The etiology of glandular cells in a urine specimen includes both benign entities (e.g., contaminating endometrial cells, cystitis glandularis) and malignant entities (e.g., adenocarcinoma).

CHECKLIST: Etiologic Considerations for the Glandular Pattern

☐ Primary Adenocarcinoma

☐ HGUC with Glandular Features

☐ Metastatic Adenocarcinoma and Infiltrating Colorectal Carcinoma

☐ Cystitis Glandularis

☐ Endometrial Cells

☐ Vesicoenteric Fistula

PRIMARY ADENOCARCINOMA

Primary adenocarcinoma of the bladder is uncommon (<2% of bladder primary cancers) and typically develops in the lateral wall or trigone of the bladder, or else arises from urachal remnants located in the bladder dome (Figures 6.167-6.181). Most commonly, the adenocarcinoma cells morphologically resemble colorectal adenocarcinoma, and invasion from outside the urinary tract should be considered. In either case, the cells have dark, elongated nuclei, and necrotic material is seen in the background. Primary adenocarcinoma may alternatively display signet ring and/or mucinous morphologies. Some HGUCs contain areas of glandular differentiation, and therefore, one must always look carefully for a second population of malignant cells. If only adenocarcinoma is present, TPS recommends a diagnosis of *Other: Carcinoma with glandular features*. This diagnosis allows for either a primary or secondary adenocarcinoma and further includes the possibility of a mixed tumor, even if the urinary tract cytology specimen does not contain a secondary component of differentiation.

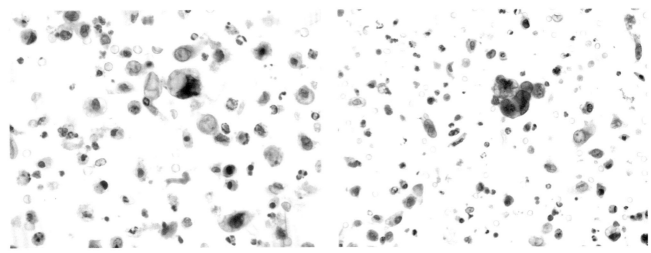

Figure 6.167. Primary adenocarcinoma. A large cell with a dark nucleus is present at the top center of the field. The cytoplasm is vacuolated. While vacuolization can occur in urothelial cells (both benign and malignant), this vacuole appears to compress the nucleus, an unusual feature. This patient was found to have a primary bladder adenocarcinoma (Pap stain).

Figure 6.168. Primary adenocarcinoma. In this alternate field, a cluster of tumor cells can be seen. The cells demonstrate many features of adenocarcinoma: anisonucleosis, three-dimensionality, irregular nuclear borders, and hyperchromasia. Some of the cells have vacuolated cytoplasm (Pap stain).

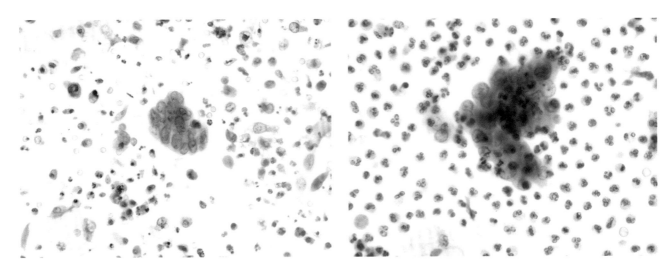

Figure 6.169. Primary adenocarcinoma. Despite having a hypochromatic appearance, the cells at center are suspicious for malignancy because they have high nuclear to cytoplasmic (N/C) ratios and irregular nuclear borders. As rare cases of high-grade urothelial carcinoma (HGUC) with hypochromasia have been described, it should remain in the differential diagnosis (Pap stain).

Figure 6.170. Primary adenocarcinoma. This patient had a clear cell carcinoma of the bladder. Note the three-dimensionality of the fragment, as well as the size variation between the nuclei. By comparison, high-grade urothelial carcinoma (HGUC) usually has coarse chromatin, is more discohesive, and does not usually form three-dimensional fragments (Pap stain).

HIGH-GRADE UROTHELIAL CARCINOMA WITH GLANDULAR FEATURES

As mentioned in the previous section, HGUC sometimes develops glandular differentiation. In a urine specimen, either the glandular or the urothelial component may predominate. To make this diagnosis, both components must be identified within the specimen. TPS recommends the diagnosis of *HGUC with glandular differentiation* in these cases.

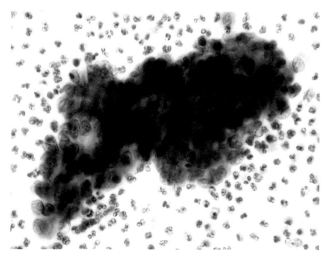

Figure 6.171. Primary adenocarcinoma. Alternate field (Pap stain).

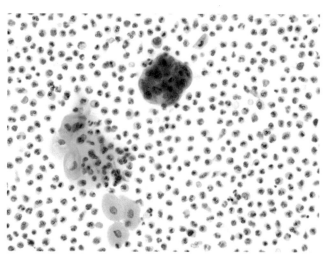

Figure 6.172. Primary adenocarcinoma. Alternate field (Pap stain).

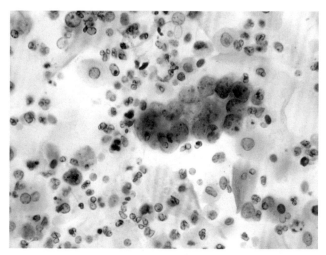

Figure 6.173. Primary adenocarcinoma. These cells form a glandular formation—the nuclei have a "figure 8" arrangement around two central lumens. The cells have high nuclear to cytoplasmic (N/C) ratios and irregular nuclear borders. This patient was subsequently diagnosed with micropapillary carcinoma of the bladder (Pap stain).

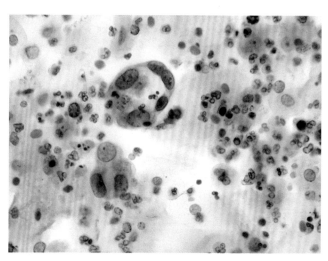

Figure 6.174. Primary adenocarcinoma. Alternate field (Pap stain).

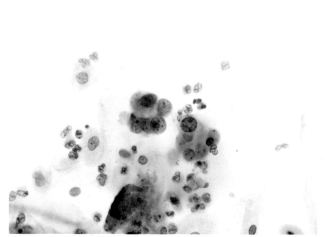

Figure 6.175. Primary adenocarcinoma. Alternate field (Pap stain).

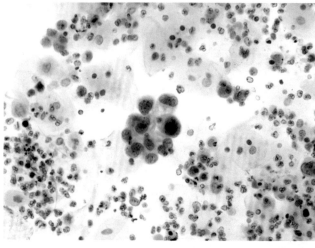

Figure 6.176. Primary adenocarcinoma. Alternate field (Pap stain).

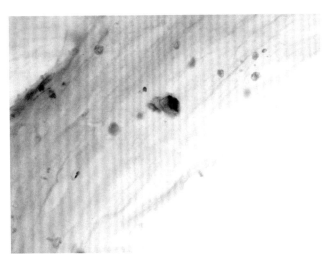

Figure 6.177. Primary adenocarcinoma. A degenerating cell is embedded in a background of thick mucous material. The cell has a large, dark nucleus with irregular borders. This patient was subsequently diagnosed with a urachal adenocarcinoma (Pap stain).

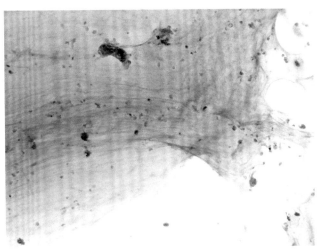

Figure 6.178. Primary adenocarcinoma. Alternate field (Pap stain).

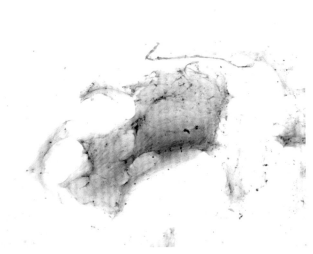

Figure 6.179. Primary adenocarcinoma. The presence of abundant, thick mucous material suggests the presence of a mucin-producing neoplasm, even if the specimen is acellular (Pap stain).

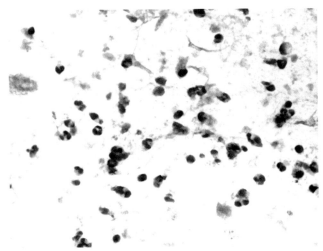

Figure 6.180. Primary adenocarcinoma. The field shows numerous degenerated cells in a background of mucin. The patient had an adenocarcinoma with a signet ring morphology, which is difficult to identify in these degenerated cells. It is likely that the mucinous background interfered with cellular preservation and specimen preparation (Pap stain).

METASTATIC ADENOCARCINOMA AND INFILTRATING COLORECTAL CARCINOMA

Adenocarcinoma arising in adjacent organs may directly invade or metastasize to the urinary tract; the cytomorphology typically resembles the morphology seen at the primary site.[55] In most instances, the patient has a known history of malignancy. The most common extraurinary adenocarcinomas with glandular differentiation to appear in the urine include colorectal, uterine, ovarian, and breast carcinomas (Figures 6.182-6.192). In instances of gynecologic tract malignancies, contamination of the urinary stream in voided urine specimens should be excluded. Prostate carcinoma is the most common extraurinary carcinoma seen in urinary tract specimens and is discussed under the "Prominent Nucleoli Pattern" (Figures 6.193-6.203).

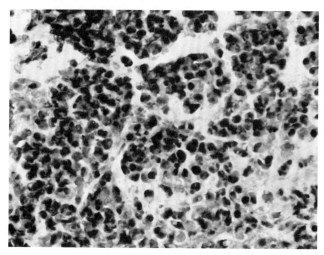

Figure 6.181. Primary adenocarcinoma. This field is from a corresponding cell block section from the same specimen in the previous figure. The same findings can be seen: numerous tumor cells in various states of degeneration. A few cells are better preserved and show an eccentrically placed dark nucleus compressed by an intracytoplasmic mucin vacuole (H&E).

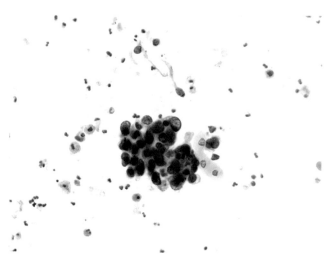

Figure 6.182. Endometrial adenocarcinoma. Endometrial cells (benign or malignant) may contaminate the urinary stream during specimen collection. They appear as they do in Pap test specimens—cells with dark nuclei and high nuclear to cytoplasmic (N/C) ratios that form small clusters with hobnailed edges. Even benign-appearing endometrial cells are cause for concern in a postmenopausal patient (Pap stain).

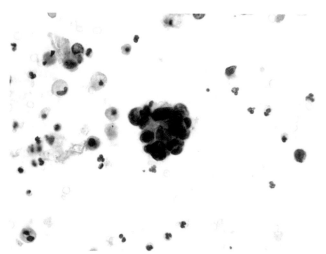

Figure 6.183. Endometrial adenocarcinoma. The cells form a three-dimensional cluster and are hyperchromatic with irregular nuclear borders and nuclear size variation. These are diagnostic of an adenocarcinoma, although determining a site of origin may require ancillary studies or a known history of cancer (Pap stain).

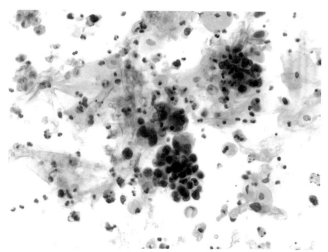

Figure 6.184. Endometrial adenocarcinoma. Alternate field (Pap stain).

CYSTITIS GLANDULARIS

The urothelial lining may undergo glandular metaplasia in response to chronic inflammation, and this alteration is known as cystitis glandularis. It appears in urinary tract specimens as bland-appearing, columnar cells or as groups of cells with vacuolated cytoplasm and eccentrically placed nuclei. The literature to date does not contain any rigorous studies defining the cytomorphology of cystitis glandularis, and thus, its identification may lack sensitivity and specificity. Furthermore, at present, there is little clinical significance attached to this finding, and it is currently recommended that this finding not be reported in urinary tract specimens.

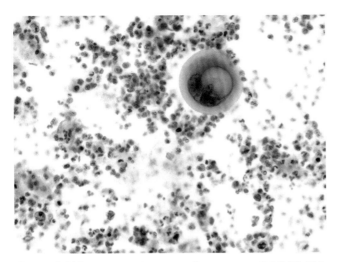

Figure 6.185. Mixed malignant Mullerian tumor (MMMT). This odd cell is large and has dense cytoplasm with an enlarged, dark nucleus. The patient had a known history of MMMT (Pap stain).

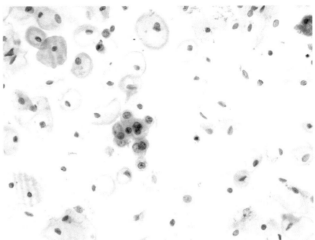

Figure 6.186. Mixed malignant Mullerian tumor. Adenocarcinoma cells are present in a loose cluster (center). The cells are the size of urothelial cells and may be mistaken for such (Pap stain).

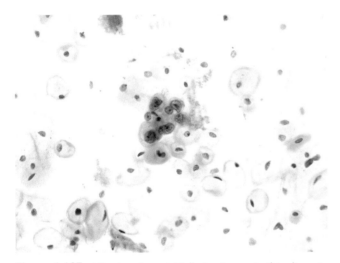

Figure 6.187. Mixed malignant Mullerian tumor. In this alternate field, the adenocarcinoma cells have more prominent hyperchromasia and anisonucleosis (Pap stain).

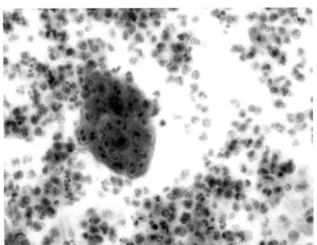

Figure 6.188. Mixed malignant Mullerian tumor. In this patient, the tumor cells have overtly malignant features. The cells form a three-dimensional cluster and have high nuclear to cytoplasmic (N/C) ratios, prominent nucleoli, and markedly irregular nuclear borders. The formation of a "ball" of cells is more suggestive of an adenocarcinoma than a high-grade urothelial carcinoma (HGUC) (Pap stain).

ENDOMETRIAL CELLS

Voided urine specimens from women are prone to contamination from the gynecologic tract, including by endometrial cells. The endometrial cells seen in urine specimens resemble those seen on a Pap test: small hyperchromatic cells with high N/C ratios present in small clusters with hobnailed borders.[63] These hyperchromatic crowded groups share significant overlap with RTCs. Endometrial groups are more likely to be associated with neutrophils and are more likely to contain vacuolated cells. They do not have to be reported in premenopausal women, but postmenopausal women should be referred to a gynecologist for further evaluation. If menopausal history is not known, The Bethesda System for Reporting Cervical Cytology currently recommends reporting even benign-appearing endometrial cells in all patients at the age of 45 years and above in Pap tests, and it is reasonable to apply this guideline to urine specimens as well.[64]

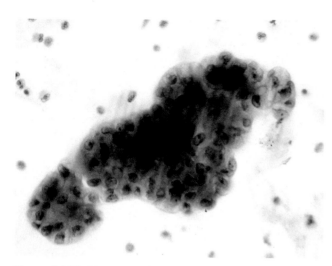

Figure 6.189. Metastatic adenocarcinoma. This patient had a gallbladder adenocarcinoma that was distantly metastatic to the urothelial tract. While the nuclear to cytoplasmic (N/C) ratios are low, the cells have irregular nuclear borders and great variation in nuclear size (Pap stain).

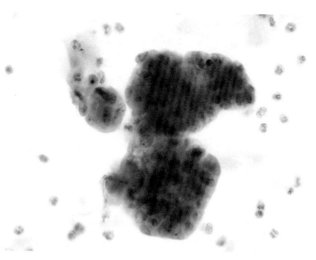

Figure 6.190. Metastatic adenocarcinoma. Alternate field (Pap stain).

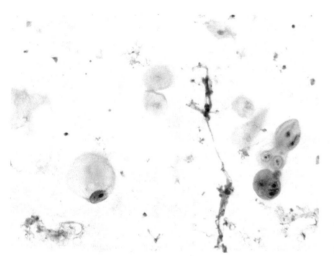

Figure 6.191. Metastatic adenocarcinoma. The patient's known breast cancer has found its way to the urinary tract. Several tumor cells can be seen, some vacuolated and one multinucleated. All the nuclei contain a distinctive red nucleolus (Pap stain).

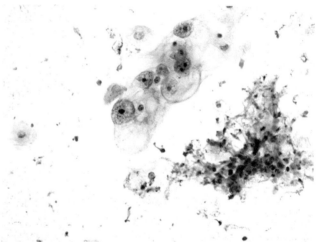

Figure 6.192. Metastatic adenocarcinoma. Alternate field (Pap stain).

VESICOENTERIC FISTULA

A vesicoenteric fistula occurs rarely but may result in the presence of bland-appearing glandular cells in a urine specimen. As the name suggests, this entity describes an abnormal connection between the gastrointestinal tract and the bladder. Patients with a vesicoenteric fistula may have a history of Crohn disease or recent surgery in the area. Other cytologic findings besides the bland glandular cells which suggest the possibility of such a fistula include the presence of vegetable material, bacteria, and acute inflammatory cells (Figures 6.204-6.206).[65] It is important to note, however, that these findings may be seen in a patient with cystitis glandularis who has submitted voided urine contaminated by vegetable/fecal matter. In the second instance, a catheterized specimen helps to exclude the possibility of contaminating fecal vegetable material.

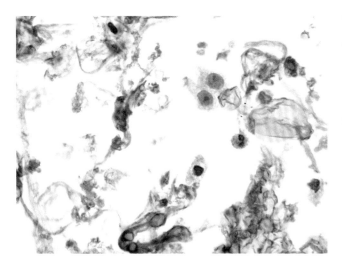

Figure 6.193. Prostate carcinoma. Two carcinoma cells can be seen, each with an enlarged nucleus, prominent nucleolus, and abundant foamy cytoplasm (Pap stain).

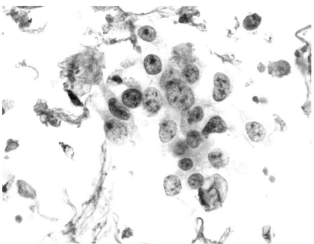

Figure 6.194. Prostate carcinoma. While some of the tumor cells have prominent nucleoli, other cells have coarse chromatin that resembles high-grade urothelial carcinoma (HGUC). The presence of abundant foamy cytoplasm favors prostate carcinoma, but ancillary immunostains may be required to confirm the diagnosis (Pap stain).

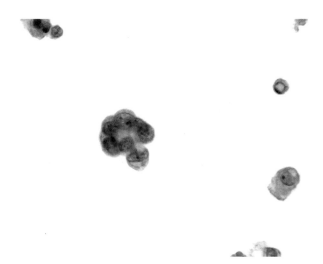

Figure 6.195. Prostate carcinoma. The tumor cells form an acinar arrangement (Pap stain).

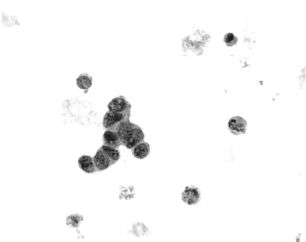

Figure 6.196. Prostate carcinoma. Alternate field (Pap stain).

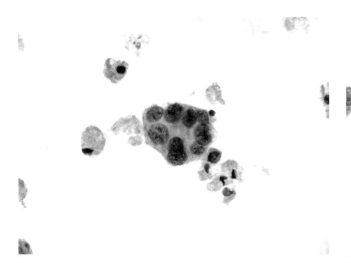

Figure 6.197. Prostate carcinoma. Alternate field (Pap stain).

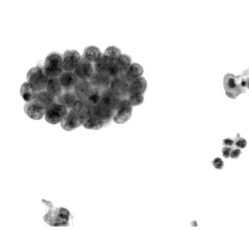

Figure 6.198. Prostate carcinoma. The cells have a morular arrangement. Endometrial cells can form into a similar arrangement. The cells do not have prominent nucleoli and while the cytomorphology is compatible with an adenocarcinoma, an origin would have to be confirmed with immunostains or by patient history (Pap stain).

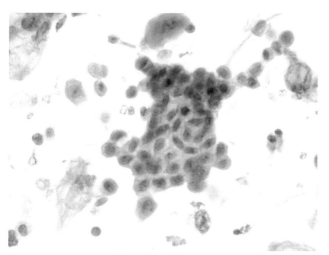

Figure 6.199. Prostate carcinoma. This monolayer sheet contains large nuclei with regular borders and small nucleoli. Without more information, these cells may be incorrectly assumed to be urothelial in origin (Pap stain).

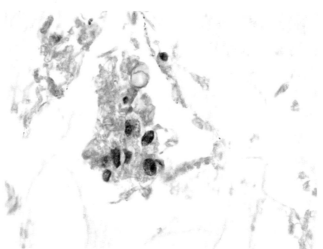

Figure 6.200. Prostate carcinoma. The preparation of a cell block from residual specimen allows for the performance of confirmatory immunohistochemical studies (H&E).

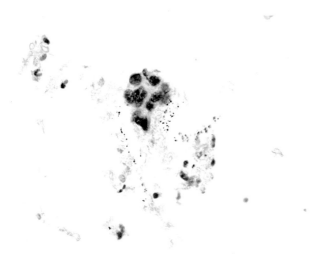

Figure 6.201. Prostate carcinoma. NKX3.1 is a sensitive and specific marker for prostate carcinoma and is not expressed in urothelial carcinoma (NKX3.1 immunostain).

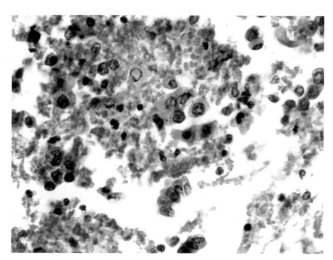

Figure 6.202. Prostate carcinoma. A different cell block preparation specimen containing prostate carcinoma cells (H&E).

Figure 6.203. Prostate carcinoma. An example of PSA-positive prostate carcinoma cells in cell block material (PSA immunostain).

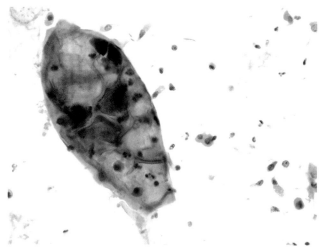

Figure 6.204. Vegetable material. Vegetable material can contaminate the urinary stream during specimen collection. The material can be varied in appearance but often has geometric shapes and thick cell walls. In this case, the patient had Crohn disease and a fistula tract formed between the bladder and the rectum. The columnar cells seen likely represent glandular cells from the gastrointestinal tract (Pap stain).

Figure 6.205. Vegetable material. Alternate field (Pap stain).

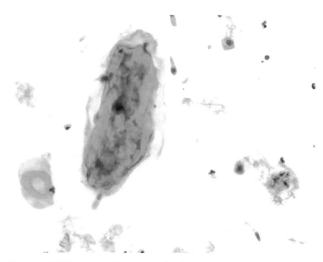

Figure 6.206. Vegetable material. Alternate field (Pap stain).

OTHER

CHEMOTHERAPY CHANGES

Chemotherapy-related changes in urine have not been well-described in the literature and may overlap with BCG-related changes (described above). Specimens usually contain numerous multinucleated giant cells, the majority of which are binucleated and likely represent reactive umbrella cells.[66] Cytoplasm is typically abundant in these umbrella cells, and the nuclei are round with regular borders, which helps to distinguish them from the irregular nuclei of HGUC. Degenerated HGUC cells may be seen post treatment and, in the setting of recent chemotherapy, should not be categorized as suspicious or atypical unless viable malignant cells are seen.

VEGETABLE MATERIAL

Voided urine specimens may be contaminated by fecal vegetable material. In catheterized specimens containing vegetable material, a vesicoenteric fistula should be excluded[67] (Figures 6.204-6.206). Vegetable material may occasionally resemble parasites and/or ova that can also contaminate a urinary stream (or, in the case of *Schistosoma haematobium*, arise within the urinary tract) in infected individuals.

SAMPLE NOTE: VEGETABLE MATERIAL

Negative for High Grade Urothelial Carcinoma. See note.

Note: The specimen contains vegetable material, bacteria, acute inflammation, and glandular cells. In the setting of Crohn disease, these findings may indicate the presence of a vesicoenteric fistula. A catheterized specimen may help exclude the possibility that the vegetable material is an extraurinary contaminant.

PEARLS & PITFALLS

While TPS is useful for stratifying a patient's risk for HGUC, it is not designed to report urinary tract specimens submitted for other reasons. For instance, a patient complaining of cloudy urine or other urinary symptoms may provide a specimen with abundant spermatozoa, indicating retrograde ejaculation. Some features, such as the presence of crystals, red blood cells, casts, etc. are not necessary to report for patients undergoing surveillance or screening for urothelial carcinoma. This recommendation is to prevent distraction from the key diagnosis; however, these features may be important to report in nonsurveillance, nonscreening patients. It is, therefore, important to be aware of each specimen's indication and report such features accordingly.

CRYSTALS

Crystals and crystalloids are a common finding in urinary tract specimens (Figures 6.207-6.209). Specimens submitted to exclude HGUC typically do not need an assessment of urine crystals in the diagnostic report. The formation of crystals can be associated with urolithiasis. Patients with urolithiasis may experience hematuria, which in turn may lead to a urinary tract specimen collection to exclude urothelial carcinoma as the cause of the hematuria. Urolithiasis can also cause reactive changes in urothelial cells which may be overinterpreted as *AUC*.

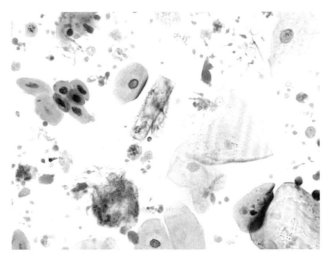

Figure 6.207. Crystals. Crystals and crystalloids can form in the urinary tract under a variety of conditions. They can be increased in patients with urolithiasis, which can cause reactive atypia in urothelial cells (Pap stain).

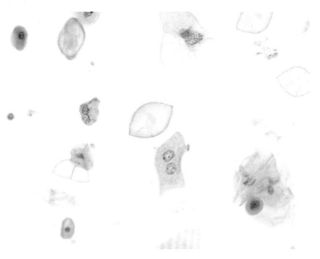

Figure 6.208. Crystals. Several uric acid crystals are seen along with two umbrella cells (Pap stain).

SPERMATOZOA

Spermatozoa may be seen in small or large numbers in male patients (Figures 6.210 and 6.211). The finding is often associated with retrograde ejaculation, which can occur in patients with chronic diseases such as diabetes. The spermatozoa can be engulfed by macrophages, forming spermiophages. Spermiophages can contain numerous dark, small spermatozoa nuclei, with numerous spermatozoa tails projecting from the cytoplasm (Figures 6.212 and 6.213).

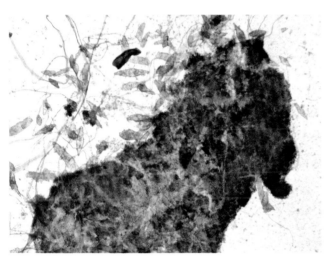

Figure 6.209. Crystals. Numerous uric acid crystals are seen along a large collection of acute inflammatory cells (Pap stain).

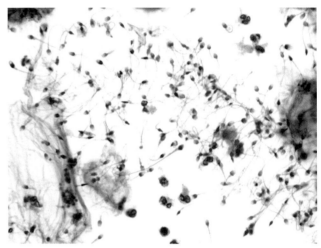

Figure 6.210. Spermatozoa. The presence of spermatozoa in urine is associated with retrograde ejaculation, which can occur in patients with diabetes and other chronic illnesses (Pap stain).

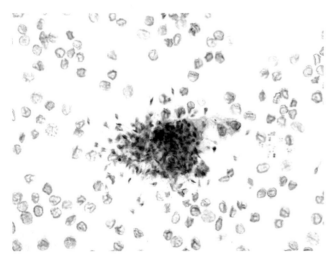

Figure 6.211. Spermatozoa. Alternate field (Pap stain).

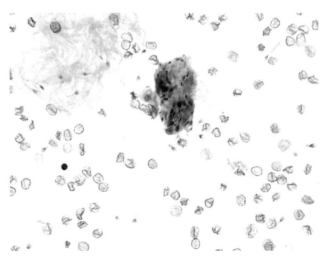

Figure 6.212. Spermatozoa. Spermatozoa are sometimes engulfed by macrophages (spermiophages), which can create a strange appearance (Pap stain).

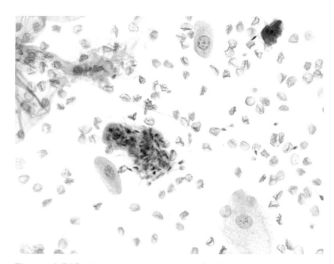

Figure 6.213. Spermatozoa. Alternate field (Pap stain).

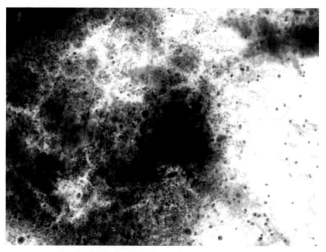

Figure 6.214. *Schistosoma haematobium* ova. The ovum has a golden appearance on the Pap stain and is associated with heavy granular debris and inflammation. Over time, this inflammatory process can result in primary bladder carcinoma, most commonly squamous cell carcinoma of the bladder (Pap stain).

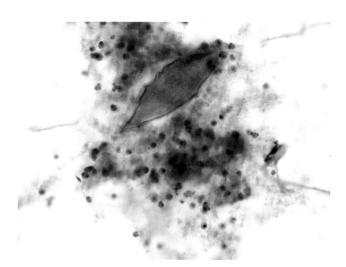

Figure 6.215. *Schistosoma haematobium* ova. Other species are not found in the urinary tract. *S. haematobium* is additionally differentiated by having a terminal spine, as seen here (Pap stain).

BUGS

SCHISTOSOMA HAEMATOBIUM

S. haematobium may be seen both in patients from areas endemic for the parasite and in international travelers who have spent time in those areas. Urinary tract cytology is not a sensitive test for infection with *S. haematobium*. The most common diagnostic finding of *S. haematobium* is the presence of ova, which are rare. The ova are not necessarily intact and are therefore difficult to recognize (Figures 6.214 and 6.215). When present, the ova are often accompanied by an inflammatory response with accompanying granular debris.[68]

NEAR MISSES

BK POLYOMAVIRUS MISTAKEN FOR HIGH-GRADE UROTHELIAL CARCINOMA

Changes secondary to BK polyomavirus include extremely high N/C ratios and hyperchromasia. These cells have been labeled as "decoy cells" owing to their similarity with HGUC (Figures 6.216-6.219). If the changes are consistent with BK virus (rare cells with marginated and/or "ground glass" chromatin), the findings may be reported under the *NHGUC* category. If the findings cannot be comfortably distinguished from degenerated HGUC cells, the recommendation is to use the *AUC* category.[54]

SMALL CELL CARCINOMA MISTAKEN FOR INFLAMMATORY CELLS

Small cell carcinoma usually appears as a predominantly dispersed population of small cells, which may blend in with the background (Figures 6.220-6.224). At low magnification, the cells may be mistaken for inflammatory cells. If a high-grade urothelial cell component is not present, the dispersed small cell carcinoma cells may be overlooked during a search for larger HGUC cells. In a specimen with numerous dispersed cells, always examine the cells at high magnification to exclude small cell carcinoma. This practice is particularly important in patients with a history of prostate cancer, who may present with a transformed component invading the urinary tract.

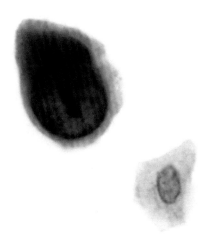
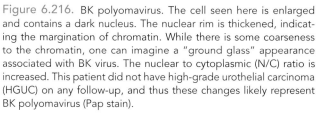
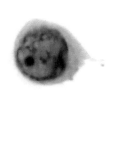

Figure 6.216. BK polyomavirus. The cell seen here is enlarged and contains a dark nucleus. The nuclear rim is thickened, indicating the margination of chromatin. While there is some coarseness to the chromatin, one can imagine a "ground glass" appearance associated with BK virus. The nuclear to cytoplasmic (N/C) ratio is increased. This patient did not have high-grade urothelial carcinoma (HGUC) on any follow-up, and thus these changes likely represent BK polyomavirus (Pap stain).

Figure 6.217. BK polyomavirus. The chromatin pattern has a "ground glass" appearance and aside from one dark inclusion, the chromatin is not coarse. The nuclear membranes appear round and regular. Some chromatin clumps appear to strand across the nucleus, providing a partial "spider web" appearance sometimes seen in BK polyomavirus. The patient did not have high-grade urothelial carcinoma (HGUC) on follow-up, and thus these changes likely represent BK polyomavirus (Pap stain).

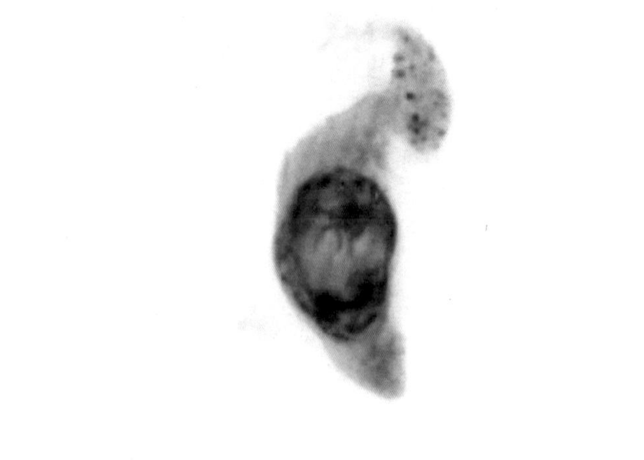

Figure 6.218. High-grade urothelial carcinoma (HGUC) with BK-like changes. This patient had HGUC on follow-up. The nucleus is enlarged, and the cell is large; despite not having a nuclear to cytoplasmic (N/C) ratio above 0.7, this cell is concerning for HGUC. The nuclear border is irregular, but the chromatin has a "ground glass" appearance with marginated chromatin. Some studies have identified HGUC cells infected with BK virus, suggesting a possible link between the two (Pap stain).

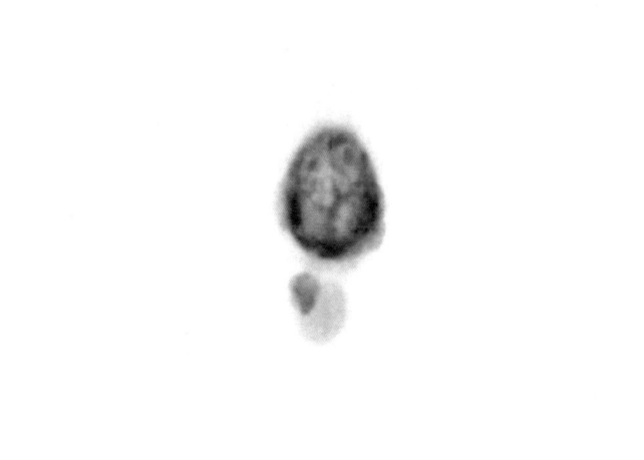

Figure 6.219. High-grade urothelial carcinoma (HGUC) with BK-like changes. The cell is degenerating and the cytoplasm is indistinct. The nucleus is large with smooth borders, and the chromatin has a "spider web" appearance sometime seen in cells infected with BK polyomavirus. This patient had HGUC on follow-up biopsy, indicating that this cell is likely an HGUC cell and not simply one demonstrating changes secondary to BK polyomavirus infection (Pap stain).

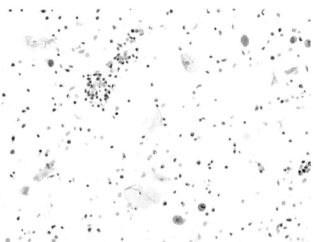

Figure 6.220. Small cell carcinoma. At low magnification, the numerous cells in the background could represent inflammatory cells or degenerated urothelial cells. Small cell carcinoma is rarely seen in urinary tract specimens and thus can be easily missed if a specimen is not carefully examined at the proper magnification (Pap stain).

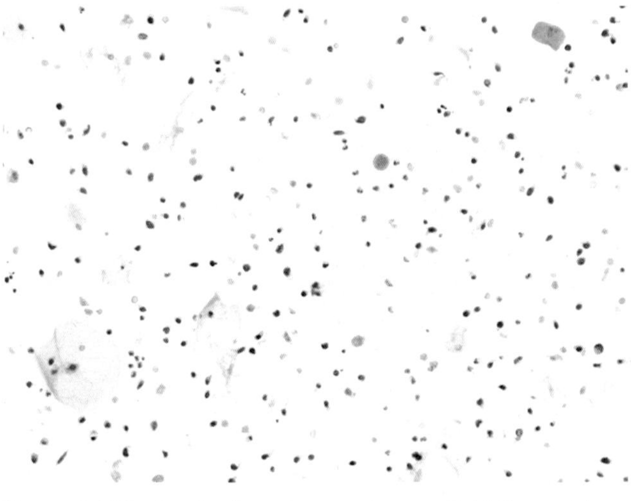

Figure 6.221. Small cell carcinoma. Alternate field (Pap stain).

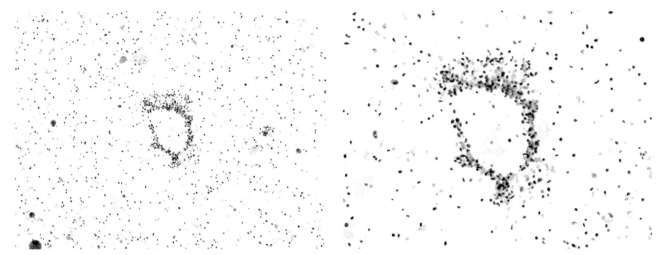

Figure 6.222. Small cell carcinoma. The small cell carcinoma cells can form loose clusters in liquid-based preparations—one clue at low magnification that these cells may not simply be inflammatory cells. Liquid-based preparations often reduce many of the features seen in small cell carcinoma (necrosis, molding, chromatin streak artifact) that are otherwise seen in conventional smears and tissue sections (Pap stain).

Figure 6.223. Small cell carcinoma. Higher magnification of Figure 6.222. Note that geographic necrosis can be seen as cells with intact nuclei alternating with "blue blobs," which represent cellular necrosis. The "blue blobs" are also dispersed in the background, where they can be difficult to interpret out of context (Pap stain).

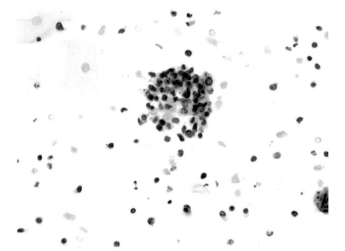

Figure 6.224. Small cell carcinoma. Alternate field. At this magnification, the neuroendocrine quality of the chromatin can be appreciated. The cells lack the thin rim of cytoplasm seen in lymphocytes and have more variation in nuclear size and shape than would be seen in a population of lymphocytes (Pap stain).

References

1. Prather J, Arville B, Chatt G, et al. Evidence-based adequacy criteria for urinary bladder barbotage cytology. *J Am Soc Cytopathol*. 2015;4(2):57-62.

2. van Hoeven KH, Artymyshyn RL. Cytology of small cell carcinoma of the urinary bladder. *Diagn Cytopathol*. 1996;14(4):292-297.

3. VandenBussche CJ. A review of the Paris system for reporting urinary cytology. *Cytopathology*. 2016;27(3):153-157.

4. Barkan GA, Wojcik EM, Nayar R, et al. The Paris system for reporting urinary cytology: the quest to develop a standardized terminology. *Acta Cytol*. 2016;60(3):185-197.

5. Kurtycz DF, Barkan GA, Pavelec DM, et al. Paris interobserver reproducibility study(PIRST). *J Am Soc Cytopathol* 2018;7(4):174-184.

6. Owens CL, Vandenbussche CJ, Burroughs FH, Rosenthal DL. A review of reporting systems and terminology for urine cytology. *Cancer Cytopathol.* 2013;121(1):9-14.

7. Onur I, Rosenthal DL, VandenBussche CJ. Benign-appearing urothelial tissue fragments in noninstrumented voided urine specimens are associated with low rates of urothelial neoplasia. *Cancer Cytopathol.* 2015;123(3):180-185.

8. Onur I, Rosenthal DL, VandenBussche CJ. Atypical urothelial tissue fragments in noninstrumented voided urine specimens are associated with low but significantly higher rates of urothelial neoplasia than benign appearing urothelial tissue fragments. *Cancer Cytopathol.* 2015;123(3):186-192.

9. McCroskey Z, Pambuccian SE, Kleitherms S, et al. Accuracy and interobserver variability of the cytologic diagnosis of low-grade urothelial carcinoma in instrumented urinary tract cytology specimens. *Am J Clin Pathol.* 2015;144(6):902-908.

10. Kern WH. The cytology of transitional cell carcinoma of the urinary bladder. *Acta Cytol.* 1975;19(5):420-428.

11. Raab SS, Lenel JC, Cohen MB. Low grade transitional cell carcinoma of the bladder. Cytologic diagnosis by key features as identified by logistic regression analysis. *Cancer.* 1994;74(5):1621-1627.

12. Zhang ML, Rosenthal DL, VandenBussche CJ. The cytomorphological features of low-grade urothelial neoplasms vary by specimen type. *Cancer Cytopathol.* 2016;124(8):552-564.

13. Murphy WM, Soloway MS, Jukkola AF, Crabtree WN, Ford KS. Urinary cytology and bladder cancer. The cellular features of transitional cell neoplasms. *Cancer.* 1984;53(7):1555-1565.

14. De Berardinis E, Busetto GM, Giovannone R, Antonini G, Di Placido M, Gentile V. Recurrent transitional cell carcinoma of the bladder: a mixed nested variant case report and literature review. *Can Urol Assoc J.* 2012;6(2):E57-E60.

15. Sternberg I, Rona R, Olsfanger S, Lew S, Leibovitch I. The clinical significance of class III (suspicious) urine cytology. *Cytopathology.* 2011;22(5): 329-333.

16. Ton Nu TN, Kassouf W, Ahmadi-Kaliji B, Charbonneau M, Auger M, Brimo F. The value of the "suspicious for urothelial carcinoma" cytology category: a correlative study of 4 years including 337 patients. *Cancer Cytopathol.* 2014;122(11):796-803.

17. Piaton E, Decaussin-Petrucci M, Mege-Lechevallier F, Advenier AS, Devonec M, Ruffion A. Diagnostic terminology for urinary cytology reports including the new subcategories 'atypical urothelial cells of undetermined significance' (AUC-US) and 'cannot exclude high grade' (AUC-H). *Cytopathology.* 2014;25(1):27-38.

18. VandenBussche CJ, Sathiyamoorthy S, Owens CL, Burroughs FH, Rosenthal DL, Guan H. The Johns Hopkins Hospital template for urologic cytology samples: parts II and III: improving the predictability of indeterminate results in urinary cytologic samples: an outcomes and cytomorphologic study. *Cancer Cytopathol.* 2013;121(1):21-28.

19. Wang Y, Auger M, Kanber Y, Caglar D, Brimo F. Implementing the Paris System for Reporting Urinary Cytology results in a decrease in the rate of the "atypical" category and an increase in its prediction of subsequent high-grade urothelial carcinoma. *Cancer Cytopathol.* 2018;126(3):207-214.

20. Hassan M, Solanki S, Kassouf W, et al. Impact of implementing the Paris System for Reporting Urine Cytology in the performance of urine cytology: a correlative study of 124 cases. *Am J Clin Pathol.* 2016;146(3):384-390.

21. Straccia P, Bizzarro T, Fadda G, Pierconti F. Comparison between cytospin and liquid-based cytology in urine specimens classified according to the Paris System for Reporting Urinary Cytology. *Cancer Cytopathol.* 2016;124(7):519-523.

22. Fite JJ, Rosenthal DL, VandenBussche CJ. When words matter: a "suspicious" urinary tract cytology diagnosis improves patient follow-up among nonurologists. *Cancer Cytopathol.* 2018;126(4):282-288.

23. Brimo F, Vollmer RT, Case B, Aprikian A, Kassouf W, Auger M. Accuracy of urine cytology and the significance of an atypical category. *Am J Clin Pathol.* 2009;132(5):785-793.

24. Hang JF, Charu V, Zhang ML, VandenBussche CJ. Digital image analysis supports a nuclear-to-cytoplasmic ratio cutoff value of 0.5 for atypical urothelial cells. *Cancer Cytopathol.* 2017;125(9):710-717.

25. Zhang ML, Guo AX, VandenBussche CJ. Morphologists overestimate the nuclear-to-cytoplasmic ratio. *Cancer Cytopathol.* 2016;124(9):669-677.

26. Wojcik EM. What should not be reported as atypia in urine cytology. *J Am Soc Cytopathol.* 2015;4(1): 30-37.

27. Rosenthal DL, Vandenbussche CJ, Burroughs FH, Sathiyamoorthy S, Guan H, Owens C. The Johns Hopkins Hospital template for urologic cytology samples: part I-creating the template. *Cancer Cytopathol.* 2013;121(1):15-20.

28. Muus Ubago J, Mehta V, Wojcik EM, Barkan GA. Evaluation of atypical urine cytology progression to malignancy. *Cancer Cytopathol.* 2013;121(7):387-391.

29. Mokhtar GA, Al-Dousari M, Al-Ghamedi D. Diagnostic significance of atypical category in the voided urine samples: a retrospective study in a tertiary care center. *Urol Ann.* 2010;2(3):100-107.

30. Kapur U, Venkataraman G, Wojcik EM. Diagnostic significance of 'atypia' in instrumented versus voided urine specimens. *Cancer.* 2008;114(4):270-274.

31. Bhatia A, Dey P, Kakkar N, Srinivasan R, Nijhawan R. Malignant atypical cell in urine cytology: a diagnostic dilemma. *CytoJournal.* 2006;3:28.

32. Deshpande V, McKee GT. Analysis of atypical urine cytology in a tertiary care center. *Cancer.* 2005;105(6):468-475.

33. Barasch S, Choi M, Stewart J, Das K. Significance of atypical category in voided urine specimens prepared by liquid-based technology: experience of a single institution. *J Am Soc Cytopathol.* 2014;3:118-125.

34. Cowan ML, VandenBussche CJ. The Paris System for Reporting Urinary Cytology: early review of the literature reveals successes and rare shortcomings. *J Am Soc Cytopathol.* 2018;7(4):185-194.

35. VandenBussche CJ, Allison DB, Gupta M, Ali SZ, Rosenthal DL. A 20-year and 46,000-specimen journey to Paris reveals the influence of reporting systems and passive peer feedback on pathologist practice patterns. *Cancer Cytopathol.* 2018;126(6):381-389.

36. Abbas F, Civantos F, Benedetto P, Soloway MS. Small cell carcinoma of the bladder and prostate. *Urology.* 1995;46(5):617-630.

37. Hoda RS, Loukeris K, Abdul-Karim FW. Gynecologic cytology on conventional and liquid-based preparations: a comprehensive review of similarities and differences. *Diagn Cytopathol.* 2013;41(3):257-278.

38. Pedersen N, Pedersen MW, Lan MS, Breslin MB, Poulsen HS. The insulinoma-associated 1: a novel promoter for targeted cancer gene therapy for small-cell lung cancer. *Cancer Gene Ther.* 2006;13(4):375-384.

39. Travis WD. Update on small cell carcinoma and its differentiation from squamous cell carcinoma and other non-small cell carcinomas. *Mod Pathol.* 2012;25(suppl 1):S18-S30.

40. Pant-Purohit M, Lopez-Beltran A, Montironi R, MacLennan GT, Cheng L. Small cell carcinoma of the urinary bladder. *Histol Histopathol.* 2010;25(2):217-221.

41. Mincione GP, Grechi G. Urinary cytology of rhabdomyosarcoma in children. Report of two cases located in the urinary bladder and in the prostate. *Pathologica.* 1983;75(1040):797-801.

42. Mitchell CS, Yeo TA. Noninvasive botryoid extension of Wilms' tumor into the bladder. *Pediatr Radiol.* 1997;27(10):818-820.

43. Renshaw AA, Madge R, Granter SR. Intracytoplasmic eosinophilic inclusions (Melamed-Wolinska bodies). Association with metastatic transitional cell carcinoma in pleural fluid. *Acta Cytol.* 1997;41(4):995-998.

44. Ajit D, Dighe SB, Desai SB. Cytology of Ileal conduit urine in bladder cancer patients: diagnostic utility and pitfalls. *Acta Cytol.* 2006;50(1):70-73.

45. Cimino-Mathews A, Ali SZ. The clinicopathologic correlates of cellular atypia in urinary cytology of ileal neobladders. *Acta Cytol.* 2011;55(5):449-454.

46. Cowan ML, Rosenthal DL, VandenBussche CJ. Improved risk stratification for patients with high-grade urothelial carcinoma following application of the Paris System for Reporting Urinary Cytology. *Cancer.* 2017;125(6):427-434.

47. Renshaw AA, Gould EW. High-grade urothelial carcinoma in urine cytology with jet black and smooth or glassy chromatin. *Cancer Cytopathol.* 2018;126(1):64-68.

48. Alexandroff AB, Jackson AM, O'Donnell MA, James K. BCG immunotherapy of bladder cancer: 20 years on. *Lancet.* 1999;353(9165):1689-1694.

49. Takashi M, Schenck U, Koshikawa T, Nakashima N, Ohshima S. Cytological changes induced by intravesical bacillus Calmette-Guerin therapy for superficial bladder cancer. *Urol Int.* 2000;64(2):74-81.

50. Reploeg MD, Storch GA, Clifford DB. Bk virus: a clinical review. *Clin Infect Dis.* 2001;33(2):191-202.

51. Ramos E, Drachenberg CB, Portocarrero M, et al. BK virus nephropathy diagnosis and treatment: experience at the University of Maryland Renal Transplant Program. *Clin Transpl.* 2002:143-153.

52. Crabbe JG. "Comet" or "decoy" cells found in urinary sediment smears. *Acta Cytol.* 1971;15(3):303-305.

53. Barkan GA, Tabatabai L, Sturgis C, Kurtycz DF, Souers RJ, Nayar R. In preparation for the Paris System for Reporting Urinary Tract Cytopathology (TPSRUTC): observations from the 2014 supplemental questionnaire of the College of American Pathologists (CAP) cytopathology interlaboratory comparison program (CICP). *Mod Pathol.* 2015;28(2S):82A.

54. Allison DB, Olson MT, Lilo M, Zhang ML, Rosenthal DL, VandenBussche CJ. Should the BK polyomavirus cytopathic effect be best classified as atypical or benign in urine cytology specimens? *Cancer Cytopathol.* 2016;124(6):436-442.

55. Bardales RH, Pitman MB, Stanley MW, Korourian S, Suhrland MJ. Urine cytology of primary and secondary urinary bladder adenocarcinoma. *Cancer.* 1998;84(6):335-343.

56. Sangoi AR, Karamchandani J, Kim J, Pai RK, McKenney JK. The use of immunohistochemistry in the diagnosis of metastatic clear cell renal cell carcinoma: a review of PAX-8, PAX-2, hKIM-1, RCCma, and CD10. *Adv Anat Pathol.* 2010;17(6):377-393.

57. Gurel B, Ali TZ, Montgomery EA, et al. NKX3.1 as a marker of prostatic origin in metastatic tumors. *Am J Surg Pathol.* 2010;34(8):1097-1105.

58. Chang A, Amin A, Gabrielson E, et al. Utility of GATA3 immunohistochemistry in differentiating urothelial carcinoma from prostate adenocarcinoma and squamous cell carcinomas of the uterine cervix, anus, and lung. *Am J Surg Pathol.* 2012;36(10):1472-1477.

59. Mostafa MH, Sheweita SA, O'Connor PJ. Relationship between schistosomiasis and bladder cancer. *Clin Microbiol Rev.* 1999;12(1):97-111.

60. Serretta V, Pomara G, Piazza F, Gange E. Pure squamous cell carcinoma of the bladder in western countries. Report on 19 consecutive cases. *Eur Urol.* 2000;37(1):85-89.

61. Owens CL, Ali SZ. Atypical squamous cells in exfoliative urinary cytology: clinicopathologic correlates. *Diagn Cytopathol.* 2005;33(6):394-398.

62. Hattori M, Nishimura Y, Toyonaga M, Kakinuma H, Matsumoto K, Ohbu M. Cytological significance of abnormal squamous cells in urinary cytology. *Diagn Cytopathol.* 2012;40(9):798-803.

63. Sherman ME, Dasgupta A, Schiffman M, Nayar R, Solomon D. The Bethesda Interobserver Reproducibility Study (BIRST): a web-based assessment of the Bethesda 2001 system for classifying cervical cytology. *Cancer.* 2007;111(1):15-25.

64. Nayar R, Wilbur DC. *The Bethesda System for Reporting Cervical Cytology: Definitions, Criteria, and Explanatory Notes.* 3rd ed. New York City: Springer; 2015.

65. Daniels IR, Bekdash B, Scott HJ, Marks CG, Donaldson DR. Diagnostic lessons learnt from a series of enterovesical fistulae. *Colorectal Dis.* 2002;4(6):459-462.

66. Renshaw AA, Gould EW. High-grade urothelial carcinoma on urine cytology resembling umbrella cells. *Acta Cytol.* 2018;62(1):62-67.

67. Rathert P, Roth S. *Indications for Urinary Cytology. Urinary Cytology: Manual and Atlas.* Berlin, Heidelberg: Springer Berlin Heidelberg; 1993:9-13.

68. Clements MH, Oko T. Cytologic diagnosis of schistosomiasis in routine urinary specimens. A case report. *Acta Cytol.* 1983;27(3):277-280.

CHAPTER OUTLINE

THE UNREMARKABLE PAP TEST

SUPERFICIAL SQUAMOUS CELLS

Superficial squamous cells are polygonal in shape with small, angulated nuclei that are slightly darker than intermediate cell nuclei. Not only are superficial cells the largest cells in the normal maturation process, but they also have the smallest nuclei, resulting in the lowest nuclear to cytoplasmic (N/C) ratio (Figure 7.1).[1,2] The cytoplasm of superficial squamous cells is abundant, stains pink (eosinophilic) on the Pap stain, and has a translucent quality. In contrast, parabasal cells possess a cytoplasm that is denser and opaque. Estrogen promotes the maturation of squamous cells into superficial squamous cells, and as a result, they are often rare or absent in high-progesterone or low-estrogen states (such as in women who are pregnant, postmenopausal, or taking antiestrogen drugs).[3]

KEY FEATURES of Superficial Squamous Cells
- The cells are polygonal in shape with abundant cytoplasm.
- The cytoplasm is most often pink and translucent.
- The nuclei contain dark chromatin and have angulated borders.

INTERMEDIATE CELLS

Intermediate cells retain the polygonal shape of superficial squamous cells but are slightly smaller with blue, cyanophilic cytoplasm.[1,2] The cytoplasm of intermediate cells is denser and less translucent than that of superficial squamous cells but not as opaque as the cytoplasm of parabasal cells. Intermediate cells are associated with progesterone and predominate during the high-progresterone states of pregnancy and the second phase of the menstrual cycle (Figures 7.2 and 7.3).[3]

The nuclei of intermediate cells are the "reference nuclei" used for comparison in The Bethesda System for Reporting Cervical Cytology (TBS) (Table 7.1) for Pap test interpretation. Familiarity with normal intermediate cell nuclei is crucial for Pap test interpretation, as they are used as the standard for nuclear size as well as for chromatin staining and texture. Intermediate cell nuclei are between the size of superficial squamous cell and parabasal cell nuclei and are approximately the size of a neutrophil. The chromatin of intermediate cell nuclei is evenly distributed and finely granular, in contrast to the darker nuclei of superficial squamous cells. The Pap test in women of reproductive age typically shows a combination of predominantly superficial and intermediate cells because these cells are the closest to the surface and are most easily exfoliated during instrumentation (Figures 7.4 and 7.5)[3].

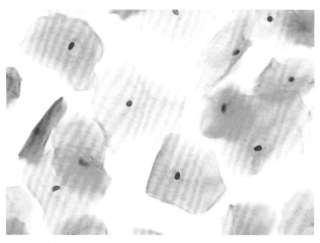

Figure 7.1. Superficial cells. Superficial cells have abundant polygonal pink cytoplasm and small pyknotic nuclei (Pap stain).

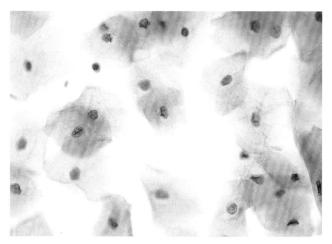

Figure 7.2. Intermediate cells showing abundant blue cytoplasm. An intermediate cell nucleus is approximately the size of a red blood cell. The chromatin is vesicular (open). Intermediate cells are the cells of reference for comparison of nuclear size and chromatin characteristics (Pap stain).

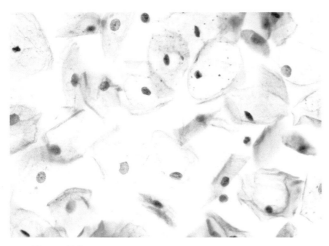

Figure 7.3. Intermediate cells. Separate field (Pap stain).

TABLE 7.1: The 2014 Bethesda System for Reporting Cervical Cytology

General Categorization	Interpretation
Negative for intraepithelial lesion or malignancy (NILM)	Nonneoplastic findings and organisms
Other	Endometrial cells in a woman ≥45 years old
Epithelial cell abnormality	**Squamous Cells** Atypical squamous cells • of undetermined significance (ASC-US) • cannot exclude HSIL (ASC-H) Low-grade squamous intraepithelial lesion (LSIL) High-grade squamous intraepithelial lesion (HSIL) Squamous cell carcinoma **Glandular cells** Atypical glandular cells Atypical endocervical cells Atypical endometrial cells Atypical endocervical cells, favor neoplastic Atypical glandular cells, favor neoplastic Endocervical adenocarcinoma in situ (AIS) Adenocarcinoma • endocervical • endometrial • extrauterine • not otherwise specified (NOS)
Other malignant neoplasms	(Further specified by the pathologist; for instance, "Metastatic Melanoma" does not fit into the above categories.)

KEY FEATURES of Intermediate Squamous Cells

• The intermediate squamous cell nucleus is used as a reference to determine if nuclear enlargement is present and to compare with the chromatin characteristics of a particular cell of interest.

• These cells are polygonal in shape.

• The cytoplasm in typically cyanophilic.

• The chromatin is finely granular, in contrast to the dark nuclei of superficial cells.

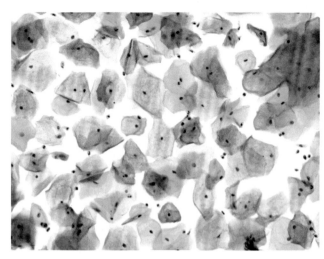

Figure 7.4. Superficial and intermediate cells. A separate specimen demonstrating a mixture of superficial and intermediate cells (Pap stain).

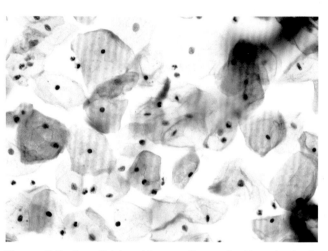

Figure 7.5. Superficial and intermediate cells. Note the background neutrophils, which are approximately the size of the intermediate cell nucleus, whereas the superficial cell nuclei are smaller (Pap stain).

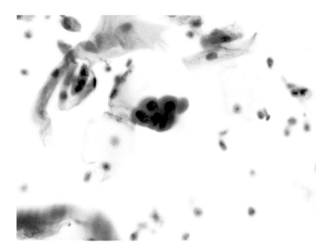

Figure 7.6. Small cluster of parabasal cells. The cells have round and dense cytoplasm. Their nuclei are also round to oval with smooth nuclear borders (Pap stain).

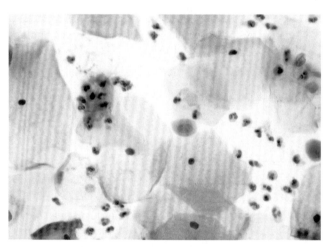

Figure 7.7. Parabasal cell. The cell is round, and the cytoplasm is dense compared with that of nearby intermediate cells. The nucleus is round with smooth nuclear membranes. The bland appearance of the nucleus distinguishes it from a dysplastic cell, which would appear more hyperchromatic and have nuclear membrane irregularities (Pap stain).

PARABASAL CELLS

Parabasal cells are the smallest squamous cells routinely seen on the Pap test. Parabasal cells are round to oval with dense, blue cytoplasm and distinct cell borders. The nuclei (50 μm²) are usually larger than the nuclei of intermediate cells, but most parabasal cells will still have an N/C ratio below 0.5. The nuclei often appear round to oval with evenly distributed chromatin.[1,2] Parabasal cells predominate in low-estrogen environments and are the predominant cell type in atrophic specimens, such as those from children, postmenopausal women, and postpartum women (Figures 7.6-7.12).[3]

KEY FEATURES of Parabasal Cells

- These cells are small and round to oval in shape
- The cytoplasm is dense and blue in color.
- The nuclei are round to oval with smooth nuclear contours.
- The nuclei are larger than the nuclei of intermediate cells but usually still have an N/C ratio below 0.5.

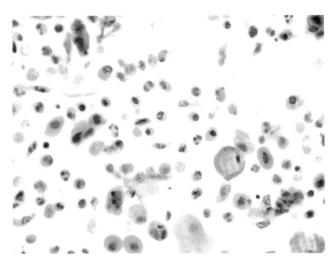

Figure 7.8. Atrophy. The field shows predominantly parabasal cells in a singly dispersed pattern. The cells have low nuclear to cytoplasmic (N/C) ratios but appear hyperchromatic with mild nuclear contour irregularities (Pap stain).

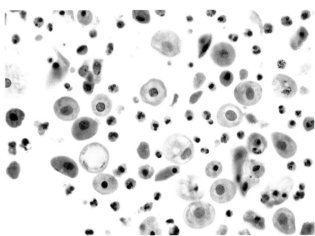

Figure 7.9. Atrophy. Numerous singly dispersed parabasal cells are seen with low nuclear to cytoplasmic (N/C) ratios and regular nuclear contours. The background shows inflammation and "blue blobs" (degenerated cells) (Pap stain).

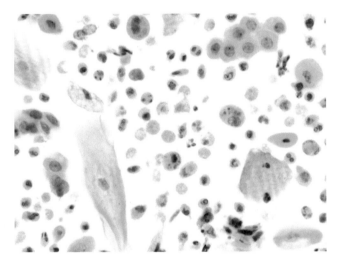

Figure 7.10. Atrophy. Separate field (Pap stain).

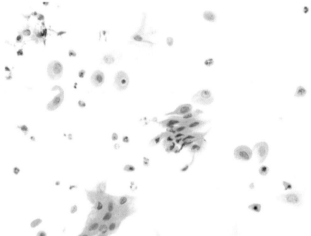

Figure 7.11. Atrophy. Separate field. Some parabasal cells are seen in small tissue fragments; nuclei remain evenly spaced and organized within the fragments (Pap stain).

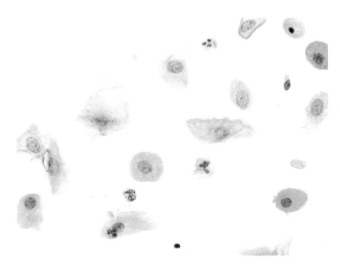

Figure 7.12. Atrophy. Separate field (Pap stain).

BENIGN ENDOCERVICAL CELLS

Endocervical cells are columnar cells that are typically at least twice as long as they are wide. Endocervical cells can occur singly, as strips ("picket fence" appearance), or in sheets ("honeycomb" arrangement) (Figures 7.13-7.15)[1,2] Endocervical cells contain abundant, mucinous cytoplasm that appears blue-gray on the Pap stain. The nuclei are typically uniform, basally oriented, and oval to round with fine chromatin. Not uncommonly, however, reactive states induce changes leading to nuclear pleomorphism. In such states, the nuclear size can be quite variable and the picket fence or honeycomb arrangement of the cells may be disturbed. The presence of endocervical cells is not required for a specimen to be considered adequate but is nevertheless an important finding in the Pap test because it indicates that the transformation zone was sampled. As a result, the presence or absence of endocervical cells should be noted in Pap test specimens.

KEY FEATURES of Benign Endocervical Cells

* Endocervical cells are columnar in shape.
* The nucleus is round to oval in shape and is located in the basal portion of the cell.

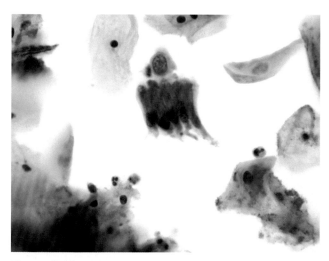

Figure 7.13. Endocervical cells. A strip of endocervical cells lying on their side; these tall columnar cells form a "picket fence" arrangement (Pap stain).

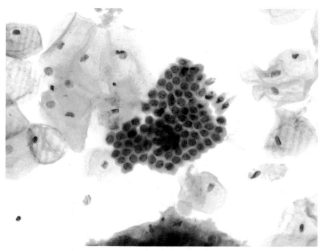

Figure 7.14. Endocervical cells. Endocervical cells standing *en face*; while their columnar shape cannot be appreciated in this single plane, the even distribution of their nuclei within this monolayer ("honeycomb" arrangement) can be appreciated (Pap stain).

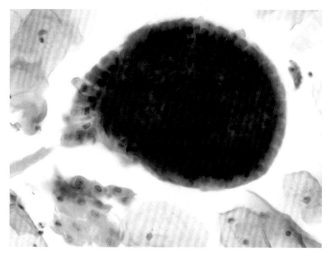

Figure 7.15. Endocervical cells. Large endocervical tissue fragments may form three-dimensional spherical structures that may emulate endometrial cell clusters. However, the cells at the periphery are tall and columnar with predominantly basely located nuclei, consistent with an endocervical origin. The underlying core represents stroma (Pap stain).

- Depending on the orientation of the cells, they most display a picket fence or a honeycomb arrangement.
- Reactive endocervical cell may have significant nuclear enlargement and anisonucleosis.

BENIGN ENDOMETRIAL CELLS

Shedding from the endometrial cavity or sampling of the lower uterine segment (LUS) results in the presence of endometrial cells on the Pap test. Depending on both the context and the morphology, the significance of endometrial cells ranges from incidental and benign to worrisome for adenocarcinoma. The term *"exodus"* is used to describe the characteristic appearance of endometrial cell groups that have spontaneously exfoliated (normally seen on days 6-10 of the menstrual cycle) (Figures 7.16 and 7.17).[1,2] Normal endometrial cells exfoliate as three-dimensional groups composed of small cells. These cells have scant, sometimes vacuolated, cytoplasm and round, hyperchromatic nuclei with rare nucleoli (Figure 7.18)[1,2] A characteristic feature of exfoliated endometrial cells known as the "double-contour" pattern refers a three dimensional structure with a dark center containing histiocytes and stromal cells surrounded by a second layer of hobnailed endometrial cells.

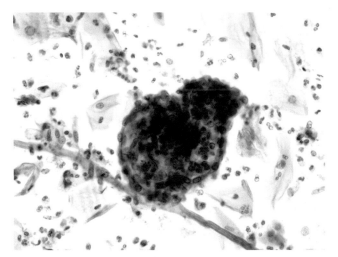

Figure 7.16. Endometrial cells. Endometrial cells form the classic "double-contour" structure in which a thin layer of hobnailed glandular cells overlie stromal cells (Pap stain).

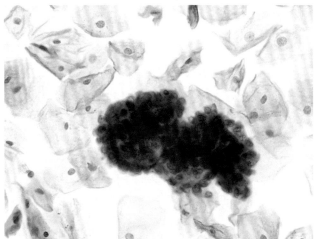

Figure 7.17. Endometrial cells. Separate field demonstrating an irregularly shaped "double-contour" structure (Pap stain).

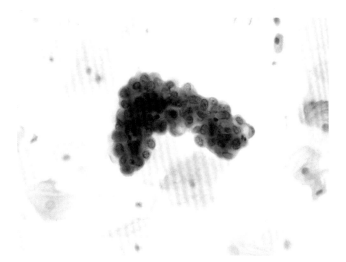

Figure 7.18. Endometrial cells. Cluster of small cells with scant cytoplasm and high nuclear to cytoplasmic (N/C) ratios. Some cells have vacuolated cytoplasm, and a rare neutrophil is associated with the cluster. While the nuclei have mild contour irregularities, they are uniform in size and have small, indistinct nucleoli (Pap stain).

Neutrophils often accompany endometrial cells; these neutrophils may be within the cytoplasm of individual cells or present as a collection associated with the endometrial cells. Sampling of the LUS often results in large, hyperchromatic fragments containing endometrial cells and stromal cells. These fragments may form three-dimensional tubular and/or glandular structures that help establish their origin.

KEY FEATURES of Benign Endometrial Cells

- Benign endometrial cells are most often present as tight three-dimensional groups.
- The cytoplasm is scant and vacuolated which results in a high N/C ratio and may contain intracytoplasmic neutrophils.
- Three-dimensional groups may contain a "double contour" pattern with hobnailed cells at edge and darker stromal cells in the center.

PEARLS & PITFALLS

Benign endometrial cells appear as hyperchromatic crowded groups of cells, which brings up the differential diagnosis of high-grade squamous intraepithelial lesion (HSIL), squamous cell carcinoma, or endocervical adenocarcinoma in situ (AIS). Endometrial cells are considered a normal finding through days 6-10 of the menstrual cycle, and it is recommended that the cervical Pap test should be avoided during this time period. Endometrial cells may be difficult to avoid in patients with irregular menses, including perimenopausal patients. Numerous endometrial cells can obscure the cervical cells of interest, resulting in an inadequate or suboptimal specimen. Ideally, Pap test specimens should be collected during the middle of the menstrual cycle to avoid this potential obscuring factor. For patients with irregular menses, the Pap test should be avoided if menstrual blood is visualized during the pelvic examination prior to specimen collection.

FAQ: What is The Bethesda System for Reporting Cervical Cytology (TBS)?

Answer: The worldwide implementation of the Pap test has dramatically reduced the incidence of cervical cancer and is considered to be one of the greatest successes in women's health.[4] However, a significant amount of practice variability and a lack of quality control measures initially limited the test's utility.[5] As a result, standardized reporting terminology and management guidelines were developed to ensure uniformity and reproducibility of Pap test reporting. TBS was established in 1988 and has undergone several revisions, most recently in 2014. The name "Bethesda" refers to Bethesda, Maryland, which was the location of the meeting which established the system.[5,6] Table 7.1 summarizes the current standardized diagnostic nomenclature.

HYPERCHROMATIC CROWDED GROUP PATTERN

"Hyperchromatic crowded group" (HCG) is a term coined by DeMay and describes a pattern of three-dimensional groups of cells with high N/C ratios and nuclear overlap within the group.[7] HCG has been defined by some authors as dark crowded groups of more than 15 cells that can be seen at 10× screening magnification. The differential diagnosis of an HCG is broad and includes benign endocervical cells, benign endometrial cells, severely atrophic squamous cells, HSIL, and adenocarcinoma. Endocervical cells are the most common cause of HCGs; however, HSIL and adenocarcinoma should always be included in the differential when a HCG is present.[8]

REPARATIVE CHANGES ("REPAIR")

The term reparative changes (or simply "repair") refers to reactive changes induced by many different factors including infection, hormonal changes, trauma, and radiation therapy. The cytomorphologic features of repair were first described by Bibbo in 1971.[9] Despite the well described cytomorphologic features, reparative changes are a diagnostic challenge with a low concordance rate among pathologists.[10] Reactive changes are the most common cause of a false-positive diagnosis of HSIL.[11] For this reason, cytotechnologists are required to refer all Pap test specimens containing reactive changes to a cytopathologist, regardless of how strongly the cytotechnologist favors the changes are benign.

Reparative changes may occur in both squamous and glandular cells. Reactive squamous and endocervical cells share similar features; however, nuclear enlargement may be more pronounced in endocervical cells. The reactive nuclei are round or oval and have smooth, regular contours. The chromatin is usually vesicular and uniformly distributed, which lends a hypochromatic appearance to the nuclei. In some cases, mild hyperchromasia can also be seen. Prominent nucleoli are commonly present, and occasional binucleation or multinucleation may be seen.[2,6,9] The cytoplasmic changes include polychromasia (a "two-tone" cytoplasmic staining pattern), cytoplasmic vacuolization, and small, uniform perinuclear halos that lack peripheral cytoplasmic thickening (the absence of a hard cytoplasmic rim around the halos).[2,6,9] One of the main cytomorphologic features of repair is the architectural arrangement: the cells are arranged in flat monolayer sheets. In addition, the cells have a streaming appearance with maintained polarity ("school of fish" appearance) (Figures 7.19-7.22). Polarization is one of the most helpful features in differentiating benign reactive changes from dysplasia.

KEY FEATURES of Reparative Changes ("Repair")

• Nuclear enlargement can be 1.5-2 times the size of an intermediate cell.

• Nuclear membranes are round and smooth.

• Chromatin is pale and uniformly granular.

• Prominent single or multiple nucleoli may be present.

• Clusters of cells retain their polarity ("streaming" or "school of fish" appearance).

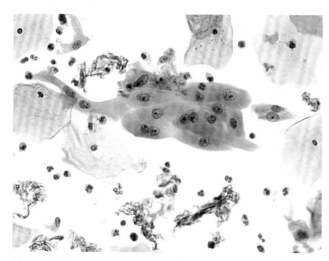

Figure 7.19. Repair. These reactive cells have formed a monolayer, meaning the cells lie flat within one plane. The cells fit together like a jigsaw and have uniformly sized nuclei; prominent nucleoli and binucleation can be seen (Pap stain).

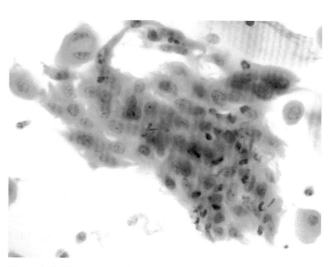

Figure 7.20. Repair. The cells are oriented in one direction ("streaming"). While the nuclei are enlarged, they are uniform in size and have regular nuclear contours. Many of the cells contain small nucleoli (Pap stain).

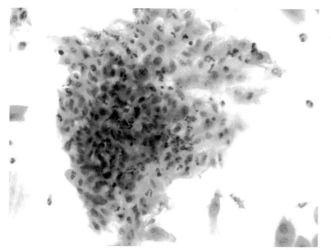

Figure 7.21. Repair. The cells within this fragment are arranged in a "streaming" (or "school of fish") pattern. Note that there is an underlying organization of nuclei and cells within this architecture. Numerous neutrophils are associated with the fragment, a reminder that the changes seen may be reactive (Pap stain).

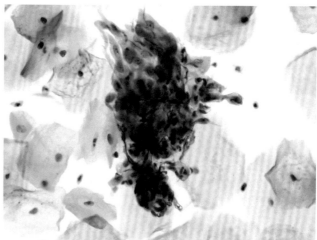

Figure 7.22. Repair. Although this fragment appears hyperchromatic, note that at the edges of the fragment, the cells have smooth nuclear membranes, uniform nuclei, and small nucleoli. Other cells in the fragment are difficult to assess due to the crushed and folded nature of the fragment, which may have resulted from forceful brushing during procurement (Pap stain).

PEARLS & PITFALLS

The presence of prominent nucleoli in squamous cells most likely represents reactive and/or reparative changes rather than HSIL. Nucleoli are typically not present in HSIL and therefore, when seen in squamous cells, indicate either a reactive process or an invasive squamous cell carcinoma. The identification of other cells in the specimen with reparative changes would favor the cells in question to be reactive. Squamous cell carcinoma cells should have markedly atypical features that do not overlap with reactive changes.

REACTIVE ENDOCERVICAL CELLS

Benign endocervical cells are the most common cause of HCGs. Normal endocervical cells are mucin-producing columnar cells with basally located nuclei and luminal cytoplasm. Depending on the orientation of the cells in the group, the cytoplasm may be in a different plane of focus than the nuclei, which imparts an HCG appearance (Figures 7.23-7.28). The nuclei are oval

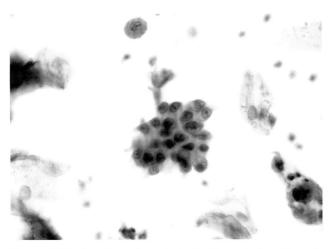

Figure 7.23. Reactive endocervical cells. The majority of the cells have uniform hypochromatic nuclei with smooth nuclear membranes and distinct nucleoli. The well-organized, honeycomb architecture seen here is a feature of benign and reactive endocervical cells (Pap stain).

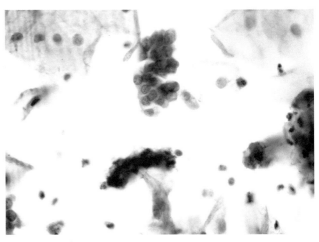

Figure 7.24. Reactive endocervical cells. The cluster is a slightly crowded, but the nuclei are small and have bland chromatin. Nuclear membranes are smooth in the majority of the cells (Pap stain).

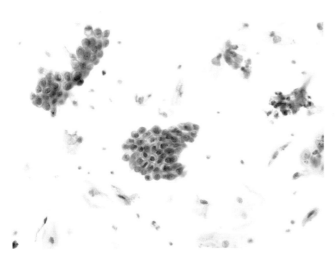

Figure 7.25. Reactive endocervical cells. The field demonstrates endocervical cells "standing up" in honeycomb fragments as well as cells that are "lying down" in which their columnar morphology is more obvious (Pap stain).

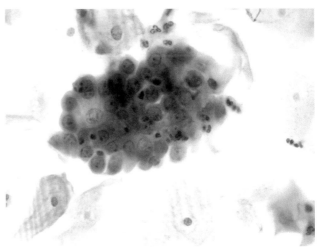

Figure 7.26. Reactive endocervical cells. The cluster is slightly crowded, and the cells show mild variation in nuclear size. The nuclei are several times larger than the nearby intermediate cell nuclei, which is allowed in reactive, benign endocervical cells. Clues for a reactive process include open chromatin (hypochromasia), nucleoli seen in some of the cells, and the associated neutrophilic infiltrate (Pap stain).

to round and typically have prominent nucleoli, though the presence of nucleoli is not always helpful, as it is a feature of both reactive lesions and malignancy. While nucleoli may be an unreliable feature, the chromatin of reactive cells should lack the hyperchromasia that would be expected in a high-grade lesion.

BENIGN ENDOMETRIAL CELLS

Benign endometrial cells are a frequent cause of HCGs. When endometrial cells shed and are detected in the Pap test, they are most often present in three-dimensional clusters, contain degenerative changes, and may be associated with intracytoplasmic neutrophils. At low magnification, these clusters appear as round balls of cells. At high magnification, the nuclei tend to be located at the periphery while the cytoplasm and accompanying neutrophils, histiocytes, and stromal components tend to be in the center of the cluster. The cytoplasm lacks the mucin seen in endocervical cells, but it may contain cytoplasmic vacuoles. The nuclei are small and round to oval or irregular. One consideration when evaluating a group of endometrial cells as part of an HCG is whether they are benign or atypical (Figures 7.29 and 7.30). Atypical endometrial cells usually have larger nuclei and additional nuclear atypia, such as anisonucleosis, hyperchromasia, and prominent nucleoli.[1,2]

FAQ: How can endometrial cells be differentiated from endocervical cells?

Answer: Endometrial cells are slightly smaller than endocervical cells and lack cytoplasmic mucin. Unremarkable endocervical glands tend to form flat, honeycomb-like structures; however, reactive endocervical cells tend to be present in three-dimensional clusters. Endocervical cells are more likely to have their nuclei located in the center of tissue fragments and their cytoplasm at the periphery. In contrast, endometrial cells are more likely to have rounded nuclei at the periphery of cellular clusters. Endometrial clusters are often closely associated with neutrophils (including intracytoplasmic neutrophils) and may contain stromal components in the center of the cluster ("double-contour" appearance). In some instances, a definitive distinction may be impossible.

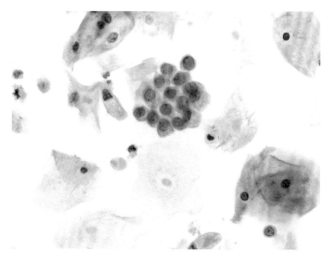

Figure 7.27. Reactive endocervical cells. Separate field (Pap stain).

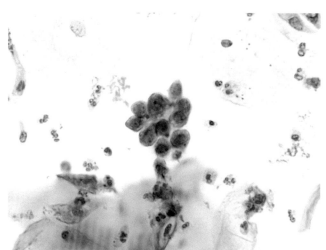

Figure 7.28. Reactive endocervical cells. The cells have a high nuclear to cytoplasmic (N/C) ratio because the cells are "standing up" and their cytoplasm is in several planes. The honeycomb arrangement and foamy cytoplasm helps identify these as endocervical cells and not a high-grade squamous intraepithelial lesion (HSIL), which would be in the differential diagnosis of cells with high N/C ratios (Pap stain).

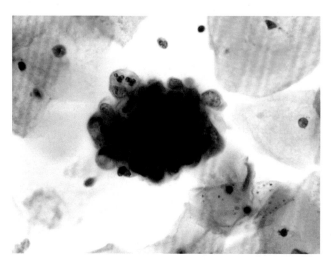

Figure 7.29. Endometrial cells. The presence of intracytoplasmic neutrophils (top left edge of fragment) is a clue to endometrial origin but does not necessarily indicate a pathologic process (Pap stain).

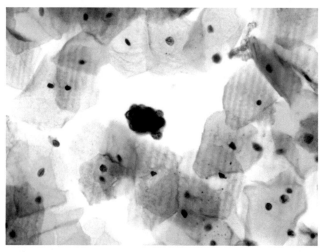

Figure 7.30. Endometrial cells. This small tight cluster of small hyperchromatic cells with high nuclear to cytoplasmic (N/C) ratios is characteristic of endometrial cells. Note the hobnailed borders of the cluster, which is are commonly seen and distinguishes endometrial cells from endocervical cells (Pap stain).

ATROPHY

In low-estrogen states, such as those that occur naturally in peri- and postmenopausal women or iatrogenically in those undergoing antiestrogen therapy, the squamous epithelium lining in the cervix thins and contains a decreased amount of superficial and intermediate cells. As a result, parabasal cells predominate in Pap tests from these women. Other associated changes may be seen, such as increased inflammation, histiocytes, parakeratosis, degenerated cells, and granular debris. In atrophy, the basal cells may have an increased N/C ratio secondary to focal nuclear enlargement. In addition, features such as hyperchromasia and nuclear membrane irregularities can be seen in benign atrophic samples, which may cause concern for squamous dysplasia.[2,12]

In cases of severe atrophy, squamous cells may exfoliate in sheets to form HCGs (Figures 7.31-7.35). Atrophic squamous cells have dense cytoplasm and enlarged nuclei (2-3 times the size of an intermediate cell nucleus) with high N/C ratios. The round uniform nuclei, retained polarity, and association with background single parabasal cells are a clue to the benign nature of a cluster of basal cells.[13–15] In challenging cases, it may not be possible to distinguish atrophic cells from an HSIL. In this instance, the *Atypical squamous cells, cannot exclude HSIL (ASC-H)* category should be utilized.

An additional challenging problem in atrophic smears is the occasional presence of granular debris, acute inflammation, and apoptotic bodies. These findings mimic the tumor diathesis seen in squamous cell carcinoma (SqCC)[16] (Figures 7.36 and 7.37). However, benign atrophy lacks the level of cytologic atypia seen in SqCC.

FAQ: Can I diagnose HSIL in a background of atrophy?

Answer: Distinguishing dysplasia within atrophic smears can be one of the most challenging diagnostic problems on the Pap test. Numerous atypical single cells with high N/C ratios, hyperchromasia, marked nuclear membrane irregularities, and nuclear pleomorphism would support a diagnosis of HSIL, regardless of an otherwise atrophic background in the Pap test (Figures 7.38 and 7.39).

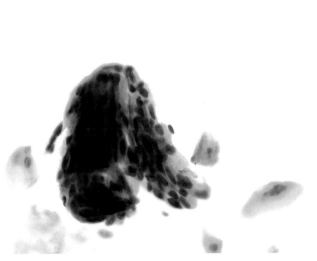

Figure 7.31. Atrophy. This fragment has a syncytial appearance as the borders between cells are difficult to identify. The nuclei are small and uniform in size but are dark and have mild nuclear border irregularities. However, the nuclei in this fragment are well organized, and some cells have a reassuring amount of cytoplasm (Pap stain).

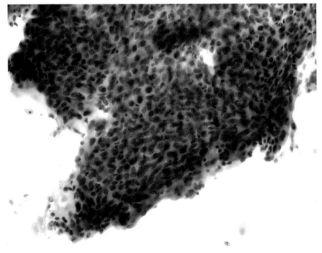

Figure 7.32. Atrophy. The numerous squamous cells in this large fragment have indistinct cellular borders, making assessment of the nuclear to cytoplasmic (N/C) ratio difficult. The cells have uniform, oval-shaped nuclei with regular nuclear contours. At the edges of the fragment, the nuclei contain bland chromatin and the cells lack hyperchromasia, in contrast to what would be seen in a high-grade squamous intraepithelial lesion (HSIL) (Pap stain).

Figure 7.33. Atrophy. These cells are loosely cohesive and have dense squamoid cytoplasm. The nuclei are somewhat dark but are uniform in size and have only mild nuclear contour irregularities; the nuclear to cytoplasmic (N/C) ratios are low. These features would not suggest a high-grade squamous intraepithelial lesion (HSIL) (Pap stain).

Figure 7.34. Atrophy. Separate field (Pap stain).

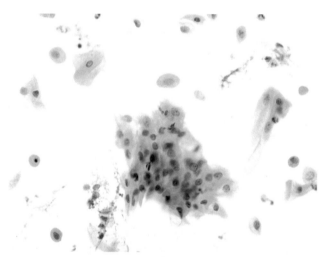

Figure 7.35. Atrophy. Separate field (Pap stain).

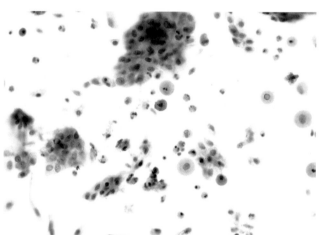

Figure 7.36. Atrophy. A single, small dyskeratotic cell can be seen in the center of the field. This cell and its pink cytoplasm, along with the presence of degenerated cells ("blue blobs") and granular material in the background, may cause initial concern for a keratinizing squamous cell carcinoma (Pap stain).

TUBAL METAPLASIA

Occasionally, endocervical cells undergo tubal metaplasia and adopt the characteristics of the glandular cells lining the fallopian tubes. Most notably, these cells are columnar and characteristically contain a terminal bar with cilia at the luminal end. As a response to injury, these cells become enlarged and crowded, which can simulate the palisading appearance typical of adenocarcinoma in situ (AIS). The nuclei, however, typically have fine, granular chromatin rather than the hyperchromasia of AIS. Fortunately, the presence of terminal bars and/or cilia is a reassuring finding and identifies the cells in question as benign (Figures 7.40 and 7.41).[2]

ADENOCARCINOMA IN SITU

Endocervical adenocarcinoma is less common than SqCC, and the vast majority of endocervical adenocarcinomas are associated with high-risk HPV infections.[17] Adenocarcinoma in situ (AIS) is the precursor lesion of invasive endocervical adenocarcinoma and is often seen with a concomitant dysplastic squamous lesion. Patients with AIS are often asymptomatic young

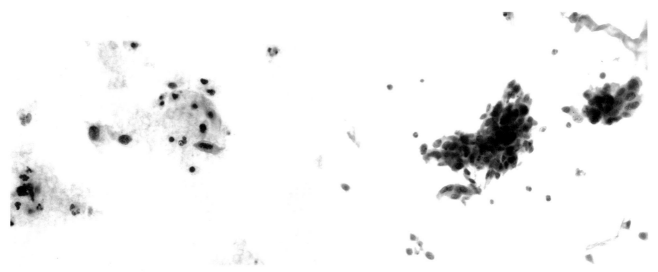

Figure 7.37. Keratinizing squamous cell carcinoma. Note the necrotic debris attached to viable tumor cells ("clinging diathesis") as well as present in the background. A single keratinizing cell with pink cytoplasm and an irregularly shaped, dark nucleus can be seen in the center of the field (Pap stain).

Figure 7.38. High-grade squamous intraepithelial lesion (HSIL). The lesional cells form hyperchromatic crowded groups. The cells have high nuclear to cytoplasmic ratios, which is concerning despite the small nuclear sizes. The chromatin has a powdery quality but is dark (Pap stain).

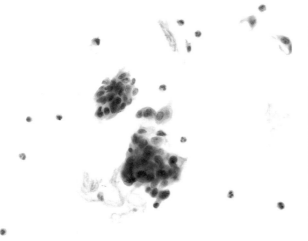

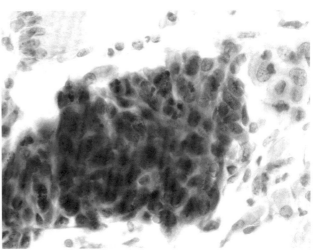

Figure 7.39. High-grade squamous intraepithelial lesion (HSIL) in a background of atrophy. The lesional cells are hyperchromatic and contain minimal cytoplasm. The nuclei also have irregular shapes (Pap stain).

Figure 7.40. Tubal metaplasia. This fragment contains crowded, dark cells with enlarged nuclei and high nuclear to cytoplasmic (N/C) ratios. However, at the fragment edges, the columnar nature of the cells can be seen along with terminal bars and cilia. Once tubal metaplasia is identified in a specimen, one must consider whether other hyperchromatic crowded groups in a the specimen simply represent tubal metaplasia lacking identifiable cilia versus a second cell type. HSIL is often in the differential diagnosis (Pap stain).

women, usually of reproductive age. The most common diagnosis on a Pap test of a woman with a subsequent diagnosis of AIS is *Atypical glandular cells* (AGCs). The Pap test is not the most sensitive test for the diagnosis of AIS and is only able to detect 38-50% of AIS cases.[18] The high false-negative rate is attributed to both difficulty in adequately sampling the endocervical canal and the challenges in recognizing the subtle cytomorphologic features of AIS.

AIS cells are columnar and have enlarged, hyperchromatic nuclei with altered polarity and pseudostratification. Inconspicuous nucleoli may be seen on some preparations, although typically the chromatin has a powdery or coarse appearance. The cells may be arranged in rosettes in some instances. Other important features include an increased N/C ratio, "feathering" (nuclei protruding from tissue fragment edges of HCGs), mitotic figures, and apoptosis (Figure 7.42-7.62). Although "feathering" is a classic diagnostic feature of

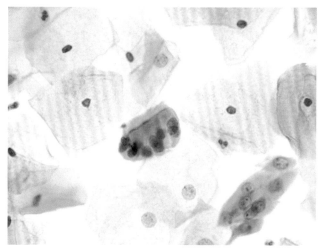

Figure 7.41. Tubal metaplasia. A strip of endocervical cells with basally oriented nuclei and ciliated terminal bars. Finding a field such as this can be reassuring if other fields contain metaplastic cells that appear more hyperchromatic and lack definitive cilia or terminal bars (Pap stain).

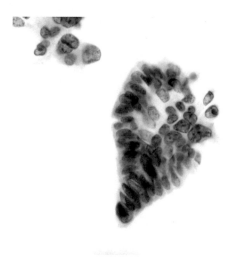

Figure 7.42. Adenocarcinoma in situ (AIS). The cells show nuclear enlargement and increased nuclear to cytoplasmic ratios. The chromatin is even but coarsely granular, giving a hyperchromatic appearance (Pap stain).

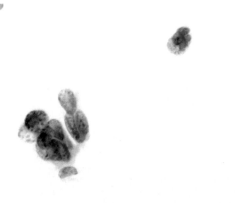

Figure 7.43. Adenocarcinoma in situ (AIS). The neoplastic cells in this small cluster have high nuclear to cytoplasmic ratios and overlapping nuclei. These cells show the classic cytomorphology for AIS, but benign endometrial cells are often in the differential. If only a small cluster of cells is seen, a diagnosis of *Atypical glandular cells* (AGC) may be appropriate (Pap stain).

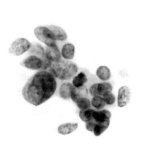

Figure 7.44. Adenocarcinoma in situ (AIS). Note the marked variation in size and nuclear overlap seen in these cells (Pap stain).

AIS, it is not always seen and can be overinterpreted in benign, reactive glandular cells. The identification of feathering should raise suspicion for AIS, but a definitive diagnosis requires additional features.[19]

KEY FEATURES of Adenocarcinoma In Situ

- Columnar cells can be present in sheets, strips, or rosette formations.
- Nuclei are often irregularly stratified between adjacent cells ("pseudostratified" appearance), crowded, and overlapping.
- Nuclei are enlarged and display hyperchromasia with powdery or coarse chromatin.
- Nuclei may project out ("feather") from fragment edges.
- The cells have round to oval nuclei and small/inconspicuous nucleoli.
- Mitoses and apoptosis may be seen

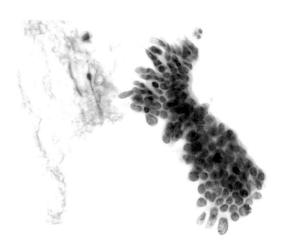

Figure 7.45. Adenocarcinoma in situ (AIS). While the cells appear well organized within the tissue fragment, the projection of elongated nuclei beyond the fragment edge (creating a ragged appearance i.e., "feathering") is a feature of AIS (Pap stain).

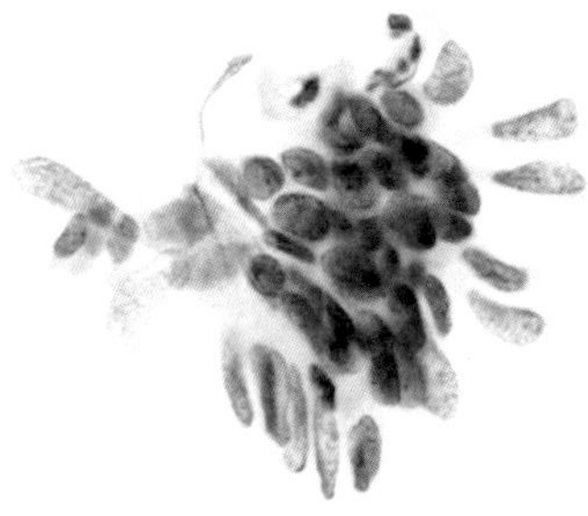

Figure 7.46. Adenocarcinoma in situ (AIS). This group of cells demonstrates the "feathering" morphology often seen in AIS (Pap stain).

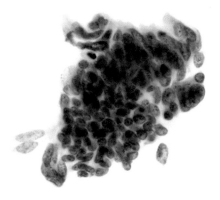

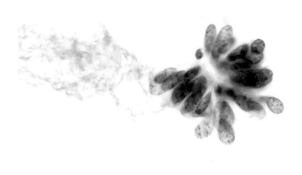

Figure 7.47. Adenocarcinoma in situ (AIS). The cells have powdery, dark chromatin, anisonucleosis, and irregular nuclear contours. The nuclei palisade in some areas and are disorganized in other areas within the fragment (Pap stain).

Figure 7.48. Adenocarcinoma in situ (AIS). Separate field containing the distinctive "feathering" morphology (Pap stain).

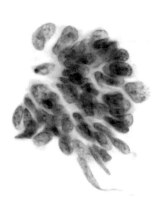

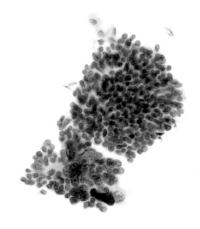

Figure 7.49. Adenocarcinoma in situ (AIS). The cells are disorganized and have nuclear contour irregularities and anisonucleosis (Pap stain).

Figure 7.50. Adenocarcinoma in situ (AIS). Compare this fragment with the organized honeycomb pattern found in reactive endocervical cells. Here, the organized honeycomb arrangement is disrupted and nuclei project out from the fragment edges (Pap stain).

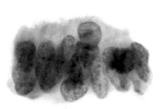

Figure 7.51. Adenocarcinoma in situ (AIS). These columnar cells have elongated nuclei. Unlike what is seen in benign endocervical cells, the nuclei are located at different levels within the cytoplasm and appear pseudostratified (Pap stain).

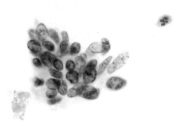

Figure 7.52. Adenocarcinoma in situ (AIS). Separate field (Pap stain).

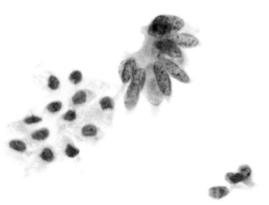

Figure 7.53. Adenocarcinoma in situ (AIS). Several AIS cells (upper right) are seen adjacent to a small cluster of benign endocervical cells (lower left). Note how the AIS cells have enlarged nuclei, high nuclear to cytoplasmic (N/C) ratios, and a distinctive chromatin pattern (Pap stain).

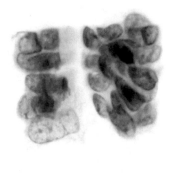

Figure 7.54. Adenocarcinoma in situ (AIS). Note the irregular stratification of the nuclei within columnar cytoplasm (Pap stain).

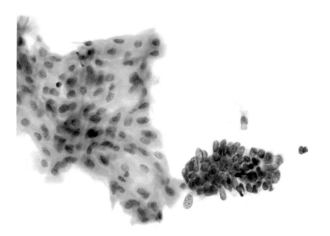

Figure 7.55. Adenocarcinoma in situ (AIS). A fragment of AIS (lower right) can be seen adjacent to benign squamous epithelial cells (left). The AIS nuclei are only slightly larger but are more pleomorphic, contain scant cytoplasm, and have darker chromatin (Pap stain).

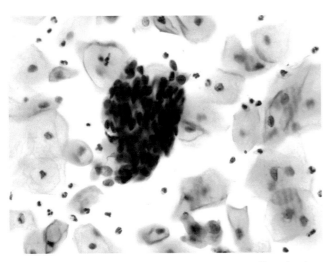

Figure 7.56. Adenocarcinoma in situ (AIS). AIS cells with elongated nuclei form a hyperchromatic crowded group that shares significant cytomorphologic overlap with a high-grade squamous intraepithelial lesion (HSIL). As a result, patients with a diagnosis of HSIL on the Pap test are occasionally found to have AIS on follow-up biopsy (Pap stain).

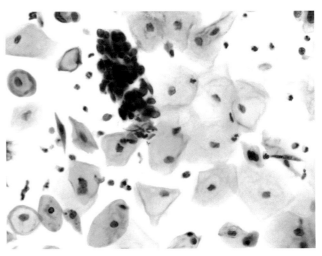

Figure 7.57. Adenocarcinoma in situ (AIS). Separate field (Pap stain).

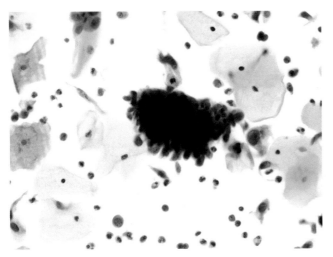

Figure 7.58. Adenocarcinoma in situ (AIS). This group is hyperchromatic and crowded to a level where the cytomorphology is difficult to assess. Note the feathering at the periphery of the cluster (Pap stain).

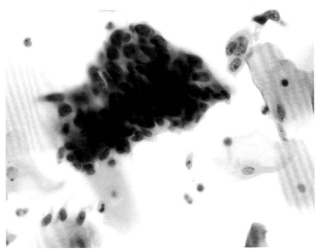

Figure 7.59. Adenocarcinoma in situ (AIS). Note the columnar cytoplasm at the periphery of the cluster (Pap stain).

ENDOCERVICAL ADENOCARCINOMA

Despite of the success of the Pap test in decreasing the incidence of SqCCs, the incidence of cervical adenocarcinoma has not decreased and, for unknown reasons, may be increasing in the United States.[17,20] There are several subtypes of endocervical adenocarcinoma, the most common of which is the usual type that is HPV driven. Rarer subtypes of endocervical adenocarcinoma, such as mucinous adenocarcinoma, gastric-type adenocarcinoma (also known as "minimal deviation adenocarcinoma" or "adenoma malignum"), and endometrioid carcinoma of the cervix, are HPV negative.[21,22]

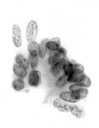

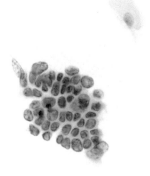

Figure 7.60. Adenocarcinoma in situ (AIS). Separate field (Pap stain).

Figure 7.61. Adenocarcinoma in situ (AIS). Note the marked variation in nuclear size (Pap stain).

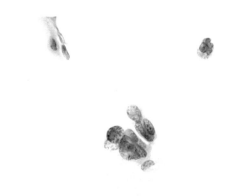

Figure 7.62. Adenocarcinoma in situ (AIS). These rare AIS cells demonstrate palisading and feathering. Note the powdery appearance to the chromatin, which contains small coarse granules as well as smaller speckles (Pap stain).

Endocervical adenocarcinoma and AIS have some overlapping cytomorphologic features, especially in the case of a well-differentiated adenocarcinoma (Figures 7.63-7.66). Adenocarcinoma may form three-dimensional structures that are not seen in AIS. AIS cells are typically uniform in size, with nuclei that are significantly less pleomorphic than those seen in adenocarcinoma. Adenocarcinoma often have greater variation in nuclear size, irregularly coarse chromatin (or sometimes chromatin clearing), and marked nuclear contour irregularities. Prominent nucleoli may be seen in adenocarcinoma and are not a feature of AIS. Features of invasive adenocarcinoma include the presence of necrosis (which may be seen as "clinging diathesis" on liquid-based preparations) and an increased number of scattered single atypical cells.[2,6,23] These features are suggestive of invasive adenocarcinoma rather than AIS, but the distinction can be difficult and an excisional procedure may be necessary for a definitive diagnosis.

Figure 7.63. Endocervical adenocarcinoma. This cluster of cells is hyperchromatic with marked nuclear size variation and nuclear crowding; the three-dimensional nature of the cells suggests carcinoma rather than AIS or high-grade squamous intraepithelial lesion (HSIL). The chromatin is coarse and unevenly distributed. The patient's surgical pathology follow-up showed invasive endocervical adenocarcinoma (Pap stain).

Figure 7.64. Endocervical adenocarcinoma. Note the marked overlapping of the cells and background of fibrinous material, which also clings to some of the cells ("clinging diathesis"). Compared with adenocarcinoma in situ (AIS), nuclei are larger and have marked nuclear contour irregularities and coarser chromatin. The patient's surgical pathology follow-up showed invasive endocervical adenocarcinoma (Pap stain).

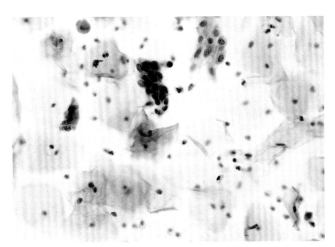

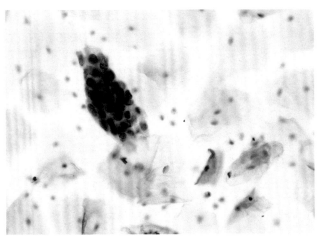

Figure 7.65. Endocervical adenocarcinoma. The cells are forming a hyperchromatic crowded group. Note that at the periphery the cells have a wispy cytoplasm characteristic of endocervical origin. Although patient's surgical pathology follow-up showed invasive endocervical adenocarcinoma, it would be appropriate to render a diagnosis of *Atypical glandular cells* (AGCs), as the atypia is not as dramatic as seen in the previous figures (Pap stain).

Figure 7.66. Endocervical adenocarcinoma. The cells have dark chromatin and irregular nuclear membranes. At the edges of the fragments, cytoplasm can be seen, indicating glandular differentiation. While the fragment is concerning for an adenocarcinoma, a diagnosis of *Atypical glandular cells* (AGCs) may be most appropriate (Pap stain).

KEY FEATURES of Endocervical Adenocarcinoma

- Abnormal cells are often present in three-dimensional structures and/or singly dispersed.
- Nuclei are crowded, overlapping, enlarged, and hyperchromatic with coarse chromatin and prominent nucleoli.
- Nuclear pleomorphism and nuclear membrane irregularities increase with grading.
- Clinging diathesis is indicative of invasion and is characterized by necrotic debris attached to the periphery of a group of malignant cells.

ENDOMETRIAL ADENOCARCINOMA

Endometrial adenocarcinoma is the most common malignancy of the gynecologic tract. Endometrial cancer predominantly affects postmenopausal women in their sixth decade. The most common clinical presentation is postmenopausal vaginal bleeding.[21,24] While endometrial cancers can be detected on the cervical Pap test, sensitivity is poor, and the Pap test is not considered a screening test for endometrial adenocarcinoma. The presence of endometrial carcinoma on a Pap test is associated with more advanced disease.[21,25]

There are several subtypes of endometrial adenocarcinoma. The most common subtype is endometrioid adenocarcinoma, which has been associated with hyperestrogenism.[21,24] The cytomorphologic features of endometrial adenocarcinoma depend on the adenocarcinoma type as well as the carcinoma's degree of differentiation (Figures 7.67-7.71). Most commonly, carcinoma appears as tight groups of haphazardly arranged, hyperchromatic cells with pleomorphic nuclei. The cells contain variable amounts of cytoplasm, and scattered large cytoplasmic vacuoles are frequently seen. The presence of nucleoli is variable and ranges from inconspicuous to prominent, with prominent nucleoli generally associated with higher grade neoplasms. Intracytoplasmic aggregates of neutrophils are commonly present ("bag of polys").[6,26–29] In the case of a poorly differentiated carcinoma, the differential diagnosis includes endocervical adenocarcinoma and nonkeratinizing SqCC. While endometrial carcinomas are HPV negative, HPV testing may be positive due to the presence of a separate HPV-related lesion in the cervix; furthermore, HPV may not be detected in some squamous cell and endocervical carcinomas. Given the abundant opportunities for misdiagnosis, HPV status should not be used to determine the origin of a poorly differentiated carcinoma on a Pap test specimen.

KEY FEATURES of Endometrial Adenocarcinoma

- Necrotic granular debris may be present in the background, indicating an invasive process, also known as diathesis.
- The malignant cells may form three-dimensional clusters.
- Vacuolated cytoplasm may be scant or abundant.
- Nuclei are enlarged and hyperchromatic with coarse chromatin; nuclear pleomorphism increases with nuclear grade.
- Cytoplasmic neutrophils may be indicative of an endometrial origin.

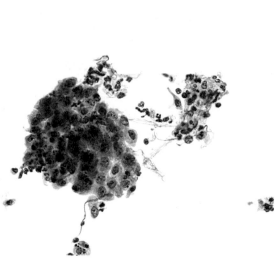

Figure 7.67. Endometrial adenocarcinoma. This fragment is three-dimensional and contains cells with enlarged nuclei, coarse chromatin, highly irregular nuclear contours, and high nuclear to cytoplasmic (N/C) ratios—all features of carcinoma. Some cells have a columnar shape and foamy cytoplasm, indicating a glandular origin. The presence of neutrophils within the fragment suggests but does not confirm an endometrial origin (Pap stain).

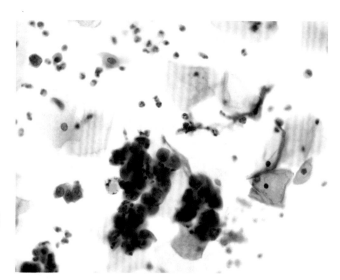

Figure 7.68. Endometrial adenocarcinoma. This loosely cohesive cluster contains cells with large, irregular-shaped nuclei with coarse chromatin. Note the presence of intracytoplasmic neutrophils, which is characteristic of endometrial origin (Pap stain).

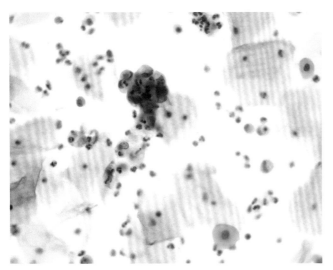

Figure 7.69. Endometrial adenocarcinoma. Separate field. Note the subtle clinging necrosis at the periphery of the cluster, associated with neutrophils. Reactive endometrial cells arising from endometrial polyps and other benign processes can also appear quite atypical; in equivocal cases. As a result, it may be appropriate to render a diagnosis of *Atypical glandular cells* (AGCs) (Pap stain).

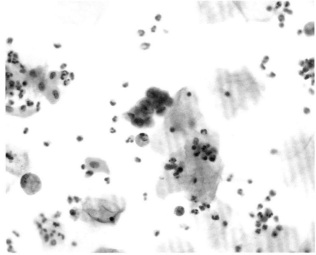

Figure 7.70. Endometrial adenocarcinoma. A small cluster of neoplastic endometrial cells with prominent nucleoli and intracytoplasmic neutrophils are seen in the center of this field (Pap stain).

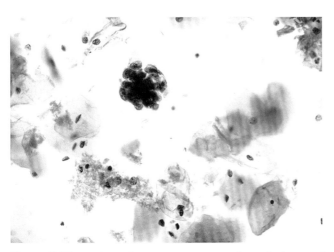

Figure 7.71. High-grade serous carcinoma. A small cluster of malignant cells surround a psammoma body. The presence of psammoma bodies raises the possibility of a serous neoplasm. The patient's surgical pathology follow-up showed a high-grade serous carcinoma of the ovary (Pap stain).

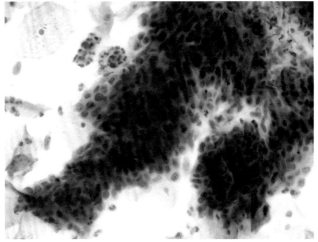

Figure 7.72. High-grade squamous intraepithelial lesion (HSIL). The cells have high nuclear to cytoplasmic (N/C) ratios, anisonucleosis, and nuclear membrane irregularities. The cytoplasm is dense, favoring a squamous rather than glandular origin (Pap stain).

HIGH-GRADE SQUAMOUS INTRAEPITHELIAL LESION

High-grade squamous intraepithelial lesions (HSILs) contain cells in which high-risk HPV (hrHPV) has become integrated within the genome. High-risk HPV types are detected in >90% of patients with HSIL using conventional methods. This rate increases to >95% when multiple methods of detection are used.[30] Consequently, it is likely that essentially all HSIL are caused by HPV infection. While in some women HSIL may clear without treatment, HSIL is considered a precursor lesion of SqCC.[21] HSIL is asymptomatic; usually the lesion is detected during routine cytology screening with the Pap test or colposcopy.

HSIL has many different morphologic appearances, which contribute to false-negative and false-positive Pap test diagnoses. In many instances, three-dimensional fragments of HSIL form HCGs (Figures 7.38-7.39 and 7.72-7.74). Examination of three-dimensional, crowded clusters is challenging as the cells of interest shield one another from examination. Cells within a fragment have high N/C ratios and marked nuclear membrane irregularities

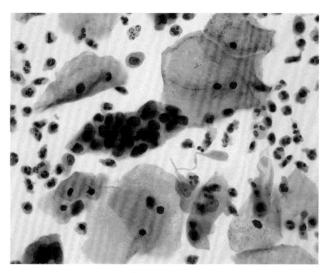

Figure 7.73. High-grade squamous intraepithelial lesion (HSIL). The cells are hyperchromatic with high nuclear to cytoplasmic (N/C) ratios and marked nuclear border irregularities. The nuclei are also disorganized within the tissue fragment, a finding not seen in benign squamous metaplasia or reparative changes (Pap stain).

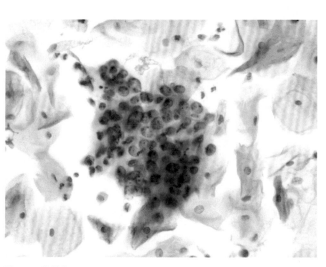

Figure 7.74. High-grade squamous intraepithelial lesion (HSIL). The chromatin in these cells is irregularly distributed. The nuclei are enlarged and overlapping with great variation in size (Pap stain).

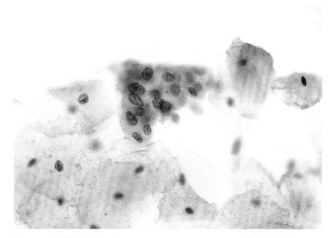

Figure 7.75. High-grade squamous intraepithelial lesion (HSIL). The cells have highly irregular nuclear contours, which is further evidenced by the presence of nuclear grooves (Pap stain).

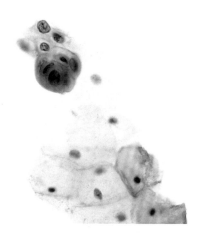

Figure 7.76. High-grade squamous intraepithelial lesion (HSIL). These atypical squamous cells in this cluster demonstrate high nuclear to cytoplasmic (N/C) ratios, irregular nuclear membranes, and irregularly distributed chromatin (Pap stain).

coupled with a disorderly arrangement (Figures 7.75-7.80). If HSIL cannot be excluded after examining HCGs, one should carefully examine the entire specimen for singly dispersed HSIL cells (See the "Dispersed Atypical Pattern") or smaller fragments in which the cytomorphology can be better assessed. Careful examination increases the likelihood of determining the nature of HCGs, whether it is dysplastic or a benign mimicker. If uncertainty continues to exist despite thorough examination, a diagnosis of ASC-H may be most appropriate.

KEY FEATURES of High-Grade Squamous Intraepithelial Lesion

- The lesional ells have scant cytoplasm and high N/C ratios.
- Nuclei are hyperchromatic an contain coarse chromatin with variable nuclear size and shape.
- Nuclear membranes are irregularities with prominent indentations.
- Cells can be distributed singly, form sheets, or syncytial aggregates.

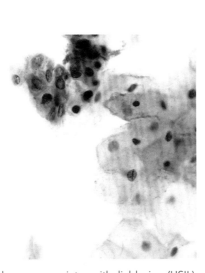

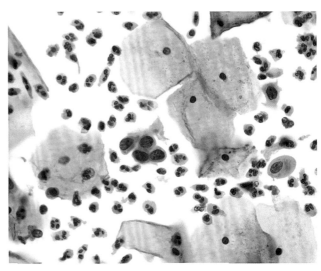

Figure 7.77. High-grade squamous intraepithelial lesion (HSIL). A cluster of atypical squamous cells with high nuclear to cytoplasmic (N/C) ratios, markedly irregular nuclear membranes, and coarse chromatin is seen adjacent to benign squamous cells (Pap stain).

Figure 7.78. Atypical squamous cells, cannot exclude high-grade squamous intraepithelial lesion (ASC-H). These atypical squamous cells have high nuclear to cytoplasmic (N/C) ratios, hyperchromasia, and nuclear membrane irregularities. The cells have dense cytoplasm and a small gap can be seen where the cells meet, suggesting that these cells may be atypical metaplastic cells. Although patient's surgical pathology follow-up showed high-grade squamous intraepithelial lesion (HSIL), a diagnosis of ASC-H would not be inappropriate (Pap stain).

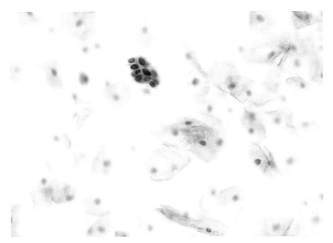

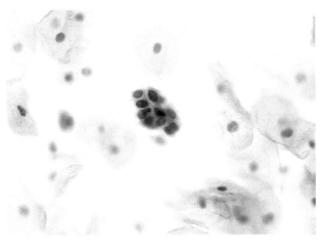

Figure 7.79. Atypical squamous cells, cannot exclude high-grade squamous intraepithelial lesion (ASC-H). A small cluster of hyperchromatic cells with high nuclear to cytoplasmic (N/C) ratios and irregular nuclear membranes is seen. If this is the only finding on a Pap test, a diagnosis of ASC-H may be most appropriate (Pap stain).

Figure 7.80. Atypical squamous cells, cannot exclude a high-grade squamous intraepithelial lesion (ASC-H). Previous field at higher magnification (Pap stain).

NONKERATINIZING SQUAMOUS CELL CARCINOMA

Cervical cancer remains one of the main causes of death in women worldwide. Cervical cancer disproportionally affects women who do not have access to adequate screening programs and/or follow-up.[31] HPV infection is implicated in 95% of cervical SqCC cases, and HPV types 16 and 18 are the most common subtypes identified. Persistent high-risk HPV infection is the main risk factor for cervical cancer.[32] Factors which predispose a patient to persistent HPV infection include immunodeficiency states (such as infection with human immunodeficiency virus, HIV), a history of smoking, multiparity, long-term oral contraceptive use, chronic pelvic inflammation, and concurrent sexually transmitted diseases.[21]

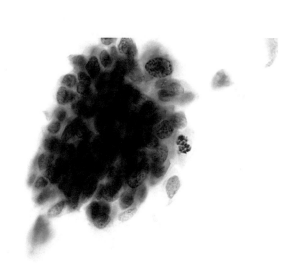

Figure 7.81. Squamous cell carcinoma (SqCC). As is typically seen in carcinoma, the cells form a three-dimensional tissue fragment. The cells are hyperchromatic and have coarse chromatin, anisonucleosis, and irregular nuclear borders. The cytoplasm is polygonal and dense, favoring a squamous rather than glandular differentiation (Pap stain).

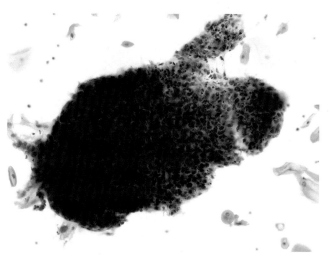

Figure 7.82. Squamous cell carcinoma (SqCC). This large fragment contains malignant cells with high N/C ratios, irregular nuclear borders, and anisonucleosis. Granular debris and neutrophils are present along some edges, suggesting the presence of necrosis. The amount of atypia is beyond what is seen in most high-grade squamous intraepithelial lesions (Pap stain).

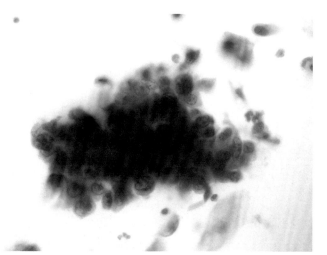

Figure 7.83. Squamous cell carcinoma (SqCC). This small fragment contains cells with enlarged nuclei. The nuclei are different shapes and sizes and have coarse chromatin. The fragment is also three-dimensional, a characteristic more commonly seen in carcinomas as compared to high-grade squamous intraepithelial lesions (Pap stain).

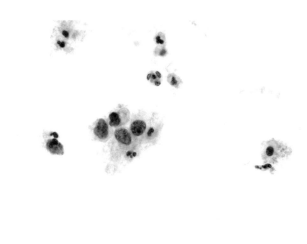

Figure 7.84. Squamous cell carcinoma (SqCC). Rare atypical cells with hyperchromasia, convoluted nuclear membranes, and coarse chromatin. The presence of clinging diathesis suggests these cells likely represent a lesion more aggressive than a high-grade squamous intraepithelial lesion (HSIL) (Pap stain).

SqCC can have keratinizing and nonkeratinizing forms.[6] TBS does not require SqCC to be further subtyped into keratinizing and nonkeratinizing forms, although this descriptive information may be useful when reviewing future specimens. Keratinizing SqCC does not fall under the differential of the HCG Pattern and is detailed further below (See the "Keratinizing Pattern"). Nonkeratinizing SqCC can form syncytial aggregates and HCGs (Figures 7.81-7.85). The chromatin pattern is one key distinguishing feature between SqCC and HSIL. SqCCs often contain irregularly distributed chromatin that forms a coarse and/or clumpy pattern. The presence of tumor diathesis in the background (which may be present primarily as "clinging diathesis" in liquid-based preparations) is also helpful in favoring SqCC over HSIL.[2,6,33] In cases when HSIL is undoubtedly present but some additional worrisome features suggest an undersampled SqCC, a diagnosis of HSIL can be provided with a note indicating that an invasive process cannot be excluded.

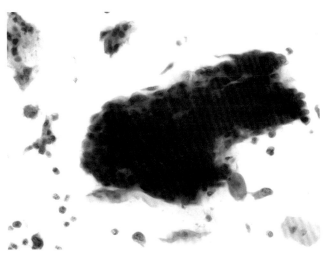

Figure 7.85. Squamous cell carcinoma (SqCC). The cells in this fragment have very dark nuclei and form a three-dimensional structure. The cells also have high N/C ratios, irregular nuclear contours, and anisonucleosis. The high level of atypia seen in this fragment, combined with the three-dimensional structure formed by these cells, favor a squamous cell carcinoma over a high-grade squamous intraepithelial lesion (Pap stain).

KEY FEATURES of Nonkeratinizing Squamous Cell Carcinoma

- Hyperchromatic crowded groups contain malignant cells with prominent nucleoli and/or unevenly distributed, coarse chromatin.
- The malignant cells are pleomorphic and have dense, squamous cytoplasm and/or high N/C ratios (basaloid appearance).
- Tumor diathesis (necrotic debris) may be present as "clinging diathesis" in liquid-based preparations (necrotic debris adherent to cells).
- HCG contain cells with prominent nucleoli and/or irregular chromatin distribution.

SAMPLE NOTE: HIGH-GRADE SQUAMOUS INTRAEPITHELIAL LESION, CANNOT EXCLUDE SQUAMOUS CELL CARCINOMA

Adequacy: The specimen is satisfactory for evaluation. The transformation zone component is present.

Interpretation: High-grade squamous intraepithelial lesion (HSIL). See note.

Note: An invasive process cannot be entirely excluded.

GLANDULAR PATTERN

While the Pap test focuses primarily on the detection of squamous lesions, glandular cells are often present in Pap test specimens and may represent benign background cells as well as clinically important lesions. Therefore, the glandular component of a Pap test cannot be ignored and should be assessed as carefully as the squamous component. The presence or absence of glandular cells, specifically endocervical cells, is reported as a quality indicator in Pap test specimens, although the presence of glandular cells is not required for specimen adequacy. In some instances, cells with squamous differentiation may have a glandular appearance, and this should be kept in mind when developing a differential diagnosis for atypical-appearing glandular cells.

CHECKLIST: Etiologic Considerations for the Glandular Pattern

☐ Reactive Endocervical Cells

☐ Intrauterine Device (IUD) Changes

☐ Glandular Cells Status Post Hysterectomy

☐ Atypical Glandular Cells

☐ Atypical Endocervical Cells

☐ Atypical Endocervical Cells, Favor Neoplastic

☐ Atypical Endometrial Cells

☐ Adenocarcinoma In Situ (AIS)

☐ Endocervical And Endometrial Adenocarcinoma

☐ High-Grade Squamous Intraepithelial Lesion (HSIL)

☐ Metastatic Adenocarcinoma

☐ Colorectal Adenocarcinoma

REACTIVE ENDOCERVICAL CELLS

The presence of reactive endocervical cells is a nonspecific finding. Endocervical cells may demonstrate marked reactive changes, resulting in strikingly enlarged nuclei. On occasion, reactive endocervical cells may even become multinucleated (described below under the "Multinucleated Pattern"). In contrast to AIS and adenocarcinoma, reactive endocervical cells are more regularly organized within tissue fragments with retained polarity, maintain ample cytoplasm and a low N/C ratio, and retain round nuclei with regular contours. Reactive nuclei may display marginated chromatin and/or a distinctive nucleolus—findings that are not seen in AIS (which has powdery or coarse chromatin) (Figures 7.23-7.28).

INTRAUTERINE DEVICE (IUD) CHANGES

Both endometrial and/or endocervical cells demonstrate reactive changes in women with an intrauterine device (IUD). The altered cells have cytoplasm containing large vacuoles, which gives a signet ring–like appearance to the cells. The cells may be present singly or arranged in small clusters (5-15 cells) (Figures 7.86 and 7.87).[34,35] IUD-related changes are not limited to the glandular cells and may be seen in the squamous component as well. The alterations in the squamous epithelium may also be related to the inflammation and *Actinomyces* that sometimes accompanies an IUD.

GLANDULAR CELLS STATUS POST HYSTERECTOMY

A cervical Pap test from a woman with a history of a total hysterectomy may occasionally contain bland glandular cells resembling endocervical cells. This finding should not cause one to suspect a specimen mix-up or the presence of a glandular neoplasm. While the origin of these cells is unknown, it has been speculated that they may arise from vulvar glands or represent metaplastic changes.[36] These cells should not be reported as endocervical cells and do not indicate the presence of transformation zone sampling.

ATYPICAL GLANDULAR CELLS

The Pap test was developed primarily as a screening test for squamous intraepithelial lesions. Despite the increased sensitivity of liquid-based cytology in detecting glandular

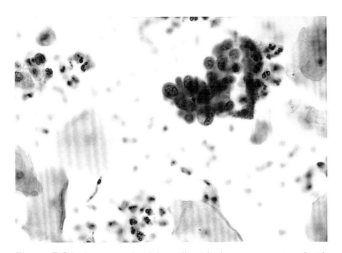

Figure 7.86. Reactive glandular cells with changes associated with intrauterine device (IUD) use. Some of the glandular cells in this cluster have enlarged, hyperchromatic nuclei and cytoplasmic vacuolization. If the patient does not have history of IUD, consideration should be given to a diagnosis of *Atypical glandular cells* (AGCs) (Pap stain).

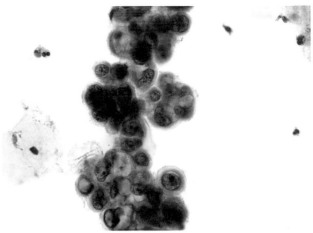

Figure 7.87. Reactive glandular cells with changes associated with intrauterine device (IUD) use. This unusually large cluster of endometrial cells contains cells with nuclear enlargement, prominent nucleoli, and cytoplasmic vacuoles. Owing to the cellularity of the cluster, the specimen was interpreted as *Atypical glandular cells* (AGCs). However, the patient was only found to have benign findings on follow-up (Pap stain).

lesions,[29,37] the overall sensitivity for the detection of glandular atypia remains modest.[18,25] TBS recommends subclassification of AGC whenever possible into one of the following categories:

- Atypical endocervical cells;
- Atypical endometrial cells;
- AGC, not otherwise specified (NOS);
- AGC, favor neoplastic; and
- Atypical endocervical cells, favor neoplastic.[6]

Practically speaking, the AGC category is used to describe cells with glandular differentiation containing atypia that falls short of AIS and adenocarcinoma but in which a glandular lesion cannot be excluded. The most common follow-up result in a premenopausal woman with AGC is HSIL. There are several reasons for this, including the existence of HSIL with glandular morphology, the increased prevalence of HSIL as compared with AIS and adenocarcinoma, and because HSIL is more likely to be sampled during subsequent workup.[38–42] The coexistence of both a squamous intraepithelial lesion and AGC on a Pap test specimen has been associated with the presence of a squamous, not glandular, lesion on follow-up colposcopy.[38–42]

In instances in which the cells are not distinctive of either an endocervical or endometrial cell origin, a diagnosis of "AGC, NOS" or "AGC, favor neoplastic" can be made. The "favor neoplastic" categories are used sparingly, as they will often result in a surgical excision without an intervening positive colposcopy result (Table 7.2). An "atypical endometrial cells, favor neoplastic" category does not exist due to the low predictive value of atypical endometrial cells on Pap test for endometrial neoplasia.

ATYPICAL ENDOCERVICAL CELLS

Atypical endocervical cells are defined by TBS as endocervical-type cells with nuclear abnormalities that exceed the nuclear alterations seen in reactive or reparative changes but do not show unequivocal features of adenocarcinoma.[6] The cells form either a honeycomb or picket fence arrangement with mild nuclear overlapping, crowding and pseudostratification. Nuclei are enlarged with mild variation in nuclear size and shape as well as mild hyperchromasia and chromatin irregularity (Figure 7.88).

TABLE 7.2: American Society for Colposcopy and Cervical Pathology (ASCCP) 2012 Consensus Guidelines for the Management of Atypical Glandular Cells (AGC) categories

Diagnosis	Initial Management	Diagnostic Excisional Procedure If No Disease Found on Colposcopy?
Atypical endocervical cells	Colposcopy with endocervical sampling Endometrial sampling (at risk patients[a])	No
Atypical endometrial cells	Colposcopy with endocervical sampling Endometrial sampling (all patients)	No
Atypical glandular cells (AGC), not otherwise specified (NOS)	Colposcopy with endocervical sampling Endometrial sampling (at risk patients[a])	No
AGC, favor neoplastic	Colposcopy with endocervical sampling Endometrial sampling (at risk patients[a])	Yes
Atypical endocervical cells, favor neoplastic	Colposcopy with endocervical sampling Endometrial sampling (at risk patients[a])	Yes

[a]At-risk patients are those above the age of 35 years or with other risk factors for endometrial neoplasia.

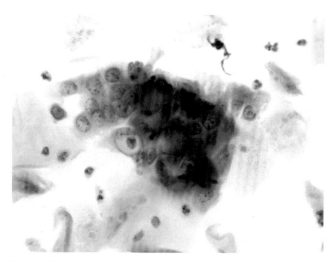

Figure 7.88. Reactive endocervical cells. The cells have uniform nuclei and ample, foamy cytoplasm. The edge of the fragment contains columnar cells with basally located nuclei, indicating that these are likely benign endocervical cells. Some cells have cytoplasmic vacuoles, a feature that can be seen in reactive endocervical cells as well as endometrial cells. In this case, the square and columnar cell shapes are not compatible with an endometrial origin (Pap stain).

ATYPICAL ENDOCERVICAL CELLS, FAVOR NEOPLASTIC

"Atypical endocervical cells, favor neoplastic" is a diagnostic phrase defined by TBS as cells with "morphology, either quantitatively or qualitatively, that falls just short of an interpretation of endocervical adenocarcinoma in situ or invasive adenocarcinoma."[6] The patient's surgical pathology follow-up usually shows a more significant lesion than patients with a diagnosis of atypical endocervical cells.[43] Importantly, according to the ASCCP guidelines, the clinical management of the "favor neoplastic" category differs greatly from that of other AGC categories. Patients with a diagnosis of AGC, favor neoplastic may receive definitive surgical treatment without an intervening positive biopsy (Table 7.2).

ATYPICAL ENDOMETRIAL CELLS

According to TBS, the distinction between benign endometrial cells and atypical endometrial cells is based primarily on increased nuclear size but a specific size criterion is not defined (Figures 7.89-7.92).[6] The diagnosis of atypical endometrial cells on a Pap test specimen is frequently associated with benign conditions such as IUD changes, endometritis, or endometrial polyps. However, the diagnosis of AGC may also indicate the presence of endometrial hyperplasia or adenocarcinoma and thus requires further clinical evaluation.[42,44]

FAQ: Does this atypical HCG represent HSIL or AIS?

Answer: Given the glandular appearance of some HSIL cells, it can be challenging to completely exclude the possibility of AIS in some specimens. While HSIL is the likely outcome in such a scenario, a diagnosis of atypical endocervical cells results in a more complete work up of the patient, requiring both colposcopy with endocervical sampling as well as endometrial sampling in some patients (Table 7.2). If HSIL is felt to be present and AIS cannot be excluded, two diagnoses can be rendered at once. Because both lesions are caused by high-risk HPV infection, they may be seen concomitantly.

SAMPLE NOTE: ATYPICAL HYPERCHROMATIC GROUPS WITH GLANDULAR FEATURES

Adequacy: The specimen is satisfactory for evaluation. The transformation zone component is present.

Interpretation: High-grade squamous epithelial lesion (HSIL). Atypical endocervical cells. See note.

Note: The presence of atypical, hyperchromatic cells with glandular morphology suggest the possibility of HSIL with glandular involvement. However, a concomitant glandular lesion, such as AIS, cannot be excluded.

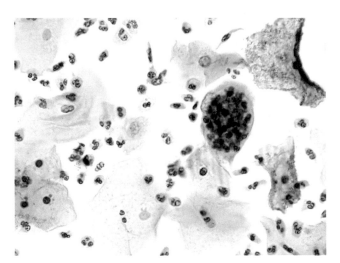

Figure 7.89. Atypical endometrial cell. An atypical endometrial cell is seen with abundant cytoplasm that is filled with neutrophils ("bag of polys"). The presence of cytoplasmic neutrophils suggests an endometrial origin but does not definitively indicate malignancy or neoplasia. However, a large number of neutrophils are more concerning (Pap stain).

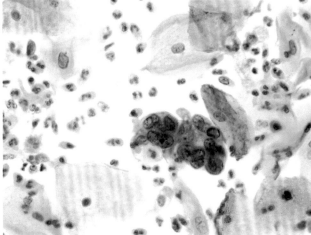

Figure 7.90. Atypical endometrial cells. Endometrial cells with hyperchromasia, coarse chromatin, enlarged nuclei, anisonucleosis, and irregular nuclear borders. The nuclear to cytoplasmic (N/C) ratios are enlarged. One cell has a large cytoplasmic vacuole containing a neutrophil, strongly suggesting an endometrial origin (Pap stain).

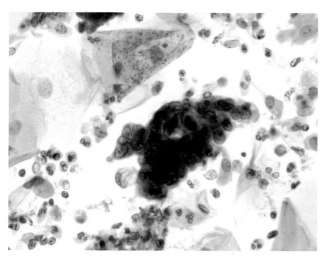

Figure 7.91. Atypical endometrial cells. This group of endometrial cells contains crowded, dark nuclei with irregular borders. The cells are not overtly malignant and could represent benign endometrial cells, perhaps arising from an endometrial polyp. If features are concerning but not diagnostic of a neoplasm, a diagnosis of *Atypical glandular cells* is often appropriate (Pap stain).

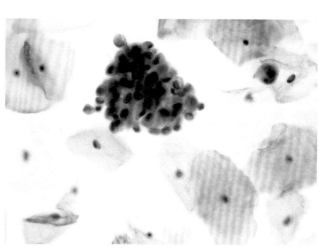

Figure 7.92. Atypical endometrial cells. Hyperchromatic endometrial cells with pleomorphic nuclei. The nuclear contours are irregular, and nucleoli can be seen. To be diagnostic of adenocarcinoma, the group would need to be more three-dimensional and contain cells with larger nuclei and greater nuclear size variation (Pap stain).

ADENOCARCINOMA IN SITU

While adenocarcinoma in situ (AIS) often falls under the differential of HCG and is more fully described in the "Hyperchromatic Crowded Group Pattern", the elongated nuclei and columnar shape of AIS cells are often recognized as glandular cells. AIS cells may form glandular arrangements such as pseudorosettes and are typically more monotonous appearing than adenocarcinoma cells, regardless of adenocarcinoma cell origin (endocervical or endometrial). When compared with reactive endocervical cells, AIS cells have darker nuclei and powdery or coarser chromatin. AIS cells have higher N/C ratios than benign, reactive endocervical cells. The nuclei in AIS have altered polarity and nuclei that project away from tissue fragment edges ("feathering"), whereas benign, reactive endocervical cells have basally located nuclei encased by rectangular cytoplasm. In contrast to HSIL with its streaming or haphazard nuclei, AIS often contains areas of palisaded nuclei.

ENDOCERVICAL AND ENDOMETRIAL ADENOCARCINOMA

Poorly differentiated adenocarcinomas lack cytomorphologic clues that elucidate their origin. In endometrial and endocervical adenocarcinomas, the background may contain necrotic debris, which may only be seen as "clinging diathesis" in liquid-based preparations and contrasts from the "clean background" seen in metastatic adenocarcinomas, such as from the ovary. Without helpful morphologic clues, ancillary studies and/or clinicoradiologic correlation may be required to determine the primary site. Poorly differentiated adenocarcinomas exhibit many, if not all, of the following features: large cell size, large nuclear size, anisonucleosis, high N/C ratio, irregular nuclear contours, coarse chromatin (with or without prominent nucleoli), hyperchromasia, and a three-dimensional growth pattern. In such instances, a poorly differentiated SqCC may also enter into the differential diagnosis.

In contrast, well and moderately differentiated adenocarcinomas may exhibit features of either endometrial or endocervical origin, and this information should be conferred to the clinical team. Endometrial adenocarcinomas are classically associated with intracytoplasmic neutrophils, cytoplasmic vacuolization, and cellular clusters with hobnailed borders. Adenocarcinoma cells with a more columnar appearance are more suggestive of endocervical origin. The cytomorphologic features of these two entities are covered in more detail under the "Hyperchromatic Crowded Group Pattern."

HIGH-GRADE SQUAMOUS INTRAEPITHELIAL LESION

High-grade squamous intraepithelial lesion (HSIL) is cytomorphologically diverse and can have a glandular appearance; some experts have postulated that HSIL involving endocervical glands may have a more glandular appearance on the Pap test (Figures 7.93 and 7.94). Regardless of what causes this appearance, HSIL may emulate glandular lesions when it presents as HCGs with predominantly oval to spindle shaped nuclei with ragged "tufts" at the edges. This pattern of HSIL has cells with small nuclei but high N/C ratios, and the differential diagnosis is often AIS. Adenocarcinoma, in which cells often have larger nuclei with more prominent anisonucleosis, is typically less favored in this setting. As previously discussed, glandular-appearing HSIL may be diagnosed as AGC, and most AGC diagnoses are associated with a follow-up diagnosis of HSIL on tissue biopsy. Notably, the presence of HSIL in a specimen increases the risk of concomitant AIS due to the patient's exposure to persistent high-risk HPV infection. Once a diagnosis of HSIL has been established, all suspicious HCGs should be examined closely to exclude concomitant AIS. If AGCs are present concurrently with HSIL but morphologically or quantitatively fall short of a diagnosis of AIS, two separate diagnoses (of both HSIL and AGC) should be rendered.[42,45]

METASTATIC ADENOCARCINOMA

Any malignancy can metastasize to the cervix, but the most common metastases are from the ovary, followed by the breast and gastrointestinal tract.[21] In contrast to the necrotic background and/or "clinging diathesis" seen in both primary invasive carcinoma and secondary cervical involvement by adjacent carcinomas, metastatic carcinomas will usually present as overtly malignant cells in a paradoxically clean background. The patient will almost always have an established history of a known high-stage carcinoma. The cells have the features of a poorly differentiated carcinoma: large cells with large nuclei, irregular nuclear borders, coarse chromatin and/or prominent nucleoli, high N/C ratios, hyperchromasia, and anisonucleosis. The cells may be present singly or as three-dimensional fragments (Figures 7.95 and 7.96). Lobular carcinoma from the breast and signet ring adenocarcinoma from the gastrointestinal tract classically appear as large, atypical but monotonous single cells at low magnifications.

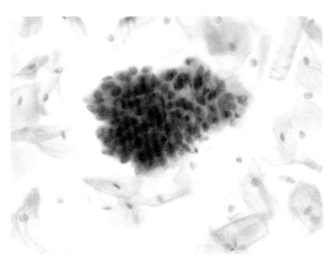

Figure 7.93. High-grade squamous intraepithelial lesion (HSIL) with a glandular appearance. The nuclei in this fragment are palisaded in some areas. Some nuclei are elongated and appear to project away from the tissue fragment edge as is often seen in adenocarcinoma in situ (AIS). However, this patient only had HSIL and not AIS on follow-up (Pap stain).

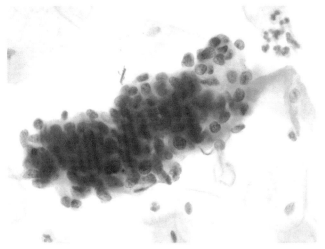

Figure 7.94. High-grade squamous intraepithelial lesion (HSIL) with a glandular appearance. Separate field (Pap stain).

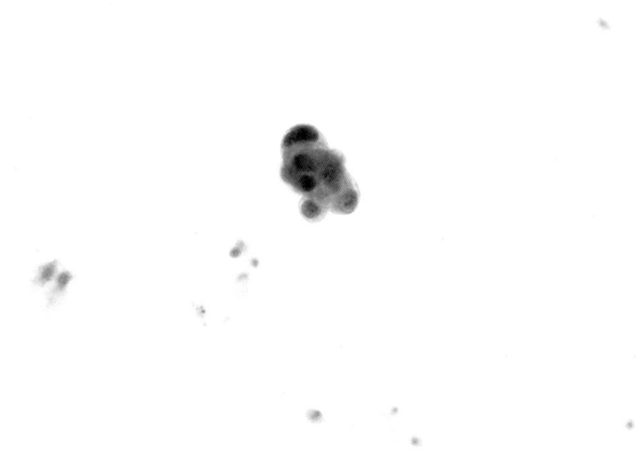

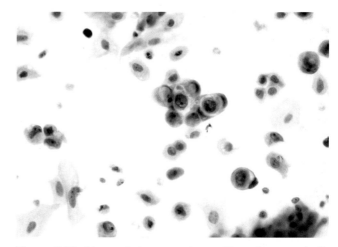

Figure 7.95. Atypical glandular cells (AGCs). AGCs with pleomorphic and dark nuclei form a small cluster. While the hobnailed edges of the cluster may suggest an endometrial origin, on follow-up, the patient was diagnosed with metastatic clear cell carcinoma of the ovary. Note that the background is clean, a feature associated with metastatic rather than locally invasive disease (Pap stain).

Figure 7.96. Metastatic breast carcinoma. The cells are markedly atypical with prominent nucleoli, enlarged dark nuclei, and a cell-in-cell arrangement ("cannibalism"). The patient follow-up revealed metastatic lobular breast carcinoma (Pap stain).

PEARLS & PITFALLS

While rare, carcinomas from other sites can metastasize to the gynecologic tract and shed cells that are subsequently sampled on a cervical Pap test. In many cases, this will be a high-grade serous carcinoma derived from the ovary/fallopian tubes. In contrast to primary carcinomas of the cervix and endometrium and locally invasive carcinomas such as colorectal and urothelial carcinoma, necrosis will be absent, resulting in the presence of overtly malignant cells in a "clean" background. This is important to note to the clinical team, as it can prompt additional workup to locate the source of the primary tumor, especially as most carcinomas identified on the Pap test are assumed to be derived from the cervix or endometrium. If the specimen is cellular, any residual material can be used to create a cell block that can be used to perform immunostains to determine a site of origin.

SAMPLE NOTE: ADENOCARCINOMA IN A CLEAN BACKGROUND

Adequacy: The specimen is satisfactory for evaluation. The transformation zone component is present.

Interpretation: Adenocarcinoma. See note.

Note: Necrotic material is not present in the background. This finding suggests the possibility of a metastatic adenocarcinoma (such as from the ovary) rather than a primary or locally invasive adenocarcinoma.

COLORECTAL ADENOCARCINOMA

Colorectal adenocarcinoma can be seen on the Pap test either due to direct extension into or metastasis to the gynecologic tract.[6,21] Because of the inherently necrotic nature of colorectal adenocarcinoma, metastatic colorectal adenocarcinoma is the exception to the rule that

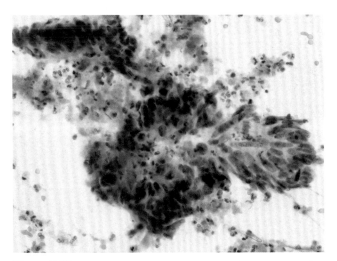

Figure 7.97. Colorectal adenocarcinoma. The classic cytomorphologic features include elongated, cigar-shaped nuclei, nuclear palisading, hyperchromasia, and necrosis. In liquid-based preparations, the amount of necrosis in the background is often reduced, and necrosis is seen as necrotic debris attached to the cells in a specimen ("clinging diathesis") (Pap stain).

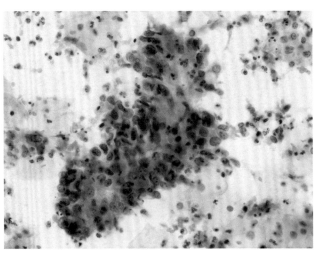

Figure 7.98. Colorectal adenocarcinoma. Separate field (Pap stain).

metastatic disease often presents with a clean background. Instead, necrotic debris typically accompanies metastatic colorectal adenocarcinoma. The cells have the classic appearance of colorectal adenocarcinoma found in other cytology specimens: columnar with elongated ("cigar shape"), hyperchromatic nuclei in a background of dirty necrosis (Figures 7.97 and 7.98). The amount of necrosis is reduced in liquid-based preparations as compared with conventional smear specimens.

KERATINIZING PATTERN

The keratinizing pattern refers to unusual patterns of keratinization in a Pap test specimen. While all epithelial cells contain keratin, nondysplastic keratinizing lesions, some dysplastic lesions, and keratinizing SqCCs possess increased amounts of keratin. In most instances, the correct classification of these entities relies on the assessment of the level of nuclear atypia seen in a specimen.

CHECKLIST: Etiologic Considerations for the Keratinizing Pattern

☐ Hyperkeratosis

☐ Parakeratosis

☐ Atypical Parakeratosis

☐ Keratinizing High-Grade Squamous Intraepithelial Lesion (HSIL)

☐ Keratinizing Squamous Cell Carcinoma

HYPERKERATOSIS

Hyperkeratosis is a pattern in which otherwise benign-appearing mature squamous cells are seen along with anucleate keratinaceous fragments, and it is a nonspecific finding on the Pap test. Some hyperkeratotic cells may have a round, empty, pale-staining area in place

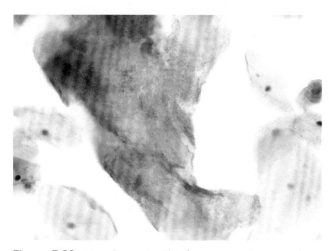

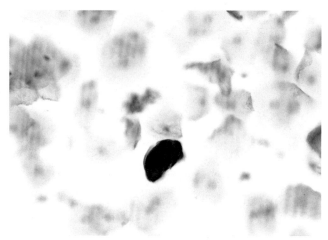

Figure 7.99. Hyperkeratosis. This fragment contains anucleate squamous cells and correlates with hyperkeratosis. Contrast this fragment with malignant keratinaceous fragments seen in squamous cell carcinoma, which are dense, irregularly shaped, and orange (Pap stain).

Figure 7.100. Atypical parakeratosis. A small cluster of cells with high nuclear to cytoplasmic (N/C) ratios and irregularly distributed nuclei. The cells have dense, orange-staining cytoplasm and could represent either reactive or dysplastic changes.

of the nucleus ("ghost nucleus"), which may be an artifact due to poor stain penetration through the increased amount of cytoplasmic keratin (Figure 7.99). This finding in isolation should be interpreted as negative. In benign hyperkeratosis, the cytoplasmic fragments resemble benign superficial epithelial cells in texture and shape.

Both anucleate keratinaceous fragments as well as "ghost nuclei" can be seen in keratinizing SqCC. However, the keratinaceous fragments associated with keratinizing SqCCs often have highly irregular shapes, with rigid irregular cytoplasmic extensions and the occasional formation of characteristic "tadpole" cells. Furthermore, the "ghost nuclei" in SqCC also have irregular shapes.[6]

PARAKERATOSIS

Parakeratosis is another nonspecific reactive state of the superficial squamous epithelium. Parakeratosis in the Pap test appears as fragments of superficial squamous cells containing nuclei closer in size to intermediate cell nuclei. Squamous pearl formations may also be seen. These pearls are not indicative of dysplasia so long as the associated nuclei remain uniform with regular nuclear contours and bland chromatin.

Parakeratosis can also be associated with HPV infection. In the presence of parakeratosis, close examination for atypia is indicated. Parakeratosis and/or squamous pearls with associated nuclear atypia indicate an underlying squamous intraepithelial lesion. If a parakeratotic group of cells contains atypical features (as described below in the "Atypical Parakeratosis" section), a diagnosis of *Atypical squamous cells of undetermined significance* (ASC-US) or LSIL may be more appropriate.[46,47]

ATYPICAL PARAKERATOSIS

Atypical parakeratosis refers to the presence of parakeratosis and concomitant nuclear atypia. The atypical cells should possess large nuclei with at least mild anisonucleosis and mild nuclear contour irregularities (Figure 7.100). Atypical parakeratosis is often associated with the presence of a concomitant, more serious lesion and such specimens warrant careful inspection to ensure a high-grade lesion is not overlooked.[48]

KERATINIZING HIGH-GRADE SQUAMOUS INTRAEPITHELIAL LESION

Keratinizing HSIL is a rare variant of HSIL in which the dysplastic cells have dense pink- or orange-staining keratinaceous cytoplasm with irregular shapes and variable

N/C ratios (Figures 7.101-7.105). The keratinizing lesional cells are often seen along with nonkeratinizing HSIL cells which may impart the appearance of two populations. Distinguishing keratinizing HSIL from keratinizing SqCC is difficult and may not be possible, as they share many of the same features including irregular cell shapes, pyknotic nuclei, and atypical keratinaceous fragments.[2,6,33] Keratinizing HSIL cells lack nucleoli and accompanying necrosis, but the absence of these features is insufficient to completely exclude SqCC. The presence of conventional HSIL in the same specimen also does not exclude SqCC, as SqCC arises from HSIL.[45]

KERATINIZING SQUAMOUS CELL CARCINOMA

Keratinizing squamous cell carcinoma (SqCC) produces thick, atypical keratin that may stain deeply pink and sometimes an unusual orange color ("Halloween orange"). Individually dispersed cells are inevitably present and intact fragments of carcinoma may or may not be

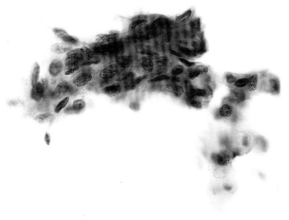

Figure 7.101. Keratinizing high-grade squamous intraepithelial lesion (HSIL). The cells are pleomorphic and have high nuclear to cytoplasmic (N/C) ratios and nuclear membrane irregularities. Some of the cells have keratinized cytoplasm. A squamous cell carcinoma cannot be excluded but would be more likely to have a background of necrosis or "clinging diathesis" (Pap stain).

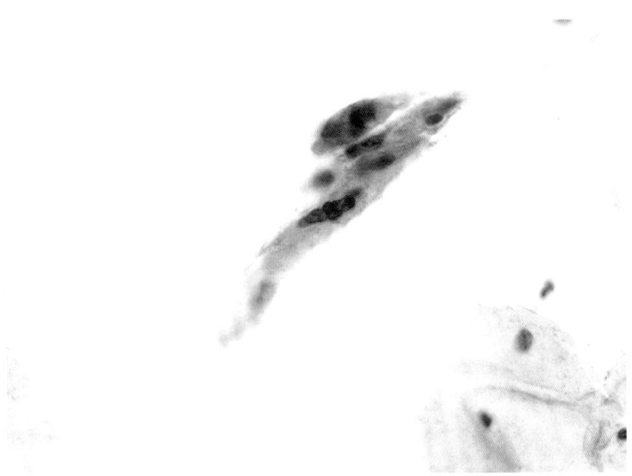

Figure 7.102. Keratinizing high-grade squamous intraepithelial lesion (HSIL). A small fragment of highly atypical keratinizing cells. On follow-up tissue biopsy, the patient was found to have HSIL (Pap stain).

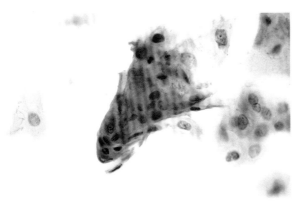

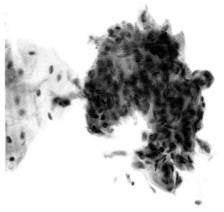

Figure 7.103. Keratinizing high-grade squamous intraepithelial lesion (HSIL). The cells have high nuclear to cytoplasmic (N/C) ratios, enlarged nuclei, and irregular nuclear contours (Pap stain).

Figure 7.104. Keratinizing high-grade squamous intraepithelial lesion (HSIL). It is difficult to believe the cells in this fragment are not overtly malignant, but the patient had only HSIL on follow-up. The cells have high nuclear to cytoplasmic (N/C) ratios and marked variation in nuclear size (Pap stain).

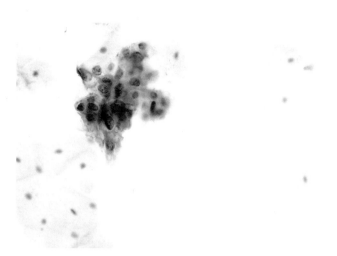

Figure 7.105. Keratinizing high-grade squamous intraepithelial lesion (HSIL). Separate field (Pap stain).

Figure 7.106. Keratinizing squamous cell carcinoma. Highly atypical single cells in a background of diathesis (tumor necrosis and associated inflammation). Some cells have small, dark, pyknotic nuclei. The surgical follow-up was invasive keratinizing squamous cell carcinoma (Pap stain).

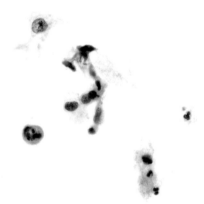

Figure 7.107. Keratinizing squamous cell carcinoma. Separate field (Pap stain).

Figure 7.108. Keratinizing squamous cell carcinoma. Note how deeply pink the cytoplasm of the keratinized cells stains, an indication of atypical keratin production (Pap stain).

seen. The cells have variable sizes and shapes, often with irregular cytoplasmic projections. Bizarre cellular shapes are not uncommon ("tadpole cells" and/or spindled cells). The nuclei are often pyknotic (small and ink black), resulting in paradoxically low N/C ratios. Nucleoli may be present and, if so, are a specific feature differentiating SqCC from HSIL. Irregularly shaped pale areas or "ghost nuclei" may be seen, which represent poorly stained nuclei. The background contains necrosis as well as irregularly shaped anucleate fragments of keratin (Figures 7.106-7.111). Hypercellularity and tumor diathesis are additional features that are variably present but when seen, favor an SqCC over keratinizing HSIL.[2,6,33]

MULTINUCLEATED CELL PATTERN

Multinucleated cells may appear in Pap test specimens and can be striking in their appearance. The etiology and morphology of multinucleated cells are quite diverse. While the varied morphologies help distinguish between most entities, some entities are similar in appearance and must be separated through the identification of subtle features.

Figure 7.109. Keratinizing squamous cell carcinoma. Keratinizing carcinoma cells often have rigid, irregular cytoplasmic projections not seen in benign processes. In this case, the malignant cell has the appearance of a tadpole ("tadpole cell"). Atypical nuclei may or may not be identifiable, but their presence can contribute to a definitive diagnosis (Pap stain).

Figure 7.110. Keratinizing squamous cell carcinoma. Separate field (Pap stain).

Figure 7.111. Keratinizing squamous cell carcinoma. Separate field (Pap stain).

CHECKLIST: Etiologic Considerations for the Multinucleated Cells Pattern

☐ Multinucleated (Reactive) Endocervical Cells

☐ Radiation Changes

☐ Syncytiotrophoblasts

☐ Herpes Simplex Virus

☐ Low-Grade Squamous Intraepithelial Lesion (LSIL)

☐ Carcinosarcoma/Malignant Mixed Mullerian Tumor (MMMT)

MULTINUCLEATED (REACTIVE) ENDOCERVICAL CELLS

Reactive endocervical cells sometimes become multinucleated. The nuclei are slightly enlarged but maintain their round shape and regular contours. Additionally, the reactive cells usually maintain their cytoplasmic shape, with a cytoplasmic tail (either tapered or rectangular) adjacent to the nuclei (Figure 7.112). The nuclei are usually uniform within a given cell but may become crowded and aggregate together. Multiple nuclei closely packed together can cause concern for HSV infection; however, the chromatin pattern of reactive endocervical cells lacks the "ground glass" appearance seen in HSV. The specimen usually contains abundant reactive endocervical cells in the background with a range of appearances, including many that are more easily recognized as reactive.

RADIATION CHANGES

Patients with a previous history of cervical SqCC may have received radiation treatment. Radiation may induce longstanding atypia in squamous cells in subsequent Pap test specimens, and these changes may persist well beyond the duration of the therapy itself. While these cells have enlarged nuclei, they also have a corresponding increase in the amount of cytoplasm, resulting in a nearly normal N/C ratio.[49] The cytoplasmic alterations include the presence of vacuoles and/or polychromasia (a "two-tone" cytoplasmic staining pattern). The cytoplasmic vacuoles are well demarcated and may displace the nucleus, causing a signet ring appearance. Nuclear changes include nuclear vacuolization, multinucleation, hyperchromasia, and wrinkling of nuclear membranes. Bizarre cellular shapes can be seen (Figures 7.113-7.119).[49] The primary differential diagnosis in these cases is recurrent SqCC, which can be difficult to completely exclude by cytomorphology alone. Recurrent SqCC is typically more proliferative, resulting in a hypercellular specimen. The presence of necrosis and/or nucleoli, while helpful in differentiating SqCC from HSIL, can be seen following radiation therapy and is therefore less helpful in this setting.[50] In difficult cases, a biopsy or other additional tissue sampling may be required for definitive classification.

SYNCYTIOTROPHOBLASTS

Syncytiotrophoblasts are cells derived from the placenta. They are large multinucleated cells with cytoplasmic extensions ("tails") (Figures 7.120-7.122).[2] These cells may be seen in a Pap test specimen during pregnancy or immediately following pregnancy. While their presence at one time was thought to indicate a threatened pregnancy, the presence of syncytiotrophoblasts is now understood to be incidental. The main differential diagnosis is multinucleated giant cells (histiocytes), which are more commonly seen in Pap test specimens

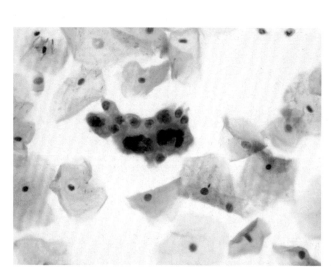

Figure 7.112. Multinucleated endocervical cells. Occasionally endocervical cells may become multinucleated. The differential diagnosis often includes herpes simplex virus infection. In this case, the foamy cytoplasm and lack of nuclear molding and "ground glass" chromatin both support an endocervical cell origin (Pap stain).

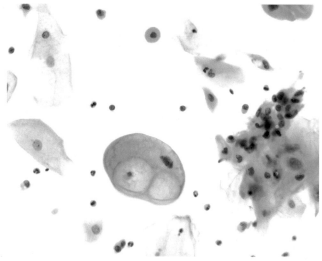

Figure 7.113. Treatment effect. An enlarged mature squamous cell with multiple intracytoplasmic vacuoles. The nuclear to cytoplasmic (N/C) ratio is low. The patient had previous history of radiation therapy (Pap stain).

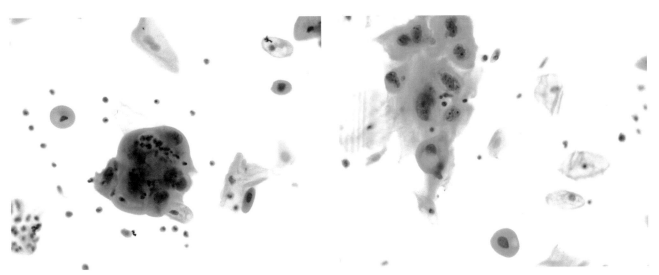

Figure 7.114. Treatment effect. The cells are enlarged but have abundant cytoplasm, which contains small vacuoles. Several cells are binucleated (Pap stain).

Figure 7.115. Treatment effect. A fragment of squamous cells, some of which are multinucleated, have anisonucleosis and coarse chromatin. Despite the increased nuclear sizes, the cells are also enlarged, contributing to normal nuclear to cytoplasmic (N/C) ratios. The patient had a previous history of radiation therapy (Pap stain).

Figure 7.116. Treatment effect. Separate field (Pap stain).

Figure 7.117. Treatment effect. The cells in this fragment are enlarged and have enlarged nuclei, but the streaming nature is reminiscent of reparative change. The patient had a recent history of radiation therapy, which is likely responsible for these changes (Pap stain).

and also have no known clinical significance. Nuclei in syncytiotrophoblasts are typically centrally located, whereas those in multinucleated giant cells tend to be peripherally located (Figure 7.123).

HERPES SIMPLEX VIRUS

Cells infected by herpes simplex virus (HSV) are enlarged; they classically exhibit the features of multinucleation, nuclear molding, marginated chromatin, and "ground glass" nuclei. Molding occurs when a nucleus pushes into an adjacent nucleus, altering the otherwise round shape of the adjacent nucleus (Figures 7.124-7.127).[51] Reactive multinucleated endocervical cells can sometimes be mistaken for HSV infection. However, the nuclei of endocervical cells do not have the characteristic "ground-glass" appearance seen in HSV infected cells.

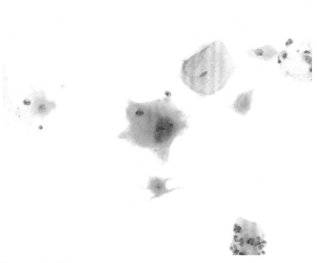

Figure 7.118. Treatment effect. This cell has an enlarged, hypochromatic nucleus with smooth nuclear contours and abundant cytoplasm (Pap stain).

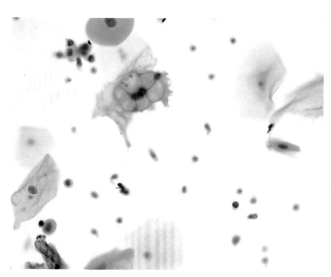

Figure 7.119. Treatment effect. Note the multiple intracytoplasmic vacuoles present in this odd-appearing cell. The patient had a previous history of radiation therapy (Pap stain).

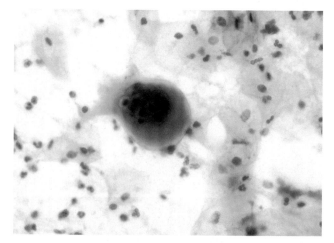

Figure 7.120. Syncytiotrophoblast. This large, multinucleated cell has a short, wide tail ("cytoplasmic extension") and dense cytoplasm. The nuclei tend to concentrate in the center of the cell, in contrast to the random and more peripheral distribution of nuclei seen in multinucleated giant cell histiocytes (Pap stain).

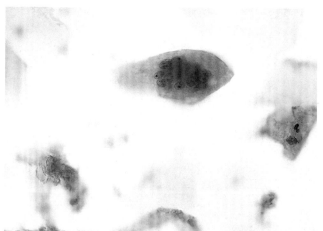

Figure 7.121. Syncytiotrophoblast. Separate field (Pap stain).

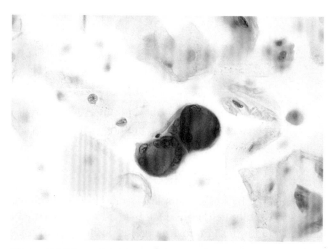

Figure 7.122. Multinucleated giant cell histiocytes. The nuclei are monomorphic and distributed at the periphery of the cell. The cells have small nucleoli, which can also be seen in syncytiotrophoblasts (Pap stain).

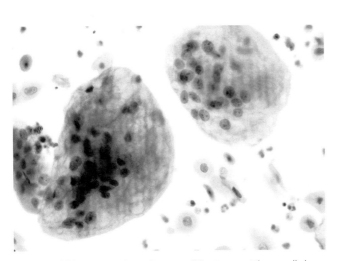

Figure 7.123. Multinucleated giant cell histiocytes. These cells have numerous, uniform nucleoli which are randomly distributed throughout the cell, with some nuclei present at the periphery of the cell (Pap stain).

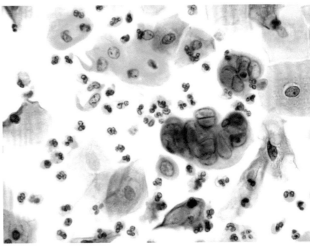

Figure 7.124. Herpes simplex virus. Multinucleated cells with nuclear molding and margination of the chromatin (the 3 M's). The chromatin has a smudged, ground glass appearance (Pap stain).

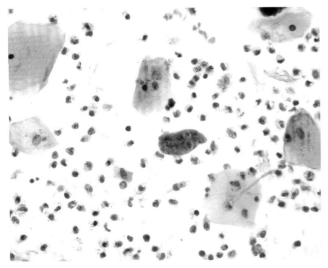

Figure 7.125. Herpes simplex virus. While the infected cell (center) is multinucleated with nuclear molding, the chromatin does not have the typical "ground glass" appearance Instead, the nuclei contain Cowdry bodies (large intranuclear inclusions) (Pap stain).

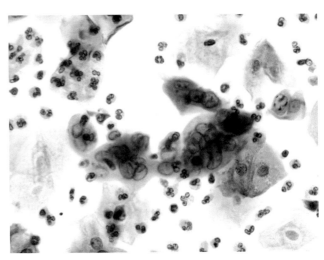

Figure 7.126. Herpes simplex virus. Separate field (Pap stain).

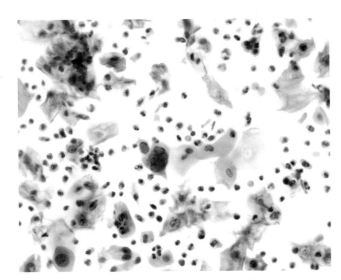

Figure 7.127. Herpes simplex virus. Separate field (Pap stain).

LOW-GRADE SQUAMOUS INTRAEPITHELIAL LESION

Binucleation is a common feature of low-grade squamous intraepithelial lesion (LSIL) cells, and in some cases, multinucleation may be seen. Multinucleated LSIL cells are easily recognizable. They either display a classic koilocytic appearance (discussed below in the "Perinuclear Halo Pattern") or may simply have nuclear enlargement and accompanying nuclear contour irregularities, resulting in a diagnosis of either LSIL or ASC-US (depending on the level of atypia present). Multinucleation in the absence of any atypical features (nuclear enlargement, nuclear membrane irregularities, and/or hyperchromasia) may be seen in reactive squamous cells and, in isolation, should not qualify a specimen for a diagnosis of ASC-US.

KEY FEATURES of Low-Grade Squamous Intraepithelial Lesion

- Nuclei are enlarged and at least 3 times the size of a normal intermediate cell nucleus.
- Binucleation and multinucleation may be present.
- Nuclei are hyperchromatic with irregular nuclear contours.
- The presence of a sharp perinuclear cytoplasmic clearing (perinuclear halo) is characteristic.

CARCINOSARCOMA/MALIGNANT MIXED MULLERIAN TUMOR

Carcinosarcoma/malignant mixed Mullerian tumor (MMMT) is a biphasic tumor composed of both malignant epithelial and sarcomatous components that is rarely seen in cervical Pap test specimens.[21] It is rarely seen on Pap test specimens but when seen confers a worse prognosis. When seen, the most common component present is the epithelial component, which has the appearance of a high-grade carcinoma.[6] The mesenchymal component is rarely identified on the Pap test, most likely because the mesenchymal cells do not shed as readily as the epithelial cells. When present, the mesenchymal cells can have diverse forms and often have enlarged nuclei with complex shapes, sometimes with multinucleation.

DISPERSED ATYPICAL CELL PATTERN

The dispersed atypical cell pattern describes the presence of an unusual appearing population of cells in the Pap test that exists as singly dispersed cells. These cells may represent a "foreign" population of cells (e.g., lymphoma cells) or an altered population of cells usually found on a Pap test (e.g., singly dispersed HSIL cells). A dispersed population of cells causes diagnostic difficulties because their true nature may only be determined at high magnification and also because the cells may be difficult to identify if they are present in low numbers in a specimen.

CHECKLIST: Etiologic Considerations for the Dispersed Atypical Cell Pattern

☐ Atrophy

☐ Low-Grade Squamous Intraepithelial Lesion (LSIL)

☐ Atypical Squamous Cells of Undetermined Significance (ASC-US)

☐ High-Grade Squamous Intraepithelial Lesion (HSIL) With Single Cell Pattern ("Litigation Cells")

☐ Intrauterine Device (IUD) Cells

☐ Melanoma

☐ Small Cell Carcinoma

ATROPHY

Atrophy occurs in women with decreased estrogen levels and is most commonly seen in postmenopausal women. Superficial cells are deceased in number and may not be present at all, while intermediate and parabasal cells predominate. Parabasal cells can be seen in tissue fragments and/or as single, dispersed cells. The benign parabasal cells can have increased N/C ratios, hyperchromasia, and mild nuclear contour irregularities. Thus, it can be challenging to completely exclude HSIL in atrophic smears. A diagnosis of ASC-US or ASC-H may be appropriate, depending on the degree of atypia and the patient's history of HPV infection and dysplasia. However, one study has demonstrated that only 6% of postmenopausal women with a diagnosis of ASC-H had HSIL on follow-up biopsy,[15] suggesting that ASC-H is overdiagnosed in specimens from these patients.

LOW-GRADE SQUAMOUS INTRAEPITHELIAL LESION

While LSIL may exist in small tissue fragments, single cells may have sufficient atypical features to merit a diagnosis of LSIL. This may include the presence of single koilocytes (covered in more detail below in the "Perinuclear Halo Pattern") or cells without perinuclear halos but sufficiently enlarged nuclei (Figures 7.128 and 7.129). The nucleus should be at least 3 times the size of a normal intermediate cell nucleus and contain other forms of nuclear atypia (hyperchromasia, nuclear contour irregularities, and/or bi- or multinucleation). LSIL nuclei can become quite large and thus, large nuclear size alone does not suggest HSIL; in fact, HSIL cells often have smaller nuclei and much higher N/C ratios than LSIL cells due to a smaller cell size.

ATYPICAL SQUAMOUS CELLS OF UNDETERMINED SIGNIFICANCE

Singly dispersed squamous cells with atypical features that fall short of an LSIL diagnosis may be diagnosed as *Atypical squamous cells of undetermined significance* (ASC-US). However, the atypical squamous cells must have a nucleus at least 2.5 times the size of a normal intermediate cell nucleus. In addition to an increase in nuclear size, the nucleus should contain at least mild hyperchromasia or nuclear border irregularities. In general, only rare atypical cells are seen in specimens diagnosed as ASC-US, as the presence of numerous atypical cells should either be sufficient for a diagnosis of LSIL or are likely reactive in nature. Reactive changes (especially secondary to *Candida* spp., which may not be seen due to sampling limitations) can result in the presence of rare squamous cells with enlarged nuclei, though these cells usually lack other atypical nuclear features.

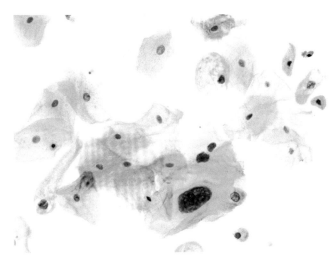

Figure 7.128. Low-grade squamous intraepithelial lesion (LSIL). This mature squamous cell has a markedly enlarged hyperchromatic nucleus (more than three times the size of the nuclei of the surrounding intermediate cells). This finding is sufficient for a diagnosis of LSIL even in the absence of a koilocytic halo (Pap stain).

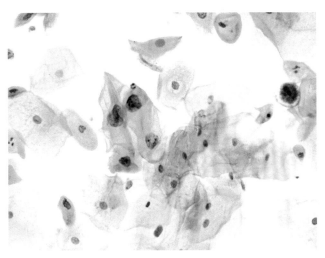

Figure 7.129. Low-grade squamous intraepithelial lesion (LSIL). Several cells have enlarged and hyperchromatic nuclei when compared with the background intermediate cells. Nuclear contour irregularities are also seen (Pap stain).

HIGH-GRADE SQUAMOUS INTRAEPITHELIAL LESION WITH SINGLE CELL PATTERN ("LITIGATION CELLS")

HSIL cells can be present exclusively as single atypical cells with elevated N/C ratios, hyperchromasia, and nuclear border irregularities. These cells have dense cyanophilic cytoplasm and closely resemble parabasal and/or metaplastic cells (Figures 7.130-7.133). They have been given the name "litigation cells" because they are easily overlooked (due to their singly dispersed nature and because only rare cells may be present in a specimen). When only a few of these atypical cells are seen in the absence of other diagnostic features of HSIL, a diagnosis of ASC-H may be warranted. When numerous cells are seen, a diagnosis of HSIL can be made, though some cytopathologists prefer to see the atypical cells present both as single cells as well as in tissue fragments before making a diagnosis of HSIL.

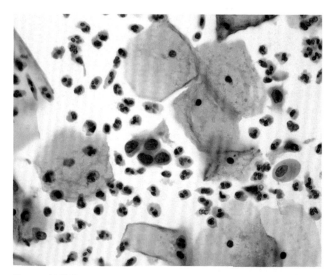

Figure 7.130. Atypical squamous cells, cannot exclude high-grade squamous intraepithelial lesion (ASC-H). The four cells in this group have high nuclear to cytoplasmic ratios, hyperchromasia, and nuclear membrane irregularities. The cells are very small compared with cells from low-grade squamous intraepithelial lesion (LSIL) lesions. The cytoplasm is dense, with small "windows" between the cells, indicating that these may be metaplastic cells. In this case, the follow-up biopsy showed high-grade squamous intraepithelial lesion (HSIL) (Pap stain).

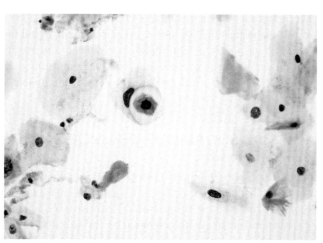

Figure 7.131. Atypical squamous cells, cannot exclude high-grade squamous intraepithelial lesion (ASC-H). The two cells in the center form a cell-in-cell arrangement. The engulfed cell is markedly atypical with orangeophilic cytoplasm and an "ink black" hyperchromatic nucleus (Pap stain).

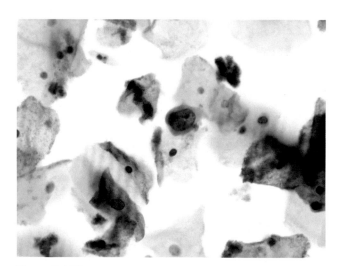

Figure 7.132. Atypical squamous cells, cannot exclude high-grade squamous intraepithelial lesion (ASC-H). This single cell in the center of field has an elevated nuclear to cytoplasmic (N/C) ratio and an irregularly shaped nucleus. A diagnosis of ASC-H would be appropriate for these changes, despite the atypia being less severe as compared with other examples in this chapter (Pap stain).

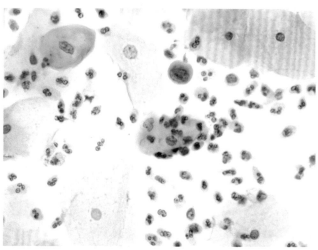

Figure 7.133. Atypical squamous cells, cannot exclude high-grade squamous intraepithelial lesion (ASC-H). Rare squamous cells with high nuclear to cytoplasmic ratios, hyperchromasia, and irregular nuclear contours are seen in a background of acute inflammation (Pap stain).

FAQ: How do I report the presence of cells concerning for HSIL in the presence of an LSIL?

Answer: In some Pap tests, LSIL cells are seen together with a separate population of squamous cells with atypical features suspicious for HSIL. While some laboratories have previously reported this finding as "low-grade squamous intraepithelial lesion, cannot exclude HSIL (LSIL-H)," TBS recommends against this single combined diagnosis and instead recommends providing a diagnosis of both LSIL and ASC-H.[52–54] Despite being an indeterminate diagnosis, an ASC-H diagnosis generally prompts more aggressive clinical triage management, with most patients receiving colposcopy regardless of HPV status.

INTRAUTERINE DEVICE (IUD) CELLS

While IUD cells often have vacuolated cytoplasm and a glandular appearance (as discussed in greater detail in the "Glandular Pattern"), IUD cells sometimes appear as dispersed hyperchromatic cells with high N/C ratios (Figures 7.134 and 7.135). These cells are usually only present in small numbers, and it is not uncommon to only see a single IUD cell of this type in a specimen. The cells may be misdiagnosed as ASC-H due to overlapping features (in particular, hyperchromasia and elevated N/C ratio) between these IUD cells and the "litigation cells" discussed in the preceding section. The presence of other cells with more classic IUD-associated changes (such as cytoplasmic vacuolization) and/or a history of IUD are reassuring. The presence of a nucleolus argues against dysplasia because nucleoli are not seen in cells with high-grade dysplasia (ASC-H, HSIL).

MELANOMA

The cytologic features of melanoma seen on the Pap test are similar to those of melanoma in other sites. The neoplastic cells are enlarged and have round eccentric nuclei with regular borders. The cells are usually discohesive, singly distributed, and contain ample cytoplasm with low N/C ratios (Figures 7.136 and 7.137). Melanin pigment may

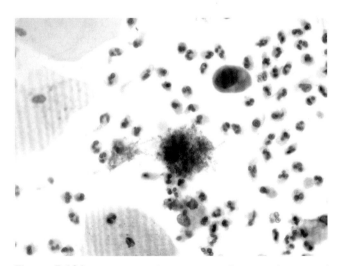

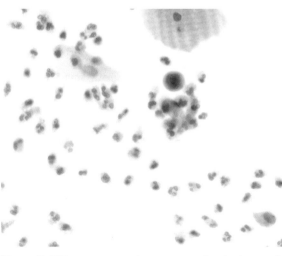

Figure 7.134. Intrauterine device (IUD) cells. A single atypical cell can be seen at the top right corner of the field. The cell has a prominent nucleolus, dark chromatin, and a nuclear to cytoplasmic (N/C) ratio of around 0.5. While high-grade squamous intraepithelial lesion (HSIL) may be on the differential diagnosis, HSIL cells do not have nucleoli. The presence of cytoplasmic vacuoles is also uncommon for HSIL (Pap stain).

Figure 7.135. Intrauterine device (IUD) cells. The large cell in the center is a perfect mimic for a singly dispersed high-grade squamous intraepithelial lesion (HSIL) cell ("litigation cell") given the dense "squamoid" appearance to its cytoplasm. Other more convincing IUD cells were seen in this specimen, and the patient had a benign follow-up (Pap stain).

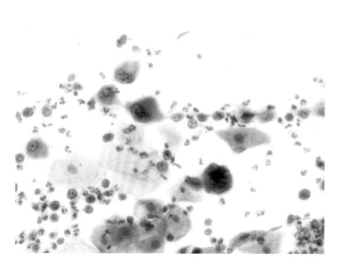

Figure 7.136. Melanoma. Several singly dispersed melanoma cells can be seen on this conventional smear. The cells have abundant, granular cytoplasm, prominent nucleoli, and eccentrically placed nuclei. Some cells are multinucleated. These features are suggestive of melanoma even in the absence of melanin pigment (Pap stain).

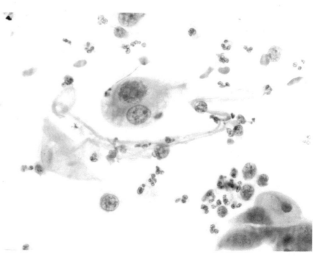

Figure 7.137. Melanoma. A single, large binucleate cell with abundant cytoplasm is in the center of the field. Intranuclear inclusions can be seen in melanoma but are nonspecific. The field also contains several much smaller melanoma cells with minimal cytoplasm; note that the chromatin pattern in these cells matches that of the two nuclei in the much larger cell (Pap stain).

be seen in the cytoplasm and allow for a definitive diagnosis. The presence of binucleation, intranuclear inclusions, and/or prominent nucleoli may also suggest the possibility of melanoma. Malignant melanomas are more commonly metastatic rather than primary to the gynecologic tract; when metastatic melanoma is present, a history is usually known. Melanoma is determined to arise from the gynecologic tract in 5-10% of the cases encountered on Pap test specimens. If cellularity is sufficient, an additional preparation can be made for confirmatory immunostains using melanoma-associated markers (e.g., HMB-45, Melan-A, SOX10, S-100 protein).

SMALL CELL CARCINOMA

Small cell carcinoma of the cervix is a rare gynecologic malignancy and is morphologically similar to small cell carcinoma of the lung and other sites.[21] The neoplastic cells have scant cytoplasm, high N/C ratios, salt-and-pepper chromatin, and nuclear molding (Figures 7.138 and 7.139). Apoptotic bodies and mitoses are frequently seen.[55,56] The characteristic crush artifact described on other preparations is diminished on liquid-based preparations. In liquid-based preparations, the visibility of background necrosis is reduced, though tumor necrosis it may be seen primarily as "clinging diathesis." Before assuming that a small cell carcinoma is primary to the cervix, it is important to exclude metastatic small cell carcinoma from other sites such as the lung; a history of lung cancer is usually known in this instance. The majority of primary small cell carcinomas of the cervix are HPV positive (usually HPV 18), which is not the case in small cell carcinoma of the lung.[57]

PERINUCLEAR HALO PATTERN

A cervical Pap test specimen may contain cells with a distinctive pale area surrounding the nucleus ("perinuclear halo" or "perinuclear clearing") that is sharply delineated from the rest of the cytoplasm by a crisp cytoplasmic border. Perinuclear halos are found in reactive squamous cells, the classic koilocytes of LSIL, following Trichomonas infection, and the glycogen-rich navicular cells associated with pregnancy. Superficial and intermediate squamous cells may occasionally have folded cytoplasm that gives the appearance of a perinuclear halo ("false halos").

KOILOCYTES

Koilocytes are considered pathognomonic for HPV infection and are the classical cells representing LSIL. They are superficial or intermediate cells with large, well-defined cytoplasmic halos and atypical nuclei (Figures 7.140-7.152). Koilocytes may be seen singly or in small fragments of up to 10-20 cells. When well developed, the perinuclear halo is characteristic and appears as an optically clear perinuclear area surrounded by a crisp cytoplasmic interface. The nuclei exhibit changes consistent with LSIL (enlargement, hyperchromasia, irregular nuclear borders, and/or binucleation). When distinct koilocytic clearing is present but the atypical nuclear features are missing, the best diagnosis may be ASC-US. If the perinuclear clearing is not classic and well-defined, and atypical nuclear features are also absent, one should hesitate before rendering a diagnosis of ASC-US or LSIL.

INFLAMMATORY HALOS ("TRICHOMONAS HALOS")

Inflammatory halos are small, uniform, round perinuclear halos usually involving the majority of superficial and intermediate cells in a Pap test specimen (Figures 7.143-7.155). They are classically associated with *Trichomonas* infection, though *Trichomonas* organisms may not be seen along with inflammatory halos, either due to the nonspecific nature of these halos or lack of organisms due to clearance or recent treatment.[2] Inflammatory halos are commonly associated with a background of increased acute inflammation as well as reactive epithelial changes; these findings should prompt a careful search for *Trichomonas* organisms. Unlike the halos seen in navicular cells and koilocytes, inflammatory halos are more diffusely and uniformly seen through out the squamous cells in a specimen and do not have thickened borders.

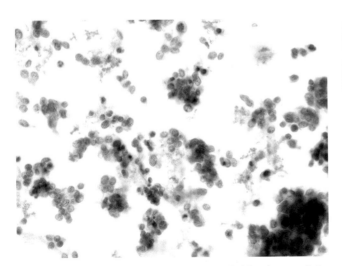

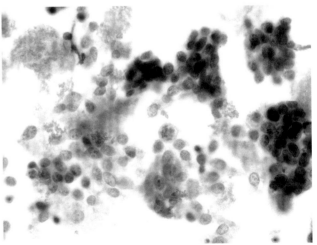

Figure 7.138. Small cell carcinoma. The field is hypercellular and contains predominantly neoplastic cells. Despite the name, the cells can look deceivingly large on cytologic preparations; the near-absence of cytoplasm is one clue to the diagnosis. The cells also have a "salt-and-pepper" neuroendocrine chromatin pattern. Degenerated blood and granular debris (diathesis) is seen in the background and clinging to the neoplastic cells (Pap stain).

Figure 7.139. Small cell carcinoma. Separate field at higher magnification. Primary small cell carcinoma is rarely seen in the cervix but is associated with high-risk human papillomavirus (HPV) infection (Pap stain).

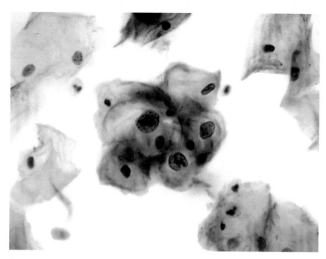

Figure 7.140. Low-grade squamous intraepithelial lesion (LSIL). These cells have abundant cytoplasm but also enlarged nuclei. The nuclei are dark and have nuclear contour irregularities. While the cytoplasm appears pale in some areas, perinuclear "halos" are not well defined for these cells to be considered true koilocytes. Regardless, the cells are diagnostic of LSIL (Pap stain).

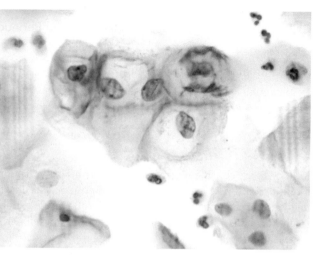

Figure 7.141. Low-grade squamous intraepithelial lesion (LSIL). At least one cell in this fragment has a well-defined perinuclear halo, though all the cells have enlarged nuclei with irregular borders and are also diagnostic of LSIL (Pap stain).

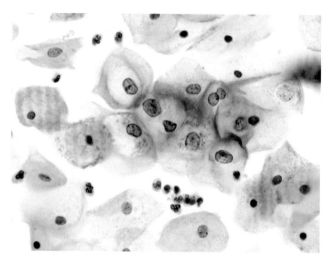

Figure 7.142. Low-grade squamous intraepithelial lesion (LSIL). Several cells in this fragment have well-defined areas of perinuclear clearing. More specific features include an irregularly shaped halo (rather than round) and a thickened interface between the cleared area and the rest of the cytoplasm (Pap stain).

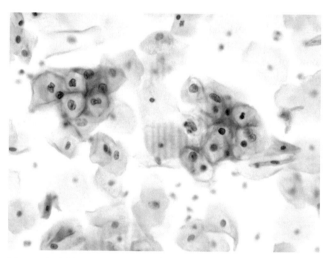

Figure 7.143. Low-grade squamous intraepithelial lesion (LSIL). The field contains two fragments of well-defined koilocytes. Other features of nuclear atypia are present: enlargement, irregular nuclear contours, hyperchromasia, and binucleation (Pap stain).

NAVICULAR CELLS (GLYCOGENATED CELLS)

Navicular cells are boat-shaped intermediate cells with thickened, yellowish halos containing glycogen (Figures 1.156-1.158).[1,2,34] This phenomenon is more often seen during pregnancy, although it can be seen during the second phase of the menstrual cycle and in patients using medroxyprogesterone acetate for contraception. Navicular cells can be difficult to differentiate from koilocytes. Koilocytes tend to have optically clear halos and some form of nuclear atypia; navicular cell nuclei may have reactive changes but not the atypical nuclear features seen in koilocytes (enlarged, hyperchromatic, "raisinoid" nuclei).

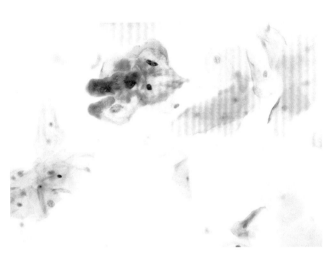

Figure 7.144. Low-grade squamous intraepithelial lesion (LSIL). Note the peripheral thickening of the cytoplasm, which is characteristic of koilocytes (Pap stain).

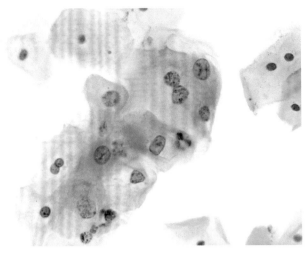

Figure 7.145. Low-grade squamous intraepithelial lesion (LSIL). A separate field containing a fragment of dysplastic cells in which nuclear enlargement was the primary diagnostic feature (Pap stain).

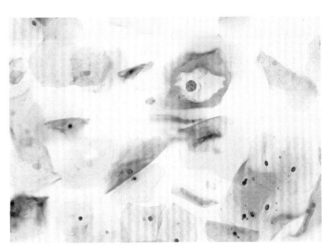

Figure 7.146. Koilocytes. Superficial cells with enlarged nuclei and large perinuclear halos. Note that the cytoplasm is clear around the nuclei and thickened at the periphery. Koilocytes are the hallmark of human papillomavirus (HPV) infection. However, if only single cells or rare cells with koilocytic changes are seen, most people would diagnose the specimen as *Atypical squamous cells of undetermined significance* (ASC-US) (Pap stain).

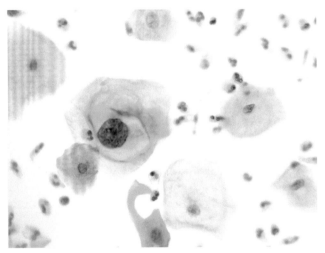

Figure 7.147. Low-grade squamous intraepithelial lesion (LSIL). This intermediate cell has a very large nucleus that is also dark and irregularly shaped. This serves as a reminder that large nuclear size can be diagnostic of LSIL even in the absence of koilocytes (Pap stain)

BUGS

HUMAN PAPILLOMAVIRUS

Human papillomavirus (HPV) is a double-stranded DNA virus belonging to the papillomavirus family.[58] Numerous subtypes have been identified over the years. Certain subtypes have been designated as "high-risk" based on whether a particular subtype has been associated with carcinogenesis. Approximately 15 types are currently considered oncogenic (HPV types 16, 18, 31, 33, 35, 39, 45, 51, 52, 56, 58, 59, 68, 73, 82).[59] HPV 16 is associated with 55-60% of all cervical cancers, while HPV 18 is associated with 25-35% of all cervical cancers.[60,61] In most cases, an HPV infection is transient and the patient clears the infection on their own. In some instances, an infection may persist; a causal link between persistent

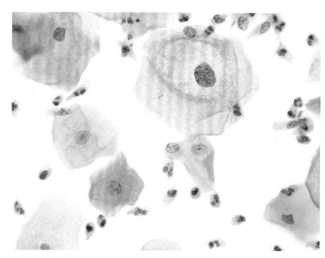

Figure 7.148. Koilocyte. This cell has an enlarged nucleus and a poorly defined perinuclear halo. While it is likely representative of a low-grade squamous intraepithelial lesion (LSIL), if seen alone in a specimen, *Atypical squamous cells of undetermined significance* (ASC-US) might be a better diagnosis (Pap stain).

Figure 7.149. Koilocyte. This superficial cell has enlarged nuclei, binucleation, and a well-defined perinuclear halo. The features are diagnostic of a low-grade squamous intraepithelial lesion (LSIL) (Pap stain).

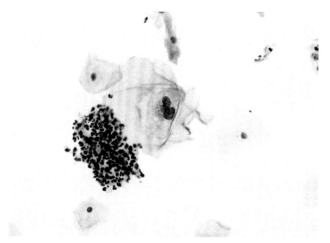

Figure 7.150. Koilocyte. This cell has two dark and enlarged nuclei. The perinuclear halo is poorly developed and has an indistinct border with the rest of the cytoplasm. Careful examination of the rest of the specimen may reveal better developed koilocytes (Pap stain).

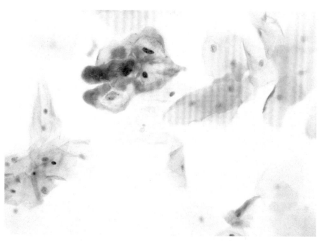

Figure 7.151. Low-grade squamous intraepithelial lesion (LSIL). This small fragment of mature squamous cells demonstrates nuclear enlargement, perinuclear halos, and hyperchromasia (Pap stain).

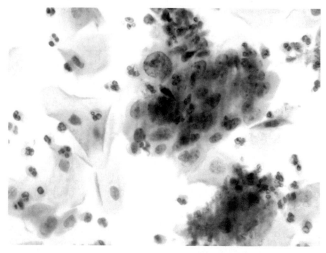

Figure 7.152. Low-grade squamous intraepithelial lesion (LSIL). This fragment of LSIL contains cells with enlarged nuclei and anisonucleosis. Enlarged nuclear size is often associated with LSIL, whereas high-grade squamous intraepithelial lesion (HSIL) should be associated with high nuclear to cytoplasmic (N/C) ratio (Pap stain).

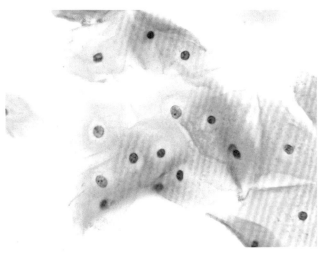

Figure 7.153. Inflammatory halos. Numerous mature squamous cells showing small perinuclear halos. In addition to being small, the halos are also uniform and round and have indistinct borders with the rest of the cytoplasm. Although they are commonly known as "Trichomonas halos" (or "Trich halos"), they can sometimes be seen in other reactive conditions (Pap stain).

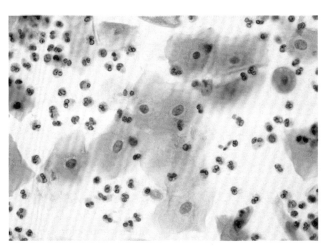

Figure 7.154. Inflammatory halos. Some of these superficial cells show mild nuclear enlargement. However, they are hypochromatic and uniform in size. The background contains numerous acute inflammatory cells; these findings together should prompt a careful search for *Trichomonas* organisms (Pap stain).

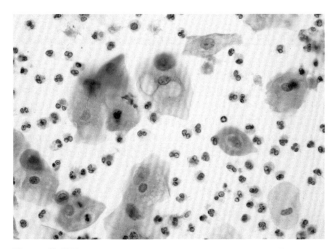

Figure 7.155. Inflammatory halos (Pap stain). Separate field.

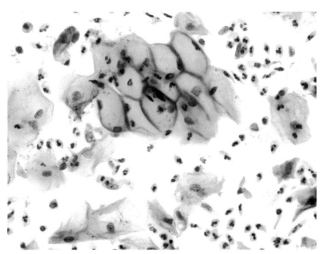

Figure 7.156. Glycogenated cells. The nuclei in these cells lack any atypia or enlargement. This suggests against these cells being koilocytes, with the accumulation of cytoplasmic glycogen being the most likely cause of these "halos" (Pap stain).

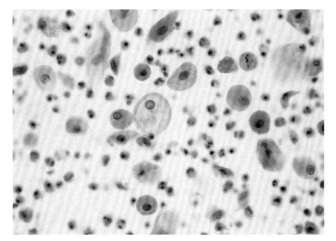

Figure 7.157. Glycogenated cells. The cell in the center of the field has a large, round perinuclear vacuole with a delicate interface with the rest of the cytoplasm. The nucleus is not enlarged compared to other cells, favoring against dysplasia.

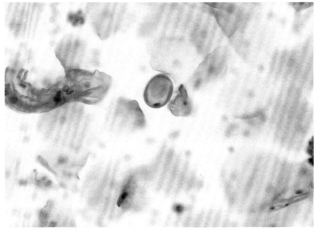

Figure 7.158. Glycogenated cells. The faint yellow coloring inside this vacuole is not always identified but is associated with glycogen accumulation (Pap stain).

infection with high-risk HPV and the development of SqCC is well accepted.[62] Current models of onogenesis and HPV infection attribute tumor development to increased expression of the viral oncoproteins E6 and E7 in infected cells, which leads to activation of the cell cycle and inhibition of apoptosis.[59]

TRICHOMONAS VAGINALIS

Trichomonas vaginalis is a protozoan parasite of the genital tract. Infected women usually present with green-yellow malodorous vaginal discharge.[63,64] *Trichomonas vaginalis* is a pear-shaped microorganism with eccentrically placed pale nuclei. Eosinophilic (red on Pap stain) cytoplasmic granules, when seen, may aid in identification. The organism's flagella are rarely seen on the Pap test.[2,63,64] Other clues to the diagnosis include background reactive cellular changes (squamous cells with small perinuclear inflammatory halos) and an abundant neutrophilic infiltrate.[2] The organisms may cluster together and look like detached cytoplasmic fragments at low magnification. Examination at high magnification may reveal an eccentrically placed nucleus and reddish cytoplasmic granules (Figures 7.159 and 7.161). Cytoplasmic fragments from degenerated epithelial cells, especially those associated with increased acute inflammation, may appear as small blue blobs and be mistaken for *Trichomonas* organisms. *Trichomonas* is often seen concurrently with *Leptothrix* bacteria, which are long, thin bacterial organisms distinct from usual vaginal flora.

FUNGAL ORGANISMS MORPHOLOGICALLY CONSISTENT WITH *CANDIDA* SUBSPECIES

Candida subspecies are common microorganisms seen on the cervical Pap test. They are associated with multiple conditions, including pregnancy, diabetes, and immunodeficiency.[63,64] *Candida* are polymorphous and may be present as pseudohyphae (elongated pinkish filamentous structures) and/or small budding yeast. Pseudohyphae frequently pierce mature and intermediate squamous cells, resulting in a "shish kebab" appearance (Figures 7.162-7.165).[2,63,64] These flattened squamous cells stacked together on their side

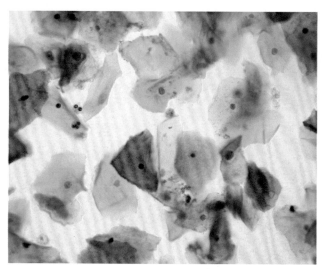

Figure 7.159. *Trichomonas vaginalis.* The center of the field contains a *Trichomonas* organism showing an elliptical nucleus, red cytoplasmic granules, and a cytoplasmic extension that might represent a flagellum. These features are not always easily identified, but the red cytoplasmic granules are usually the most readily identifiable feature and strongly suggest *Trichomonas* (Pap stain).

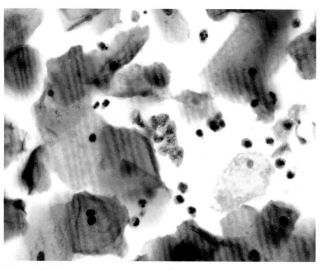

Figure 7.160. *Trichomonas vaginalis.* Numerous *Trichomonas vaginalis* organisms have clustered together, often known as a "trich party" (Pap stain).

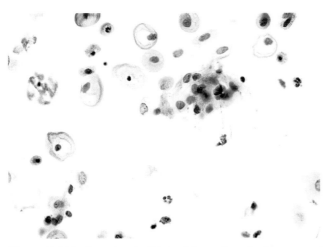

Figure 7.161. Cytoplasmic "blobs." Several small, degenerated "blue blobs" can be seen in the field, some with cytoplasmic granules. While these could be degenerated *Trichomonas* organisms, they could also represent degenerated neutrophils and are often seen in the background of increased acute inflammation. The diagnosis of *Trichomonas* should be made when intact cells are seen, with the pale-staining nucleus being the most specific feature for identification (Pap stain).

can be identified at low magnification, which frequently allows for the identification of *Candida* during closer examination. *Candida* infection often induces reactive epithelial changes, including hyperkeratosis and nuclear enlargement. When *Candida* is present, reactive changes such as mild nuclear enlargement may simulate ASC-US.

FAQ: In the setting of *Candida*, are these atypical changes reactive or do they represent LSIL?

Answer: Infection with *Candida* spp. often results in enlarged nuclei seen in single squamous cells or squamous cells in fragments. The nuclei may vary in size but should maintain regular nuclear contours, lack hyperchromasia compared with background cells, and lack the perinuclear halos that are characteristic of koilocytes. LSIL and *Candida* spp. can coexist in a specimen, so while the presence of *Candida* spp. should raise one's threshold for making a diagnosis of ASC-US, cells meeting the criteria of LSIL can be diagnosed as such. *Candida* spp. should not cause nuclear membrane irregularities, hyperchromasia, or koilocytic changes. Increased nuclear size, anisonucleosis, and bi- or multinucleation are less specific features for LSIL.

SHIFT IN VAGINAL FLORA SUGGESTIVE OF BACTERIAL VAGINOSIS

A shift in vaginal flora occurs when the predominant aerobic microorganisms (*Lactobacillus* spp.) are replaced by anaerobic microorganisms such as *Gardnerella vaginalis*, among others. Patients present with vaginal discharge, itching, pain, and odor.[63,64] Shift in flora suggestive of bacterial vaginosis is characterized by the presence of "clue cells," which are superficial or intermediate squamous cells covered with coccobacilli[2,63,64] (Figures 7.166 and 7.167). The background is clean and without significant inflammation, and there is an absence of lactobacilli.

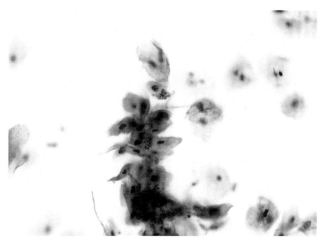

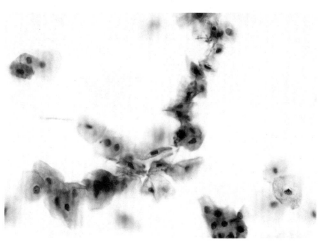

Figure 7.162. *Candida* spp. *Candida* spp. pseudohyphae will characteristically pierce through superficial squamous epithelial cells, giving the "shish kebab" appearance. This structure can be easily recognized at low magnification and prompt a closer examination of the field to confirm the presence of the organism (Pap stain).

Figure 7.163. *Candida* spp. Separate field (Pap stain).

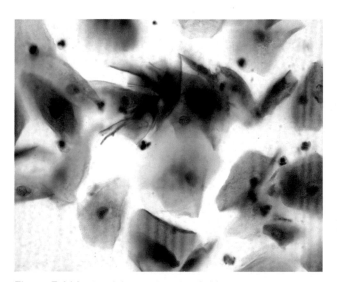

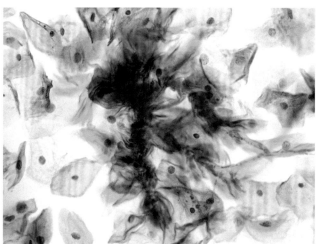

Figure 7.164. *Candida* spp. Separate field (Pap stain).

Figure 7.165. *Candida* spp. Separate field (Pap stain).

ACTINOMYCES

Actinomyces species are gram-positive, filamentous bacteria that form clusters of thin, delicate, radiating filaments.[63,65] They are seen at low magnification as purple "cotton balls" (Figures 7.168-7.170). *Actinomyces* is classically associated with the use of an IUD, and the diagnosis should be questioned in patients without an IUD.[65] The finding should be interpreted in conjunction with the patient's clinical findings, as the diagnosis may require IUD removal. An aggregate of lactobacilli can have a similar "cotton ball" appearance. Close examination of the aggregate edges at high magnification should reveal whether the organisms are truly filamentous or simply rod-shaped bacteria in chains.

HERPES SIMPLEX VIRUS

Herpes simplex virus (HSV)–infected cells have a characteristic appearance on the Pap test.[63,64] HSV-infected squamous cells are enlarged, multinucleated cells with molded nuclei and "ground glass" chromatin[51]. Chromatin is also typically marginated, resulting in the

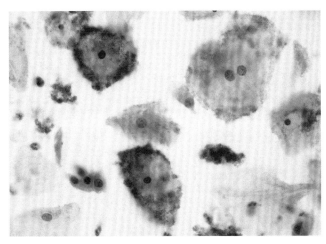

Figure 7.166. Clue cells. Mature squamous cells covered with bacteria have a "shag carpet" appearance. When found throughout the specimen, this finding is associated with bacterial vaginosis (Pap stain).

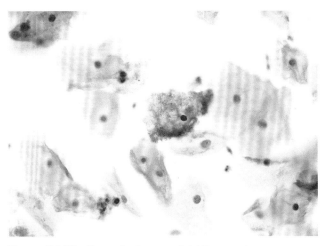

Figure 7.167. Clue cells. Separate field (Pap stain).

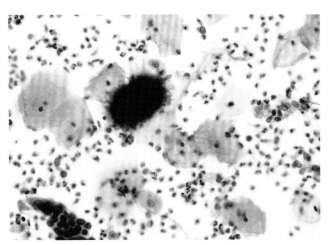

Figure 7.168. *Actinomyces*. *Actinomyces* is seen at low power as purple-red staining "dust-balls." The organisms are filamentous and care must be taken not to mistake rod-shaped bacteria with a linear growth pattern as *Actinomyces* (Pap stain).

Figure 7.169. *Actinomyces*. Separate field. The diagnosis should be questioned in patients without a history of intrauterine device (IUD) use (Pap stain).

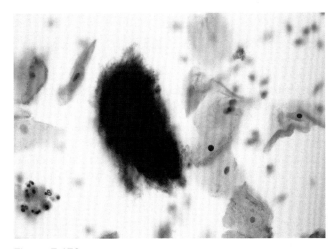

Figure 7.170. *Actinomyces*. Separate field (Pap stain).

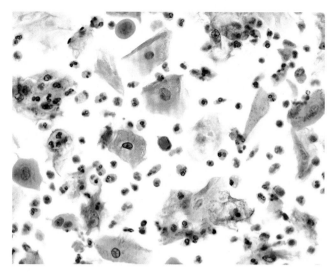

Figure 7.171. Herpes simplex virus (HSV). The cell in the center of the field has a high nuclear to cytoplasmic (N/C) ratio and a "ground glass" appearance to its chromatin. In this case, multinucleation and molding are absent, making the diagnosis more challenging (Pap stain).

mnemonic three M's: multinucleation, molding, and chromatin margination (Figures 7.124-7.127).[51] HSV-infected cells may also present as single mononucleated cells (Figure 7.171) with high N/C ratios. HSV infection is further discussed under the "Multinucleated Cell Pattern."

KEY FEATURES of Herpes Simplex Virus
- The infected cells may be multinucleated.
- Nuclear contours are compressed by adjacent nuclei, referred to as "molding".
- Chromatin is often marginated, resulting in a thickened, dark nuclear rim.
- The nuclei within infected cells has a "ground glass" chromatin appearance.

CYTOMEGALOVIRUS

Cytomegalovirus (CMV)–infected cells are rarely seen on the Pap test.[63,64] The infected cells are usually of endocervical origin. Paradoxically, this finding is not more common in immunocompromised patients. CMV-infected cells are enlarged and have both nuclear and cytoplasmic inclusions. The most characteristic finding is the prominent eosinophilic nuclear inclusion with marginated chromatin ("owl's eye").[66]

NEAR MISSES

HIGH-GRADE SQUAMOUS INTRAEPITHELIAL LESION WITH SINGLE CELL PATTERN ("LITIGATION CELLS")

"Litigation cells," or "ASC-H cells," are singly dispersed HSIL cells. Owing to their small size and sometimes scarce nature, a specimen may contain only one or two of these cells that are easily missed. The specimen may be reviewed during the "5 year look back" in which negative Pap tests preceding a new HSIL diagnosis must be reviewed. During this look back, the "litigation cells" may be found. The term "litigation cells" refers to the fact that, when these cells are missed, a patient may receive a reassuring Pap test result and develop SqCC before the next screening interval, a situation which may lead to litigation. To avoid missing "litigation cells", a pathologist must become familiar with the morphology of

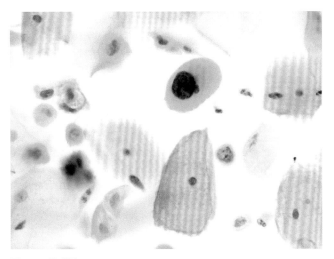

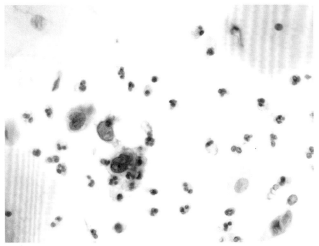

Figure 7.172. Litigation cell. This cell has dense cytoplasm and a large, dark nucleus. The nuclear to cytoplasmic (N/C) ratio is low compared with what is seen in most high-grade squamous intraepithelial lesion (HSIL) cells, but low-grade squamous intraepithelial lesion (LSIL) cells rarely demonstrate such dark chromatin or this quality of cytoplasm. The patient had HSIL on follow-up biopsy (Pap stain).

Figure 7.173. Litigation cells. Several small cells with high nuclear to cytoplasmic (N/C) ratios and irregular nuclear borders can be seen in a background of neutrophils and mature squamous cells. Singly dispersed high-grade squamous intraepithelial lesion (HSIL) cells are often small, making them more easily missed compared with lower grade lesions (Pap stain).

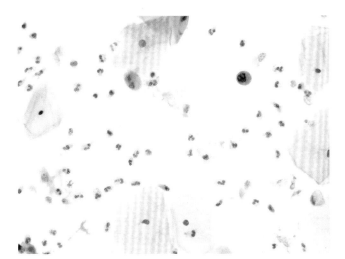

Figure 7.174. Litigation cell. The cell in the top right hand corner of the field has dense, metaplastic cytoplasm and an enlarged, dark nucleus with an irregular shape. Such a finding requires close examination of the specimen for similar cells (Pap stain).

these cells. The cells have dense, metaplastic cytoplasm, dark chromatin, irregular nuclear borders, and elevated N/C ratios compared with bystander parabasal cells (Figures 7.171-7.174). Specimens must be screened carefully for these cells, as they are easily missed at low magnification.

RADIATION CHANGES

Most patients with recent radiation therapy to the pelvis have had a history of SqCC, creating a diagnostic dilemma of whether any atypical squamous cells seen in a specimen are representative of radiation changes, recurrent SqCC, or a combination of the two. Acute radiation changes include cellular enlargement, multinucleation, and cytoplasmic vacuolization. Late changes include nuclear enlargement, coarse chromatin, and the presence of nucleoli. Changes are usually present up to 6 months following radiation but may persist for 30 years or more.[67] If benign, these cells will usually have regular nuclear contours, evenly distributed chromatin, and maintained N/C ratios, whereas recurrent carcinoma cells have high N/C ratios and abnormal chromatin patterns (Figures 7.175-7.179). In general, a higher threshold for a diagnosis of recurrent SqCC is recommended in a patient with a history of radiation therapy. The assessment of such specimens is not always straightforward and expert opinion may be required.

OVERDIAGNOSIS

Because the Pap test is largely considered a "screening test," most patients will not receive definitive treatment (e.g. cone biopsy, hysterectomy, radiation therapy) before receiving a confirmatory diagnosis on biopsy or curettage following colposcopy. However, the Pap test can also be considered a diagnostic test in certain scenarios. It is important to be aware of the ASCCP guidelines and when a Pap test diagnosis may trigger a potentially unnecessary surgical excision without an intervening tissue diagnosis. For instance, diagnoses of SqCC, adenocarcinoma, AIS, and AGCs, favor neoplasia and may result in a diagnostic excisional

Figure 7.175. Radiation effect. These cells have enlarged nuclei containing bland chromatin and abundant cytoplasm. The cells have a tissue culture–like appearance and seem to be crawling away from the fragment (Pap stain).

Figure 7.176. Radiation effect. Epithelioid histiocytes containing carrot-shaped or indented hyphen–shaped nuclei form a cluster in the center of the field (Pap stain).

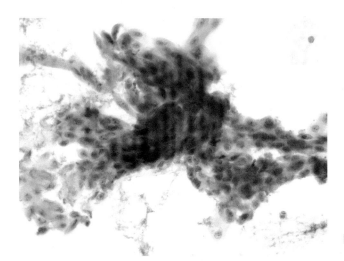

Figure 7.177. Radiation effect. These cells appear to stream within the tissue fragment, similar to what is seen in repair. The nuclei are enlarged, but so are the cells, causing the cells to have near-normal nuclear to cytoplasmic (N/C) ratios. Note the prominent nucleoli present in some of the cells (Pap stain).

Figure 7.178. Radiation effect. This markedly atypical cell has multiple, enlarged nuclei but also abundant cytoplasm. The cytoplasm has numerous, slender projections, giving a tissue culture–like appearance (Pap stain).

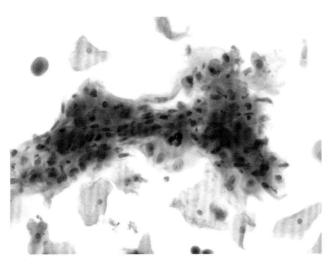

Figure 7.179. Radiation effect. This large fragment appears disorderly, but the cells have low nuclear to cytoplasmic (N/C) ratios. The nuclei are dark, but many are not much larger than the nucleus of the bystander intermediate cells (Pap stain).

procedure if colposcopy fails to identify a lesion, although many clinicians prefer to have a confirmatory biopsy first. If a patient receives multiple and consecutive diagnoses of HSIL on a Pap test specimen, they may undergo conization or LEEP even if no disease is found following colposcopy—this is because colposcopy is imperfect and may fail to sample the HSIL found on a Pap test specimen.

References

1. Herzberg AJ, Dominic SR, Silverman JF. Color Atlas of Normal Cytology. Philadelphia: Churchill Livingstone.

2. Demay RM. *The Pap Test*. American Society of Clinical Pathology; 2005.

3. McEndree B. Clinical application of the vaginal maturation index. *Nurse Pract*. 1999;24(9):48, 51-2, 55-6.

4. Vu M, Yu J, Awolude OA, Chuang L. Cervical cancer worldwide. *Curr Probl Cancer*. 2018;42(5):457-465.

5. Nayar R, Wilbur DC. The Bethesda system for reporting cervical cytology: a historical perspective. *Acta Cytologica*. 2017;61(4–5):359-372.

6. Nayar R, Wilbur DC. *The Bethesda System for Reporting Cervical Cytology: Definitions, Criteria and Explanatory Notes*. 3rd ed. New York: Springer; 2015.

7. Demay RM. Hyperchromatic crowded groups: pitfalls in pap smear diagnosis. *Am J Clin Pathol*. 2000(114 suppl):S36-S43.

8. Chivukula M, Austin RM, Shidham VB. Evaluation and significance of hyperchromatic crowded groups (HCG) in liquid-based paps. *CytoJournal*. 2007;4:2.

9. Bibbo M, Keebler CM, Wied GL. The cytologic diagnosis of tissue repair on the female genital tract. *Acta Cytol*. 1971;15(2):133-137.

10. Colgan TJ, Woodhouse SL, Styer PE, et al. Reparative changes and the false-positive/false-negative papanicolaou test: a study from the college of American pathologists interlaboratory comparison program in cervicovaginal cytology. *Arch Pathol Lab Med*. 2001;125(1):134-140.

11. Crothers BA, Booth CN, Darragh TM, et al. False-positive papanicolaou (PAP) test rates in the College of American Pathologists PAP education and PAP proficiency test programs: evaluation of false-positive responses of high-grade squamous intraepithelial lesion or cancer to a negative reference diagnosis. *Arch Pathol Lab Med*. 2014;138(5):613-619.

12. Crothers BA, Booth CN, Darragh TM, et al. Atrophic vaginitis: concordance and interpretation of slides in the college of American pathologists cervicovaginal interlaboratory comparison program in gynecologic cytopathology. *Arch Pathol Lab Med*. 2012;136(11):1332-1338.

13. Abati A, Jaffurs W, Wilder AM. Squamous atypia in the atrophic cervical vaginal smear: a new look at an old problem. *Cancer*. 1998;84(4):218-225.

14. Johnston EI, Logani S. Cytologic diagnosis of atypical squamous cells of undetermined significance in perimenopausal and postmenopausal women: lessons learned from human papillomavirus DNA testing. *Cancer*. 2007;111(3):160-165.

15. Saad RS, Dabbs DJ, Kordunsky L, et al. Clinical significance of cytologic diagnosis of atypical squamous cells, cannot exclude high grade, in perimenopausal and postmenopausal women. *Am J Clin Pathol*. 2006;126(3):381-388.

16. Selvaggi SM. Atrophic vaginitis versus invasive squamous cell carcinoma on ThinPrep cytology: can the background be reliably distinguished? *Diagn Cytopathol*. 2002;27(6):362-364.

17. Wang SS, Sherman ME, Hildesheim A, et al. Cervical adenocarcinoma and squamous cell carcinoma incidence trends among white women and black women in the United States for 1976-2000. *Cancer*. 2004;100(5):1035-1044.

18. Zhao C, Crothers BA, Tabatabai ZL, et al. False-negative interpretation of adenocarcinoma in situ in the College of American pathologists gynecologic PAP education program. *Arch Pathol Lab Med*. 2017;141(5):666-670.

19. Biscotti CV, Gero MA, Toddy SM, et al. Endocervical adenocarcinoma in situ: an analysis of cellular features. *Diagn Cytopathol*. 1997;17(5):326-332.

20. Adegoke O, Kulasingam S, Virnig B. Cervical cancer trends in the United States: a 35-year population-based analysis. *J Womens Health (Larchmt)*. 2012;21(10):1031-1037.

21. Kurman RJ, Carcangiu ML, Herrington CS, Young RH. *WHO Classification of Tumours of Female Reproductive Organs*. 4th ed.: IARC; 2014.

22. Pirog EC, Lloveras B, Molijn A, et al. HPV prevalence and genotypes in different histological subtypes of cervical adenocarcinoma, a worldwide analysis of 760 cases. *Mod Pathol*. 2014;27(12):1559-1567.

23. Conrad RD, Liu AH, Wentzensen N, et al. Cytologic patterns of cervical adenocarcinomas with emphasis on factors associated with underdiagnosis. *Cancer Cytopathol*. 2018;126(11):950-958.

24. Sorosky JI. Endometrial cancer. *Obstet Gynecol*. 2012;120(2 Pt 1):383-397.

25. Serdy K, Yildiz-Aktas I, Li Z, Zhao C. The value of papanicolaou tests in the diagnosis of endometrial carcinoma: a large study cohort from an academic medical center. *Am J Clin Pathol*. 2016;145(3):350-354.

26. Patel C, Ullal A, Roberts M, et al. Endometrial carcinoma detected with SurePath liquid-based cervical cytology: comparison with conventional cytology. *Cytopathology*. 2009;20(6):380-387.

27. Zhou J, Tomashefski J Jr, Khiyami A. Diagnostic value of the thin-layer, liquid-based Pap test in endometrial cancer: a retrospective study with emphasis on cytomorphologic features. *Acta Cytol*. 2007;51(5):735-741.

28. Zhou J, Tomashefski JF Jr, Khiyami A. ThinPrep Pap tests in patients with endometrial cancer: a histo-cytological correlation. *Diagn Cytopathol*. 2007;35(7):448-453.

29. Schorge JO, Hossein Saboorian M, Hynan L, et al. ThinPrep detection of cervical and endometrial adenocarcinoma: a retrospective cohort study. *Cancer*. 2002;96(6):338-343.

30. Ge Y, Christensen P, Luna E, et al. Aptima human papillomavirus E6/E7 mRNA test results strongly associated with risk for high-grade cervical lesions in follow-up biopsies. *J Low Genit Tract Dis*. 2018;22(3):195-200.

31. Deleted in review

32. Cancer Genome Atlas Research Netwok, Albert Einstein College of Medicine, Analytical Biological Services, et al. Integrated genomic and molecular characterization of cervical cancer. *Nature*. 2017;543(7645):378-384.

33. Clark SB, Dawson AE. Invasive squamous-cell carcinoma in ThinPrep specimens: diagnostic clues in the cellular pattern. *Diagn Cytopathol*. 2002;26(1):1-4.

34. Kobayashi TK, Casslen B, Stormby N. Cytologic atypias in the uterine fluid of intrauterine contraceptive device users. *Acta Cytol*. 1983;27(2):138-141.

35. Risse EK, Beerthuizen RJ, Vooijs GP. Cytologic and histologic findings in women using an IUD. *Obstet Gynecol*. 1981;58(5):569-573.

36. Tambouret R, Pitman MB, Bell DA. Benign glandular cells in posthysterectomy vaginal smears. *Acta Cytologica*. 1998;42(6):1403-1408.

37. Bai H, Sung CJ, Steinhoff MM. ThinPrep Pap Test promotes detection of glandular lesions of the endocervix. *Diagn Cytopathol*. 2000;23(1):19-22.

38. Zhao C, Austin RM, Pan J, et al. Clinical significance of atypical glandular cells in conventional pap smears in a large, high-risk U.S. west coast minority population. *Acta Cytol*. 2009;53(2):153-159.

39. Zhao C, Florea A, Onisko A, et al. Histologic follow-up results in 662 patients with Pap test findings of atypical glandular cells: results from a large academic womens hospital laboratory employing sensitive screening methods. *Gynecol Oncol.* 2009;114(3):383-389.

40. Miller RA, Mody DR, Tams KC, et al. Glandular lesions of the cervix in clinical practice: a cytology, histology, and human papillomavirus correlation study from 2 institutions. *Arch Pathol Lab Med.* 2015;139(11):1431-1436.

41. Patadji S, Li Z, Pradhan D, et al. Significance of high-risk HPV detection in women with atypical glandular cells on Pap testing: analysis of 1857 cases from an academic institution. *Cancer Cytopathol.* 2017;125(3):205-211.

42. Pradhan D, Li Z, Ocque R, et al. Clinical significance of atypical glandular cells in Pap tests: an analysis of more than 3000 cases at a large academic women's center. *Cancer Cytopathol.* 2016;124(8):589-595.

43. DeSimone CP, Day ME, Tovar MM, et al. Rate of pathology from atypical glandular cell Pap tests classified by the Bethesda 2001 nomenclature. *Obstet Gynecol.* 2006;107(6):1285-1291.

44. Chen L, Booth CN, Shorie JA, et al. Atypical endometrial cells and atypical glandular cells favor endometrial origin in Papanicolaou cervicovaginal tests: correlation with histologic follow-up and abnormal clinical presentations. *CytoJournal.* 2014;11:29.

45. Selvaggi SM. Cytologic features of high-grade squamous intraepithelial lesions involving endocervical glands on ThinPrep cytology. *Diagn Cytopathol.* 2002;26(3):181-185.

46. Steinman S, Smith D, Chandler N, et al. Morphologic, patient and interpreter profiles of high-risk human papillomavirus-positive vs.-negative cases of atypical squamous cells of undetermined significance. *Acta Cytol.* 2008;52(3):279-285.

47. Kir G, Sarbay BC, Seneldir H. The significance of parakeratosis alone in cervicovaginal cytology of Turkish women. *Diagn Cytopathol.* 2017;45(4):297-302.

48. Abramovich CM, Wasman JK, Siekkinen P, et al. Histopathologic correlation of atypical parakeratosis diagnosed on cervicovaginal cytology. *Acta Cytol.* 2003;47(3):405-409.

49. Powers CN. Radiation treatment effects in cervical cytology. *Diagn Cytopathol.* 1995;13(1):75-80.

50. Padilha CML, Araújo MLC Jr, Souza SAL, et al. Cytopathologic evaluation of patients submitted to radiotherapy for uterine cervix cancer. *Rev Assoc Méd Bras.* 2017;63(4):379-385.

51. Naib ZM, Nahmias AJ, Josey WE. Cytology and histopathology of cervical herpes simplex infection. *Cancer.* 1966;19(7):1026-1031.

52. Hunter C, Duggan MA, Duan Q, et al. Cytology and outcome of LSIL: cannot exclude HSIL compared to ASC-H. *Cytopathology.* 2009;20(1):17-26.

53. Shidham VB, Kumar N, Narayan R, Brotzman GL. Should LSIL with ASC-H (LSIL-H) in cervical smears be an independent category? A study on SurePath™ specimens with review of literature. *CytoJournal.* 2007;4:7.

54. Difurio MJ, Mailhiot T, Sundborg MJ, Nauschuetz KK. Comparison of the clinical significance of the Papanicolaou test interpretations LSIL cannot rule out HSIL and ASC-H. *Diagn Cytopathol.* 2010;38(5):313-317.

55. Satoh T, Takei Y, Treilleux I, et al. Gynecologic Cancer InterGroup (GCIG) consensus review for small cell carcinoma of the cervix. *Int J Gynecol Cancer.* 2014;24(9 suppl 3):S102-S108.

56. Howitt BE, Kelly P, McCluggage WG. Pathology of neuroendocrine tumours of the female genital tract. *Curr Oncol Rep.* 2017;19(9):59.

57. Xing D, Zheng G, Schoolmeester JK, et al. Next-generation sequencing reveals recurrent somatic mutations in small cell neuroendocrine carcinoma of the uterine cervix. *Am J Surg Pathol.* 2018;42(6):750-760.

58. Van Doorslaer K, Li Z, Xirasagar S, et al. The papillomavirus episteme: a major update to the papillomavirus sequence database. *Nucleic Acids Res.* 2017;45(D1):D499-D506.

59. Stanley M. Pathology and epidemiology of HPV infection in females. *Gynecol Oncol.* 2010;117(2 suppl):S5-S10.

60. de Sanjose S, Quint WG, Alemany L, et al. Human papillomavirus genotype attribution in invasive cervical cancer: a retrospective cross-sectional worldwide study. *Lancet Oncol.* 2010;11(11):1048-1056.

61. Munoz N, Bosch FX, de Sanjosé S, et al. Epidemiologic classification of human papillomavirus types associated with cervical cancer. *N Engl J Med.* 2003;348(6):518-527.

62. Boshart M, Gissmann L, Ikenberg H, et al. A new type of papillomavirus DNA, its presence in genital cancer biopsies and in cell lines derived from cervical cancer. *EMBO J.* 1984;3(5):1151-1157.

63. Fitzhugh VA, Heller DS. Significance of a diagnosis of microorganisms on pap smear. *J Low Genit Tract Dis.* 2008;12(1):40-51.

64. Powers CN. Diagnosis of infectious diseases: a cytopathologist's perspective. *Clin Microbiol Rev.* 1998;11(2):341-365.

65. Gupta PK, Hollander DH, Frost JK. Actinomycetes in cervico-vaginal smears: an association with IUD usage. *Acta Cytol.* 1976;20(4):295-297.

66. Gideon K, Zaharopoulos P. Cytomegalovirus endocervicitis diagnosed by cervical smear. *Diagn Cytopathol.* 1991;7(6):625-627.

67. Shield P, Daunter B, Wright R. Post-irradiation cytology of cervical cancer patients. *Cytopathology.* 1992;3(3):167-182.

SPECIMEN PREPARATION AND ADEQUACY

8

CHAPTER OUTLINE

INADEQUATE PATTERNS

Several patterns can result in inadequate or nondiagnostic specimens. Some samples have defined criteria for adequacy based on a reporting system, whereas others without a reporting system may only have evidence-based criteria.[1-5] Many specimens, however, lack evidence-based criteria and rely on a laboratory's practice or a pathologist's judgment. It is important to assess each specimen for adequacy before rendering a diagnosis because an "inadequate" diagnosis informs the clinical team that the specimen was non-informative. A "negative" diagnosis provided on an inadequate sample would be falsely reassuring.

CHECKLIST: Etiologic Considerations for the Inadequate Patterns

☐ Obscuring Pattern
☐ Virtually Acellular Pattern
☐ Paucicellular Pattern
☐ Missed Lesion Pattern
☐ Insufficient for Ancillary Studies Pattern

OBSCURING PATTERN

The obscuring pattern occurs when bystander cells and/or background elements are present in great numbers and interfere with the microscopic assessment of potentially diagnostic cells in a specimen. Red blood cells, inflammatory cells, and debris are common elements that may obscure a specimen (Figures 8.1-8.8). In specimens that are only partially obscured, a diagnosis should be provided, and the specimen should not be regarded as inadequate. In inadequate specimens, the obscuring elements generally entirely cover areas of interest and the presence of nonobscured elements cannot be determined.

VIRTUALLY ACELLULAR PATTERN

The virtually acellular pattern refers to specimens which contain no cells, or very few cells that do not result in a specific diagnosis. Because most inadequate specimens contain at least bystander cells (such as red blood cells), the absence of cells can indicate that a specimen was not properly transferred to the collection container or material was lost during

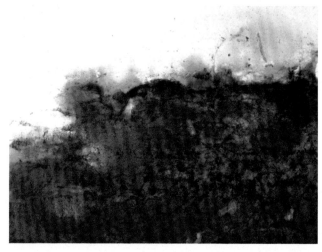

Figure 8.1. Obscuring blood. A large number of red blood cells along with proteinaceous serum components have been fixed to form a thick layer at the bottom of the field. It is difficult to determine whether any cells of interest may be caught within this material (Pap stain).

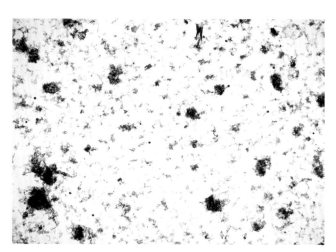

Figure 8.2. Obscuring degenerated blood. The field contains degenerated blood. The cells entrapped in this material cannot be adequately assessed, and thus the material may be considered inadequate due to obscuring blood. If atypical cells of interest can be visualized outside of the obscuring material, the specimen can be considered adequate (Pap stain).

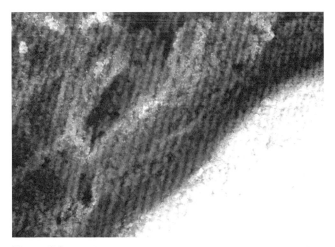

Figure 8.3. Obscuring blood. The field contains a thick layer of red blood cells, both intact and degenerated. It is uncertain whether the field contains only blood or may contain cells of interest within the blood that cannot be assessed (Pap stain).

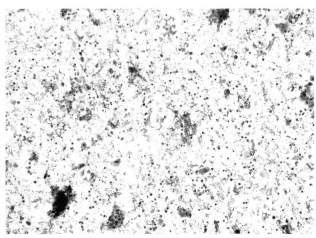

Figure 8.4. Obscuring blood. The specimen contains degenerated blood that has covered some cells, interfering with their visual assessment. As the majority of cells can be assessed, this specimen may be considered "suboptimal" owing to obscuring blood rather than completely inadequate. While most specimen types do not have defined criteria, Pap test specimens should be considered inadequate if more than 75% of the specimen is obscured by blood or inflammation (Pap stain).

Figure 8.5. Obscuring blood. The field contains intact red blood cells as well as clot material that has covered and obscured a cell (Pap stain).

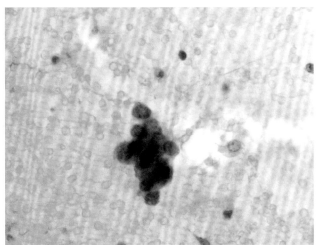

Figure 8.6. Small cell carcinoma obscured by blood. These cells appear much larger than the background red blood cells, are hyperchromatic, and have high nuclear to cytoplasmic (N/C) ratios. Despite the obscuring blood, they should be regarded as at least atypical, which would make the specimen adequate for a diagnosis. However, the obscuring blood may prevent a definitive diagnosis of malignancy in such situations (Pap stain)

processing in the laboratory. The absence of cells in some specimens (such as cerebrospinal fluids and some voided urine specimens) can be a normal finding and should not cause the specimen to be called inadequate.

PAUCICELLULAR PATTERN

The paucicellular pattern refers to specimens that are not virtually acellular but contain only rare cells that are not sufficient in number (Figures 8.9-8.11). If atypical cells possibly representing a lesion are seen, the specimen should be regarded as adequate and a diagnosis should be provided. For some specimens (such as the Pap test), the number of

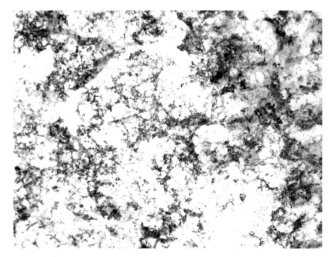

Figure 8.7. Obscuring blood. This thyroid specimen was spray-fixed with alcohol, causing an uneven distribution and suboptimal staining of the background red blood cells. Any epithelial cells of interest are further obscured by blending in with the background cells (Pap stain).

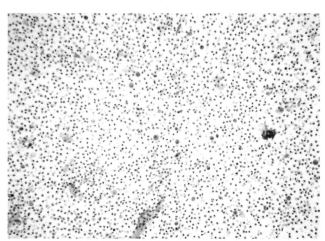

Figure 8.8. Obscuring inflammation. The presence of abundant inflammatory cells is a common reason for a specimen to be considered inadequate. In some specimens, the presence of inflammation is diagnostic (e.g., the aspiration of an abscess) but may still obscure important cells (e.g., an inflamed cyst in which the lining cells are obscured thus preventing a definitive diagnosis) (Pap stain).

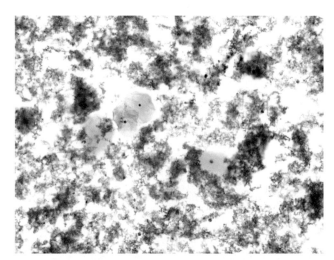

Figure 8.9. Inadequate squamous component (Pap test). The density of squamous cells in this specimen is low, and the specimen is also obscured by blood. For conventional smears, at least 8000-12,000 squamous cells must be present; for liquid-based smears, at least 5000 squamous cells must be seen (Pap stain).

Figure 8.10. Inadequate squamous component in a cervical Pap specimen. Only granular debris and inflammatory cells are seen, indicating that the squamous lining was not adequately sampled. Most cytology specimens do not have a defined number of cells required for adequacy, and adequacy assessment depends on the pathologist's judgment (Pap stain).

cells required for adequacy has been defined (Table 8.1). Other specimens do not have evidence-based definitions of adequacy, such as the number of lymphocytes that should be seen from a lymph node aspiration.

MISSED LESION PATTERN

The missed lesion pattern refers to specimens that may contain abundant cellularity, but predominantly contain bystander cells rather than lesional cells (Figures 8.12-8.17). This pattern is often seen in endoscopic procedures targeting a mass on imaging studies, such as a lymph node or a possible neoplasm. In a bronchoscopic procedure, the specimen may contain predominantly bronchial respiratory epithelial cells, cartilage, and macrophages but lack any lymphocytes or atypical epithelial cells. The missed lesion pattern is never seen in exfoliative cytology samples because exfoliative cytology is performed without the expectation that a lesion will necessarily be sampled.

SAMPLE NOTE: MISSED LESION PATTERN

Nondiagnostic. Bronchial respiratory cells and fragments of cartilage. See note.

Note: The material is not representative of the mass lesion seen on imaging studies.

Figure 8.11. Inadequate squamous component in a cervical Pap specimen. Squamous cells are absent at low magnification, meaning the specimen is likely inadequate. This is often due to poor sampling during specimen procurement but may also be caused if an ulcerated area was sampled (Pap stain).

TABLE 8.1: Criteria for Adequacy According to Reporting System Guidelines

Specimen Type	Inadequate if[a]
Pap test, conventional smear	Less than 8000-12,000 squamous cells or more than 75% of cells obscured by inflammation or bacteria
Pap test, liquid-based preparation	Less than 5000 squamous cells or more than 75% of cells obscured by inflammation or bacteria
Thyroid fine-needle aspiration (FNA)	Less than six groups of 10 follicular cells in the absence of abundant colloid or numerous lymphocytes

[a]Specimens are always adequate if any atypical findings are present, including a single atypical cell.

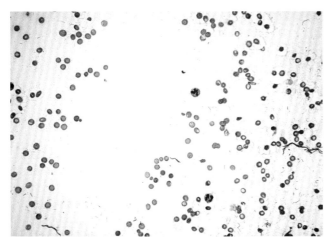

Figure 8.12. Missed lesion. This fine-needle aspiration (FNA) of a soft tissue lesion yielded only blood components. FNA procedures typically target a mass lesion seen grossly or on imaging studies; if the findings do not explain the presence of a mass lesion, the specimen should be considered inadequate (Diff-Quik stain).

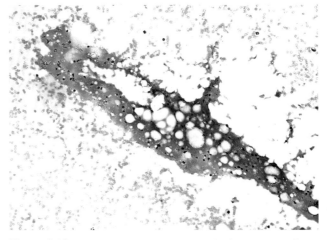

Figure 8.13. Missed lesion. Adipocytes and inflammatory cells are trapped in clot material. In this case, a lipoma was not suspected and this material was assumed to be from benign soft tissue rather than lesional cells (Diff-Quik stain).

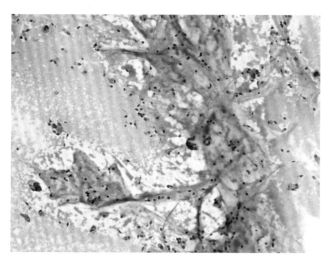

Figure 8.14. Missed lesion. An ultrasound-guided endobronchial fine-needle aspiration of a mass lesion was attempted, yielding this smear of mucin and bronchial respiratory epithelial cells. Because only background elements are seen, the specimen should be considered nondiagnostic (Diff-Quik stain).

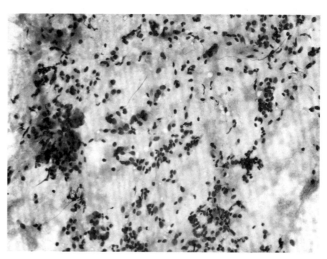

Figure 8.15. Missed lesion. The field contains predominantly benign bronchial respiratory epithelial cells, as evidenced by their columnar shape and oval nuclei as well as occasionally identified cilia and terminal bars. There is no definitive evidence of lesional cells, making this specimen nondiagnostic (Diff-Quik stain).

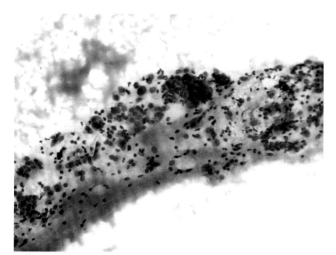

Figure 8.16. Missed lesion. Clot material containing pulmonary alveolar macrophages, inflammatory cells, and bronchial respiratory epithelial cells. The cells were entrapped in blood which clotted in the needle before being smeared on the slide. If any cells are interpreted as atypical, the specimen could be considered adequate; otherwise, the material does not appear to represent a mass lesion and should be considered nondiagnostic.

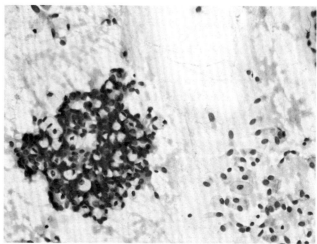

Figure 8.17. Missed lesion. The fragment on the left contains benign goblet cells and bronchial respiratory epithelial cells. The scattered cells on the right are mostly ciliated bronchial respiratory epithelial cells and rare macrophages. These are all benign elements sampled from the airway, and there is no indication that a mass lesion was sampled (Diff-Quik stain).

INSUFFICIENT FOR ANCILLARY STUDIES PATTERN

This pattern refers to specimens in which lesional cells are present and a diagnosis can be provided, but the number or proportion of lesional cells is insufficient for the performance of ancillary studies, such as a next-generation sequencing panel or immunohistochemical studies. In many instances, the diagnostic material may be present on one preparation (such as a conventional smear) but not on the material preferred for ancillary testing (such as a cell block preparation).

SUBOPTIMAL PATTERNS

Several patterns may impact the assessment of a specimen, and their identification can help identify issues with specimen procurement, transport, storage, and preparation. The identification of such patterns also allows the cytopathologist to review a specimen with increased caution and provide a diagnosis on the context of the specimen's limitations. For instance, the recognition that a urinary tract specimen has degenerated cells may result in cytologic atypia being regarded as likely benign and secondary to degeneration, rather than being representative of a malignant process.

CHECKLIST: Etiologic Considerations for the Suboptimal Patterns

☐ Paucicellular Pattern

☐ Low-Volume Pattern

☐ Air-Drying Artifact

☐ Poorly Preserved Pattern

☐ Clot Artifact Pattern

☐ Staining Artifact Pattern

PAUCICELLULAR PATTERN

The paucicellular pattern refers to specimens which contain some but less than the desired number of cells of interest. Generally, this number varies depending on specimen type and preparation and often relies on the subjective impression of the reviewing pathologist rather than well-established, evidence-based cut-off values (Table 8.2). Paucicellular specimens may prevent a definitive diagnosis of malignancy due to the lack of sufficient cells for such a diagnosis or, in the absence of any atypical cells, may suggest that a benign diagnosis has an increased risk of being falsely negative. It is often useful to indicate in the diagnosis that the specimen is a "scant specimen" or an "extremely scant specimen" so the clinician can know that the diagnosis was provided on limited material.

LOW-VOLUME PATTERN

Because cytologic specimens are ultimately concentrated, the volume of a specimen usually cannot be determined by microscopic examination. However, this number should be recorded by the laboratory and reviewed at the time a diagnosis is rendered. Studies have indicated that low-volume specimens can be associated with decreased sensitivity in certain

TABLE 8.2: Published Criteria Associated With Increased False-Negative Rates

Specimen Type	Increased False-Negative Rate Associated With
Pleural effusion	Specimen volume of less than 75 mL
Ascites fluid	Specimen volume of less than 80 mL
Voided urine (SurePath)	Specimen volume less than 25 mL
Voided urine (ThinPrep)	Specimen volume less than 25 mL
Voided urine (Cytospin)	Specimen volume less than 30 mL
Urinary tract barbotage (ThinPrep)	20 well-visualized, well-preserved urothelial cells per 10 high-power fields
Instrumented urinary tract specimens	Less than 10 or more than 50 urothelial cells per 10 high-power fields

specimen types, such as pleural effusion specimens (Table 8.2).[3,6-8] In many cases, however, it is uncertain whether these evidence-based cut-offs are sufficient to merit labeling a specimen as inadequate, or simply suboptimal.[9]

FAQ: Is this urinary tract specimen an adequate specimen?

Answer: Very little data exist regarding adequacy in urinary tract specimens.[3-5,8] It is generally accepted that a washing/barbotage specimen should contain some number of urothelial cells, whereas a voided urine specimen may be dilute and, thus, relatively acellular. Generally, it is best to regard samples as "less than optimal" rather than nondiagnostic. Less than optimal specimens have the following varying parameters depending on the specimen type and laboratory preparation: voided urine specimens less than 25 mL in volume; washing/barbotage specimens containing less than 20 urothelial cells per 10 high-power fields (HPF) (ThinPrep preparations) or less than 10 urothelial cells per 10 HPF (Cytospin preparations).

SAMPLE NOTE: LESS THAN OPTIMAL URINARY TRACT SPECIMEN

Negative for high-grade urothelial carcinoma. See note.

Note: The specimen is less than optimal due to its low volume (<25 mL) and the scantiness of the urothelial component. Less than optimal specimens have diminished sensitivity for the detection of high-grade urothelial carcinoma.

Reference:
VandenBussche CJ, Rosenthal DL, Olson MT. Adequacy in voided urine cytology specimens: the role of volume and a repeat void upon predictive values for high-grade urothelial carcinoma. *Cancer Cytopathol.* 2016;124(3):174-180.

SAMPLE NOTE: LESS THAN OPTIMAL PLEURAL FLUID SPECIMEN

Diagnosis: Scant specimen. Rare mesothelial cells, histiocytes, and lymphocytes. See note.

Note: The volume of the submitted specimen was 50 mL. Studies have shown that volumes less than 75 mL are associated with an increased rate of false-negative diagnoses. If a pleural effusion recurs, we recommend submitting a repeat specimen containing more than 75 mL for cytologic analysis.

Reference:
Rooper LM, Ali SZ, Olson MT. A minimum fluid volume of 75 mL is needed to ensure adequacy in a pleural effusion: a retrospective analysis of 2540 cases. *Cancer Cytopathol.* 2014;122(9):657-665.

AIR-DRYING ARTIFACT PATTERN

Air-drying artifact occurs primarily in alcohol-fixed conventional smears. Once smeared, slides must be immediately placed in alcohol, otherwise the smeared material will immediately be exposed to air and begin to dry. While Diff-Quik and similar stains are designed for specimens that have been fixed to the slide by air-drying, the Pap stain is optimized for cells that have been alcohol-fixed to the slide. Immediate exposure to alcohol results in rapid fixation of cells which allows cells to maintain their shape. During the air-drying process, cells flatten as they fix to the slide. This process causes cells to become larger and results in cellular contents to be less densely distributed within compartments. Subsequent staining with the Pap stain results in a pale stain, with severely air-dried specimens resulting in large, pale-staining cells (Figures 8.18-8.23).

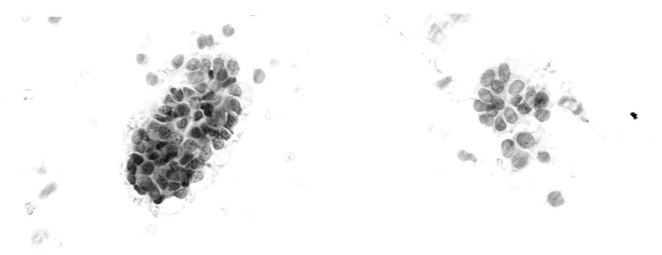

Figure 8.18. Air-drying artifact. The cells in the center tissue fragment retained moisture before being fixed in alcohol, while the adjacent cells and cells in the background were allowed to air-dry before being placed in fixative. The air-dried cells flattened out on the glass slide, making them appear larger and causing them to be pale-staining (Pap stain).

Figure 8.19. Air-drying artifact. In this adjacent field, the cells of interest display some air-drying artifact. Compared with the better preserved cells in the previous figure, here the same cells appear larger and their staining is paler (Pap stain).

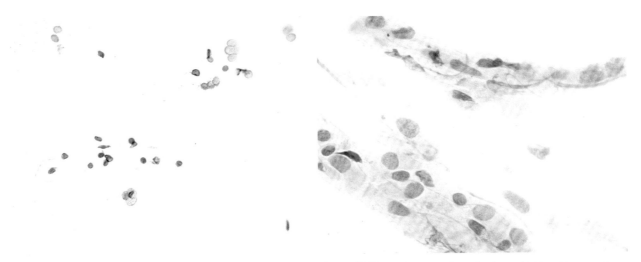

Figure 8.20. Air-drying artifact. All the cyan-staining cells seen here are red blood cells, although they appear as different shapes and sizes. The cells at the top right-hand corner underwent air-drying and thus appear larger and paler than the cells at the center of the field (Pap stain).

Figure 8.21. Air-drying artifact. This bronchial brushing specimen demonstrated significant air-drying artifact. The cilia form indistinct red blobs, and both the nuclei and cytoplasm of these cells appear pale. Air-drying artifact is more common during procedures in which the proceduralist is not a pathologist, as they do not see the impact of delayed specimen fixation in alcohol (Pap stain).

KEY FEATURES of Air-Drying Artifact Pattern

- Cells appear to be increased in size, including an increased footprint of cell cytoplasm and nucleus.
- Chromatin and cytoplasmic quality become less detailed
- Air-dried cells have a paler appearance.

POORLY PRESERVED PATTERN

The poorly preserved pattern is seen when the cells of interest in a given specimen have degenerated to a degree that their cytomorphologic features cannot be properly assessed. There are several opportunities for cells to become degenerated before examination, and the pattern will depend on the specimen type and step at which the cells became degenerated.

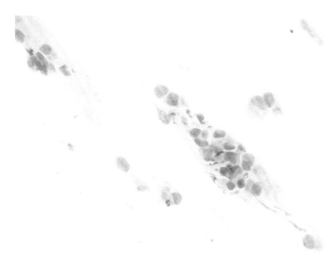

Figure 8.22. Air-drying artifact. Separate field (Pap stain).

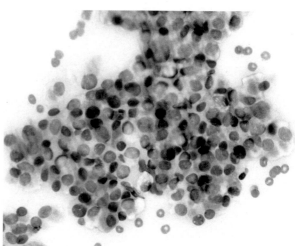

Figure 8.23. Air-drying artifact. This smear was created from the fine-needle aspiration of a benign thyroid nodule. The cells seen are benign thyroid follicular cells on a slide which was not immediately fixed in alcohol following the smearing procedure. The nuclei appear large and are overlapping, with some oval shapes, possibly resulting in an unnecessary diagnosis of *Atypia of Undetermined Significance (AUS)* (Pap stain).

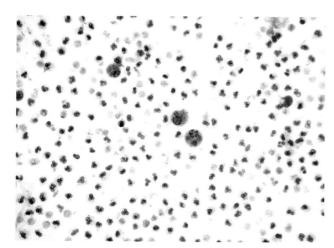

Figure 8.24. Poorly preserved cells. Several degenerated urothelial cells can be seen in a background of acute inflammation. The cells have abundant, granular cytoplasm and small nuclei with karyorrhexis. The small, round cyanophilic cytoplasmic inclusions are known as Melamed-Wolinska bodies and are thought to be condensed lysosomes (Pap stain).

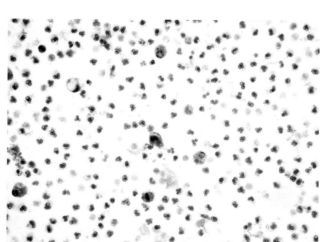

Figure 8.25. Poorly preserved cells. Several degenerated urothelial cells can be seen. Although some nuclei appear quite dark and have markedly irregular borders, the nuclei are simply condensed into a small space and do not contain the increased DNA content that would otherwise be seen in degenerated high-grade urothelial carcinoma cells (Pap stain).

Cells may become degenerated in vivo. This process is especially true in cerebrospinal fluid and voided urine specimens, where cells have naturally exfoliated into fluids and may remain for long periods of time before procurement. The cells are exposed to body temperatures and will begin to degenerate. Similarly, freshly procured specimens will begin to degenerate when kept at room temperature. Degenerative changes include expanded, granular and/or vacuolated cytoplasm, bare/extruded nuclei, pyknosis, indistinct nuclear-cytoplasmic interface, and poor chromatin detail (Figures 8.24-8.28).

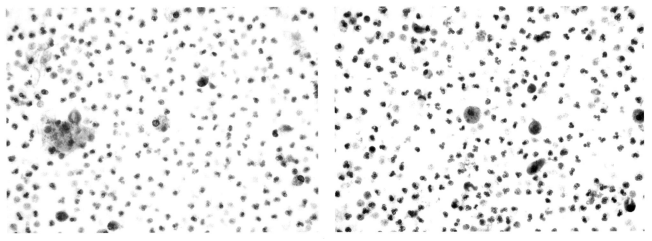

Figure 8.26. Poorly preserved cells. Separate field (Pap stain).   Figure 8.27. Poorly preserved cells. Separate field (Pap stain).

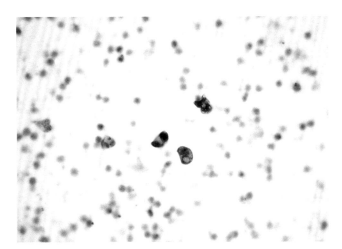

Figure 8.28. Poorly preserved cells. In poorly preserved cells, the interface between the nucleus and cytoplasm cannot be appreciated at high magnification. At low magnification, the degenerated nucleus may appear dark and cause concern (Pap stain).

KEY FEATURES of Poorly Preserved Pattern
- The nuclear-cytoplasmic interface becomes poorly defined.
- Cytoplasmic borders become less distinct.
- The cytoplasm becomes expanded, with or without vacuolization.
- The background may contain extruded or "bare" nuclei.
- Condensed, pyknotic nuclei may be seen.
- Cytoplasmic elements become condensed.

CLOT ARTIFACT PATTERN

Clot artifact occurs on conventional smears in specimens contaminated with blood. Blood will quickly begin to clot and may clot inside a fine-needle aspiration (FNA) needle if not immediately discharged onto a glass slide and smeared. If a specimen is not smeared quickly enough, clots will begin to form as well. This phenomenon is seen more frequently in endoscopic procedures owing to the increased time needed to transfer specimen from the procedure to the glass slide. Another common setting is in an outpatient office in which a clinician performs FNA and also needs to smear slides; in this case, the clinician may not have time to smear the slide before the clot forms, or he or she may transfer several passes to the slides and smear the slides at the end of the procedure.

Clot artifact is noticeable because a rust-colored clot material will be present in clumps and contain the majority of lesional cells. Clot material will attach to lesional cells and exert physical forces as the clot forms, causing alterations in cellular and nuclear shapes (Figures 8.29-8.42). The formation of clot around lesional cells may also slow alcohol fixation, resulting in some amount of air-drying artifact. Clot material may also limit stain penetration, causing staining artifacts (see below).

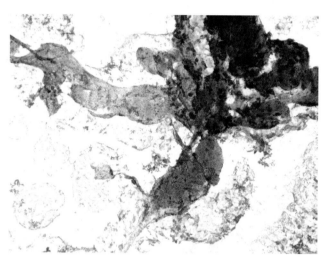

Figure 8.29. Clot artifact. This thyroid was spray-fixed with alcohol following smearing, resulting in an uneven distribution of cells on the glass slide. In addition, the specimen began to clot before it was smeared, causing thick areas that entrap and obscure the cells of interest (Pap stain).

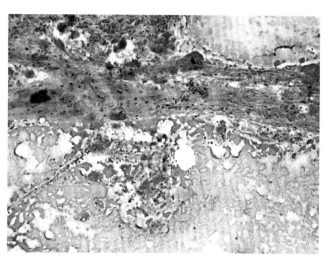

Figure 8.30. Clot artifact. Cystic macrophages and benign thyroid follicular cells are entrapped in clot material. Instead of having their usual round and regular nuclei, the follicular cells in the clot material have elongated nuclei, a feature seen in papillary thyroid carcinoma (Diff-Quik stain).

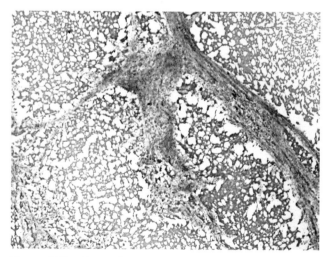

Figure 8.31. Clot artifact. The presence of a clot is suggested by streaming, thickened areas on the slide which in this case appear more red (due to entrapped red blood cells) and blue (due to thickened serum and/or colloid) than the background (Diff-Quik stain).

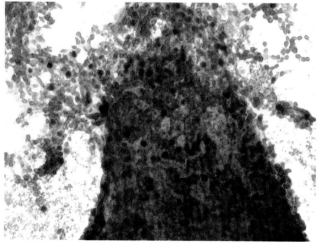

Figure 8.32. Clot artifact. Benign follicular cell nuclei are entrapped along with intact red blood cells in clot material. At the edges of the fragment, the nuclei stain differently than the red blood cells. Within the thickened clot, the epithelial cells are obscured and poorly stained and are difficult to distinguish from the adjacent red blood cells (Pap stain).

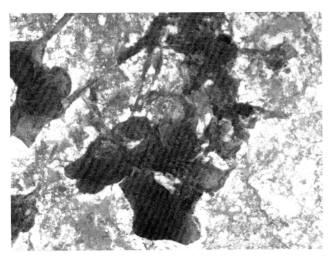

Figure 8.33. Clot artifact. The clot material in this smear from a thyroid fine-needle aspiration (FNA) forms a papillary formation, causing concern for an obscured papillary thyroid carcinoma (Pap stain).

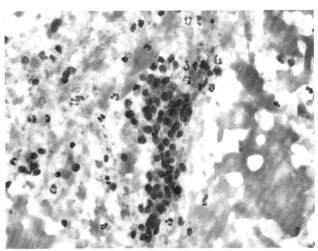

Figure 8.34. Clot artifact. Benign follicular cells entrapped in clot material have indistinct cytoplasm and artifactually enlarged, elongated nuclei. Unfortunately, this can result in an indeterminate diagnosis even though benign thyroid follicular cells caught in clot material rarely have a more reassuring appearance (Diff-Quik stain).

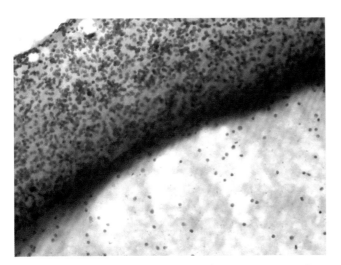

Figure 8.35. Clot artifact. This fine-needle aspiration (FNA) from a mediastinal lymph node began to clot in the needle before being aspirated onto the glass slide. The majority of lymphocytes are trapped within the clot material; note how the lymphocytes outside the clot are easier to examine (Diff-Quik stain).

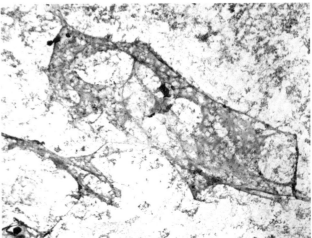

Figure 8.36. Clot artifact. This clot was forming as the slide was smeared, causing a weblike structure in this field. This can potentially be mistaken for mucin or myxoid matrix material (Pap stain).

STAINING ARTIFACT PATTERN

The staining artifact pattern refers to specimens in which the staining process has improperly stained the cells in a specimen. This artifact most commonly occurs in large, three-dimensional fragments; in this case, some stain components may not penetrate into the middle of the fragments, causing an unusual coloring to cells in the center of a fragment while cells at the edges of a fragment stain properly. This result can cause the center of tissue fragments on the Pap stain to appear pink, whereas cells stained by Diff-Quik appear to lose cellular and nuclear details (Figures 8.43 and 8.44).

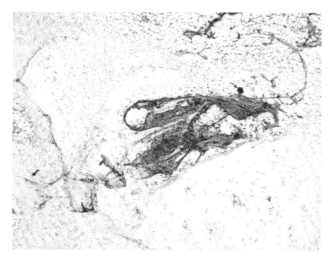

Figure 8.37. Clot artifact. A weblike clot has been smeared across this field and contains the majority of lymphocytes aspirated from a lymph node. Lymphocytes are essentially absent outside the clot material (Pap stain).

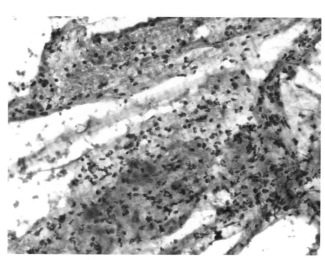

Figure 8.38. Clot artifact. Clot material often concentrates neutrophils from the blood. Here, a mixture of lymphocytes, rare bronchial respiratory epithelial cells, and neutrophils are trapped in the clot material (Diff-Quik stain).

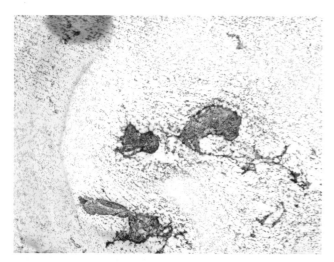

Figure 8.39. Clot artifact. These small clots containing lymphocytes can give the impression of epithelial tissue fragments at low magnification (Diff-Quik stain).

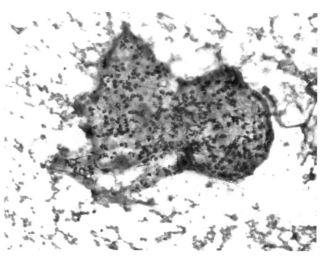

Figure 8.40. Clot artifact. Higher magnification of the previous field (Diff-Quik stain).

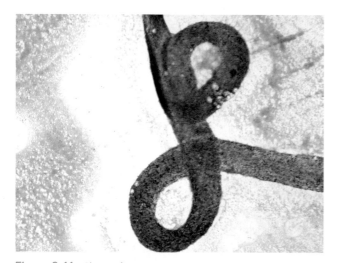

Figure 8.41. Clot artifact. A worm-like clot has formed in the needle, resulting in a concentration of lymphocytes within the clot rather than evenly distributed throughout the slide (Diff-Quik stain).

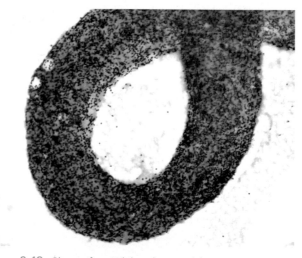

Figure 8.42. Clot artifact. While suboptimal for examination, the cells within the clot can clearly be identified as small lymphocytes intermixed with rare adipocytes, both normal components of the targeted lymph node (Diff-Quik stain).

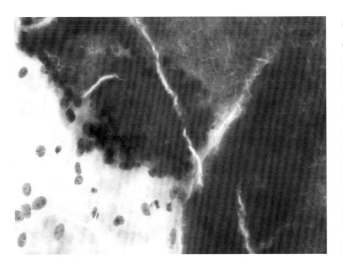

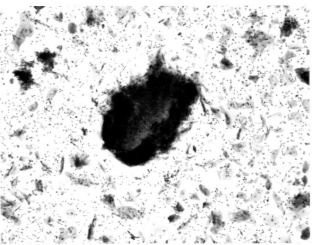

Figure 8.43. Stain artifact. This conventional smear was not allowed to completely dry before the Diff-Quik stain was applied. The cells at the edge were able to dry and stain appropriately; the eosin-containing solution did not have enough time to displace the water and stain the centrally located cells (Diff-Quik stain).

Figure 8.44. Stain artifact. This large fragment was not penetrated properly by all the stain components of the Pap stain, resulting in an even stain around the fragment edges and a predominantly red stain in the center of the fragment. This phenomenon can sometimes be mistaken for the true orangeophilic stain seen in keratinizing cells. This artifact is rarely seen in ThinPrep preparations, as large three-dimensional fragments are more likely to be removed (Pap stain).

Staining artifact can also be seen when an area of a slide is not exposed to one or more stain components. This staining irregularity can be caused by an improper manual stain technique, an automatic stainer malfunction, or the presence of interfering substances (Figures 8.45 and 8.46).

PEARLS & PITFALLS

Cytology specimens are limited and typically cannot provide the same amount of information as small tissue biopsy specimens or larger resection specimens. While it is important to provide an assessment of adequacy to the clinician, a "nondiagnostic" diagnosis should be avoided if a descriptive diagnosis can be provided instead. A definitive diagnosis of malignancy or a diagnosis completely excluding malignancy may not be possible, but even small details can help guide the clinical team.

FAQ: Should I call a suboptimal specimen atypical and be done with it?

Answer: A suboptimal specimen alone is not a sufficient cause to provide an indeterminate (or "atypical") diagnosis. An atypical diagnosis should be provided to indicate that the patient is at an increased risk of dysplasia or neoplasia. If cytologic atypia seen is due to a suboptimal specimen, these concerns should be noted in the diagnosis and possibly directly related to the clinical team, who may decide to obtain a new specimen as the best course of action. Making a diagnosis of "atypical cells" without further qualification in such a circumstance may result in a patient undergoing a more invasive procedure unnecessarily.

OTHERS

LIQUID-BASED PREPARATION PATTERN

It has become more common for liquid-based preparations (LBPs) to replace conventional smear preparations. LBPs allow for specimens to be collected more easily by clinicians and prevents issues with conventional smears (such as air-drying artifact) when a dedicated

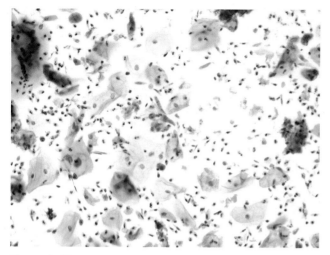

Figure 8.45. Stain artifact. An area on this slide was not exposed evenly to all components of the Pap stain, resulting in aberrant pink staining. Unlike the previous example, this is not due to the specimen but rather due to improper stain technique or the presence of an interfering factor on this area of the slide (Pap stain).

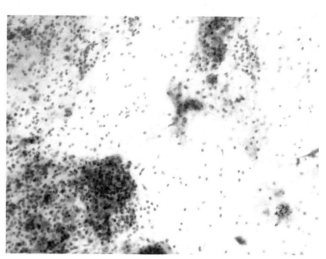

Figure 8.46. Stain artifact. Uneven staining resulting in uneven colorization throughout the field (Pap stain).

TABLE 8.3: Some Cytomorphologic Differences in Liquid-Based Preparations, as Compared With Conventional Preparations

Conventional Smears	Liquid-Based Preparations
Air-drying artifact more likely	No air-drying artifact
Increased cellularity (entire specimen may be smeared on a single slide)	Decreased cellularity (residual material remains)
Maintains tissue fragments of all sizes	Large tissue fragments less likely to be transferred to the slide (ThinPrep > SurePath)
Increased background elements (debris, blood, etc.)	Decreased background elements, resulting in a "clean" background (ThinPrep > SurePath)
Tumor diathesis in background	Tumor diathesis primarily seen attached to intact cells ("clinging diathesis")
Maintained cell cohesion (e.g., preserved "molding" of small cell carcinoma)	Cells more likely to be dispersed (e.g., loss of "molding" in small cell carcinoma)
Increased smearing (crush) artifact (e.g., "lymphoid tangles" in lymphocyte populations)	Decreased smearing (crush) artifact

technician, pathologist, or cytotechnologist is not present to create the smears. However, LBPs can result in certain artifacts that are not present in conventional smears, and some diagnostically useful artifacts found in conventional smears are not seen in LBPs (Table 8.3).[10-15]

SMEARING ARTIFACT PATTERN

The creation of conventional smears requires cells to be smeared onto glass slides. The forces exerted on cells during the smearing process can disrupt cytomorphology. Lymphocytes and small round blue cell neoplasms (such as small cell carcinoma) are particularly fragile, resulting in the "streaking" of chromatin in the direction of the smear (Figures 8.47-8.52).[11] These artifacts are reduced or not seen in LBPs.

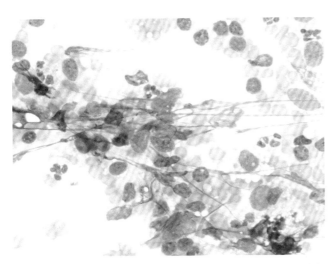

Figure 8.47. Smearing artifact. Lymphoid cells have more delicate chromatin which has a tendency to "streak" in the direction a specimen was smeared. These are sometimes known as "lymphoid tangles" and are not usually seen on liquid-based preparations (Diff-Quik stain).

Figure 8.48. Smearing artifact. Prominent lymphoid tangles are seen surrounded by dispersed lymphoid cells (Pap stain).

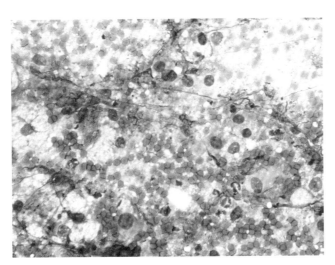

Figure 8.49. Smearing artifact. Lymphoid tangles are seen intermixed with epithelioid histiocytes in a fine-needle aspiration (FNA) specimen sampling a necrotizing granuloma. Lymphoid tangles are often seen more prominently in granulomatous inflammation, a situation in which the artifact helps rather than hinders a diagnosis (Diff-Quik stain).

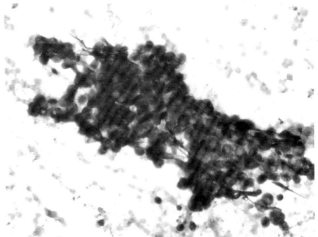

Figure 8.50. Smearing artifact. Small cell carcinoma, demonstrating nuclear molding as well as the "chromatin streaking" artifact, both of which help in making a cytomorphologic diagnosis. Both features are reduced or absent in liquid-based preparations (Diff-Quik).

BRUSHING ARTIFACT PATTERN

The use of a brush to spread cells onto a slide results in additional physical forces to be exerted on these cells.[16] Cells are more likely to be disrupted from fragments, causing the presence of smaller fragments as well as singly dispersed cells. Cells may also be stretched by the brushing process, causing alterations in cell shape (Figures 8.53-8.58).

WASHING ARTIFACT PATTERN

Washings (lavages and barbotages) are sometimes taken from the urinary tract, respiratory tract, gastrointestinal tract, bile duct, and peritoneal cavity. While washings do not typically disrupt cellular morphology to the degree of brushings, washings often disrupt large amounts of benign lining epithelial cells such as urothelial fragments (urinary tract) and mesothelial sheets (peritoneal washings) (Figures 8.59-8.62).[16] These numerous large fragments may be misinterpreted as neoplastic; if properly recognized as benign, they may outnumber and obscure lesional cells, causing a missed or suboptimal diagnosis.

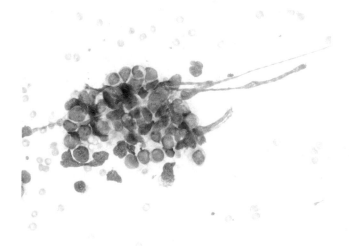

Figure 8.51. Smearing artifact. Small cell carcinoma, separate field (Diff-Quik stain).

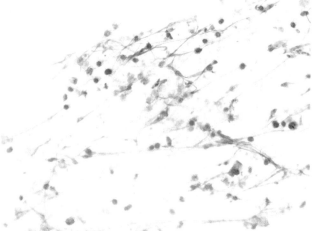

Figure 8.52. Smearing artifact. Small cell carcinoma with prominent chromatin streaking. The cells can be distinguished from lymphocytes because they are slightly larger, have round to oval nuclei that lack angulation, and have little to absent cytoplasm (Pap stain).

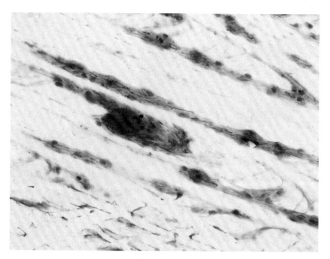

Figure 8.53. Brushing artifact. This bronchial brushing specimen was created by the brushing of cells onto the slide. While the act of brushing to forcibly exfoliate cells can exert physical forces that alter morphology, these bronchial respiratory cells were likely brushed too forcibly onto the glass slide (Diff-Quik stain).

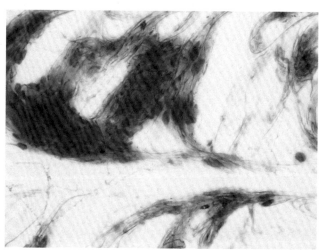

Figure 8.54. Brushing artifact. The forces of the brushing have caused the cells to have enlarged and elongated nuclei and their columnar shape has been lost. Their cilia are no longer identifiable as such (Diff-Quik stain).

NEAR MISS

CLOGGED THINPREP FILTER

ThinPrep technology uses a proprietary filter that under most circumstances selects for cells of interest and selects against large, uninterpretable fragments. In bloody specimens, blood components may preferentially stick to the filter and reduce the number of lesional cells attached to the filter (reducing the number of lesional cells transferred to the specimen slide). Unfortunately, bloody diathesis is sometimes seen in patients with cervical carcinoma, resulting in a decreased number of evaluable lesional cells and an increased chance of a falsely negative diagnosis.[17] Diagnosis is further hampered by the presence of obscuring material. Specimens may contain a thin peripheral "ring" of bloody

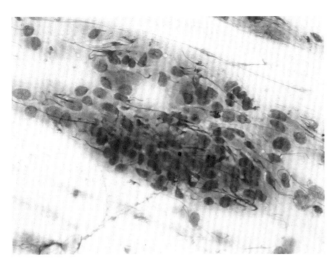

Figure 8.55. Brushing artifact. Separate field (Diff-Quik stain).

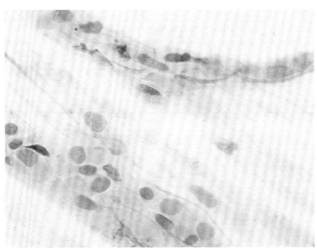

Figure 8.56. Brushing artifact. This brushing specimen contains bronchial respiratory epithelial cells and suffers from two artifacts. The first is the brushing artifact, causing the cells to be elongated and misshapen. The second is an air-drying artifact, causing the cells to be further enlarged and pale-stained (Pap stain).

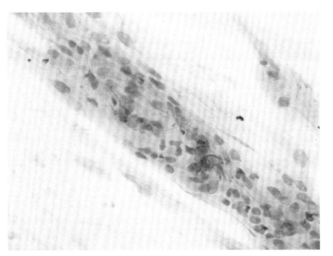

Figure 8.57. Brushing artifact. Separate field (Pap stain).

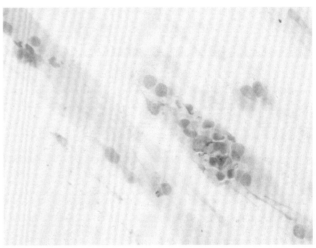

Figure 8.58. Brushing artifact. Separate field (Pap stain).

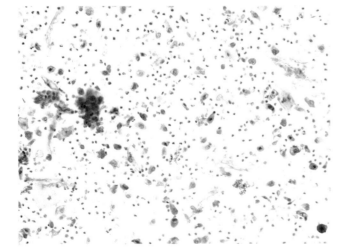

Figure 8.59. Washing artifact. The use of a washing or barbotage to forcibly exfoliate cells does not usually dramatically alter their cytomorphology. However, this process can result in the sampling of large numbers of benign cells that would not otherwise be seen in a naturally exfoliated specimen (such as voided urine). The increased cellularity may cause suspicion for a neoplasm (Pap stain).

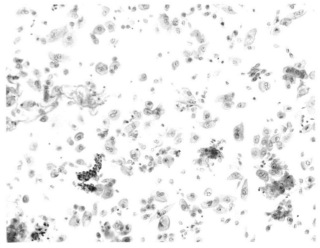

Figure 8.60. Washing artifact. This specimen contains numerous umbrella cells, seen as large cells with abundant, granular cytoplasm and one to two nuclei. It would be unusual to see cells in such great numbers in a voided urine specimen (Pap stain).

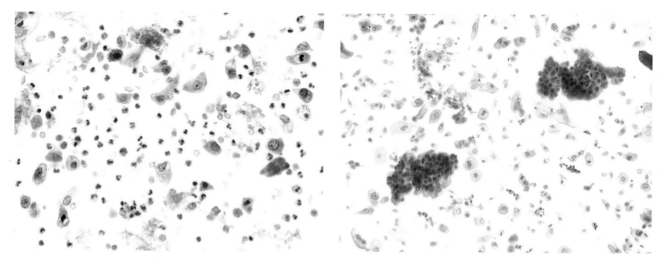

Figure 8.61. Washing artifact. Separate field (Pap stain).

Figure 8.62. Washing artifact. This urinary tract washing specimen contains two medium-sized tissue fragments of benign urothelial cells. It is unusual to see such fragments in voided urine specimens, although they may occur in patients with urolithiasis. The presence of urothelial tissue fragments may cause concern for a papillary urothelial neoplasm (Pap stain).

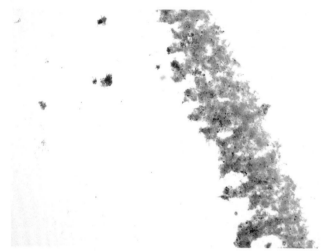

Figure 8.63. Clogged ThinPrep filter. This Pap test specimen contains abundant blood and granular debris, which clogged the filter and blocked transfer of material to the glass slide, except in the peripheral area of the ThinPrep circle. This results in a dramatic decrease in the number of cells of interest that can be examined (Pap stain).

Figure 8.64. Clogged ThinPrep filter. Separate field. Note the presence of cells trapped in the red debris which can be examined at higher magnification (Pap stain).

diathesis containing rare malignant cells, with rare to absent material in the center of the ring (Figures 8.63-8.66). In specimens containing blood or degenerated blood in which material is not evenly distributed throughout the ThinPrep circle, treatment with glacial acetic acid can improve cellular yield.[18]

OVERINTERPRETING BACKGROUND BENIGN CELLS

If an inadequate specimen is called adequate, the clinician and patient will be falsely reassured, and a repeat specimen may not be taken. This practice can result in delay of treatment that can be harmful to the patient. This scenario commonly arises when

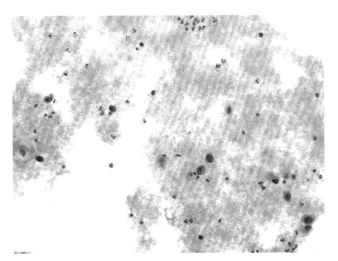

Figure 8.65. Clogged ThinPrep filter. At higher magnification, markedly atypical cells can be seen with dark, enlarged nuclei and low nuclear to cytoplasmic (N/C) ratios. This patient was found to have a squamous cell carcinoma (Pap stain).

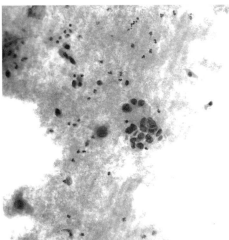

Figure 8.66. Clogged ThinPrep filter. Separate field. Note the highly atypical, keratinizing cells, as well as the small fragment of cells that is diagnostic of at least high-grade squamous intraepithelial lesion (Pap stain).

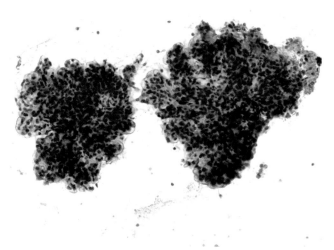

Figure 8.67. Glomeruli. Two glomeruli are seen in this touch preparation. Their papillary structure may be confused for a papillary renal cell carcinoma during on site evaluation. One clue is the empty "rings" (empty capillaries) seen at the edges of the fragments, which are characteristic of glomeruli (Pap stain).

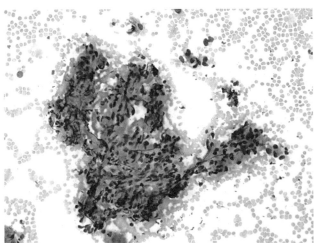

Figure 8.68. Glomerulus. This patient had glomerulonephritis in addition to a renal mass on imaging studies. This glomerulus has become unfolded and contains lymphoid tangles, making it difficult to identify as a nonneoplastic background component (Diff-Quik stain).

benign background cells are mistakenly identified as lesional: for instance, misinterpreting reactive hepatocytes as a metastatic adenocarcinoma or glomeruli as a papillary neoplasm (Figures 8.67 and 8.68). This specific pitfall does not occur for exfoliative specimens, in which a lesion does not necessarily have to be present for a specimen to be considered adequate. Commonly misinterpreted benign elements are listed in Table 8.4.

SMALL CELL CARCINOMA ON LIQUID-BASED PREPARATIONS

Small cell carcinoma is often considered a morphologic diagnosis on surgical pathology specimens. Small cell carcinoma is characterized by several cytomorphologic features on conventional smears, which include the presence of nuclear molding, chromatin smearing, geographic necrosis, and background necrosis. In LBPs, some of these features may be present, especially if the carcinoma cells are present in tissue fragments. However, in some instances the cells may present as a population of discohesive single cells (Figure 8.69). At low magnification, the cells may resemble a population of inflammatory cells. The amount of molding and necrosis is reduced, and chromatin smearing is often absent. At high magnification, these cells may be identified by their small size, minimal to absent cytoplasm, irregular nuclear borders, and anisonucleosis. Intact necrotic cells may also be seen scattered in the background, appearing as "blue blobs" (Figure 8.70).

TABLE 8.4: Commonly Overinterpreted Benign Components During Fine-Needle Aspiration (FNA) at Various Sites

Organ	Background Cells
Liver	Reactive hepatocytes
Kidney	Renal tubular cells Glomeruli
Pancreas	Gastrointestinal contamination (especially gastric epithelium) Benign acinar cells Reactive ductal epithelium
Lung	Reactive bronchial respiratory epithelial cells Pulmonary alveolar macrophages Type II pneumocytes
Lymph node	Germinal center cells Histiocytes

Figure 8.69. Small cell carcinoma. Small cell carcinoma cells are present singly throughout the field. At this low magnification, they may resemble inflammatory cells. Liquid-based preparations reduce certain cytomorphologic features of small cell carcinoma, including nuclear molding, geographic necrosis, background necrosis, and chromatin smearing (Pap stain).

Figure 8.70. Small cell carcinoma. Examination at higher magnification may reveal small clusters of small cell carcinoma that contain diagnostic features. One example is the presence of several necrotic "blue blobs" associated with viable carcinoma cells (Pap stain).

References

1. Nayar R, Wilbur DC. The pap test and Bethesda 2014. *Acta Cytol.* 2015;59(2):121-132.

2. Ali SZ, Cibas ES. *The Bethesda System for Reporting Thyroid Cytopathology: Definitions, Criteria, and Explanatory Notes*: Springer; 2017.

3. VandenBussche CJ, Rosenthal DL, Olson MT. Adequacy in voided urine cytology specimens: the role of volume and a repeat void upon predictive values for high-grade urothelial carcinoma. *Cancer Cytopathol.* 2016;124(3):174-180.

4. Renshaw AA, Gould EW. Evidence-based adequacy criteria for instrumented urine cytology using cytospin preparations. *Diagn Cytopathol.* 2018;46(6):520-521.

5. Prather J, Arville B, Chatt G, et al. Evidence-based adequacy criteria for urinary bladder barbotage cytology. *J Am Soc Cytopathol.* 2015;4(2):57-62.

6. Rooper LM, Ali SZ, Olson MT. A minimum fluid volume of 75 mL is needed to ensure adequacy in a pleural effusion: a retrospective analysis of 2540 cases. *Cancer Cytopathol.* 2014;122(9):657-665.

7. Rooper LM, Ali SZ, Olson MT. A specimen volume of ≥ 80 mL improves cytologic sensitivity for malignant ascites: a retrospective analysis of 2665 cases. *J Am Soc Cytopathol.* 2016;5(5):301-305.

8. Rezaee N, Tabatabai ZL, Olson MT. Adequacy of voided urine specimens prepared by ThinPrep and evaluated using the Paris system for reporting urinary cytology. *J Am Soc Cytopathol.* 2017;6(4):155-161.

9. Renshaw AA, Gould EW. Adequacy criteria for voided urine cytology using cytospin preparations. *Cancer Cytopathol.* 2019;127(2):116-119.

10. Hoda RS, VandenBussche C, Hoda SA. *Liquid-based specimen collection, preparation, and morphology*. In: *Diagnostic Liquid-Based Cytology*: Springer; 2017:1-12.

11. Bavikatty NR, Michael CW. Cytologic features of small-cell carcinoma on ThinPrep®. *Diagn Cytopathol.* 2003;29(1):8-12.

12. Renshaw AA, Young NA, Birdsong GG, et al. Comparison of performance of conventional and ThinPrep gynecologic preparations in the College of American Pathologists Gynecologic Cytology Program. *Arch Pathol Lab Med.* 2004;128(1):17-22.

13. Belsley NA, Tambouret RH, Misdraji J, Muzikansky A, Russell DK, Wilbur DC. Cytologic features of endocervical glandular lesions: comparison of SurePath, ThinPrep, and conventional smear specimen preparations. *Diagn Cytopathol.* 2008;36(4):232-237.

14. Tulecke MA, Wang HH. ThinPrep® for cytologic evaluation of follicular thyroid lesions: correlation with histologic findings. *Diagn Cytopathol.* 2004;30(1):7-13.

15. Biscotti CV, Hollow JA, Toddy SM, Easley KA. ThinPrep versus conventional smear cytologic preparations in the analysis of thyroid fine-needle aspiration specimens. *Am J Clin Pathol.* 1995;104(2):150-153.

16. Nodi L, Balassanian R, Sudilovsky D, Raab SS. Improving the quality of cytology diagnosis: root cause analysis for errors in bronchial washing and brushing specimens. *Am J Clin Pathol.* 2005;124(6):883-892.

17. Chacho MS, Mattie ME, Schwartz PE. Cytohistologic correlation rates between conventional Papanicolaou smears and ThinPrep cervical cytology: a comparison. *Cancer Cytopathol.* 2003;99(3):135-140.

18. Agoff SN, Dean T, Nixon BK, Ingalls-Severn K, Rinker L, Grieco VS. The efficacy of reprocessing unsatisfactory cervicovaginal ThinPrep specimens with and without glacial acetic acid: effect on Hybrid Capture II human papillomavirus testing and clinical follow-up. *Am J Clin Pathol.* 2002;118(5):727-732.

CHAPTER 1. FINE-NEEDLE ASPIRATION OF THE THYROID

1-1. **Which of the following is true regarding the diagnosis for this thyroid FNA specimen?**

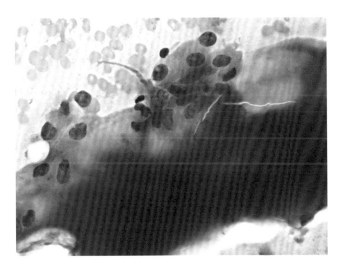

A. Although there is cytologic atypia, the presence of abundant colloid is a reassuring finding that favors categorization as atypia of undetermined significance (AUS).

B. This diagnosis is often associated with *RAS* mutations.

C. *BRAF* mutations are found in approximately 45% of these cases.

D. Rare intranuclear pseudoinclusions should not be interpreted as features of papillary thyroid carcinoma in this lesion displaying Hurthle cell features.

1-2. **Which of the following would be the least reasonable approach when encountering this finding on thyroid FNA?**

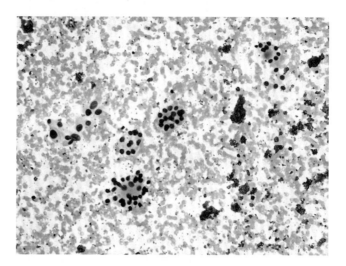

    A. Repeat fine-needle aspiration

    B. Molecular testing

    C. Thyroid lobectomy

    D. Near-total thyroidectomy

1-3. **These cells were seen in one field of a thyroid FNA specimen. What additional finding would explain the morphology of these cells?**

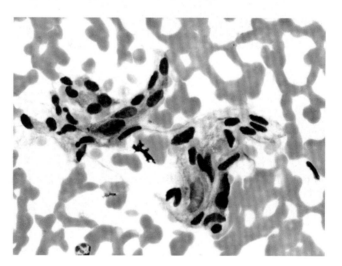

    A. Cystic macrophages

    B. Elevated cyst fluid parathyroid hormone

    C. Intranuclear pseudoinclusions

    D. "Bubble gum" colloid

1-4. **Which of the following is true regarding the presence of numerous lymphocytes seen on a thyroid FNA?**

    A. In the absence of thyroid follicular cells, the specimen should be considered nondiagnostic.

    B. The patient has an increased risk of lymphoma.

    C. A definitive diagnosis of papillary thyroid carcinoma is not possible.

    D. The additional presence of multinucleated giant cells is a reassuring finding.

1-5. **Which of the following is (are) the most reliable feature(s) for identifying papillary thyroid carcinoma in a cystic background?**

    A. The presence of cells with numerous, small cytoplasmic vacuoles.

    B. The presence of cells with enlarged nuclei and irregular nuclear contours.

    C. The presence of cells with high N/C ratios and overlapping nuclei.

    D. The presence of cells with enlarged nuclei in an absence of colloid.

1-6. **These cells were identified on a thyroid FNA specimen. What would be the most reasonable panel of immunostains to perform?**

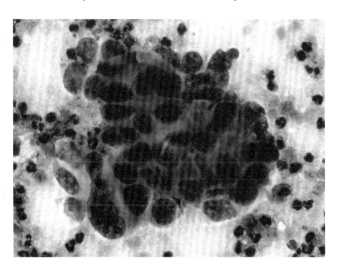

    A. TTF-1, thyroglobulin, and napsin A

    B. TTF-1, napsin A, and Pax-8

    C. Calcitonin, thyroglobulin, and synaptophysin

    D. TTF-1, napsin A, and GATA-3

1-7. **This finding was identified on the FNA of an indeterminate thyroid nodule. Which of the following is true?**

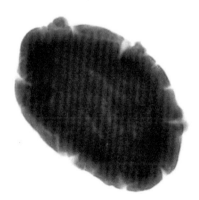

    A. Even in the absence of atypical cells, a diagnosis of at least Suspicious for Papillary Thyroid Carcinoma is indicated.

    B. The finding is reassuring and is consistent with a benign nodule.

    C. The patient has elevated serum calcitonin levels.

    D. This finding is less likely to be seen on liquid-based preparations than conventional smears.

1-8. **What is the most common neoplasm to metastasize to the thyroid gland?**
   A. Lung adenocarcinoma
   B. Colorectal adenocarcinoma
   C. Medulloblastoma
   D. Renal cell carcinoma

CHAPTER 2. SALIVARY GLAND AND CERVICAL LYMPH NODES

2-1. **Which of the following salivary gland lesions is most likely to produce the fine-needle aspiration findings from the image seen here?**

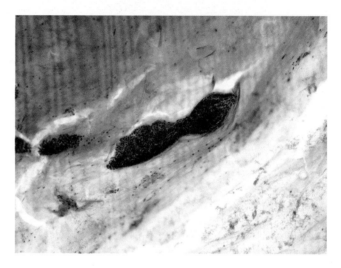

   A. Warthin tumor
   B. Pleomorphic adenoma
   C. Secretory carcinoma
   D. Low-grade mucoepidermoid carcinoma

2-2. **Which of the following statements is FALSE regarding parotid gland lesion seen here?**

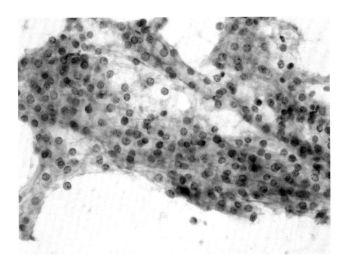

    A. These neoplasms are often bilateral and associated with smoking.

    B. Even though approximately 1/3 of cases locally recur, the 5-year survival approaches 90%.

    C. The presence of tumor-associated lymphoid proliferation (TALP) can mimic lymph node involvement.

    D. Immunochemical staining for DOG1 is likely to be positive.

2-3. **What is the most diagnostically useful feature present on this fine-needle aspiration smear from a salivary gland mass?**

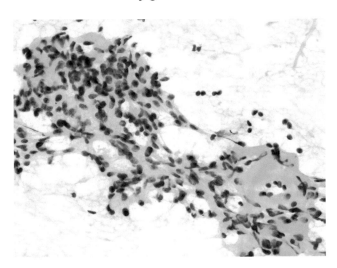

    A. Metachromatic fibrillary chondromyxoid material

    B. Dense, light green mucopolysaccharide material surrounded by basaloid cells

    C. Amyloid deposition

    D. Keratinization

2-4. **What is the best diagnosis based on the following field from an FNA of a parotid mass?**

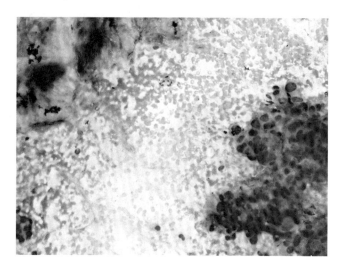

A. Low-grade mucoepidermoid carcinoma

B. Salivary duct carcinoma

C. Pleomorphic adenoma

D. Carcinoma ex pleomorphic adenoma

2-5. **Which of the following gene fusions is commonly associated with the diagnosis below?**

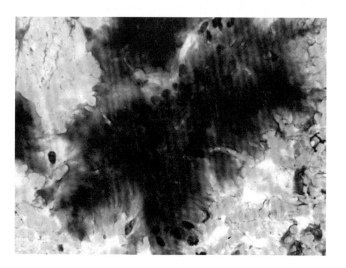

A. *CRTC1-MAML2*

B. *PLAG1*

C. *MYB-NFIB*

D. *ETV6-NTRK3*

CHAPTER 3. PULMONARY

3-1. **Which of the following mutations must be tested in all lung adenocarcinomas?**

    A. *EGFR, KRAS, ALK*

    B. *EGFR, ALK, ROS1*

    C. *EGFR, KRAS, ROS1*

    D. *KRAS, ALK, ROS1*

3-2. **Which of the following statements is true regarding this FNA from a lung tumor?**

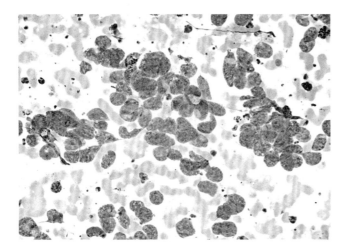

    A. Immunohistochemistry is required to make a definitive diagnosis.

    B. Patients with these tumors have a relatively good prognosis compared with other primary lung tumors.

    C. These tumors typically have high N/C ratios, necrosis, and few mitotic figures.

    D. Distinguishing these tumors from other primary lung tumors has important therapeutic implications.

3-3. **Which of the following statements is true regarding this FNA from a lung nodule?**

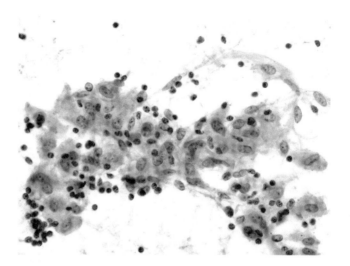

A. Microbiological workup should be performed to rule out an infectious etiology.

B. This lesion demonstrates a second population of enlarged, malignant cells.

C. The lungs are an uncommon primary site for this lesion.

D. A definitive diagnosis can usually be made on cytology alone.

3-4. **Which of the following statements is true regarding this finding, seen in a bronchoalveolar lavage (BAL) specimen?**

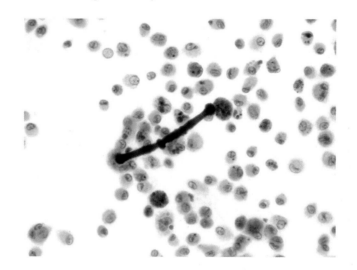

A. It is a nonspecific finding and further workup is not indicated.

B. The specimen does not meet adequacy criteria.

C. The finding should be reported, as it may be associated with a malignant process.

D. Microbiological workup should be performed to rule out an infectious etiology.

3-5. **These cells were identified from the FNA of a lung lesion. Which of the following is true?**

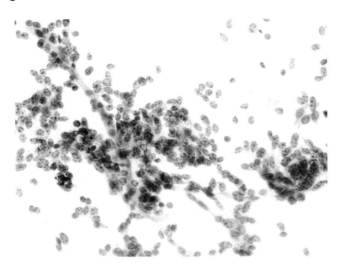

A. A Ki-67 proliferation index is expected to be highly elevated (>90%).

B. The presence of these cells in a lymph node does not change the prognosis.

C. Napsin A is expected to be negative in these cells.

D. A silver stain should be ordered to exclude the presence of organisms.

3-6. **An FNA of a pulmonary nodule produced these cells. The morphology seen here is classically associated with which of the following?**

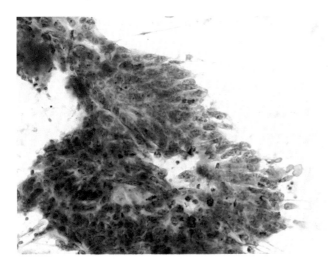

A. Lung adenocarcinoma

B. Atypical carcinoid tumor

C. Metastatic adenocarcinoma

D. Mesothelioma

CHAPTER 4. HEPATOPANCREATOBILIARY

4-1. **Which of the following statements is true regarding the lesion seen below?**

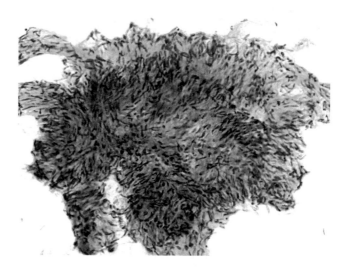

    A. The liver is the most common primary site for this lesion.

    B. The majority of these lesions are malignant.

    C. Pleomorphism is a common morphologic feature of this lesion.

    D. Immunohistochemistry is essential to make a definitive diagnosis.

4-2. **Which of the following statements is true regarding this pancreatic fine-needle aspiration sample?**

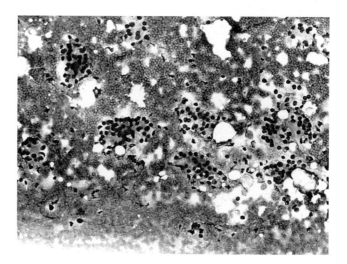

    A. The finding is benign, and no intervention is indicated based on this sample.

    B. The lesion is immunoreactive for synaptophysin and chromogranin.

    C. Positive staining with trypsin helps to confirm the diagnosis.

    D. The differential diagnosis includes adenocarcinoma.

4-3. **A cystic lesion in the head of the pancreas is aspirated. Which of the following statements is NOT true regarding this lesion?**

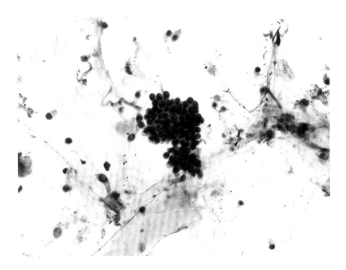

A. This lesion has high-risk features that have important clinical implications.

B. Cytology is not a reliable modality for grading these lesions.

C. A cyst fluid CEA level of 2000 ng/mL is compatible with this lesion.

D. Invasive adenocarcinoma is in the differential for this lesion.

4-4. **A fine-needle aspiration of a liver nodule was performed. Which of the following statements is LEAST LIKELY to be true regarding this lesion?**

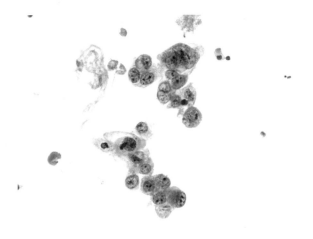

A. The cells are malignant, but a definitive diagnosis cannot be made based on these cytomorphologic features alone.

B. Albumin in situ hybridization would be helpful in this case.

C. Glypican-3 would be a helpful immunostain in this case.

D. This is most likely a primary liver lesion.

4-5. **What is true about this finding in a pancreatic FNA?**

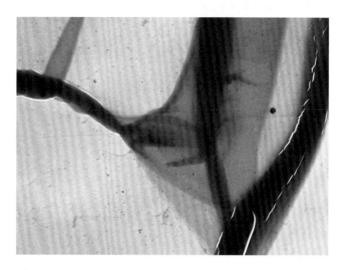

    A. In the absence of epithelial cells, the specimen should be considered nondiagnostic.

    B. The finding is diagnostic of a neoplastic process.

    C. The specimen is expected to have low levels of CEA and amylase.

    D. This finding is characteristic of fluid taken from a serous cystadenoma.

4-6. **The FNA of a pancreatic tail mass demonstrated this finding. What immunopanel would be the most useful to characterize this mass?**

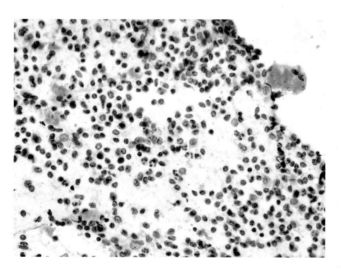

    A. CD8 and CD45

    B. Synaptophysin and chromogranin

    C. β-catenin and CD10

    D. BCL10 and trypsin

CHAPTER 5. SEROUS EFFUSION CYTOPATHOLOGY

5-1. **Atypical epithelial cells were found on a cell block preparation made from an ascites fluid specimen. After a panel of immunostains were performed, the atypical cells were found to be positive for MOC-31 and negative for calretinin. What additional finding would strongly suggest these cells are malignant?**

   A. Diffuse nuclear staining for Pax-8.
   B. Patchy nuclear staining for estrogen receptor (ER).
   C. Diffuse nuclear staining for p53.
   D. Diffuse membranous staining for BerEP4.

5-2. **A pleural fluid specimen was submitted to the cytopathology laboratory. A BAP-1 immunostain was performed on cell block material, resulting in this finding. What is the most likely diagnosis?**

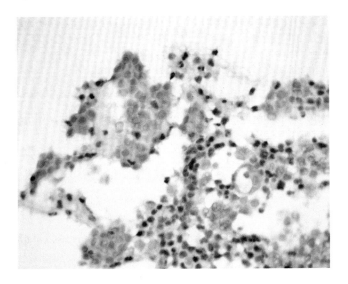

   A. Mesothelioma
   B. Involvement by a borderline serous neoplasm
   C. Metastatic lung adenocarcinoma
   D. Small cell carcinoma

5-3. **Which of the following is true about this finding in an ascites fluid specimen?**

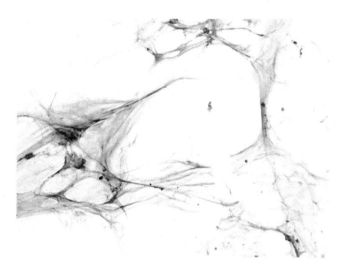

A. The finding is associated with a neoplastic process.

B. The finding is associated with an infectious process.

C. The finding is associated with iatrogenic material.

D. The finding is associated with an "empty tap."

5-4. **Which of the following is most likely to be seen as cells within tissue fragments in a serous cavity specimen?**

A. Melanoma

B. Sarcoma

C. Lobular breast carcinoma

D. Mesothelioma

5-5. **Which of the following is true regarding psammomatous calcification when seen in serous cavity specimens?**

A. The presence of psammomatous calcification is strongly associated with malignancy when found in a pelvic washing specimen.

B. The presence of abundant psammoma bodies is more commonly seen in high-grade serous carcinomas and less commonly in borderline serous neoplasms.

C. Psammoma bodies may be associated with benign mesothelial proliferations.

D. Metastatic papillary thyroid carcinoma is the most common cause of psammoma bodies in the pericardial cavity.

5-6 **Which of the following immunomarkers used during a carcinoma of unknown primary workup are both considered nuclear stains?**

A. CDX2 and CK20

B. NKX3.1 and PSA

C. HepPar1 and arginase

D. GATA-3 and ER

CHAPTER 6. URINARY TRACT

6-1. **Which is true regarding these cells seen in a voided urine specimen?**

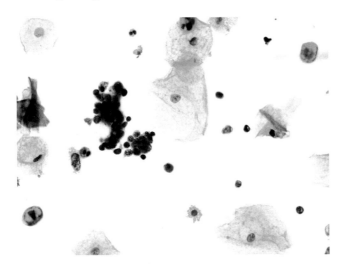

    A. These cells originate from the kidney.

    B. These cells may be associated with a history of prostate adenocarcinoma.

    C. These cells are commonly seen following treatment with BCG.

    D. These cells are associated with *Proteus* infection.

6-2. **Which of the following is best represented in this field, seen in a voided urine specimen?**

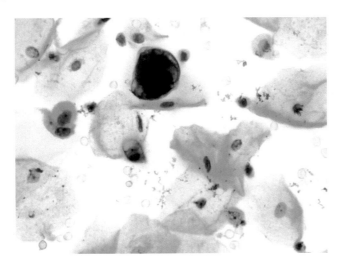

    A. BK polyomavirus

    B. High-grade urothelial carcinoma

    C. Melamed-Wolinska body

    D. Low-grade urothelial neoplasm

6-3. **Which of the following should be categorized as** *Suspicious for High-Grade Urothelial Carcinoma (SHGUC)* **according to The Paris System (TPS), when found in a voided urine specimen?**

    A. Twelve cells with coarse chromatin, markedly irregular nuclear borders, hyperchromasia, and N/C ratios of 0.6.

    B. Six cells with coarse chromatin, markedly irregular nuclear borders, hyperchromasia, and N/C ratios of 0.8.

    C. One cell with hyperchromasia, bland chromatin, regular nuclear borders, and an N/C ratio of 0.6.

    D. Six cells with irregular nuclear borders, hyperchromasia, and N/C ratios of 0.3.

6-4. **This field was seen in an upper tract washing specimen in a patient with a filling defect in the right renal pelvis. Which of the following categories may be used, according to The Paris System (TPS)?**

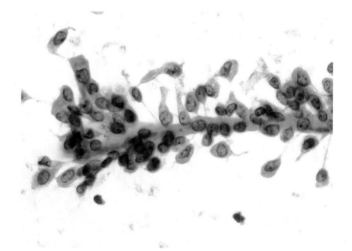

    A. *Negative for High-Grade Urothelial Carcinoma (NHGUC)*

    B. *Atypical Urothelial Cells (AUC)*

    C. *Suspicious for High-Grade Urothelial Carcinoma (SHGUC)*

    D. *High-Grade Urothelial Carcinoma (HGUC)*

6-5. **Which patient history is most compatible with this finding, seen in a voided urine specimen?**

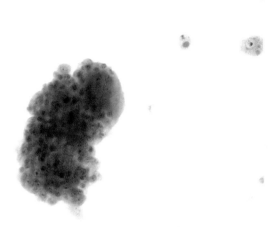

    A. A history of recent treatment with BCG.

    B. A history of untreated high-grade urothelial carcinoma.

    C. A history of incompletely resected low-grade urothelial neoplasm.

    D. A history of an unbiopsied renal cell lesion seen on imaging studies.

6-6. **A 38-year-old woman with recent onset hematuria has a voided urine specimen shown here. Which of the following is LEAST LIKELY to help identify the etiology of this finding?**

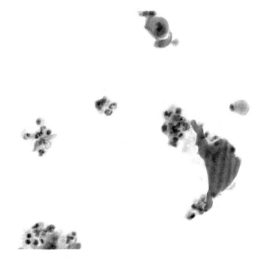

    A. A subsequent urine specimen collected through a catheter.

    B. Staining of cell block material created from residual specimen with a p40 immunostain.

    C. Referral of the patient for a Pap test.

    D. Performance of high-risk HPV studies on a cell block created from residual specimen.

CHAPTER 7. GYNECOLOGIC TRACT CYTOPATHOLOGY

7-1. **What is the most common subtype of HPV associated with invasive squamous cell carcinoma in the United States?**

   A. HPV 16
   B. HPV 18
   C. HPV 45
   D. HPV 53

7-2. **What is the most common type of cell/lesion associated with hyperchromatic crowded groups seen on cervical Pap test specimens?**

   A. Reactive endocervical cells
   B. High-grade squamous intraepithelial lesion (HSIL)
   C. Adenocarcinoma in situ (AIS)
   D. Squamous cell carcinoma

7-3. **These cells were identified on a cervical Pap test specimen. What is the best diagnosis?**

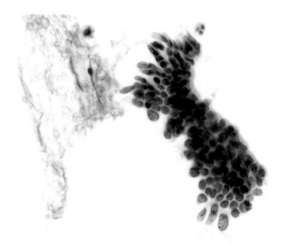

   A. High-grade squamous intraepithelial lesion (HSIL)
   B. Atypical glandular cells (AGC)
   C. Adenocarcinoma in situ (AIS)
   D. Endocervical adenocarcinoma

7-4. **What is the most common surgical pathology follow-up in a woman with the diagnosis of atypical glandular cells (AGC) made on a cervical Pap test specimen?**

   A. High-grade squamous intraepithelial lesion (HSIL)
   B. Adenocarcinoma in situ (AIS)
   C. Endometrial adenocarcinoma
   D. Endocervical adenocarcinoma

7-5. **A cervical Pap test was examined and squamous cells with enlarged nuclei were identified. Which of the following additional features would favor a diagnosis of high-grade squamous intraepithelial lesion (HSIL) over low-grade squamous intraepithelial lesion (LSIL)?**

    A. Irregular nuclear contours

    B. Severe hyperchromasia

    C. Multinucleation

    D. High N/C ratios

7-6. **This cell was seen in a cervical Pap test. Which of the following may explain this finding?**

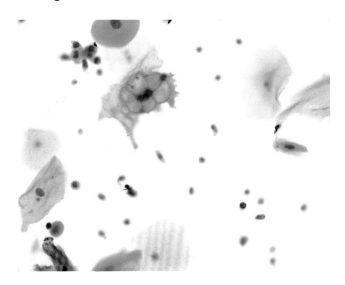

    A. The patient recently received vaccination against HPV.

    B. The patient is 6 months pregnant.

    C. The patient has a history of cervical carcinoma.

    D. The patient has a low-grade squamous intraepithelial lesion (LSIL).

7-7. **These findings were identified on a cervical Pap test specimen. Which of the following is most likely to explain these findings?**

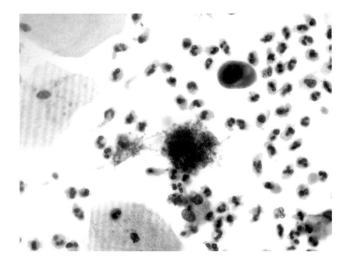

    A. High-grade squamous intraepithelial lesion (HSIL)

    B. Intrauterine device (IUD)

    C. Pregnancy

    D. Atrophic vaginitis

CHAPTER 8. SPECIMEN PREPARATION AND ADEQUACY

8-1. **A patient undergoes aspiration of a lung mass using endobronchial ultrasound (EBUS)–guided FNA. What finding on the smears would allow the specimen to be considered adequate?**

    A. Numerous bronchial respiratory epithelial cells

    B. Numerous pulmonary alveolar macrophages

    C. Numerous lymphocytes

    D. Abundant mucin-containing scattered mixed inflammatory cells

8-2 **What is observed with air-drying artifact?**

    A. Overstaining and obscured chromatin

    B. Cell shrinking and nuclear dissolution

    C. "Flame" cells

    D. Cell enlargement and pale staining

8-3. **A kidney FNA is performed, resulting in this finding in several fields. The specimen was otherwise paucicellular. What is the best diagnosis?**

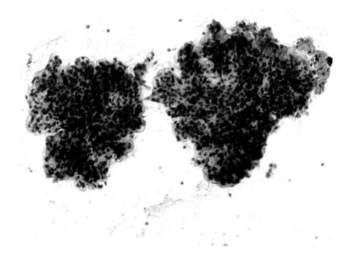

    A. Suspicious for clear cell renal cell carcinoma

    B. Suspicious for papillary renal cell carcinoma

    C. Adrenal tissue, cannot exclude an adrenal neoplasm

    D. Nondiagnostic

8-4. **What is commonly seen in benign thyroid follicular cells when they are entrapped in clot material on a conventional smear?**

    A. Nuclear enlargement and nuclear shape irregularities

    B. Nuclear "pseudo" pseudoinclusions

    C. Abundant, granular cytoplasm and prominent nucleoli

    D. Abundant, vacuolated cytoplasm

8-5. **Which of the following thyroid FNA specimens should be called inadequate?**

A. A paucicellular specimen containing 8 groups of 10 follicular cells.

B. An acellular specimen containing only abundant colloid.

C. A specimen lacking follicular cells but containing numerous polymorphous lymphocytes.

D. A specimen lacking follicular cells but containing numerous cystic macrophages.

E. A specimen containing only one group of thyroid follicular cells forming a microfollicle.

F. A specimen containing 3 groups of 10 follicular cells, all with Hurthle cell metaplasia.

G. A specimen containing 3 groups of 10 follicular cells, one of which contains an intranuclear pseudoinclusion.

8-6. **What is true about liquid-based preparations compared with conventional smears?**

A. Liquid-based preparations contain all the cells collected during fine-needle aspiration.

B. Liquid-based preparations lack the "tissue paper colloid" seen on conventional smears from benign colloid nodules.

C. Liquid-based preparations increase features of small cell carcinoma, such as nuclear molding, necrosis, and chromatin smearing artifact.

D. Colloid may have radial cracks on liquid-based preparations, causing resemblance to psammoma bodies.

SELF-ASSESSMENT ANSWERS

CHAPTER 1. FINE-NEEDLE ASPIRATION OF THE THYROID

1-1. Answer – C. *BRAF* p.V600E mutations are present in approximately 45% of papillary thyroid carcinomas (PTC), while RAS mutations are markers of thyroid neoplasms with a follicular architecture (see Table 1.4) (B). Notably, the presence of this thick, ropey "bubble gum" colloid is often associated with PTC and is not a reassuring finding in this case (A). Additionally, the entrapped follicular cells display nuclear enlargement, nuclear elongation, irregular nuclear folds, and an intranuclear pseudoinclusion present at 12 o'clock. This degree of cytologic atypia is not best categorized as atypia of undetermined significance (AUS) (A) or a follicular lesion (B). Finally, although it is true that rare intranuclear pseudoinclusions can be present in Hurthle cell neoplasms, the cytologic atypia and "bubble gum" colloid present in this case are not consistent with a Hurthle cell lesion (D).

References:

1. Xing M. BRAF mutation in papillary thyroid cancer: pathogenic role, molecular bases, and clinical implications. *Endocr Rev.* 2007;28(7):742-762.

2. Nikiforov YE, Nikiforova MN. Molecular genetics and diagnosis of thyroid cancer. *Nat Rev Endocrinol.* 2011;7:569.

1-2. Answer – D. **According to** *The Bethesda System for Reporting Thyroid Cytopathology*, a near-total thyroidectomy should be reserved for patients with aspirates that show features suspicious for or diagnostic of a malignancy (e.g., papillary thyroid carcinoma). The pattern observed in this figure is microfollicular, not papillary. If the microfollicular features present are focal or if the overall cellularity is low, the specimen may be best categorized as atypia of undetermined significance (AUS). As a result, repeating the fine-needle aspiration, performing molecular testing, or undergoing a partial thyroidectomy (depending on the radiologic features) would all be reasonable approaches (A, B, and C). If this specimen has increased cellularity with this microfollicular architecture, it would be best classified as suspicious for a follicular neoplasm (SFN)/follicular neoplasm (FN). Consequently, molecular testing or a thyroid lobectomy depending on the radiologic features would both be warranted. Therefore, the least reasonable approach for an AUS or SFN/FN diagnosis would be to perform a near-total thyroidectomy.

1-3. Answer – A. The cells pictured are cyst-lining cells in which the cytoplasm and nuclei appear elongated due to compressive forces exerted on the cells over time by the cyst fluid they contain. The cyst fluid typically contains benign colloid and/or cystic macrophages. While the elongated and enlarged nuclei seen in these cells can also be seen in papillary thyroid carcinoma, the nuclear atypia seen here is not sufficient for a diagnosis of PTC, which may have features such as intranuclear pseudoinclusions and/or "bubble gum" colloid (C, D). An elevated cyst fluid parathyroid hormone indicates that parathyroid tissue was sampled, but parathyroid tissue is rarely cystic (B).

1-4. Answer – B. Patients with lymphocytic thyroiditis are at a slightly increased risk of developing diffuse large B-cell lymphoma and extranodal marginal zone lymphoma. A specimen containing numerous lymphocytes should not be regarded as nondiagnostic, even in the absence of any follicular epithelial cells (A). Papillary thyroid carcinoma may exist in a background of lymphocytic thyroiditis. While this can make a definitive diagnosis difficult because of the reactive changes caused by thyroiditis, a definitive diagnosis of PTC can and should be made when possible (C). The presence of multinucleated giant cells can be seen in both PTC as well as lymphocytic thyroiditis but is not reassuring because they may also be present in specimens containing both processes (D).

Reference:

1. Hyjek E, Isaacson PG. Primary B cell lymphoma of the thyroid and its relationship to Hashimoto's thyroiditis. *Hum Pathol*. 1988;19(11):1315-1326.

1-5. Answer – B. Cystic papillary thyroid carcinomas (PTCs) should have the nuclear atypia seen in conventional PTC, which includes nuclear enlargement, irregular nuclear borders, and intranuclear pseudoinclusions. Cystic PTCs often contain abundant, vacuolated cytoplasm and have a histiocytoid appearance. However, the presence of cytoplasmic vacuoles is nonspecific and can be seen in cystic macrophages and other cells in the setting of a benign nodule with cystic degeneration (A). While the presence of intranuclear pseudoinclusions is the most specific atypical feature of PTC, they are not always seen, and thus nuclear enlargement and nuclear contour irregularities are often the most helpful features to identify PTC in a cystic background. The abundant, vacuolated cytoplasm results in low N/C ratios and reduces the amount of nuclear overlap (C).

1-6. Answer – B. Anaplastic thyroid carcinoma resembles conventional adenocarcinoma seen at other sites, such as lung adenocarcinoma and breast adenocarcinoma. In the absence of a patient history, metastatic adenocarcinoma should be excluded, and thus it is important to obtain material for immunohistochemical workup. Anaplastic thyroid carcinoma often loses expression of thyroglobulin and TTF-1; furthermore, TTF-1 would also be positive in metastatic lung adenocarcinoma. Therefore, the panel listed in (A) would not be as useful as a panel containing Pax-8, which is positive in approximately 76% of anaplastic thyroid carcinomas. Medullary thyroid carcinoma would be positive for calcitonin and synaptophysin but does not usually have the pleomorphic appearance seen in these cells. Panel (D) would help exclude a metastatic lung (both TTF-1 and napsin-A positive) or breast (GATA-3 positive) but would not help identify a possible primary anaplastic thyroid carcinoma, which should be high in the differential diagnosis in this case.

Reference:

1. Rivera M, Sang C, Gerhard R, Ghossein R, Lin O. Anaplastic thyroid carcinoma: morphologic findings and PAX-8 expression in cytology specimens. *Acta Cytol*. 2010;54(5):668-672.

1-7. Answer – B. The globule with cracked edges represents colloid and is an artifact seen on liquid-based ThinPrep preparations (D). The presence of colloid is reassuring because it is often associated with benign nodules. The cracked edges sometimes cause colloid globules to be misidentified as psammoma bodies, which have a strong association with papillary thyroid carcinoma (A). Medullary thyroid carcinoma produces amyloid, which has a more amorphous appearance (C).

Reference:

1. Krane JF, Nayar R, Renshaw AA. Atypia of undetermined significance/follicular lesion of undetermined significance. In: *The Bethesda System for Reporting Thyroid Cytopathology*. Springer, Cham; 2018:49-70.

1-8. Answer – D. The thyroid gland is rarely a site of metastasis, and thus most malignant nodules are assumed to be primary malignancies. However, metastases may occasionally be found on FNA of the thyroid gland. Renal cell carcinoma (most often clear cell renal cell carcinoma) is the most common metastatic tumor and may have a long latency period, which means a clinical history of renal cell carcinoma may not be available. Medulloblastoma rarely metastasizes outside the central nervous system (C). When lung and colorectal adenocarcinoma metastasize to the thyroid gland, the patient usually has a known history of high-stage cancer. Despite being common malignancies, they do not metastasize to the thyroid as frequently as renal cell carcinoma.

CHAPTER 2. SALIVARY GLAND AND CERVICAL LYMPH NODES

2-1. Answer – D. The lesion seen here is a low-grade mucoepidermoid carcinoma (MEC). The diagnostic clues include the presence of abundant extracellular mucin and a large fragment of epithelial tissue. Although at this power, it is impossible to determine the nature of the epithelium—such as mucinous, epidermoid, or intermediate type—it is clearly not entrapped or contaminated unremarkable salivary gland. Other diagnostic considerations may include neoplasms that can undergo mucinous metaplasia, such as a pleomorphic adenoma or a Warthin tumor; however, the mucinous metaplasia seen in these cases is usually limited to intracellular mucin production and would not produce the amount of extracellular mucin present in this case. Furthermore, diagnostic features of a pleomorphic adenoma or a Warthin tumor are lacking (A and B). Secretory carcinomas may have malignant cells with mucicarmine-positive vesicles, but the background is much more likely to be comprised of eosinophilic, colloid-like mucoproteinaceous secretory material instead of mucin (C).

References:

1. Taxy JB. Necrotizing squamous/mucinous metaplasia in oncocytic salivary gland tumors. A potential diagnostic problem. *Am J Clin Pathol.* 1992;97(1):40-45.

2. Guo SP, Cheuk W, Chan JKC. Pleomorphic adenoma with mucinous and squamous differentiation: a mimicker of mucoepidermoid carcinoma. *Int J Surg Pathol.* 2009;17(4):335-337.

2-2. Answer – A. The lesion seen here is an acinic cell carcinoma (ACC), characterized as malignant by its disorganized architecture and relatively monotonous cells with round, regular nuclei, punctate nucleoli, and granular cytoplasm. In contrast, Warthin tumors (WT) are comprised of oncocytic epithelium in a background of abundant lymphocytes and proteinaceous debris. WTs are benign neoplasms of the parotid gland and are often bilateral and associated with smoking (A). Most ACCs occur in the parotid gland and despite their excellent prognosis with a 5-year survival approaching 90%, up to approximately 1/3 of cases locally recur (B). Additionally, ACCs are commonly associated with tumor-associated lymphoid proliferation (TALP), which can be virtually impossible to distinguish from lymph node involvement in a fine-needle aspiration or small biopsy specimen (C). Finally, positive DOG1 expression may be helpful to confirm acinar differentiation in cases that may appear oncocytoid or secretory (D).

References:

1. Patel NR, Sanghvi S, Khan MN, Husain Q, Baredes S, Eloy JA. Demographic trends and disease-specific survival in salivary acinic cell carcinoma: an analysis of 1129 cases. *Laryngoscope.* 2014;124(1):172-178.

2. Jo VY, Krane JF. Ancillary testing in salivary gland cytology: a practical guide. *Cancer Cytopathol.* 2018;126(S8):627-642.

2-3. Answer – B. This image shows a diagnostic field for adenoid cystic carcinoma (AdCC). The key to making the diagnosis is to recognize the presence of the dense, light green mucopolysaccharide material that can be round or ropey in long strands or tubules. This material is produced by the basaloid cells which often surround or line the substance. The matrix material produced by a pleomorphic adenoma is much more fibrillary, myxoid, and less dense (A). Amyloid deposition in the salivary gland is exceedingly rare and would not be associated with the basaloid proliferation seen in this field (C). Squamous metaplasia is non-specific and can occur in a variety of salivary gland lesions, though keratinization is much rarer and may warrant consideration for a metastatic squamous cell carcinoma. However, there is no evidence of keratinization in the image shown, which most often appears as pink/orange material on the Pap stain (D).

2-4. Answer – D. The lower right-hand field contains a poorly differentiated carcinoma in three-dimensional clusters with enlarged and atypical nuclei with significant anisonucleosis. The clue that this carcinoma arose from a pleomorphic adenoma is the presence of classic metachromatic fibrillary chondromyxoid material at the upper left portion of the field (C). Although these malignant cells may have salivary duct carcinoma differentiation, the best diagnosis based on the presence of this stroma is a carcinoma ex pleomorphic adenoma (B). Finally, this stromal component should not be confused for the mucin that would be seen in a low-grade mucoepidermoid carcinoma (A).

2-5. Answer – B. This field shows the classic metachromatic fibrillary chondromyxoid material characteristic of a pleomorphic adenoma (PA) with embedded bland-appearing basaloid cells. PAs are often associated with either *PLAG1* or *HMGA2* gene fusions. *CRTC1-MAML2*, *MYB-NFIB*, and *ETV6-NTRK3* gene fusions are most often associated with mucoepidermoid carcinomas, adenoid cystic carcinomas, and secretory carcinomas, respectively (A, C, and D). See Table 2.2 for further details.

CHAPTER 3. PULMONARY

3-1. Answer – B. Per current recommendations, *EGFR*, *ALK*, and *ROS1* mutations must be tested in all lung adenocarcinomas (see Table 3.2). Patients with lung adenocarcinomas harboring certain mutations in the *EGFR* gene, *ALK* gene rearrangements, or *ROS1* gene rearrangements are eligible for targeted therapies. Thus, the current CAP/IASLC/AMP recommendations state that these three genes must be tested in all non–small cell lung carcinomas with an adenocarcinoma component. While the *KRAS* gene is a common driver mutation in lung adenocarcinomas, effective therapies targeting *KRAS* have yet to be developed (A, C, and D).

Reference:

1. Lindeman NI, Cagle PT, Aisner DL, et al. Updated molecular testing guideline for the selection of lung cancer patients for treatment with targeted tyrosine kinase inhibitors: guideline from the college of American pathologists, the international association for the study of lung cancer, and the association for molecular pathology. *J Mol Diagn.* 2018;20:129-159.

3-2. Answer – D. The lung tumor pictured is a small cell lung carcinoma. It is important to distinguish small cell carcinoma from non–small cell carcinoma, as the former is more responsive to chemotherapy, and the latter may harbor targetable driver mutations. The diagnosis of small cell carcinoma is primarily based on morphology: relatively small cells with smudgy chromatin, high N/C ratios with very scant/not appreciable cytoplasm, nuclear molding, abundant necrosis, and frequent mitotic figures (C). Positive cytoplasmic expression of neuroendocrine markers (i.e., synaptophysin, chromogranin) can be helpful in confirming the diagnosis but is not required (A). In contrast to non–small cell carcinomas, small cell carcinomas are more aggressive; they have a higher propensity to metastasize and overall worse survival (B).

3-3. Answer – A. The lung nodule pictured is a nonnecrotizing (noncaseating) granuloma. The most important initial step is to rule out an infectious etiology by performing special stains for fungi and acid-fast bacilli and correlating with microbiology cultures. The lungs and hilar lymph nodes are the most common primary sites of granulomas, both in infectious cases (e.g., tuberculosis, other mycobacterial or fungal infections) and in sarcoidosis (C). Though the differential diagnosis is focused with some classical associations, a definitive etiology cannot be determined on cytology alone and requires ancillary microbiological studies (D). In this figure, the larger cells with bland ovoid nuclei and abundant syncytial cytoplasm are histiocytes, while the smaller round cells with scant cytoplasm are associated lymphocytes; no malignant cells are present (B). However, it is worth noting that malignant processes may elicit a granulomatous response, and a careful search for malignant cells may be warranted in the appropriate clinical setting.

3-4. Answer – C. Ferruginous bodies are pictured here. This finding in a BAL specimen should always be reported, as ferruginous bodies are commonly associated with asbestos exposure, which is a risk factor for lung malignancy (A). This BAL specimen is adequate both because there are abundant pulmonary alveolar macrophages in the background (an indicator of adequate sampling of the alveolar spaces) and because there is a positive finding (B). Ferruginous bodies are not associated with any infectious etiologies (D).

3-5. Answer – C. The morphology pictured here is most compatible with a carcinoid tumor. Carcinoid tumors are positive for neuroendocrine markers (e.g., synaptophysin, chromogranin) and negative for napsin A. The cells have spindled nuclei, "speckled" neuroendocrine-type chromatin, and minimal cytoplasm. Carcinoid tumors typically have a low Ki-67 proliferation index (A). Metastatic carcinoid tumor to a lymph node confers a worse prognosis (B). There is no connection with any infectious organisms (D).

3-6. Answer – C. The cells have large, hyperchromatic nuclei arranged in a "picket fence" configuration. The findings are strongly suggestive of a metastatic colorectal carcinoma. The nuclei are too pleomorphic to represent an atypical carcinoid tumor (B). Lung adenocarcinoma can rarely have gastrointestinal differentiation, but this the less likely possibility (A). The cells appear to demonstrate glandular differentiation, which would be an unusual appearance for mesothelioma (D).

CHAPTER 4. HEPATOPANCREATOBILIARY

4-1. Answer – D. The lesion pictured is a gastrointestinal stromal tumor (GIST). Immunohistochemistry is considered essential to the diagnosis of GISTs, which are positive for CD117 and DOG1 in >95% of cases (these markers are relatively specific as well). The stomach is the most common site (60% of cases), followed by the small bowel (35% of cases), though the liver is common site of metastasis (A). Tumor site is an important risk factor: 20-25% of gastric GISTs and 40-50% of small intestinal GISTs are malignant, while most lesions do not progress (B). Morphologically, GISTs typically consist of a uniform population of spindled or epithelioid cells; pleomorphism is rare, and when present, should prompt consideration of other mesenchymal entities (C).

References:

1. Liegl B, Hornick JL, Corless CL, Fletcher CD. Monoclonal antibody DOG1.1 shows higher sensitivity than KIT in the diagnosis of gastrointestinal stromal tumors, including unusual subtypes. *Am J Surg Pathol.* 2009;33:437-446.

2. Eisenberg BL, Pipas JM. Gastrointestinal stromal tumor–background, pathology, treatment. *Hematol Oncol Clin North Am.* 2012;26:1239-1259.

4-2. Answer – A. This image depicts benign pancreatic acinar tissue, which is present as "grape-like" clusters, individual groups of acinar cells, and single acinar cells. It is important to recognize the spectrum of benign pancreatic acinar tissue to avoid overdiagnosis. Potential pitfalls in the differential diagnosis of benign acinar tissue include pancreatic neuroendocrine tumor, which is immunoreactive for synaptophysin and chromogranin (B), and acinar cell carcinoma. Both benign and malignant acinar proliferations would demonstrate cytoplasmic staining with trypsin, so the distinction is primarily based on morphology and clinical/radiologic correlation (C). Though acinar formations may resemble glands, the cells are not atypical or pleomorphic enough to raise consideration for adenocarcinoma (D).

4-3. Answer – B. The cyst lining shown here is comprised of mucinous epithelium with high-grade atypia. Studies have shown that cytology is the best modality for identifying high-risk cysts based on assessment of the presence of high-grade atypia. The identification of high-grade atypia in mucinous cysts stratifies the cyst as high-risk, which may prompt surgical resection (i.e., pancreaticoduodenectomy) with significant associated morbidity versus surveillance (A). Neoplastic mucinous cysts of the pancreas typically have cyst fluid CEA levels ≥192 ng/mL (C). On cytology, it is very difficult to distinguish high-grade atypia/dysplasia from invasive adenocarcinoma. Neoplastic mucinous cysts with high-grade dysplasia can certainly be associated with an invasive carcinoma component, which is the most important negative prognostic factor (D).

References:

1. Brugge WR, Lewandrowski K, Lee-Lewandrowski E, et al. Diagnosis of pancreatic cystic neoplasms: a report of the cooperative pancreatic cyst study. *Gastroenterology.* 2004;126:1330-1336.

2. Scourtas A, Dudley JC, Brugge WR, Kadayifci A, Mino-Kenudson M, Pitman MB. Preoperative characteristics and cytological features of 136 histologically confirmed pancreatic mucinous cystic neoplasms. *Cancer.* 2017;125:169-177.

3. Cizginer S, Turner BG, Bilge AR, Karaca C, Pitman MB, Brugge WR. Cyst fluid carcinoembryonic antigen is an accurate diagnostic marker of pancreatic mucinous cysts. *Pancreas.* 2011;40:1024-1028.

4. Pitman MB, Centeno BA, Daglilar ES, Brugge WR, Mino-Kenudson M. Cytological criteria of high-grade epithelial atypia in the cyst fluid of pancreatic intraductal papillary mucinous neoplasms. *Cancer Cytopathol.* 2014;122:40-47.

4-4. Answer – D. This image depicts loosely cohesive malignant epithelioid cells and is consistent with a poorly differentiated carcinoma. In the liver, metastatic carcinomas are more common than primary liver carcinomas (i.e., hepatocellular carcinomas and intrahepatic cholangiocarcinomas). The malignant cells have high N/C ratios, coarse chromatin, and marked pleomorphism. The cytoplasm appears somewhat foamy/vacuolated, suggesting a diagnosis of adenocarcinoma, but there are no supporting architectural features (A). Albumin in situ hybridization is a very sensitive and specific marker of hepatic origin and can be helpful in distinguishing primary versus metastatic carcinoma (B). Immunohistochemical markers of hepatocyte differentiation, such as HepPar-1, glypican-3, and arginase, can be helpful in ruling in/out poorly differentiated hepatocellular carcinoma (C).

References:

1. Ferrone CR, Ting DT, Shahid M, et al. The ability to diagnose intrahepatic cholangiocarcinoma definitively using novel branched DNA-enhanced albumin RNA in situ hybridization technology. *Ann Surg Oncol.* 2016;23:290-296.

2. Anatelli F, Chuang ST, Yang XJ, Wang HL. Value of glypican 3 immunostaining in the diagnosis of hepatocellular carcinoma on needle biopsy. *Am J Clin Pathol.* 2008;130:219-223.

3. Geramizadeh B, Seirfar N. Diagnostic value of arginase-1 and glypican-3 in differential diagnosis of hepatocellular carcinoma, cholangiocarcinoma and metastatic carcinoma of liver. *Hepat Mon.* 2015;15:e30336.

4-5. Answer – B. The field shows "clean" mucin and thus was sampled from a mucin-producing neoplasm. Contaminating "dirty" mucin from the gastrointestinal tract typically contains granular debris, inflammatory cells, and/or bacteria (A), while "clean" mucin is acellular or contains macrophages and/or mucinous epithelium. In the proper clinicoradiologic context, the findings are diagnostic of a mucin-producing neoplastic cyst. Levels of CEA are expected to be elevated (≥192 ng/mL) (C). Sampling of serous cystadenomas usually yields nonspecific findings and should not contain "clean" mucin (D).

Reference:

1. Nagula S, Kennedy T, Schattner MA, et al. Evaluation of cyst fluid CEA analysis in the diagnosis of mucinous cysts of the pancreas. *J Gastro Surg*. 2010;14(12):1997-2003.

4-6. Answer – A. The field demonstrates a dispersed population of monotonous, small cells. At this magnification, the cells have angulated nuclei and are favored to be lymphocytes. This suggests the possibility of a splenule (ectopic splenic tissue) or an intra-/peripancreatic lymph node. However, a pancreatic neuroendocrine tumor (PanNET) may be considered in the differential diagnosis. CD8 would highlight sinusoids in a splenule and CD45 would be positive in the lymphocytes. Synaptophysin and chromogranin would be positive in most PanNETs (B). Acinar cell carcinoma (positive for BCL10 and trypsin) and solid pseudopapillary neoplasm (positive for CD10 along with nuclear expression of β-catenin) are in the differential diagnosis when a dispersed population of cells are seen (C and D). However, these neoplasms typically form tissue fragments and have other cytomorphologic features not identified in this field.

CHAPTER 5. SEROUS EFFUSION CYTOPATHOLOGY

5-1. Answer – C. Diffuse nuclear staining for p53 or a complete absence of p53 nuclear staining are patterns associated with aberrant p53 expression, which is seen in high-grade serous carcinoma as well as clear cell carcinoma. Interpretation on cell block material may be challenging if the atypical cells are not present in large numbers or if the cell block material contains numerous bystander cells. Numerous benign processes within the pelvic cavity may be positive for Pax-8 and ER (such as endometriosis and endosalpingiosis), and thus these markers are not specific for a malignant process (A and B). Similar to MOC-31, BerEP4 stains epithelial cells and thus would be noninformative in this instance (D).

5-2. Answer – A. The loss of nuclear BAP-1 expression is a specific yet insensitive marker for malignant mesothelioma. The retained nuclear staining in benign, background cells can be used as an internal "positive control." At this time, BAP-1 is not used to diagnose borderline serous neoplasms, lung adenocarcinomas, or small cell carcinomas (B, C, and D).

References:

1. Cigognetti M, Lonardi S, Fisogni S, et al. BAP1 (BRCA1-associated protein 1) is a highly specific marker for differentiating mesothelioma from reactive mesothelial proliferations. *Mod Pathol*. 2015;28:1043-1057.

2. Hasteh F, Lin GY, Weidner N, Michael CW. The use of immunohistochemistry to distinguish reactive mesothelial cells from malignant mesothelioma in cytologic effusions. *Cancer Cytopathol*. 2010;118:90-96.

5-3. Answer – A. The field contains mucin and rare macrophages. This finding is associated with the clinical impression of pseudomyxoma peritonei and the aspiration of mucinous material (B, C, and D). While mucin can be associated with mucinous adenocarcinomas, low-grade mucinous neoplasms may also produce mucin, which enters into the peritoneal cavity ("disseminated peritoneal adenomucinosis").

Reference:

1. Ronnett BM, Zahn CM, Kurman RJ, Kass ME, Sugarbaker PH, Shmookler BM. Disseminated peritoneal adenomucinosis and peritoneal mucinous carcinomatosis. A clinicopathologic analysis of 109 cases with emphasis on distinguishing pathologic features, site of origin, prognosis, and relationship to "pseudomyxoma peritonei". *Am J Surg Pathol.* 1995;19(12):1390-1408.

5-4. Answer – D. While mesothelioma can rarely be seen as dispersed, single cells, it usually presents within tissue fragments. Poorly differentiated adenocarcinomas, lobular breast carcinoma, lymphomas, sarcomas, and melanomas often exist as single, dispersed cells when found in serous cavity specimens (A, B, and C).

5-5. Answer – C. Psammoma bodies may be associated with cystadenofibromas, benign mesothelial proliferations, and endosalpingiosis in pelvic cavity specimens. The presence of psammoma bodies in pleural fluid specimens, but not pelvic cavity specimens, is strongly associated with malignant processes (A). While high-grade serous carcinoma cells are sometimes associated with psammomatous calcification, psammoma bodies are usually found in greater number in borderline serous tumors (B). Metastatic papillary carcinoma rarely involves serous cavity specimens (D).

5-6. Answer – D. Of the markers listed, CDX2, NKX3.1, GATA-3, and ER are all nuclear stains. CK20 is a membranous stain, whereas PSA, HepPar1, and arginase are cytoplasmic stains (A, B, and C).

Reference:

1. Cowan ML, VandenBussche CJ. Cancer of unknown primary: ancillary testing of cytologic and small biopsy specimens in the era of targeted therapy. *Cancer Cytopathol.* 2018;126:724-737.

CHAPTER 6. URINARY TRACT

6-1. Answer – B. The cells seen are small cell carcinoma cells and may be confused with lymphocytes at low magnification. However, small cell carcinoma cells have little to absent cytoplasm and are larger and more pleomorphic than lymphocytes. Small cell carcinoma may be primary to the bladder, arise as a component of high-grade urothelial carcinoma, or arise from prostate adenocarcinoma and invade into the urinary tract. They may also be mistaken for renal tubular cells, which are usually present in small clusters and not seen singly dispersed in the background (A). Following BCG treatment, multinucleated giant cells, lymphocytes, granular debris, and epithelioid histiocytes may be seen (C). These cells are not associated with any infectious process (D).

6-2. Answer – B. The cell is large and contains a large, dark nucleus. Because the cell is degenerating, the cytoplasm is vacuolated, resulting in a low N/C ratio. However, the nucleus must contain a substantial amount of chromatin material given its size and level of hyperchromasia, and it must be regarded as at least suspicious for high-grade urothelial carcinoma. BK polyomavirus cells usually have absent to minimal cytoplasm and a nucleus with smooth contours and chromatin that appears glassy or in a "spider web" configuration (A). Melamed-Wolinska bodies are small, concentric cytoplasmic inclusions in degenerated urothelial cells and are usually red or green on the Pap stain (C). Low-grade urothelial neoplasia cells are usually found in tissue fragments and are usually not much larger than a red blood cell (D).

References:

1. Cowan ML, Rosenthal DL, VandenBussche CJ. Improved risk stratification for patients with high-grade urothelial carcinoma following application of the Paris System for Reporting Urinary Cytology. *Cancer Cytopathol.* 2017;125(6):427-434.

2. Allison DB, Olson MT, Lilo M, Zhang ML, Rosenthal DL, VandenBussche CJ. Should the BK poly-omavirus cytopathic effect be best classified as atypical or benign in urine cytology specimens? *Cancer Cytopathol.* 2016;124(6):436-442.

3. Zhang ML, Rosenthal DL, VandenBussche CJ. The cytomorphological features of low-grade urothe-lial neoplasms vary by specimen type. *Cancer Cytopathol.* 2016;124(8):552-564.

6-3. Answer – A. According to TPS, the *SHGUC* category applies when an in-sufficient number of malignant cells are found in a specimen (less than 5 in a voided urine and less than 10 in an upper tract specimen) or when any number of cells are found with atypical features more severe than seen in the *Atypical Urothelial Cells (AUC)* category but insufficient for a diagnosis of *High-Grade Urothelial Carcinoma (HGUC)*. This applies to choice A, whereas choice B describes cells sufficient for a diagnosis of *HGUC*. Choice C de-scribes a situation best diagnosed as *AUC*, whereas choice D would be con-sidered *NHGUC*.

Reference:

1. VandenBussche CJ. A review of the Paris system for reporting urinary cytology. *Cytopathol.* 2016;27(3):153-156.

6-4. Answer – A. TPS recommends that atypia associated with low-grade urothelial neoplasms be diagnosed as *NHGUC*, although the choice to make a diagnosis of *Low-Grade Urothelial Neoplasm* is allowed when a papillary lesion is seen with a true fibrovascular core and a mass lesion is identified. In this case, atypical fea-tures associated with HGUC are not seen, and thus diagnoses of *AUC*, *SHGUC*, and *HGUC* would be inappropriate because they suggest the patient is more likely to have HGUC.

References:

1. VandenBussche CJ. A review of the Paris system for reporting urinary cytology. *Cytopathol.* 2016;27(3):153-156.

2. Zhang ML, Rosenthal DL, VandenBussche CJ. The cytomorphological features of low-grade urothe-lial neoplasms vary by specimen type. *Cancer Cytopathol.* 2016;124(8):552-564.

6-5. Answer – A. The field shows a cluster of epithelioid histiocytes associated with a multinucleated giant cell. This finding may be seen in patients undergoing treat-ment with BCG. The cells do not represent a urothelial carcinoma or renal cell carcinoma, though they may be classified as atypical and concerning for neopla-sia if not identified as epithelioid histiocytes (B, C, and D).

6-6. Answer – B. The field contains an irregularly shaped keratin fragment and raises concern for a squamous lesion such as squamous cell carcinoma. Squa-mous cell carcinoma may arise in the bladder (both primary and as a compo-nent of high-grade urothelial carcinoma) or may contaminate the urinary tract stream from the gynecologic tract. An invasive squamous cell carcinoma may invade into the urinary tract from adjacent structures such as the cervix and/or anus. Because keratinizing cells have squamous differentiation, a p40 im-munostain would be positive in the atypical cells regardless of their source. Furthermore, p40 would be positive in any background benign squamous cells and urothelial cells. The use of a catheter to collect a sample can narrow down the source of atypical squamous cells to the urinary tract if the cells continue to be present in the catheterized sample (A). Patients with cervical squamous cell carcinoma usually have no record of cervical screening, and a Pap test can help confirm the presence of atypical squamous cells (C). If atypical squamous cells are positive for high-risk HPV studies, they are likely from a gynecologic or anal origin (D).

CHAPTER 7. GYNECOLOGIC TRACT CYTOPATHOLOGY

7-1. Answer – A. In the United States, HPV 16 is most commonly found in squamous cell carcinomas, followed by HPV 18 (B). HPV 45 is a less frequent high-risk subtype, and HPV 53 is not considered a high-risk subtype (C and D).

Reference:

1. Nayar R, Wilbur DC. *The Bethesda System for Reporting Cervical Cytology: Definitions, Criteria and Explanatory Notes.* 3rd ed. New York: Springer; 2015.

7-2. Answer – A. Reactive endocervical cells are commonly found on the Pap test and may form hyperchromatic crowded groups. While the other choices can also form hyperchromatic crowded groups, they are less frequently found on Pap test specimens (B, C, and D).

Reference:

1. Nayar R, Wilbur DC. *The Bethesda System for Reporting Cervical Cytology: Definitions, Criteria and Explanatory Notes.* 3rd ed. New York: Springer; 2015.

7-3. Answer – C. This image depicts AIS. The cells are hyperchromatic with enlarged nuclei and high N/C ratios. The nuclei are elongated and have pale chromatin. Nuclei protrude at the fragment edges, giving the appearance of a "feathered" fragment. This cytomorphology is distinctive of AIS, and thus a definitive diagnosis may be provided (B). While HSIL can sometimes have a glandular appearance, the nuclei are typically less uniform and do not often palisade as seen here (A). The cells shown here do not demonstrate significant pleomorphism or anisonucleosis and do not form a three-dimensional fragment which would be features that support a diagnosis of endocervical adenocarcinoma (D).

Reference:

1. Nayar R, Wilbur DC. *The Bethesda System for Reporting Cervical Cytology: Definitions, Criteria and Explanatory Notes.* 3rd ed. New York: Springer; 2015.

7-4. Answer – A. The most common lesion identified following a diagnosis of AGC is HSIL. This is in part because some HSIL lesions can have a glandular appearance on the Pap test and is also due to the relative rarity of glandular malignancies compared to the incidence of HSIL in screening populations. While there is an increased risk of adenocarcinoma following a diagnosis of AGC, AGC has a poor predictive value for adenocarcinoma (B, C, and D). Regardless, a diagnosis of AGC prompts colposcopy with endocervical sampling as well as an endometrial biopsy in patients at risk for endometrial carcinoma.

References:

1. Zhao C, Austin RM, Pan J, et al. Clinical significance of atypical glandular cells in conventional pap smears in a large, high-risk U.S. west coast minority population. *Acta Cytol.* 2009;53(2):153-159.
2. Zhao C,Florea A, Onisko A, et al. Histologic follow-up results in 662 patients with Pap test findings of atypical glandular cells: results from a large academic womens hospital laboratory employing sensitive screening methods. *Gynecol Oncol.* 2009;114(3):383-389.
3. Miller RA, Mody DR, Tams KC, et al. Glandular lesions of the cervix in clinical practice: a cytology, histology, and human papillomavirus correlation study from 2 institutions. *Arch Pathol Lab Med.* 2015;139(11):1431-1436.
4. Patadji S, Li Z, Pradhan D, et al. Significance of high-risk HPV detection in women with atypical glandular cells on Pap testing: analysis of 1857 cases from an academic institution. *Cancer Cytopathol.* 2017;125(3):205-211.
5. Pradhan D, Li Z, Ocque R, et al. Clinical significance of atypical glandular cells in Pap tests: an analysis of more than 3000 cases at a large academic women's center. *Cancer Cytopathol.* 2016;124(8):589-595.

7-5. Answer – D. The most specific feature of HSIL listed above is elevated N/C ratios. The nuclear size in HSIL is variable. Cell nuclei may show the same degree of enlargement as LSIL or may be smaller than those of intermediate cells. However, HSIL cells have less cytoplasm resulting in an increased N/C ratio. Irregular nuclear contours and severe hyperchromasia support a diagnosis of HSIL but are not specific findings (A and B). Multinucleation can be seen in reactive squamous cells, LSIL, postmenopausal atrophy, and invasive carcinoma (C).

Reference:

1. Nayar R, Wilbur DC. *The Bethesda System for Reporting Cervical Cytology: Definitions, Criteria and Explanatory Notes.* 3rd ed. New York: Springer; 2015.

7-6. Answer – C. This is often seen in patients with a history of cervical squamous cell carcinoma that has been treated with radiation therapy. The atypical cell is enlarged and has a dark, large nucleus. However, the cell also has abundant cytoplasm with prominent cytoplasmic vacuolization and irregular projections. These findings may be seen following radiation therapy and may persist for years in some patients. There are no known documented Pap test changes that are associated with recently vaccinated patients (A). The cell of interest seen here does not have the features classically associated with LSIL, such as multinucleation and a perinuclear halo (D). Similarly, the cell does not have the morphology of multinucleated syncytiotrophoblasts, which are sometimes seen in pregnant patients (B).

Reference:

1. Nayar R, Wilbur DC. *The Bethesda System for Reporting Cervical Cytology: Definitions, Criteria and Explanatory Notes.* 3rd ed. New York: Springer; 2015.

7-7. Answer – B. The field demonstrates a cluster of filamentous *Actinomyces* organisms adjacent to a cell with a large, dark nucleus. The findings are most compatible with IUD use, which may result in the presence of rare, atypical appearing "IUD cells." The presence of *Actinomyces* is rarely seen in the absence of an IUD. HSIL may present as singly dispersed cells, but these cells usually have high N/C ratios compared with the atypical cell seen in this field (A). Pregnancy may cause atypical changes in Pap test specimens but is unlikely in a patient with an IUD (C). A Pap test with atrophic vaginitis may have parabasal cells, "blue blobs," inflammation, and granular debris (D).

Reference:

1. Nayar R, Wilbur DC. *The Bethesda System for Reporting Cervical Cytology: Definitions, Criteria and Explanatory Notes.* 3rd ed. New York: Springer; 2015.

CHAPTER 8. SPECIMEN PREPARATION AND ADEQUACY

8-1. Answer – C. In order to be adequate, a fine-needle aspiration should demonstrate findings that explain a mass lesion. In the case of numerous polymorphous lymphocytes, their presence would suggest the sampling of a lymph node. The other findings could be sampled from the airway and do not indicate that the mass lesion seen on imaging studies was truly sampled (A, B, and D).

8-2. Answer – D. Air-drying artifact results when a Pap stain is applied to an air-fixed preparation. While air-fixation is appropriate prior to staining with Giemsa-like stains (such as Diff-Quik), the cells become flattened and enlarged on a glass slide. This increased surface area results in a pale stain following the Pap stain as well as loss of both nuclear and cytoplasmic details (A and B). "Flame" cells, which are characterized by magenta/pink cytoplasmic vacuoles, are sometimes seen in hyperplastic lesions such as Graves disease (C).

8-3. Answer – D. The structures seen in the figure are glomeruli and can be mistaken for neoplastic cells on a renal FNA (A, B, and C). Close examination reveals empty endothelial "rings" at the peripheral tufts of the glomeruli. Familiarity with these structures helps prevent a nondiagnostic specimen (in which a lesion does not appear to be sampled) from being called adequate.

8-4. Answer – A. Benign follicular cells trapped in clot material may appear to have enlarged, overlapping nuclei and irregular nuclear shapes when compared with similar cells free from clot material on the same slide. These changes overlap with those seen in papillary thyroid carcinoma (PTC) and are secondary to forces exerted on the cells as the clot forms. "Pseudo" pseudoinclusions refer to the presence of false intranuclear inclusions, such as when a red blood cell overlies a thyroid follicular cell; the clot artifact does not commonly cause these (B). Hurthle cells contain abundant, granular cytoplasm and prominent nucleoli (C). Hurthle cell change is reactive and takes place in vivo prior to sampling and clot formation. Cystic PTC cells may have increased amounts of vacuolated, bubbly cytoplasm, taking on a histiocytoid appearance (D).

8-5. Answer – D. A thyroid FNA specimen is adequate if it contains at least 6 groups of 10 follicular cells, abundant colloid, numerous lymphocytes, or any number of atypical follicular cells (A-C). The last three choices (E-G) describe scenarios in which *Atypia of Undetermined Significance (AUS)* should be diagnosed for a scant specimen containing only microfollicles, only Hurthle cells, or nuclear atypia, respectively. The presence of only cyst fluid is associated with a small increased risk of malignancy due to the possible presence of a cystic papillary thyroid carcinoma and should be considered inadequate for diagnosis (D).

Reference:

1. *The 2017 Bethesda System for Reporting Thyroid Cytopathology*. 2nd ed.: Springer International Publishing; 2017.

8-6. Answer – D. In liquid-based preparations, colloid may be seen as globules containing cracks, which may be mistaken for a psammoma body. Colloid can also have a "tissue paper" appearance on liquid-based preparations that is not seen in conventional smears (B). Liquid-based preparations use only a fraction of the cells in a sample; this means that some residual specimen remains and can be used for ancillary studies (A). Liquid-based preparations reduce many of the diagnostic features for small cell carcinoma seen in conventional smears, such as nuclear molding, necrosis, and chromatin streaking (C).

Reference:

1. Hoda RS. Non-gynecologic cytology on liquid-based preparations: a morphologic review of facts and artifacts. *Diagn Cytopathol*. 2007;35(10):621-634.

Note: Page numbers followed by "f" indicate figures, "t" indicate tables and "b" indicate boxes.